Cancer Treatment and Research

For other titles published in this series, go to
www.springer.com/series/5808

Pediatric and Adolescent Osteosarcoma

Edited by

Norman Jaffe MD, DSc, Dip Paed

Professor Emeritus, Children's Cancer Hospital, University of Texas M.D. Anderson Cancer Center, 1515 Holcombe Blvd., Unit #87, Houston, TX 77030-4009, USA

Øyvind S. Bruland MD, PhD

Professor of Clinical Oncology, Faculty of Medicine, University of Oslo, The Norwegian Radium Hospital, N-0310 Oslo, Norway

Stefan S. Bielack

Studienleiter, Cooperative Osteosarkomstudiengruppe COSS, Ärztlicher Direktor, Pädiatrie 5 (Onkologie, Hämatologie, Immunologie), Klinikum Stuttgart, Zentrum für Kinder- und Jugendmedizin – Olgahospital, Bismarckstr. 8, D-70176 Stuttgart, Germany

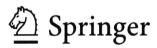

Editors

Norman Jaffe MD, DSc, Dip Paed
Professor Emeritus
Children's Cancer Hospital
University of Texas M.D.
Anderson Cancer Center
1515 Holcombe Blvd., Unit #87
Houston, TX 77030-4009
USA
njaffe@mdanderson.org

Øyvind S. Bruland MD, PhD
Professor of Clinical Oncology
Faculty of Medicine
University of Oslo
The Norwegian Radium Hospital
N-0310 Oslo, Norway
oyvind.bruland@medisin.uio.no

Stefan S. Bielack
Studienleiter, Cooperative
Osteosarkomstudiengruppe COSS
Ärztlicher Direktor, Pädiatrie 5
(Onkologie, Hämatologie, Immunologie)
Klinikum Stuttgart, Zentrum für
Kinder- und Jugendmedizin – Olgahospital
Bismarckstr. 8, D-70176 Stuttgart
Germany
coss@olgahospital-stuttgart.de

ISBN 978-1-4419-0283-2   e-ISBN 978-1-4419-0284-9
DOI 10.1007/978-1-4419-0284-9
Springer New York Dordrecht Heidelberg London

Library of Congress Control Number: 2009927708

© Springer Science+Business Media, LLC 2009
All rights reserved. This work may not be translated or copied in whole or in part without the written permission of the publisher (Springer Science+Business Media, LLC, 233 Spring Street, New York, NY 10013, USA), except for brief excerpts in connection with reviews or scholarly analysis. Use in connection with any form of information storage and retrieval, electronic adaptation, computer software, or by similar or dissimilar methodology now known or hereafter developed is forbidden.
The use in this publication of trade names, trademarks, service marks, and similar terms, even if they are not identified as such, is not to be taken as an expression of opinion as to whether or not they are subject to proprietary rights.

Printed on acid-free paper

Springer is part of Springer Science+Business Media (www.springer.com)

Dedication

It is forbidden to live in a city where there is no physician.[1]

To my patients and their parents for honoring me. They granted me the privilege to be their physician. Their serene fortitude was a paradigm of Trust, Hope and Courage. In their heroic struggles against a formidable enemy they taught me many lessons.

I give thanks to the Almighty for giving me life, strength and opportunity to see the completion of this task.

Norman Jaffe
Senior Editor

1. *Babylonian Talmud, Sunhedrin, 17b: second folio. www.myjewish learning.com/daily_life/The body/ Healthy Healing.*

Preface

Why (Another) Symposium on Osteosarcoma?

Osteosarcoma serves as a prototype for the coordinated multidisciplinary treatment of malignancy. Therapy must be carefully integrated since occasionally tactics and strategies appear as opposing forces. This is not unexpected since not infrequently, the "correct" treatment is by no means established. A fundamental principle, however, is that the plan of management must be sufficiently flexible to accommodate changing circumstances.

Major advances have been forged in the management of osteosarcoma. These have been presented and discussed in many conferences and meetings. This monograph is a compilation of the presentations delivered at the osteosarcoma conference "Pediatric and Adolescent Osteosarcoma...Progress of the Past, Prospects for the Future" held at the M.D. Anderson Cancer Center, March 6–8, 2008.

The question may rightly be asked, "Why organize another Conference on Osteosarcoma?" Two significant reasons may be advanced:

1. This was the first conference devoted exclusively to pediatric and adolescent osteosarcoma.
2. Unfortunately, we have reached a plateau in the survival and therapeutic strategies of osteosarcoma. This unfavorable situation developed within a short period after the discovery of the majority of the chemotherapeutic agents that were effective in the treatment of osteosarcoma some 30–40 years ago. At that stage, a new era in treatment was considered to have emerged. However, since that time, no major advances have been discovered or reported to combat chemoresistant metastatic osteosarcoma cells. To breach the barrier, new concepts and therapies are required.

What is the solution?
The answer may possibly be derived from some ancient Talmudic advice.

הפך בה והפך בה דכלה בה[1]

Delve in it; delve in it for everything is in it.

Knowledge may be gleaned from repeatedly examining the past and possibly exposing fresh depths of unexpected meaning. To this end authorities were invited to review their past experiences and express opinions on the impact their results could have in creating new tactics and strategies for treatment. No attempt was made to disguise controversies or differences of opinion. By necessity some overlap was inevitable, but an attempt was made to keep it to a minimum.

Mindful that therapeutic research is dependent also upon plumbing the depths of uncharted waters, selected investigators were invited to present reports of their innovative studies. The task to explore the unknown is arduous but hopefully their efforts will be fruitful and be amply rewarded. Unfortunately, time constraints limited the number of investigators who could be invited to present their elegant results. To my colleagues in this category, I offer my sincere apologies.

Contributors were permitted wide berth in an effort to provide innovative opinions and concepts. It is my earnest hope that their presentations will stimulate provocative thought for the mind that invents and the hand that crafts.

The responsibility of weighing a decision, examining a controversy, and implementing treatment is assumed by the primary physician. He or she must serve as a patient's anchor to windward and support their charge through a perilous journey. To alleviate their burden, it is hoped that the accumulated assistance derived from the experience of investigators in these diverse disciplines will be of assistance. It is in this spirit that I express a sense of deep gratitude to my distinguished colleagues and associate editors without whose help, prudent counsel, and expertise this effort would not have materialized.

לפום צערא אגרא[1]

The reward is proportional to the effort!

Houston, TX   Norman Jaffe

Reference

1. Scherman N, ed. *Ethics of the Fathers* 2007;5:578-580. Complete Artscroll Siddur. New York: Mesorah Publi shing Co.

Contents

General Aspects of Osteosarcoma

The Epidemiology of Osteosarcoma 3
Giulia Ottaviani and Norman Jaffe

The Etiology of Osteosarcoma 15
Giulia Ottaviani and Norman Jaffe

**Imaging Assessment of Osteosarcoma in Childhood
and Adolescence: Diagnosis, Staging, and Evaluating
Response to Chemotherapy** 33
Farzin Eftekhari

**Osteosarcoma Multidisciplinary Approach to the Management
from the Pathologist's Perspective** 63
 A. Kevin Raymond and Norman Jaffe

Conditions that Mimic Osteosarcoma 85
A. Kevin Raymond and Norman Jaffe

Treatment

Surgical Management of Primary Osteosarcoma 125
Alan W. Yasko

The Role of Radiotherapy in Oseosarcoma 147
Rudolf Schwarz, Oyvind Bruland, Anna Cassoni, Paula Schomberg,
and Stefan Bielack

**Osteosarcoma Lung Metastases Detection and Principles
of Multimodal Therapy** 165
Dorothe Carrle and Stefan Bielack

Contents

Surgical Treatment of Pulmonary Metastases from Osteosarcoma in Pediatric and Adolescent Patients 185
Matthew Steliga and Ara Vaporciyan

Non-Surgical Treatment of Pulmonary and Extra-pulmonary Metastases 203
Pete Anderson

Review of the Past, Impact on the Future

Adjuvant Chemotherapy in Osteosarcoma: An Odyssey of Rejection and Vindication 219
Norman Jaffe

Osteosarcoma: Review of the Past, Impact on the Future. The American Experience 239
Norman Jaffe

Osteosarcoma: The European Osteosarcoma Intergroup (EOI) Perspective 263
Alan W. Craft

The Treatment of Nonmetastatic High Grade Osteosarcoma of the Extremity: Review of the Italian Rizzoli Experience. Impact on the Future 275
Stefano Ferrari, Emanuela Palmerini, Eric L. Staals, Mario Mercuri, Bertoni Franco, Piero Picci, and Gaetano Bacci

Osteosarcoma: The COSS Experience 289
Stefan Bielack, Herbert Jürgens, Gernot Jundt, Matthias Kevric, Thomas Kühne, Peter Reichardt, Andreas Zoubek, Mathias Werner, Winfried Winkelmann, and Rainer Kotz

Treatment of Osteosarcoma. The Scandinavian Sarcoma Group Experience 309
Øyvind S. Bruland, Henrik Bauer, Thor Alvegaard, and Sigbjørn Smeland

Childhood Osteosarcoma: Multimodal Therapy in a Single-Institution Turkish Series 319
İnci Ayan, Rejin Kebudi, and Harzem Özger

International Collaboration is Feasible in Trials for Rare Conditions: The EURAMOS Experience 339
N. Marina, S. Bielack, J. Whelan, S. Smeland, M. Krailo, M.R. Sydes, T. Butterfass-Bahloul, G. Calaminus, and M. Bernstein

Contents xi

Pediatric and Adult Osteosarcoma: Comparisons and Contrasts in Presentation and Therapy 355
Robert S. Benjamin and Shreyaskumar R. Patel

Supportive Care and Quality of Life

The Role of Physical Therapy and Occupational Therapy in the Rehabilitation of Pediatric and Adolescent Patients with Osteosarcoma 367
Marissa Punzalan and Gayle Hyden

Caring for Children and Adolescents with Osteosarcoma: A Nursing Perspective 385
Margaret Pearson

Prosthetics for Pediatric and Adolescent Amputees 395
Ted B. Muilenburg

Functional, Psychosocial and Professional Outcomes in Long-Term Survivors of Lower-Extremity Osteosarcomas: Amputation Versus Limb Salvage 421
Giulia Ottaviani, Rhonda S. Robert, Winston W. Huh, and Norman Jaffe

Research and Investigation: New and Innovative Strategies

Bridging the Gap Between Experimental Animals and Humans in Osteosarcoma 439
Stephen J. Withrow and Chand Khanna

Is There a Role for Immunotherapy in Osteosarcoma? 447
David M. Loeb

Molecular Classification of Osteosarcoma 459
Ching C. Lau

Current Concepts on the Molecular Biology of Osteosarcoma 467
Richard Gorlick

How the NOTCH Pathway Contributes to the Ability of Osteosarcoma Cells to Metastasize 479
Dennis P.M. Hughes

The Role of Fas/FasL in the Metastatic Potential of Osteosarcoma and Targeting this Pathway for the Treatment of Osteosarcoma Lung Metastases 497
Nancy Gordon and Eugenie S. Kleinerman

Bone Marrow Micrometastases Studied by an Immunomagnetic Isolation Procedure in Extremity Localized Non-metastatic Osteosarcoma Patients 509

Øyvind S. Bruland, Hanne Høifødt, Kirsten Sundby Hall, Sigbjørn Smeland, and Øystein Fodstad

Strategies to Explore New Approaches in the Investigation and Treatment of Osteosarcoma 517

Su Young Kim and Lee J. Helman

History of Orthopedic Oncology in the United States: Progress from the Past, Prospects for the Future 529

William F. Enneking

Editorial Summation 573

Index 577

Contributors

Thor Alvegaard MD, PhD
Regional Cancer Registry, Lund University Hospital, SE-221 85 Lund, Sweden

Pete Anderson MD, PhD
Professor, Children's Cancer Hospital, University of Texas M.D. Anderson Cancer Center, Unit 87, Pediatrics, 1515 Holcombe Blvd., Houston, TX 77030-4009, USA
pmanders@mdanderson.org

İnci Ayan MD
Professor of Pediatrics and Pediatric Oncology, İstanbul University, Oncology Institute, Division of Pediatric Hematology Oncology & Acıbadem University, Department of Pediatrics, Division of Pediatric Hematology Oncology & Acıbadem Bakırköy and Maslak Hospitals, Director of Pediatrics and Pediatric Oncology, İstanbul, Turkey
inciayan@googlemail.com

Gaetano Bacci MD
Chemotherapy, Department of Muscoloskeletal Oncology, Istituto Ortopedico Rizzoli, Via Pupilli 1, 40136 Bologna, Italy
gaetano.baccii@ior.it

Henrik Bauer MD, PhD
Department of Orthopedic Surgery, Karolinska University Hospital, SE-171 76 Stockholm, Sweden

Robert S. Benjamin MD
Professor of Medicine Sarcoma Center, Department of Sarcoma Medical Oncology, The University of Texas M.D. Anderson Cancer Center, 1515 Holcombe Blvd., Unit 450/FC 11.3022, Houston, TX 77030-4009, USA
rbenjami@mdanderson.org

Mark Bernstein MD
Division of Pediatric Hematology-Oncology, IWK Health Centre, Dalhousie University, PO Box 9700, 5850/5980 University Avenue, Halifax, NS, Canada B3K 6R8
mark.bernstein@iwk.nshealth.ca

Stefan S. Bielack MD
Professor of Pediatric Oncology, Department of Pädiatrie 5
(Onkologie, Hämatologie, Immunologie), Klinikum Stuttgart – Olgahospital,
Bismarckstr. 8, D-70176 Stuttgart, Germany
coss@olgahospital-stuttgart.de

Øyvind S. Bruland MD
Professor of Clinical Oncology, Department of Medical Oncology and
Radiotherapy Det Norske Radiumhospital, N-0310 Oslo, Norway
oyvind.bruland@medisin.uio.no

Trude Butterfaß-Bahloul
Coordinating Center for Clinical Trials, University Hospital Muenster,
Von-Esmarch-Str. 62, 48129 Muenster, Germany
butterft@mednet.uni-muenster.de

Gabriele Calaminus MD
Department of Pediatric Oncology and Hematology, University Children's
Hospital Münster, Albert-Schweitzer-Str. 33, 48129 Münster, Germany
gabriele.calaminus@ukmuenster.de

Dorothe Carrle
Studienärztin, Cooperative Osteosarkomstudiengruppe COSS,
Klinikum Stuttgart, Zentrum für Kinder- und Jugendmedizin – Olgahospital,
Pädiatrie 5 (Onkologie, Hämatologie, Immunologie), Bismarckstr. 8,
D-70176 Stuttgart, Germany
coss@olgahospital-stuttgart.de

Anna Cassoni, MD
Radiation Oncologist, University College Hospital London, 235 Euston Road,
London NW12BU, Great Britain, annacassoni@uclh.nhs.uk

Alan Craft MD, FRCPCH, FMedSci
Director of Institute, Northern Institute for Cancer Research, Newcastle
University, Newcastle upon Tyne NE1 7RU, UK
a.w.craft@ncl.ac.uk

Farzin Eftekhari MD
Professor, Department of Diagnostic Radiology, Division of Diagnostic Imaging,
The University of Texas M.D. Anderson Cancer Center, Houston,
TX 77030-4004, USA
feftekhari@mdanderson.org

William F. Enneking MD
Distinguished Service Professor Emeritus, Departments of Orthopaedics
and Pathology, College of Medicine, University of Florida, Gainesville, FL, USA
billkingfisher@aol.com

Stefano Ferrari MD
Responsabile della Sezione di Chemioterapia, dei Tumori dell' Apparato Locomotore, Istituto Ortopedico Rizzoli, Via Pupilli 1, 40136 Bologna, Italy
stefano.ferrari@ior.it

Øystein Fodstad MD, PhD
Department of Tumorbiology, The Norwegian Radium Hospital, N-0310 Oslo, Norway

Bertoni Franco MD, PhD
Pathology, Department of Muscoloskeletal Oncology, Istituto Ortopedico Rizzoli, Via Pupilli 1, 40136 Bologna, Italy
franco.bertoni@ior.it

Richard Gorlick MD
Associate Professor of Molecular Pharmacology and Pediatrics, The Albert Einstein College of Medicine of Yeshiva University, Vice Chairman, Division Chief of Hematology-Oncology, The Children's Hospital at Montefiore, 3415 Bainbridge Avenue, Rosenthal 3rd floor, Bronx, NY 10467, USA
rgorlick@montefiore.org

Nancy Gordon MD
Postdoctoral Fellow, Division of Pediatrics, Children's Cancer Hospital, University of Texas M.D. Anderson Cancer Center, 1515 Holcombe Blvd., Unit #87, Houston, TX 77030-4009, USA
ngordon@mdanderson.org

Kirsten Sundby Hall MD, PhD
Department of Oncology, The Norwegian Radium Hospital, N-0310 Oslo, Norway

Lee J. Helman MD
Scientific Director for Clinical Research, Center for Cancer Research, National Cancer Institute, National Institutes of Health, Bethesda, MD, USA
helmanl@mail.nih.gov

Hanne Høifødt BSc
Department of Tumorbiology, The Norwegian Radium Hospital, N-0310 Oslo, Norway

Dennis P.M. Hughes MD, PhD
Assistant Professor, Children's Cancer Hospital, University of Texas M.D. Anderson Cancer Center, 1515 Holcombe Blvd., Houston, TX 77030-4009, USA
dphughes@mdanderson.org

Winston Huh MD
Assistant Professor of Pediatrics, Children's Cancer Hospital, University of Texas M.D. Anderson Cancer Center, 1515 Holcombe Blvd., Houston, TX 77030-4009, USA
whuh@mdanderson.org

Gayle Hyden BSc
Senior Occupational Therapist, Rehabilitation Services Department,
MD Anderson Cancer Center, Houston, TX 77030-4009, USA

Norman Jaffe MD, DSc, Dip Paed
Professor Emeritus, Children's Cancer Hospital, University of Texas M.D.
Anderson Cancer Center, 1515 Holcombe Blvd., Unit #87, Houston,
TX 77030-4009, USA
njaffe@mdanderson.org

Gernot Jundt MD
Professor of Pathology, Kantonspital Basel, Institut für Pathologie,
Schönbeinstrasse 40, CH-4003 Basel, Switzerland
gernot.jundt@unibas.ch

Herbert Jürgens MD
Professor of Pediatrics, Universitätsklinikum Münster, Klinik und
Poliklinik für Kinderheilkunde, Päd. Hämatologie/Onkologie,
Albert-Schweitzer-Str. 33, 48129 Münster, Germany
jurgh@uni-muenster.de

Rejin Kebudi MD
Professor of Pediatrics and Pediatric Oncology, İstanbul University,
Oncology Institute, Division of Pediatric Hematology Oncology & İstanbul
University, Cerrahpaşa Medical School, İstanbul, Turkey, Director,
Pediatric Oncology Unit, American Hospital, Istanbul, Turkey
rejinkebudi@hotmail.com

Matthias Kevric
Data Manager, Cooperative Osteosarcoma Study Group, Klinikum Stuttgart,
Zentrum für Kinder- und Jugendmedizin – Olgahospital, Pädiatrie 5
(Onkologie, Hämatologie, Immunologie), Bismarckstr. 8,
D-70176 Stuttgart, Germany
coss@olgahospital-stuttgart.de

Chand Khanna DVM, PhD
Dipl. ACVIM (Oncology), Head, Tumor and Metastasis Biology Section,
Pediatric Oncology Branch, Center for Cancer Research, National Cancer
Institute, Director, Comparative Oncology Program, Center for Cancer Research,
National Cancer Institute, 37 Convent Drive, Rm 2144, Bethesda,
MD 20892, USA
khannac@mail.nih.gov

Su Young Kim
Assistant Clinical Investigator, Center for Cancer Research,
National Cancer Institute, National Institutes of Health,
Bethesda, MD, USA

Eugenie S. Kleinerman MD
Professor and Head, Professor, Department of Cancer Biology, Mosbacher Pediatrics Chair, Division of Pediatrics, Children's Cancer Hospital, University of Texas M.D. Anderson Cancer Center, 1515 Holcombe Blvd., Unit #87, Houston, TX 77030, USA
ekleiner@mdanderson.org

Rainer Kotz MD
Professor of Orthopedics, Universitätsklinik für Orthopädie, Währinger Gürtel 18-20, A-1090 Wien, Austria
rainer.kotz@akh-wien.ac.at

Mark Krailo PhD
Department of Preventive Medicine, Keck School of Medicine, University of Southern California, Los Angeles, CA, USA
mkrailo@childrensoncologygroup.org

Thomas Kühne MD
Oberarzt, Universitätskinderspital beider Basel, Onkologie/Hämatologie, Römergasse 8, CH-4005 Basel, Switzerland
Thomas.Kuehne@ukbb.ch

Ching C. Lau MD, PhD
Associate Professor of Pediatrics, Baylor College of Medicine, Director Cancer Genomics Program, Texas Children Cancer Center, 6621 Fannin Street, MC 3-3320, Houston, TX 77030, USA
cclau@txccc.org

David M. Loeb MD, PhD
Assistant Professor, Oncology and Pediatrics, Director, Musculoskeletal Tumor Program, Johns Hopkins University, Bunting-Blaustein Cancer Research Building, Room 2M51, 1650 Orleans St., Baltimore, MD 21231, USA
LOEBDA@jhmi.edu

Neyssa Marina MD
Professor of Pediatrics, Department of Pediatrics, Division of Hematology-Oncology, Stanford University Medical Center, 1000 Welch Road, Suite 300, Palo Alto, CA 94304-1812, USA
neyssa.marina@stanford.edu

Mario Mercuri MD, PhD
Orthopedic Surgery, Department of Muscoloskeletal Oncology, Istituto Ortopedico Rizzoli, Via Pupilli 1, 40136 Bologna, Italy
mario.mercuri@ior.it

Ted B. Muilenburg CP, FAAOP
President, Muilenburg Prosthetics Inc., 3900 La Branch Houston, TX, 77004-4094, USA
ted@mpihouston.com

Giulia Ottaviani MD, PhD
Assistant and Aggregate Professor of Pathology, University of Milano,
Italy, Visiting Scientist, Children's Cancer Hospital, The University
of Texas M.D. Anderson Cancer Center, Houston, TX 77030-4009, USA
giulia.ottaviani@unimi.it

Harzem Özger MD
Professor of Traumatology and Orthopedic Surgery, Department of Traumatology
and Orthopedic Surgery, İstanbul University, İstanbul Medical School,
Istanbul, Turkey

Emanuela Palmerini MD
Chemotherapy, Department of Muscoloskeletal Oncology,
Istituto Ortopedico Rizzoli, Via Pupilli 1, 40136 Bologna, Italy
emanuela.palmerini@ior.it

Shreyaskumar R. Patel MD
Center Medical Director, Sarcoma Center, Professor of Medicine
and Deputy Chairman, Department of Sarcoma Medical Oncology,
The University of Texas M.D. Anderson Cancer Center, 1515 Holcombe Blvd.,
Unit 450/FC 11.3022, Houston, TX 77030-4009, USA
spatel@mdanderson.org

Margaret Pearson RN, MSN, CPNP, CPON
Advanced Nurse Practitioner for the Solid Tumor Service, Children's Cancer
Hospital, The University of Texas M.D. Anderson Cancer Center,
1515 Holcombe Blvd., Houston, TX 77030-4009, USA
peggyharding@sbcglobal.net

Piero Picci MD
Laboratory Research, Department of Muscoloskeletal Oncology,
Istituto Ortopedico Rizzoli, Via Pupilli 1, 40136 Bologna, Italy
piero.piccii@ior.it

Marissa Punzalan BSc
Senior Physical Therapist, Rehabilitation Services Department,
MD Anderson Cancer Center, Houston, TX 77030-4009, USA
mpunzala@mdanderson.org

Peter Reichardt MD
Klinik für Innere Medizin III (Hämatologie, Onkologie und Palliativmedizin),
Pieskower Straße 33, D-15526 Bad Saarow, Germany
peter.reichardt@helios-kliniken.de

Rhonda S. Robert PhD
Division of Pediatrics, Children's Cancer Hospital, University of Texas M.D.
Anderson Cancer Center, 1515 Holcombe Blvd., Houston,
TX 77030-4009, USA
rrobert@mdanderson.org

Contributors

A. Kevin Raymond MD
Associate Professor, Department of Pathology, The University of Texas M.D.
Anderson Cancer Center, 1515 Holcombe Blvd., Houston, TX 77030-4009, USA
kraymond@mdanderson.org

Paula Schomberg, MD
Prof. of Radiation Oncology, Department of Radiation Oncology, Mayo Clinic
Rochester, 200 First Str. S.W., MN 55905 Rochester, USA,
pschomberg@mayo.edu

Rudolf Schwarz MD
Radiation Oncologist, Department of Radiation Oncology, Medical Center
Hamburg-Eppendorf, Martinistr. 52, D-20246 Hamburg, Germany
rschwarz@uke.uni-hamburg.de

Sigbjørn Smeland MD, PhD
Director, Cancer Clinic, The Norwegian Radium Hospital, N-0310 Oslo, Norway

Eric L. Staals
Orthopedic Surgery, Department of Muscoloskeletal Oncology,
Istituto Ortopedico Rizzoli, Via Pupilli 1, 40136 Bologna, Italy
eric.staals@ior.it

Matthew A. Steliga MD
4301 W. Markham Street Little Rock AR 72205
masteliga@uams.edu

Matthew Sydes
Senior Medical Statistician, Cancer Group, MRC Clinical Trials Unit,
222 Euston Rd, London NW1 2DA, UK
matthew.sydes@ctu.mrc.ac.uk

Ara Vaporciyan MD, FACS
Associate Professor, Director, Clinical Education and Training,
Director, Oncology Cardiac & Vascular Surgery Program, University of Texas
M.D. Anderson Cancer Center, 1515 Holcombe Blvd., Houston,
TX 77030-4009, USA
avaporci@mdanderson.org

Mathias Werner MD
HELIOS Klinikum Emil von Behring GmbH, Orthopädische
Pathologie – Referenz-Zentrum, Walterhöferstraße 11, 14165 Berlin, Germany
mathias.werner@helios-kliniken.de

Jeremy Whelan MD
Department of Oncology, University College Hospital, 250 Euston Road,
London NW1 2PG, UK
jeremy.whelan@uclh.nhs.uk

Winifried Winkelmann MD
Professor of Orthopedics, Universitätsklinikum Münster, Klinik und Poliklinik für
Allgemeine Orthopädie, Albert Schweitzer Str. 33, 48129 Münster, Germany
fiegeh@uni-muenster.de

Stephen J Withrow DVM
Director, Animal Cancer Center, University Distinguished Professor,
Stuart Chair in Oncology, Colorado State University, College of Veterinary
Medicine and Biomedical Sciences, Ft Collins, CO 80523, USA
Stephen.Withrow@ColoState.EDU

Alan W. Yasko MD
Professor of Orthopaedic Surgery, Department of Orthopaedic Surgery,
Feinberg School of Medicine, Northwestern University, Chief, Orthopaedic
Oncology, Robert H. Lurie Comprehensive Cancer Center of Northwestern
University, Chicago, IL, USA
a-yasko@northwestern.edu

Andreas Zoubek MD
Assistant Professor of Pediatrics, St. Anna Kinderspital, Kinderspitalgasse 6,
A-1090 Wien, Austria
zoubek@stanna.at

General Aspects of Osteosarcoma

The Epidemiology of Osteosarcoma

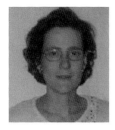

Giulia Ottaviani and Norman Jaffe

Abstract Osteosarcoma derives from primitive bone-forming mesenchymal cells and is the most common primary bone malignancy. The incidence rates and 95% confidence intervals of osteosarcoma for all races and both sexes are 4.0 (3.5–4.6) for the range 0–14 years and 5.0 (4.6–5.6) for the range 0–19 years per year per million persons. Among childhood cancers, osteosarcoma occurs eighth in general incidence and in the following order: leukemia (30%), brain and other nervous system cancers (22.3%), neuroblastoma (7.3%), Wilms tumor (5.6%), Non-Hodgkin lymphoma (4.5%), rhabdomyosarcoma (3.1%), retinoblastoma (2.8%), osteosarcoma (2.4%), and Ewing sarcoma (1.4%). The incidence rates of childhood and adolescent osteosarcoma with 95% confidence intervals areas follows: Blacks, 6.8/year/million; Hispanics, 6.5/year/million; and Caucasians, 4.6/year/million. Osteosarcoma has a bimodal age distribution, having the first peak during adolescence and the second peak in older adulthood. The first peak is in the 10–14-year-old age group, coinciding with the pubertal growth spurt. This suggests a close relationship between the adolescent growth spurt and osteosarcoma. The second osteosarcoma peak is in adults older than 65 years of age; it is more likely to represent a second malignancy, frequently related to Paget's disease. The incidence of osteosarcoma has always been considered to be higher in males than in females, occurring at a rate of 5.4 per million persons per year in males vs. 4.0 per million in females, with a higher incidence in blacks (6.8 per million persons per year) and Hispanics (6.5 per million), than in whites (4.6 per million). Osteosarcoma commonly occurs in the long bones of the extremities near the metaphyseal growth plates. The most common sites are the femur (42%, with 75% of tumors in the distal femur), the tibia (19%, with 80% of tumors in the proximal tibia), and the humerus (10%, with 90% of tumors in the proximal humerus). Other likely locations are the skull or jaw (8%) and the pelvis (8%). Cancer deaths due to bone and joint malignant neoplasms represent 8.9% of all childhood and adolescent cancer

---

G. Ottaviani (✉)
Children's Cancer Hospital, The University of Texas M.D. Anderson Cancer Center, Houston, TX, 77030-4009, USA
e-mail: giulia.ottaviani@unimi.it

deaths. Death rates for osteosarcoma have been declining by about 1.3% per year. The overall 5-year survival rate for osteosarcoma is 68%, without significant gender difference. The age of the patient is correlated with the survival, with the poorest survival among older patients. Complete surgical excision is important to ensure an optimum outcome. Tumor staging, presence of metastases, local recurrence, chemotherapy regimen, anatomic location, size of the tumor, and percentage of tumor cells destroyed after neoadjuvant chemotherapy have effects on the outcome.

Introduction

Osteosarcoma derives from primitive bone-forming mesenchymal cells and is the most common primary bone malignancy. This chapter and its companion chapter, The Etiology of Osteosarcoma, provide data from published literature in an effort to outline current concepts on the epidemiology of osteosarcoma. In our review of the literature, abstracts were identified from searches of the Web bibliographic databases, including Ovid, Medline, and PubMed, using the following combined search terms: *epidemiology, osteosarcoma, children, adolescents, survival,* and *genetics.* The updated information we present in this chapter is designed to help readers to increase their knowledge of the epidemiologic approach to osteosarcoma, to interpret and communicate research findings to patients and their families, and to enhance their own research.

Primary Osteosarcoma

Incidence

The risk of being diagnosed with cancer increases as an individual ages, and 77% of all cancers are diagnosed in persons aged 55 years and above. As a lifetime risk, the probability that an individual, over the course of a lifetime, will develop a cancer is slightly less than one in two for men and a little more than one in three for women.[1-3]

In the United States, for children aged 0–14, and adolescents aged 15–19 years, the overall incidence rate for *all cancers* is 16.5 cases per 100,000 persons per year.[1,4] The childhood and adolescent cancer incidence rate has increased from 11.5 per 100,000 persons per year in 1975, to 14.8 per 100,000 in 2004. Although this trend is recognized to be the result, in part, of improved diagnosis and reporting methods, it appears that there is a true increase in the occurrence of some childhood cancers.[2,5]

For any newborn, the risk of developing cancer by age 20 years is about one in 300 for males and one in 333 for females.[1,6] It has a peak of incidence at ages 5–14.[7] Childhood cancers account for no more than 2% of all cancers.[2]

In the United States, it is significant that all childhood and adolescent cancers combined, affect boys more frequently than girls. Children have a significantly lower incidence rate than adolescents; white children and adolescents have the highest incidence rate among all races.[4] Young people living in the Northeast of the United States have a significantly higher incidence rate compared with those in the Midwest and South census regions; this may be partially attributed to significantly higher incidence rates for central nervous system neoplasms and lymphomas in this region.[4]

In developing countries, it is more difficult to accurately measure the incidence rate because of the greater frequency of deaths from infectious diseases and malnutrition.[2,8]

According to the analysis of the Surveillance, Epidemiology and End Results (SEER) Cancer Statistics Review of the National Cancer Institute,[1] the age-adjusted incidence rate for all *bone and joint cancers* for all ages and all races is 0.9 per 100,000 persons per year, and the mortality rate is 0.4 per 100,000, with a 5-year overall survival rate of 67.9%. The median age at diagnosis for cancer of the bones and joints is 39 years, with the majority (28.7%) occurring below the age of 20 years. For children (aged 0–14 years), the incidence rate for all bone and joint cancers for both sexes is 0.7 per 100,000 persons per year, and the mortality rate is 0.1 per 100,000. For children and adolescents (aged 0–19 years), the incidence rate for all bone and joint cancers is 0.9 per 100,000 persons per year, while the mortality rate is 0.4 per 100,000.[1] Malignancies of the bone and joint, with an average annual incidence rate of 8.7 per million children and adolescents younger than 20 years, make up about 6% of childhood and adolescent cancers (Fig. 1).[3,9] The two types of malignant bone cancers that predominate in children and adolescents are osteosarcoma 1 and Ewing sarcoma, which represent about 56 and 34% of bone cancers, respectively.[10]

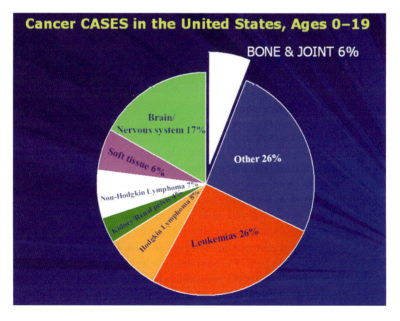

Fig. 1 Distribution of incidence by location of cancer in children and adolescents, ages 0 to 19 years, in the United States. Data are from the U.S. Cancer Statistics Working Group 2004, public-use file[3]

According to the most recent report from the U.S. Cancer Statistics Working Group,[3] the incidence rates and 95% confidence intervals for *osteosarcoma* specifically, for all races and both sexes in children and adolescents under 20 years, are 4.0 (3.5–4.6) per million persons per year for the range 0–14 years, and 5.0 (4.6–5.6) per million for the range 0–19 years. Similarly, according to SEER, the incidence rate of osteosarcoma for all races and both sexes in children and adolescents is 4.7 per million persons per year, with a positive annual percentage change of 0.2.[11]

Cancer registry data with histologic stratification indicate that osteosarcoma is the most common primary malignant tumor of the bone among people of all ages, accounting for approximately 35% of cases, followed by chondrosarcoma (25%) and Ewing sarcoma (16%).[12] Among childhood cancers, osteosarcoma is eighth in general incidence; the most common cancers, in descending order, are: leukemia (30%), brain and other nervous-system cancers (22.3%), neuroblastoma (7.3%), Wilms tumor (5.6%), non-Hodgkin lymphoma (4.5%), rhabdomyosarcoma (3.1%), retinoblastoma (2.8%), osteosarcoma (2.4%), and Ewing sarcoma (1.4%).[6]

In the United States, each year, approximately 400 new cases of osteosarcoma are diagnosed among children and adolescents younger than 20 years.[10] The specific incidence trends for osteosarcoma based on age, gender, ethnicity, and site of disease are described below.

Age

Osteosarcoma is the most frequent bone cancer occurring in children and adolescents aged 10–20 years, whereas in children younger than 10 years, the most common primary bone cancer is Ewing sarcoma.[13]

Osteosarcoma has a bimodal age distribution; the first peak occurs during adolescence, and the second occurs in older adults.[10,14–16] Osteosarcoma is rare in children younger than 5 years; only 2% of patients with osteosarcoma fall into this age group.[17] There is a steady rise in the incidence rates between 5 and 10 years, and a steeper rise occurs between 11 and 15 years, coinciding with the pubertal growth spurt. The overall peak incidence of osteosarcoma occurs at the ages of 10–14 years, after which the rates decline.[3] The second peak of incidence of osteosarcoma is in adults older than 65 years, in which it is more likely to represent a second malignancy, frequently related to Paget disease.[14,18,19]

Gender

According to the most recent publication by the U.S. Cancer Statistics Working Group,[3] the incidence rates and 95% confidence intervals of childhood and adolescent osteosarcoma are 5.0 (4.4–5.8) per million persons per year for males and 5.1 (4.4–5.8) per million for females. Nonetheless, the incidence of osteosarcoma has always been considered to be higher in males than in females,[10,13,16] and according to the most recent SEER data in 2008, it was a rate of 5.4 per million persons per year in males vs. 4.0 per million in females.[11]

Ethnicity

The National Cancer Institute SEER Study for the years 1975–1995, reported that the osteosarcoma incidence among children and adolescents younger than 20 years was higher in African Americans than in whites, with annual rates of 5.2 per million persons in African Americans, and 4.6 per million in whites.[10] More recent data from SEER demonstrate that osteosarcoma occurs more often in Asians/Pacific Islanders and in Hispanics.[13] Recently, the U.S. Cancer Statistics Working Group[3] reported a higher incidence of osteosarcoma in blacks (6.8 per million persons per year) and in Hispanics (6.5 per million) than in whites (4.6 per million).

Site

Osteosarcoma can occur in any bone. It most often occurs near the metaphyseal growth plates of the long bones of the extremities (Fig. 2). The most common sites are the femur (42%, with 75% of these tumors in the distal femur), the tibia (19%, with 80% of these tumors in the proximal tibia), and the humerus (10%, with 90% of these tumors in the proximal humerus). Other likely locations are the skull or jaw (8%), and the pelvis (8%). Only 1.25% of osteosarcomas are located in the ribs.[10,16,20–22] The most recent report from the National Cancer Data Base[23] did not provide any significant additional data, as all the three long bones of the lower extremity (the femur, the tibia, and the fibula) were grouped together. Similarly, all the long bones of the upper extremity (the humerus, the radius, and the ulna) were grouped together. Furthermore, there was no distinction between the epiphyseal, metaphyseal, and diaphyseal locations.

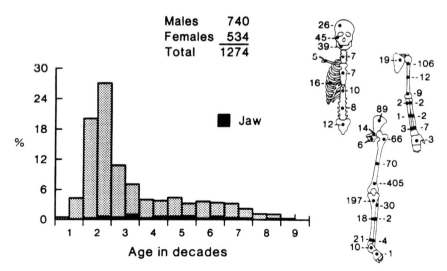

Fig. 2 Distribution of osteosarcomas by age, sex, and skeletal site of lesion for a series of 1,274 patients from the Mayo Clinic. From Dahlin and Unni,[16] by permission of Mayo Foundation for Medical Education and Research

Mortality

In the United States, *cancer*, of all types combined, is the second leading cause of death. Overall, one in every four deaths is due to cancer, according to the National Vital Statistics System.[1-3]

Cancer is the fourth most common cause of death among children and adolescents under 20 years of age, in the United States[24] About 8% of all the deaths are due to cancer between birth and 20 years of age.[1,6]

Among persons aged 1–19 in the United States, the mortality rate is 2.8 cases per 100,000.[1] The Centers for Disease Control and Prevention (CDC) reported a total of 34,500 cancer deaths among children and adolescents in the United States during the years 1990–2004.[24] A total of 2,223 childhood and adolescent cancer deaths occurred in 2004, and 12% of childhood deaths are due to cancer.[2,24] Death rates for childhood cancers have been declining by about 1.3% per year over the years 1990–2004.[24] Overall, this trend reflects the advances that have been made in cancer treatment.[4,24,25]

In 1990–2004, boys (33.1 per million persons per year) had significantly higher death rates than girls (26.1 per million) for all cancers combined; adolescents (37.9 per million) had significantly higher death rates than children (26.9 per million); whites (30.1 per million) and blacks (29.3 per million) had significantly higher death rates than both Asians/Pacific Islanders (26.4 per million) and American Indian/Alaska Natives (20.0 per million); and Hispanics (30.3 per million) had significantly higher death rates than non-Hispanics (29.1 per million).[24]

According to the most recent data from SEER, the mortality rate for all *bone and joint cancers* is 0.4 per 100,000 persons per year for both sexes, all races and all ages.[1]

Cancer deaths due to malignant neoplasms of bone and joint represent 8.9% of all childhood and adolescent cancer deaths, compared with 25.5% for the most common type of cancers, leukemias, and 25.0% for brain and other nervous-system neoplasms (Fig. 3).[24] Death rates for *osteosarcoma* have been declining by about 1.3% per year over the years 1990–2004, similar to the rate of decline for all other childhood cancers except leukemias (3.0% per year) and brain and other nervous-system neoplasms (1.0% per year).[24,26]

Survival

Overall, the treatment strategy of giving preoperative chemotherapy followed by surgery and adjuvant therapy has greatly improved the survival rates of patients with osteosarcoma, over the past decades. Prior to 1970, amputation was the only surgical treatment available for osteosarcoma, and 80% of patients died of metastatic disease, mainly of the lungs.[20-22] These historical cases led to the conclusion that more than 80% of patients without radiologic evidence of metastases at diagnosis

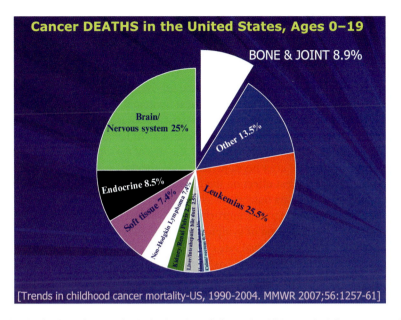

Fig. 3 Distribution of cancer deaths by location of disease in children and adolescents, ages 0 to 19 years. Data are from the Surveillance, Epidemiology and End Results (SEER) Cancer Statistics Review of the National Cancer Institute public-use file[1]

had subclinical micrometastases. This assumption was the basis for the adoption of chemotherapy protocols over the past three decades, which have led to a significant increase in the overall survival rates.[27-29]

The National Cancer Institute SEER Study for the years 1975–1995, reported that the overall *5-year survival rate* for patients with osteosarcoma diagnosed between 1974 and 1994 was 63% (59% for male patients, 70% for female patients).[10] More recent SEER data demonstrate that the survival curves for the age groups younger than 45 years were nearly identical from 1975 to 2000: greater than 65%. In contrast, the 5-year survival rate for patients 45 years and older continued to be less than 45%.[13] The National Cancer Data Base Report[23] recently described that for the single largest series of osteosarcoma cases, the relative 5-year survival rates were 60% for patients younger than 30 years, 50% for patients between 30 and 49 years, and 30% for patients, 50 years and older. The relative 5-year survival rates by subtype were 52.6% for conventional high-grade intramedullary osteosarcoma, 85.9% for parosteal osteosarcoma, 49.5% for small-cell osteosarcoma, and 17.8% for osteosarcoma in Paget's disease.[23] Based on 648 patients treated for osteosarcoma at Massachusetts General Hospital by the orthopedic oncology group, Mankin et al.[30] reported in 2004 that the overall 5-year survival rate for osteosarcoma was 68%, without a significant gender difference.

In 2002, Gatta et al.[31] reported slightly higher survival rates for osteosarcoma in the United States than in Europe; however, the difference was not significant. In 2007, Lewis et al.[32] reported an improvement in histologic response, but not in survival rate, in patients with osteosarcoma treated with intensified chemotherapy in Europe. Recently, Craft and Pritchard-Jones[33] commented on the lower overall childhood cancer survival rate in the United Kingdom compared with that in the rest of Europe.

The age of the patient is correlated with the survival data, with the poorest survival rate for older patients.[13,30] The type of surgical treatment, i.e., amputation compared with a limb-salvage procedure for nonmetastatic osteosarcoma, has no effect on the outcome.[34] Tumor stage, the presence of metastases or local recurrence, the chemotherapeutic treatment, the anatomic location, the size of the tumor, and the percentage of tumor cells destroyed after neoadjuvant chemotherapy, were considered by some researchers to have a great effect on the outcome.[14,30] The most significant variable affecting the osteosarcoma outcome was reported to be the date of diagnosis, with the improved survival rate trends mirroring the introduction of increasingly effective chemotherapy.[35] The duration of symptoms prior to the initiation of therapy has not been shown to affect the survival rates.[36]

Tumor location at presentation has been correlated with the outcome. Mankin et al.[30] reported the lowest survival rates for patients with osteosarcoma of the lumbar spine and pelvis (32%), the scapula and shoulder (45%), and the proximal femur (62%), and the higher survival rates for osteosarcoma of the proximal tibia (78%) and the distal femur (73%). Patients with primary osteosarcoma of the rib were reported to have an overall survival rate of only 15% at 5 years; 34% of patients affected by osteosarcoma of the rib presented with synchronous osteosarcoma lesions.[37]

Recently, Jeys et al.[38] reported an increased survival rate in osteosarcoma patients who underwent limb salvage and had postoperative endoprosthesis infections. The 10-year survival rate for patients with endoprosthesis infection was 84.5%, compared with 62.3% in the noninfected group; infection was an independent favorable prognostic factor, as discussed more in detail in the chapter titled "Quality of life in long-term survivors of lower extremity osteosarcomas: amputation versus limb salvage." Bramer et al.[39] reported a significantly lower survival rate in osteosarcoma patients who presented with pathologic fractures compared with the rate in patients without such fractures.

Osteosarcomas Following Treatment

Radiation-induced osteosarcomas, which develop following cancer treatment with radiation, frequently for Ewing sarcoma, have been shown in some studies to have rates of local recurrence and metastasis, and functional outcomes similar to those of patients with primary osteosarcoma.[40,41] Patients treated for radiation-induced osteosarcoma with limb-salvage procedures had functional outcomes similar to those of matched patients treated for primary osteosarcoma.[41]

A constellation of *subsequent primary cancers* was observed in osteosarcoma survivors.[42] Bacci et al.[43] reported that 2.15% of osteosarcoma patients developed a second malignant neoplasm at a median of 7.6 years (range, 1–25 years) after the

The Epidemiology of Osteosarcoma

primary osteosarcoma had been treated with neoadjuvant and adjuvant chemotherapy. The most common type of subsequent neoplasm was leukemia, followed by, in decreasing order of occurrence, breast, lung, kidney, central nervous system, soft-tissue, parotid, and colon cancers. The overall rate of second neoplasms in osteosarcoma survivors was significantly higher in females, and the latent period for subsequent hematologic tumors was shorter than that for subsequent solid tumors.[43] The risk of subsequent breast cancer was markedly increased among females previously treated for osteosarcoma; this increased risk was probably due, in part, to thoracic radiotherapy for lung metastases, although genetic predisposition also appeared to play a role. It has been reported that a family history of sarcoma is predictive of breast-cancer risk among the survivors of bone sarcoma who have not received chest radiotherapy.[44]

Jaffe et al.[45,46] reported the occurrence of single or multiple *metachronous osteosarcoma* in 4.07% of the pediatric and adolescent patients successfully treated for primary osteosarcoma. There was an increased incidence in patients who had retinoblastoma and the Li–Fraumeni syndrome. The metachronous osteosarcomas appeared as single lesions in 63.64% of cases and as multifocal in the remaining cases.[45] The interval between the discovery of the primary osteosarcoma and the first metachronous osteosarcoma ranged from 11 months to 7.33 years. The histologic variant of the metachronous osteosarcoma was concordant with that of the primary osteosarcoma in 70% of cases. A total of 45% of the patients survived for periods ranging from 20 to 50 months after the treatment of the metachronous osteosarcoma.[45]

Conclusions

Osteosarcoma is the most common bone cancer encountered in children and adolescents. It was originally reported to be more common in males than in females; however, recent reports indicate that the incidence may be equal in both sexes. The incidence is higher in African Americans than in whites. The disease most commonly occurs in the femur. The survival rate of patients with osteosarcoma has improved over the past 30 years with the introduction of multidisciplinary therapy. Patients successfully treated for osteosarcoma may develop second malignant neoplasms, including an additional osteosarcoma.

References

1. Ries LAG, Melbert D, Krapcho M, et al., eds. *SEER Cancer Statistics Review, 1975–2004, Based on November 2006 SEER Data Submission*. Bethesda, MD: National Cancer Institute. Available at: http://seer.cancer.gov/csr/1975_2004/; Accessed January 2009.
2. American Cancer Society. *Global Cancer Facts and Figures 2007*. Atlanta, GA: American Cancer Society; 2007. Available at: http://www.cancer.org/downloads/STT/Global_Cancer_Facts_and_Figures_2007_rev.pdf; Accessed January 2009.

3. U.S. Cancer Statistics Working Group. *United States Cancer Statistics: 2004 Incidence and Mortality*. Atlanta, GA: U.S. Department of Health and Human Services, Centers for Disease Control and Prevention, and National Cancer Institute; 2007. Available at: http://www.cdc. gov/cancer/npcr/npcrpdfs/US_Cancer_Statistics_2004_Incidence_and_Mortality.pdf; Accessed January 2009.
4. Li J, Thompson TD, Miller JW, et al. Cancer incidence among children and adolescents in the United States, 2001–2003. *Pediatrics*. 2008;121:e1470-e1477.
5. Steliarova-Foucher E, Stiller C, Kaatsch P, et al. Geographical patterns and time trends of cancer incidence and survival among children and adolescents in Europe since the 1970s (the ACCIS project): an epidemiological study. *Lancet*. 2004;364:2097-2105.
6. American Cancer Society. *Cancer Facts and Figures 2007*. Atlanta (GA): American Cancer Society, Inc.; 2007. Available at: http://www.cancer.org/downloads/STT/caff2007PWSecured. pdf; Accessed August 2008.
7. Minino AM, Smith BL. Deaths: preliminary data for 2000. *Natl Vital Stat Rep*. 2001;49:1-40.
8. Bryce J, Boschi-Pinto C, Shibuya K, et al. WHO estimates of the causes of death in children. *Lancet*. 2005;365:1147-1152.
9. U.S. Cancer Statistics Working Group. *United States Cancer Statistics: 2001 Incidence and Mortality*. Atlanta, GA: Centers for Disease Control and Prevention and National Cancer Institute; 2004.
10. Gurney JG, Swensen AR, Bulterys M. Malignant bone tumors. In: Ries LA, Smith MAS, Gurney JG, et al., ed. *Cancer Incidence and Survival Among Children and Adolescents: United States SEER Program 1975–1995*. Bethesda, MD: National Cancer Institute; 1999. Available at: http://seer.cancer.gov/publications/childhood/bone.pdf; Accessed August 2008.
11. Linabery AM, Ross JA. Trends in childhood cancer incidence in the U.S. (1992–2004). *Cancer*. 2008;112:416-432.
12. Fletcher CDM, Unni KK, Mertens F, eds. *World Health Organization Classification of Tumors: Pathology and Genetics of Tumors of the Soft Tissue and Bone*. Lyon: IARC Press; 2002.
13. Mascarenhas L, Siegel S, Spector L, et al. Malignant bone tumors. In: Bleyer A, O'Leary M, Barr R, et al., eds. *Cancer Epidemiology in Older Adolescents and Young Adults 15 to 29 Years of Age, Including SEER Incidence and Survival: 1975–2000 (NIH Pub. No. 06-5767)*. Bethesda, MD: National Cancer Institute; 2006:97–110. Available at: http://seer.cancer.gov/ publications/aya/8_bone.pdf; Accessed January 2009.
14. Jaffe N. Malignant bone tumors in children: incidence and etiologic considerations. In: Jaffe N, ed. *Solid Tumors in Childhood*. Littleton, MA: PSG Publishing Co; 1979:1-10.
15. Miller RW, Boice JD Jr, Curtis RE. Bone cancer. In: Schottenfeld D, Fraumeni JF, eds. *Cancer Epidemiology and Prevention*. 2nd ed. New York: Oxford University Press; 1996:971-983.
16. Dahlin DC, Unni KK, eds. *Bone Tumors: General Aspects and Data on 8,542 Cases*. 4th ed. Charles C. Thomas: Springfield, IL; 1986.
17. Hartford CM, Wodowski KS, Rao BN, et al. Osteosarcoma among children aged 5 years or younger: the St Jude Children's Research Hospital experience. *J Pediatr Hematol Oncol*. 2006;28:43-47.
18. Deyrup AT, Montag AG, Inwards CY, et al. Sarcomas arising in Paget disease of bone: a clinicopathologic analysis of 70 cases. *Arch Pathol Lab Med*. 2007;131:942-946.
19. Hansen MF, Seton M, Merchant A. Osteosarcoma in Paget's disease of bone. *J Bone Miner Res*. 2006;21(Suppl 2):P58-P63.
20. Marcove RC, Miké V, Hajeck JV, et al. Osteogenic sarcoma under the age of twenty one. A review of one hundred and forty-five operative cases. *J Bone Joint Surg Am*. 1970;52:411-423.
21. McKenna RJ, Schwinn CP, Soonh KY, et al. Sarcomata of osteogenic series (osteosarcoma, fibrosarcoma, chondrosarcoma, parosteal osteosarcoma, and sarcomata arising in abnormal bone): an analysis of 552 cases. *J Bone Joint Surg Am*. 1966;48-A:1-26.
22. Dahlin DC, Coventry MB. Osteogenic sarcoma. A study of six hundred cases. *J Bone Joint Surg Am*. 1967;49:101-110.
23. Damron TA, Ward WG, Stewart A. Osteosarcoma, chondrosarcoma, and Ewing's sarcoma: National Cancer Data Base Report. *Clin Orthop Relat Res*. 2007;459:40-47.

The Epidemiology of Osteosarcoma

24. Trends in childhood cancer mortality – United States, 1990–2004. *MMWR Morb Mortal Wkly Rep* 2007; 56:1257–1261.
25. Linet MS, Ries LA, Smith MA, et al. Cancer surveillance series: recent trends in childhood cancer incidence and mortality in the United States. *J Natl Cancer Inst*. 1999;91:1051-1058.
26. Stat bite: Childhood cancer deaths by site, 2004. *J Natl Cancer Inst* 2008; 100:165.
27. Hudson M, Jaffe MR, Jaffe N, et al. Pediatric osteosarcoma: therapeutic strategies, results and prognostic factors derived from a 10-year experience. *J Clin Oncol*. 1990;8:1988-1997.
28. Bacci G, Ferrari S, Bertoni F, et al. Long-term outcome for patients with nonmetastatic osteosarcoma of the extremity treated at the Istituto Ortopedico Rizzoli/osteosarcoma-2 protocol: an updated report. *J Clin Oncol*. 2000;18:4016-4027.
29. Pratt CB, Meyer WH, Rao BN, et al. Osteosarcoma studies at St Jude Children's Research Hospital from 1968 through 1998. *Cancer Treat Res*. 1993;62:323-6.
30. Mankin HJ, Hornicek FJ, Rosenberg AE, et al. Survival data for 648 patients with osteosarcoma treated at one Institution. *Clin Orthop Relat Res*. 2004;1:286-291.
31. Gatta G, Capocaccia R, Coleman MP, et al. Childhood cancer survival in Europe and the United States. *Cancer*. 2002;95:1767-1772.
32. Lewis IJ, Nooij MA, Whelan J, et al. Improvement in histologic response but not survival in osteosarcoma patients treated with intensified chemotherapy: a randomized phase III trial of the European Osteosarcoma Intergroup. *J Natl Cancer Inst*. 2007;99:112-128.
33. Craft AW, Pritchard-Jones K. UK childhood cancer survival falling behind rest of EU? *Lancet Oncol*. 2007;8:662-663.
34. Simon MA, Aschliman MA, Thomas N, et al. Limb salvage treatment versus amputation for osteosarcoma of the distal end of the femur. *J Bone Joint Surg Am*. 1986;68:1331-1337.
35. Foster L, Dall GF, Reid R, Wallace WH, Porter DE. Twentieth-century survival from osteosarcoma in childhood. Trends from 1933 to 2004. *J Bone Joint Surg Br*. 2007;89:1234-1238.
36. Rougraff BT, Davis K, Lawrence J. Does length of symptoms before diagnosis of sarcoma affect patient survival? *Clin Orthop Relat Res*. 2007;462:181-189.
37. Burt M. Primary malignant tumors of the chest wall. The Memorial Sloan-Kettering Cancer Center experience. *Chest Surg Clin N Am*. 1994;4:137-154.
38. Jeys LM, Grimer RJ, Carter SR, et al. Post operative infection and increased survival in osteosarcoma patients: are they associated? *Ann Surg Oncol*. 2007;14:2887-2895.
39. Bramer JA, Abudu AA, Grimer RJ, et al. Do pathological fractures influence survival and local recurrence rate in bony sarcomas? *Eur J Cancer*. 2007;43:1944-1951.
40. Bacci G, Longhi A, Forni C, et al. Neoadjuvant chemotherapy for radioinduced osteosarcoma of the extremity: The Rizzoli experience in 20 cases. *Int J Radiat Oncol Biol Phys*. 2007;67:505-511.
41. Shaheen M, Deheshi BM, Riad S, et al. Prognosis of radiation-induced bone sarcoma is similar to primary osteosarcoma. *Clin Orthop Relat Res*. 2006;450:76-81.
42. Inskip PD, Ries LAG, Cohen RJ, et al. New malignancies following childhood cancer. In: Curtis RE, Freedman DM, Ron E, et al., eds. *New Malignancies Among Cancer Survivors: SEER Cancer Registries, 1973–2000 (NIH Publ. No. 05-5302)*. Bethesda, MD: National Cancer Institute; 2006. Available at: http://seer.cancer.gov/publications/mpmono/Ch18_Childhood.pdf; Accessed August 2008.
43. Bacci G, Ferrari C, Longhi A, et al. Second malignant neoplasm in patients with osteosarcoma of the extremities treated with adjuvant and neoadjuvant chemotherapy. *J Pediatr Hematol Oncol*. 2006;28:774-780.
44. Kenney LB, Yasui Y, Inskip PD, et al. Breast cancer after childhood cancer: a report from the Childhood Cancer Survivor Study. *Ann Intern Med*. 2004;141:590-597.
45. Jaffe N, Pearson P, Yasko AW, et al. Single and multiple metachronous osteosarcoma tumors after therapy. *Cancer*. 2003;98:2457-2466.
46. Jaffe N. Metachronous skeletal osteosarcoma after therapy. *J Clin Oncol*. 2004;22:1524.

The Etiology of Osteosarcoma

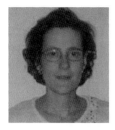

Giulia Ottaviani and Norman Jaffe

Abstract Studies to determine the etiology of osteosarcoma involve epidemiologic and environmental factors and genetic impairments. Factors related to patient characteristics include age, gender, ethnicity, growth and height, genetic and familial factors, and preexisting bone abnormalities. Rapidly proliferating cells may be particularly susceptible to oncogenic agents and mitotic errors which lead to neoplastic transformation. Genetic aberrations that accompany osteosarcoma have received increasing recognition as an important factor in its etiology. Osteosarcoma tumor cells exhibit karyotypes with a high degree of complexity which has made it difficult to determine whether any recurrent chromosomal aberrations characterize osteosarcoma. Although extremely rare, osteosarcoma has occasionally been observed in several members of the same family. No other clinical abnormalities in the proband or the affected members were reported. Pathologic examination of the tumors revealed no unusual features. Genetic testing was not available in most of these reports. The patients generally responded to conventional therapy. A genetic predisposition to osteosarcoma is found in patients with hereditary retinoblastoma, characterized by mutation of the retinoblastoma gene RB1 on chromosome 13q14. The Rothmund–Thomson syndrome is an autosomal recessive disorder with a heterogeneous clinical profile. Patients may have a few or multiple clinical features including skin rash, small stature, skeletal dysplasias, sparse or absent scalp hair, eyebrows or eyelashes, juvenile cataracts, and gastrointestinal disturbance including chronic emesis and diarrhea; its molecular basis is the mutation in the RECQL4 gene in a subset of cases. The Li–Fraumeni syndrome is an autosomal dominant disorder characterized by a high risk of developing osteosarcoma and has been found in up to 3% of children with osteosarcoma. It is associated with a germline mutation of the p53, a suppressor gene. The following three criteria must be met for a diagnosis of Li–Fraumeni syndrome: (1) A proband diagnosed with sarcoma when younger than 45 years; (2) A first-degree relative with any cancer diagnosed when younger than

---

G. Ottaviani (✉)
Children's Cancer Hospital, The University of Texas M.D. Anderson Cancer Center,
Houston, TX, 77030-4009, USA
e-mail: giulia.ottaviani@unimi.it

45 years; (3) Another first- or second-degree relative of the same genetic lineage with any cancer diagnosed when younger than 45 years or sarcoma diagnosed at any age. A second recessive p53 oncogene on chromosome 17p13.1 may also play a role in the development and progression of osteosarcoma. Osteosarcoma has also been associated with solitary or multiple osteochondroma, solitary enchondroma or enchondromatosis (Ollier's disease), multiple hereditary exostoses, fibrous dysplasia, chronic osteomyelitis, sites of bone infarcts, sites of metallic prostheses and sites of prior internal fixation. Ionizing radiation is a well-documented etiologic factor. Osteosarcoma has also been associated with the use of intravenous radium and Thorotrast. Exposure to alkylating agents may also contribute to its development ,and it is apparently independent of the administration of radiotherapy.

Introduction

Osteosarcoma may be considered to be caused by an interaction of environmental insults and genetic susceptibility (Fig. 1). Studies to determine the etiology of osteosarcoma involve epidemiologic and environmental factors, and genetic impairments. Currently, well-known risk factors associated with the development of osteosarcoma comprise ionizing radiation, alkylating agents, Paget's disease, hereditary retinoblastoma, the Li–Fraumeni familial cancer syndrome, and other chromosomal abnormalities. Discoveries regarding the etiology of osteosarcoma will enable patients to avoid the causes and prevent its occurrence. At present, however, the etiology is largely unknown.

Table 1 shows research results on risk factors for osteosarcoma, and these factors are discussed in this chapter. They have been subdivided into host factors, which

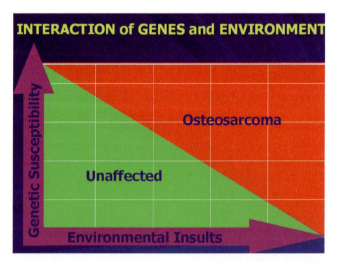

Fig. 1 Osteosarcoma is caused by the interaction of environmental insults and genetic susceptibility

The Etiology of Osteosarcoma

Table 1 Risk factors for osteosarcoma, subdivided into host and environmental factors. None of the risk factors identified can be considered a specific cause of osteosarcoma

Host factors	Comments	References
Age	Rare before 5 years; peak in adolescence, second peak in older adults	U.S. Cancer Statistics Working Group, 2007 Linabery AM et al. *Cancer* 2008;112:416–432
Gender	Rate of 5.4 per million per year in males vs. 4.0 per million in females	Linabery AM et al. *Cancer* 2008;112:416–432
Ethnicity	More frequent in African Americans and Hispanics than in whites	U.S. Cancer Statistics Working Group, 2007
Growth and height	The first peak age of onset corresponds to the adolescent growth spurt. Children with short birth lengths are at increased risk. Patients diagnosed during their growth spurts are taller than their like-aged peers, whereas patients diagnosed in adulthood have average height	Troisi R et al. *Br J Cancer* 2006;95:1603–1607 Longhi A et al. J Pediatr Hematol Oncol 2005;27:314–318
Genetic conditions	Increased risk is well documented for hereditary retinoblastoma, Li–Fraumeni syndrome, Rothmund–Thomson syndrome, Bloom and Werner syndromes	Fletcher CDM et al. *WHO Classification of Tumors.* IARC Press, Lyon, 2002 Hicks MJ et al. *J Clin Oncol* 2007;25:370–375
Paget disease	Development of osteosarcoma in ~1% of cases	Deyrup AT et al. *Arch Pathol Lab Med* 2007; 131:942–946 Hansen MF et al. *J Bone Miner Res* 2006; 21:P58–P63
Other preexisting bone abnormalities	Solitary or multiple osteochondroma, solitary enchondroma or enchondromatos.s (Ollier disease), multiple hereditary exostoses, fibrous dysplasia, chronic osteomyelitis, and sites of bone infarcts, of prostheses, and of prior internal fixation are all associated with i ncreased risk	Fletcher CDM et al. *WHO Classification of Tumors.* IARC Press, Lyon, 2002

(continued)

Table 1 (continued)

Host factors	Comments	References
Environmental factors		
Ionizing radiation, either therapeutic or inadvertent	Well-documented risk factor, responsible for ~3% of cases	Kalra S et al. *J Bone Joint Surg Br* 2007;89:808–813
Alkylating agents	Independent of radiotherapy, treatment with alkylating agents increases the risk for osteosarcoma	Le Vu B et al. *Int J Cancer* 1998; 77:370–377
Perinatal factors	Fetal x-rays are associated with increased risk. Short birth length and high birth weight are associated with elevated osteosarcoma risk. Perinatal factors were not documented to increase risk, according to the Children's Cancer Group	Buckley JD et al. Cancer 1998; 83:1440–1448 Troisi R et al. *Br J Cancer* 2006; 95:1603–1607
Viruses	As yet, there is not convincing evidence that osteosarcoma is caused by a virus or that it is contagious in the usual sense	Shah KV. *Int J Cancer* 2007; 120:215–223
Prior trauma	Prior trauma seems to account only for a very small portion of cases, if any, and it is generally considered to be coincidental	Operskalski EA et al. *Am J Epidemiol* 1987;126:118–126

are not amenable to prevention, and environmental factors, which are amenable to prevention. None of these risk factors identified can be considered a specific cause of osteosarcoma, but all of them should always be taken into account in future investigations regarding the occurrence of osteosarcoma.

Host Factors

Factors related to patient characteristics include age, gender, ethnicity, growth and height, genetic and familial factors, and preexisting bone abnormalities. Age, gender, and ethnicity are discussed briefly here; for more detail, please refer to the chapter titled "The Epidemiology of Osteosarcoma."

Age

Osteosarcoma has a bimodal age distribution, with the first peak occurring in adolescents, and the second peak in adults older than 65 years.[1-5] Osteosarcoma is rare in children younger than 5 years.[6] According to the most recent publication by the U.S. Cancer Statistics Working Group,[2] the incidence rates of osteosarcoma are 8.6 cases per million persons per year at ages 10–14 years, and 8.0 per million at ages 15–19 years.

Gender

According to the most recent Surveillance, Epidemiology and End Results (SEER) data for childhood and adolescence, osteosarcoma occurs at a rate of 5.4 per million persons per year in males vs. 4.0 per million in females.[7]

Ethnicity

The most recent data from the U.S. Cancer Statistics Working Group[2] suggest a higher incidence of osteosarcoma in African Americans (6.8 per million per year) and Hispanics (6.5 per million) than in whites (4.6 per million).

Growth

Osteosarcoma occurs more commonly at the growing ends of long bones, especially the femur, and appears to be closely related to bone growth. In dogs, giant breeds have a much higher risk of developing osteosarcoma than do small- or medium-sized breeds.[8] In humans, the first peak of osteosarcoma onset corresponds to the adolescent growth spurt, suggesting a close relationship between the rapid bone growth at the onset of puberty and osteosarcoma development.[1,9] Osteosarcoma incidence has an earlier peak in girls than in boys, which corresponds to the earlier growth spurt in girls.[10] It seems that rapidly proliferating cells might be particularly susceptible to oncogenic agents and mitotic errors, leading to their transformation into cancer cells. However, differing from the general trend, a case-control study conducted by the Children's Cancer Group[11] suggested an increased risk for osteosarcoma associated with loss of weight and height gain.

Height

In 2004, a large epidemiologic study demonstrated that osteosarcoma was more common in tall individuals.[12] This finding is supported by a report that patients with osteosarcomas diagnosed during their growth spurt are taller than their peers of the same age, whereas patients with osteosarcomas diagnosed in adulthood are of average height.[13] In contrast, other reports have claimed that there is no significant correlation between height and osteosarcoma.[14,15]

Genetic and Familial Factors

Genetic aberrations that accompany osteosarcoma have received increasing recognition as important factors in its etiology. Osteosarcoma tumor cells exhibit karyotypes with a high degree of complexity, which has made it difficult to determine whether any recurrent chromosomal aberrations characterize osteosarcoma. The application of comparative genomic hybridization to osteosarcoma tissue has disclosed several different chromosomal abnormalities, including gains of chromosome 1p, 2p, 3q, 5q, 5p, and 6p and losses of 14q (50% in the 14q11.2 region), 15q, and 16p.[16] Regions of chromosome 21 were absent in 63% of pediatric osteosarcoma cases; the most frequent loss was in the 21q11.2~21 region. These findings suggest that these chromosome 21 regions play a role in the development of osteosarcoma.[16]

Osteosarcoma in siblings has been reported in several families[17–26] (Figs. 2 and 3) and also in dogs,[27] but this occurrence is rare, affecting less than 1 in 1,000 osteosarcoma patients.[28] The disease has also been observed in parent-offspring pairs[20,29,30] and in cousins.[31] Pathologic examination of tumor cells revealed no unusual features in siblings who had osteosarcoma, although the telangiectatic variant was more frequent in familial osteosarcoma than in sporadic cases.[17,31] Genetic testing was not available in most of these family cases . The siblings affected by osteosarcoma generally responded similarly to conventional therapy, as did patients affected by sporadic osteosarcoma.

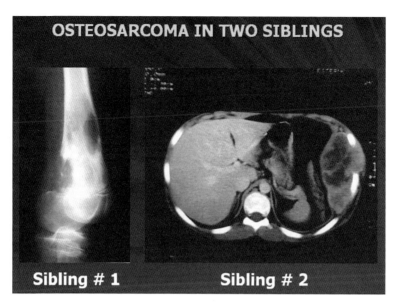

Fig. 2 An example of familial osteosarcoma. Sibling # 1 was a 11-year-old white girl who was diagnosed with telangiectatic osteosarcoma of the left femur. An anteroposterior lateral radiograph (L) shows two large, purely lytic lesions with poor margination in the distal left femur. Sibling # 2 was a 12-year-old boy diagnosed with high-grade osteosarcoma of the left rib. A computed tomography scan (R) shows a large mass (14 x 10 x 9 cm), arising from the ninth left rib, compressing the diaphragm muscle and the abdominal organs below the diaphragm. Both patients responded well to chemotherapy and treatments and are alive, 26 and 11 years after diagnosis, respectively. Family pedigree is shown in Fig. 3

At the molecular level, osteosarcoma is a puzzle of genetic alterations: the pathogenesis is based on the inactivation of tumor suppressor genes, particularly *p53* and the retinoblastoma susceptibility gene *(RB1)*, whose alterations have been observed in a significant number of the osteosarcomas screened. Loss of heterozygosity is reported in osteosarcoma in the regions of chromosomes 3q, 13q, and 18q.[32,33] Mutations in other cell cycle–regulatory genes, including amplification of the product of the murine double minute 2 *(MDM2)* and cyclin-dependent kinase 4 *(CDK4)* genes have been described in osteosarcoma.[33–36]

As could be inferred from these data on genetic mutations, the incidence of osteosarcoma is increased in several genetic disorders associated with germline alterations of tumor suppressor genes. *RB1* is located on the long arm of chromosome 13 (13q14). It functions as a tumor suppressor gene by acting as the major regulator of the progression from G1 to S phase in the cell cycle.[33,36] The frequency of *RB1* alterations in sporadic osteosarcoma has been found to be 30–75%.[36] Retinoblastoma, particularly the familial type, has been well described as frequently associated with the later development of osteosarcoma.[37,38] The strong genetic predisposition to osteosarcoma in patients with hereditary retinoblastoma is characterized by a germline mutation of *RB1*, and the higher occurrence of osteosarcoma

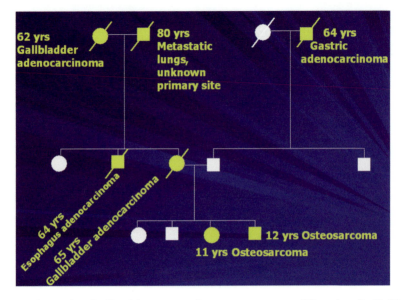

Fig. 3 Pedigree of the family with two cases of osteosarcoma among siblings described in Fig. 2. Li–Fraumeni syndrome has been suspected but not confirmed. When blood samples of the family members were analyzed, no mutation in the *p53* gene was detected. The testing was done by sequencing the coding regions in the *p53* gene. In this family, only the first two of the three criteria for establishing the diagnosis of Li–Fraumeni syndrome were met: (1) A proband diagnosed with sarcoma when younger than 45 years; (2) A first-degree relative with any cancer diagnosed when younger than 45 years; (3) Another first- or second-degree relative of the same genetic lineage with any cancer diagnosed when younger than 45 years or sarcoma diagnosed at any age. Circles represent females; squares, males. Filled circles and squares represent cancer-affected members. Circles and squares with slashes represent dead family members

in survivors of hereditary retinoblastoma supports the conclusion that a germline mutation of the gene plays a role for a germline mutation of the gene.[37,38] The prognosis for patients with *RB1* alterations seems to be poorer than that for patients without *RB1* alterations.[33]

It is estimated that 60% of retinoblastoma cases are nonhereditary and unilateral; 15%, hereditary and unilateral; and 25%, hereditary and bilateral. In the two hereditary types, autosomal dominant inheritance with nearly complete penetrance is observed.[39] The 20-year cumulative incidence of developing osteosarcoma after having been diagnosed with bilateral retinoblastoma is 12.1%.[40] The high relative risk of osteosarcoma in patients with retinoblastoma reflects the combination of genetic predisposition to multiple cancers and the secondary effects of the radiotherapy utilized for treatment of retinoblastoma.

The *p53* gene is a well-known tumor suppressor gene located on the short arm of chromosome 17 (17p). The *p53* gene codes for a nuclear phosphoprotein that increases in level in response to DNA damage and is thought to arrest progression through the cell cycle or cause apoptosis, or programmed cell death. Mutations of this gene can therefore result in tumor formation because of the loss of growth control.

The Etiology of Osteosarcoma

The *p53* gene is estimated to be defective, or it fails to express a functional protein product in more than 50% of all human cancers.[34] The amount of *p53*-positive, defective tumor cells in patients with sporadic osteosarcoma has been reported to range from 21 to 63%.[35]

The Li–Fraumeni syndrome is an autosomal dominant disorder characterized by a high risk of developing osteosarcoma, and it has been found in up to 3% of children with osteosarcomas.[41] The Li–Fraumeni syndrome is a cancer syndrome characterized by frequent familial osteosarcoma and soft-tissue sarcomas in children, breast cancer in young women, and brain tumors and other cancers in close relatives; it has an autosomal dominant inheritance and is caused by a mutation in the *p53* gene.[41–46] Given an affected parent, there is a 50% probability of affected offspring (Fig. 4). The following three criteria should be met for a diagnosis of Li–Fraumeni syndrome: (1) a proband with sarcoma diagnosed when the person is younger than 45 years; (2) having a first-degree relative, with any cancer diagnosed when the relative was younger than 45 years; and (3) another first- or second-degree relative of the same genetic lineage, with any cancer diagnosed when the person was younger than 45 years or sarcoma diagnosed at any age[41–43] (Fig. 3). In Li–Fraumeni syndrome families, germline mutations of the gene *p53* have been identified by blood tests in 50–70% of cases.[45–47]

The Rothmund–Thomson syndrome is an autosomal recessive disorder with a heterogeneous clinical profile. Patients may have a few or multiple clinical features that include a skin rash (poikiloderma); small stature; skeletal dysplasias; sparse or

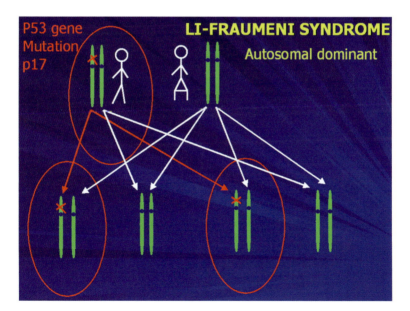

Fig. 4 Li–Fraumeni syndrome is a rare autosomal dominant hereditary disorder caused by a mutation in the *p53* gene on chromosome 17p. Given an affected parent, there is a 50% probability of affected offsprings

absent scalp hair, eyebrows, and/or eyelashes; juvenile cataracts; and gastrointestinal disturbances, including chronic emesis and diarrhea. In a subset of cases, the molecular basis for Rothmund–Thomson syndrome is a mutation in the *RECQL4* gene, which encodes a RECQ-family DNA helicase. A genotype-phenotype analysis showed that the presence of deleterious mutations in *RECQL4* was highly correlated with the development of osteosarcoma.[48–51] Ten percent of patients affected by Rothmund–Thomson syndrome develop osteosarcoma.[52] Patients with this syndrome have genomic instability, with an increased sensitivity to DNA-damaging agents, including ionizing radiation and ultraviolet radiation; they may also experience increased toxic effects of chemotherapy compared with osteosarcoma patients without the syndrome.[48–51] Osteosarcoma patients affected by this genetic syndrome should be treated with standard chemotherapy; however, they may not tolerate full doses of doxorubicin, and modifications should be made individually. Given their known genetic predisposition to cancer, they should be monitored for a second occurrence of osteosarcoma as well as for second malignant neoplasms.[51]

Two other RECQ-helicase disorders, the Bloom and Werner (adult progeria) syndromes, are also associated with an increase in osteosarcomas. Patients with Bloom syndrome present with mutations in the *BLM* (*RECQL2*) gene and are at increased risk for multiple cancers, at an earlier age and at increased frequency when compared with the general population.[53] Patients with Werner syndrome carry mutations in the *WRN* (*RECQL3*) gene, presenting an increased risk for soft-tissue sarcomas, thyroid cancer, melanomas, osteosarcoma, and other cancers. Overall, RECQ proteins may play an important role in tumor repression.[54,55]

Preexisting Bone Abnormalities

Paget's disease is a premalignant condition, as approximately 1% of patients with this disease develop osteosarcoma. Osteosarcoma in patients older than 40 years is frequently associated with Paget disease. In particular, Paget disease accounts for more than 20% of osteosarcomas in patients older than 40 years of age. Paget osteosarcoma is twice as common in men as in women, with an overall median diagnosis age of 64 years. This complication is usually observed in patients with widespread Paget disease (70%) but can occur in patients with monostotic Paget disease as well. Paget osteosarcomas are high-grade sarcomas, mostly osteoblastic or fibroblastic osteosarcomas. Telangiectatic and small-cell osteosarcomas have also been reported. The prognosis is poor, especially for patients with tumors located in the pelvic bones and the skull. Survival durations are shorter in cases of multifocal disease. Metastases are detected in 25% of osteosarcoma patients at initial presentation.[39,56,57]

Other bone conditions associated with an increased risk of osteosarcoma development are bone changes caused by radiation, solitary or multiple osteochondromas, solitary enchondroma or enchondromatosis (Ollier disease), multiple hereditary exostoses, fibrous dysplasia, and chronic osteomyelitis. Sites of bone infarcts, of prostheses, and of prior internal fixation are also at increased risk.[39,58–62]

Environmental Factors

External factors that may affect the risk for osteosarcoma are ionizing radiation, alkylating agents, perinatal factors, viruses, and trauma.

Ionizing Radiation

Osteosarcoma can develop as a result of radiation, either therapeutic or inadvertent (Fig. 5). Ionizing radiation is a well-documented etiologic factor; it is implicated in approximately 3% of osteosarcoma cases.[8] An increased incidence is likely to be seen as more patients survive long enough after primary irradiation to develop this complication. The interval between irradiation and the appearance of osteosarcoma ranges from 4 to more than 40 years (median, 12–16 years). Osteosarcoma has occurred after radiation administered for a variety of malignant as well as benign conditions.[40,63] It has been reported that, among patients with childhood cancers, those with Ewing sarcoma are at the highest risk of subsequent osteosarcoma because of the high radiation doses (41–60 Gy) usually administered to these patients.[64,65]

In a population of over 4,000 children treated for solid cancer, the 20-year cumulative incidence of developing osteosarcoma after a diagnosis of Ewing sarcoma, was reported as 6.7%.[40] Among all secondary radiation-induced sarcomas of the bone in patients of any age, osteosarcoma was the most common, and the mean age

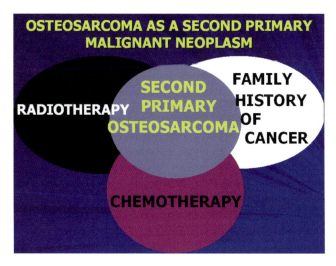

Fig. 5 Osteosarcoma as a second primary malignant neoplasm results from the interaction of predisposing factors: (1) a history of radiotherapy, (2) a history of chemotherapy, and (3) a history of cancer in a first-degree relative

of the patients at presentation was 45.6 years (range, 10–84 years). The mean latent interval between radiotherapy and diagnosis of the sarcoma was 17 years (range, 4–50 years). The median dose of radiotherapy administered was estimated at 50 Gy (mean, 49 Gy; range, 20–66 Gy). There was no correlation between the radiation dose and the time for development of a sarcoma. The pelvis was the most commonly affected site (33% of patients). Breast cancer was the most common primary tumor (19% of patients). Metastases were present at diagnosis in 21.4% of patients with sarcomas that developed as second primary malignancies.

In the past, the survival rates for patients with radiation-induced osteosarcoma were very low, as the patients' ability to undergo surgical and chemotherapeutic treatment was likely to have been compromised by prior treatment.[66] However, a recent report indicated that aggressive treatment of radiation-induced osteosarcoma would result in similar rates of local recurrence and metastasis, and similar functional outcomes, to those of patients with primary osteosarcoma.[67]

The use of intravenous radium 224 has been implicated in the development of osteosarcoma in a large percentage of patients under the age of 20 years, who were treated empirically for tuberculosis and ankylosing spondylitis. A substantial risk for osteosarcoma was documented in workers who painted watch dials with radium and in chemists who worked with radium.[68,69] Thorotrast, which contains thorium 232 and was used as a diagnostic radiocontrast agent, was also associated with the development of osteosarcoma.[70] Although an excess of osteosarcoma cases has not been reported among atomic-bomb survivors who were exposed to whole-body irradiation in Japan in 1945,[71,72] radiation exposure from the 1986 Chernobyl nuclear accident has been associated with the development of osteosarcoma.[73] No significant correlation has been found between osteosarcoma mortality and radioactivity in drinking water.[74]

Alkylating Agents

Research studies have reported that exposure to alkylating agents, including nitrogen mustards, cyclophosphamide, fosfamide, and/or anthracyclines, may contribute to the development of osteosarcoma, independently of the administration of radiotherapy.[40,64,75,76] Osteosarcoma as a second primary malignant neoplasm is particularly frequent in Ewing-sarcoma survivors because Ewing sarcoma patients undergo chemotherapy with alkylating agents combined with a high dose of radiotherapy.[40] The risk of developing a second primary osteosarcoma after a primary osteosarcoma treated by multiagent chemotherapy is lower than the risk of developing it after a primary Ewing sarcoma.[40,64] The risk of subsequent osteosarcoma rises with increasing drug exposure.[75,76] Treatment with anthracyclines has proven to decrease the interval for the development of a secondary osteosarcoma.[75] Genetic predisposition also plays a role in the development of a second primary osteosarcoma[75,76] (Fig. 5).

Perinatal Factors

Prenatal exposure to x-rays has been associated with an increased risk for osteosarcoma.[15] However, a case-control study conducted by the Children's Cancer Group found a lack of association between radiation exposure and bone cancer among 305 patients.[11] Patients and controls had had similar numbers of radiographs. The mothers of cases and controls had had similar experiences with various types of diagnostic radiographs. Fathers had had no differences in their medical and occupational exposures to radiation.

It has been reported that short birth length and high birth weight are associated with elevated osteosarcoma risk, although results have been conflicting.[11,14,15]

A case-control study conducted by the Children's Cancer Group[11] found no significant differences between the mothers of childhood osteosarcoma patients and the mothers of controls in menstrual history, rate of infertility, or pregnancy history, including the number of pregnancies, abortions, stillbirths, live births, premature births, and the frequency of toxemia. Mothers of patients and mothers of controls reported similar frequencies of viral and bacterial infections; vaccinations; kidney, heart, lung, and liver diseases; and other illnesses during pregnancy. There were also no differences in the type of delivery, the anesthetics or analgesics given during delivery, or the complications of delivery. Rates of breastfeeding and perinatal problems were not any different for cases and controls. Both cases and controls required blood transfusions at the same rates, and their exposures to infectious diseases and vaccinations were similar. No differences were found in the frequency of birth defects between cases and controls or their families. Parental smoking and alcohol histories, and frequency of household exposures to insecticides, paints, petroleum products, and other toxic agents were not different. Associations between maternal or paternal occupational exposures and osteosarcoma in offspring could not be identified.[11] The only significant difference in perinatal factors found between cases and controls was that a significantly larger number of mothers of patients had taken morning-sickness medications than had mothers of controls, though the frequency of reported morning sickness was similar for case and control mothers.[11]

Viruses

Several authors have, over the years, described a possible link between viral infection and the occurrence of osteosarcoma, especially in animals.[77–86] In hamsters, which have a low incidence of spontaneous osteosarcoma, cancers developed after inoculation of a cell-free extract obtained from human osteosarcomas.[86] Sera from patients with osteosarcoma reacted immunologically with these hamster osteosarcomas, implying that the osteosarcomas were induced by a human osteosarcoma virus.[81–83] In man, antibodies against osteosarcoma were demonstrated in 100% of patients with osteosarcoma and in 85% of their healthy family members, whereas only 29% of healthy blood donor controls possessed these antibodies.[85]

An unknown proportion of formalin-inactivated Salk poliovirus vaccine lots administered to millions of United States residents between 1955 and 1963 was contaminated with small amounts of infectious simian virus 40 (SV40), a polyomavirus of the rhesus macaque. It has been reported that osteosarcoma as well as other cancers contain SV40 DNA sequences, and it was questioned whether the SV40 infection introduced into humans by the vaccine might have contributed to the development of these cancers.[86]

Although most of these data would imply a viral etiology, there is no convincing evidence as yet that osteosarcoma is caused by a virus, or that it is contagious in the usual sense: one cannot catch it as one would a cold or the flu.

Trauma

Prior bone trauma has been suggested as a risk factor for osteosarcoma,[15] but it would account only for a very small portion of cases,[28] if any,[11] and it is generally considered to be coincidental.[3]

Conclusions

The etiology of ostesarcoma is still largely unknown. Several environmental and inherent patient characteristics, particularly genetic abnormalities, are associated with an increased occurrence of the disease. Further investigation of these factors might lead to enhanced opportunities to determine their relationships to the tumor in greater depth. This knowledge, in turn, may provide leads for developing mechanisms for prevention and better opportunities for cure.

References

1. Gurney JG, Swensen AR, Bulterys M. Malignant bone tumors. In: Ries LA, Smith MAS, Gurney JG, et al., eds. *Cancer Incidence and Survival Among Children and Adolescents: United States SEER Program 1975–1995*. Bethesda, MD: National Cancer Institute; 1999. Available at: http://seer.cancer.gov/publications/childhood/bone.pdf; Accessed August 2008.
2. U.S. Cancer Statistics Working Group. *United States Cancer Statistics: 2001 Incidence and Mortality*. Atlanta, GA: Centers for Disease Control and Prevention and National Cancer Institute; 2004.
3. Jaffe N. Malignant bone tumors in children: incidence and etiologic considerations. In: Jaffe N, ed. *Solid Tumors in Childhood*. Littleton, MA: PSG Publishing Co; 1979:1-10.
4. Miller RW, Boice JD Jr, Curtis RE. Bone cancer. In: Schottenfeld D, Fraumeni JF, eds. *Cancer Epidemiology and Prevention*. 3rd ed. New York: Oxford University Press; 1996:971-983.
5. Dahlin DC, Unni KK, eds. *Bone Tumors: General Aspects and Data on 8,542 Cases*. 4th ed. Springfield, IL: Charles C. Thomas; 1986.

The Etiology of Osteosarcoma

6. Hartford CM, Wodowski KS, Rao BN, et al. Osteosarcoma among children aged 5 years or younger: the St Jude Children's Research Hospital experience. *J Pediatr Hematol Oncol.* 2006;28:43-47.

7. Linabery AM, Ross JA. Trends in childhood cancer incidence in the U.S. (1992–2004). *Cancer.* 2008;112:416-432.

8. Tjalma RA. Canine bone sarcoma: estimation of relative risk as a function of body size. *J Natl Cancer Inst.* 1966;3:1137-1150.

9. Mascarenhas L, Siegel S, Spector L, et al. Malignant bone tumors. In: Bleyer A, O'Leary M, Barr R, et al., eds. *Cancer Epidemiology in Older Adolescents and Young Adults 15 to 29 Years of Age, Including SEER Incidence and Survival: 1975–2000 (NIH Pub. No. 06-5767).* Bethesda, MD: National Cancer Institute; 2006:97–110. Available at: http://seer.cancer.gov/publications/aya/8_bone.pdf; Accessed January 2009.

10. Price CH. Primary bone-forming tumours and their relationship to skeletal growth. *J Bone Joint Surg Br.* 1958;36:1137-1150.

11. Buckley JD, Pendergrass TW, Buckley CM, et al. Epidemiology of osteosarcoma and Ewing's sarcoma in childhood: a study of 305 cases by the Children's Cancer Group. *Cancer.* 1998;83: 1440-1448.

12. Cotterill SJ, Wright CM, Pearce MS, et al. Stature of young people with malignant bone tumors. *Pediatr Blood Cancer.* 2004;42:59-63.

13. Longhi A, Pasini A, Cicognani A, et al. Height as a risk factor for osteosarcoma. *J Pediatr Hematol Oncol.* 2005;27:314-318.

14. Troisi R, Masters MN, Joshipura K, et al. Perinatal factors, growth and development, and osteosarcoma risk. *Br J Cancer.* 2006;95:1603-1607.

15. Operskalski EA, Preston-Martin S, Henderson BE, et al. A case-control study of osteosarcoma in young persons. *Am J Epidemiol.* 1987;126:118-126.

16. dos Santos Aguiar S, de Jesus Girotto Zambaldi L, dos Santos AM, et al. Comparative genomic hybridization analysis of abnormalities in chromosome 21 in childhood osteosarcoma. *Cancer Genet Cytogenet.* 2007;175:35-40.

17. Ottaviani G, Jaffe N. Clinical and pathological study of two siblings with osteosarcoma. *Med Pediatr Oncol.* 2002;38:62-64.

18. Harmon TP, Morton KS. Osteogenic sarcoma in four siblings. *J Bone Joint Surg Br.* 1966;48:493-498.

19. Robbins R. Familial osteosarcoma. Fifth reported occurrence. *JAMA.* 1967;202:1055.

20. Epstein LI, Bixler D, Bennett JE. An incident of familial cancer, including 3 cases of ostogenic sarcoma. *Cancer.* 1970;25:889-891.

21. Swaney JJ. Familial osteogenic sarcoma. *Clin Orthop.* 1973;97:64-68.

22. Miller CW, McLaughlin RE. Osteosarcoma in siblings. Report of two cases. *J Bone Joint Surg Am.* 1977;59:261-262.

23. Mulvihill JJ, Gralnick HR, Whang-Peng J, et al. Multiple childhood osteosarcomas in an American Indian family with erythroid macrocytosis and skeletal anomalies. *Cancer.* 1977;40:3115-3122.

24. Colyer RA. Osteogenic sarcoma in siblings. *Johns Hopkins Med J.* 1979;145:131-135.

25. Hillmann A, Ozaki T, Winkelmann W. Familial occurrence of osteosarcoma. A case report and review of the literature. *J Cancer Res Clin Oncol.* 2000;126:497-502.

26. Chin KR, Mankin HJ, Gebhardt MC. Primary osteosarcoma of the distal femur in two consecutive brothers. *Clin Orthop Relat Res.* 2001;382:191-196.

27. Norrdin RW, Powers BE, Torgersen JL, et al. Characterization of osteosarcoma cells from two sibling large-breed dogs. *Am J Vet Res.* 1989;50:1971-1975.

28. Glass AG, Fraumeni JF Jr. Epidemiology of bone cancer in children. *J Natl Cancer Inst.* 1970;44:187-199.

29. Longhi A, Benassi MS, Molendini L, et al. Osteosarcoma in blood relatives. *Oncol Rep.* 2001;8:131-136.

30. Ji J, Hemminki K. Familial risk for histology-specific bone cancers: an updated study in Sweden. *Eur J Cancer.* 2006;42:2343-2349.

31. Nishida J, Abe M, Shiraishi H, et al. Familial occurrence of telangiectatic osteosarcoma: cousin cases. *J Pediatr Orthop*. 1994;14:119-122.
32. Hansen MF. Genetic and molecular aspects of osteosarcoma. *J Musculoskelet Neuronal Interact*. 2002;2:554-560.
33. Patiño-García A, Piñeiro ES, Díez MZ, et al. Genetic and epigenetic alterations of the cell cycle regulators and tumor suppressor genes in pediatric osteosarcomas. *J Pediatr Hematol Oncol*. 2003;25:362-367.
34. Levesque AA, Eastman A. p53-based cancer therapies: is defective p53 the Achilles heel of the tumor? *Carcinogenesis*. 2007;28:13-20.
35. Kaseta MK, Khaldi L, Gomatos IP, et al. Prognostic value of bax, bcl-2, and p53 staining in primary osteosarcoma. *J Surg Oncol*. 2008;97:259-266.
36. Gebhardt MC. Molecular biology of sarcomas. *Orthop Clin North Am*. 1996;27:421-429.
37. Jensen RD, Miller RW. Retinoblastoma: epidemiologic characteristics. *N Engl J Med*. 1971;285:307-311.
38. Draper GJ, Sanders BM, Kingston JE. Second primary neoplasms in patients with retinoblastoma. *Br J Cancer*. 1986;53:661-671.
39. Fletcher CDM, Unni KK, Mertens F, eds. *World Health Organization Classification of Tumors: Pathology and Genetics of Tumors of the Soft Tissue and Bone*. Lyon: IARC Press; 2002.
40. Le Vu B, de Vathaire F, Shamsaldin A, et al. Radiation dose, chemotherapy and risk of osteosarcoma after solid tumours during childhood. *Int J Cancer*. 1998;77:370-377.
41. McIntyre JF, Smith-Sorensen B, Friend SH, et al. Germline mutations of the p53 tumor suppressor gene in children with osteosarcoma. *J Clin Oncol*. 1994;12:925-930.
42. Li FP, Fraumeni JF Jr. Soft-tissue sarcomas, breast cancer, and other neoplasms: a familial syndrome? *Ann Intern Med*. 1969;71:747-752.
43. Li FP, Fraumeni JF Jr, Mulvihill JJ, et al. A cancer family syndrome in twenty-four kindreds. *Cancer Res*. 1988;48:5358-5362.
44. Plon SE, Malkin D. Childhood cancer and heredity. In: Pizzo PA, Poplack DG, eds. *Principles and Practices of Pediatric Oncology*. 5th ed. Philadelphia: Lippincott Williams and Wilkins; 2006:14-37.
45. Malkin D, Li FP, Strong LC, et al. Germ line p53 mutations in a familial syndrome of breast cancer, sarcomas, and other neoplasms. *Cancer*. 1990;250:1233-1238.
46. Birch JM, Hartley AL, Tricker KJ, et al. Prevalence and diversity of constitutional mutations in the p53 gene among 21 Li–Fraumeni families. *Cancer Res*. 1994;54:1298-1304.
47. Frebourg T, Barbier N, Yan Y, et al. Germ-line p53 mutations in 15 families with Li–Fraumeni syndrome. *Am J Hum Genet*. 1995;56:608-615.
48. Kitao S, Shimamoto A, Goto M, et al. Mutations in RECQL4 cause a subset of cases of Rothmund–Thomson syndrome. *Nat Genet*. 1999;22:82-84.
49. Sim FH, Devries EM, Miser JS, et al. Case report 760: Osteoblastic osteosarcoma (grade 4) with Rothmund–Thomson syndrome. *Skeletal Radiol*. 1992;21:543-545.
50. Wang LL, Levy ML, Lewis RA, et al. Clinical manifestations in a cohort of 41 Rothmund–Thomson syndrome patients. *Am J Med Genet*. 2001;102:11-17.
51. Hicks MJ, Roth JR, Kozinetz CA, et al. Clinicopathologic features of osteosarcoma in patients with Rothmund–Thomson syndrome. *J Clin Oncol*. 2007;25:370-375.
52. Beghini A, Larizza L. Rothmund–Thomson syndrome (RTS). Atlas Genet Cytogenet Oncol Haematol. Milan, Italy; 2001. http://atlasgeneticsoncology.org/Kprones/RothmundID10021. html; Accessed January 2009.
53. German J. Bloom's syndrome: XX – The first 100 cancers. *Cancer Genet Cytogenet*. 1997;93:100-106.
54. Goto M, Miller RW, Ishikawa Y, et al. Excess of rare cancers in Werner syndrome (adult progeria). *Cancer Epidemiol Biomarkers Prev*. 1996;5:239-246.
55. Ishikawa Y, Miller RW, Machinami R, et al. Atypical osteosarcomas in Werner Syndrome (adult progeria). *Jpn J Cancer Res*. 2000;91:1345-1349.
56. Marcove RC, Miké V, Hajeck JV, et al. Osteogenic sarcoma under the age of twenty one. A review of one hundred and forty-five operative cases. *J Bone Joint Surg Am*. 1970;52:411-423.

The Etiology of Osteosarcoma   31

57. McKenna RJ, Schwinn CP, Soonh KY, et al. Sarcomata of osteogenic series (osteosarcoma, fibrosarcoma, chondrosarcoma, parosteal osteosarcoma, and sarcomata arising in abnormal bone): an analysis of 552 cases. *J Bone Joint Surg Am.* 1966;48-A:1-26.

58. Rockwell MA, Enneking WF. Osteosarcoma developing in solitary enchondroma of the tibia. *J Bone Joint Surg Am.* 1971;53:341-344.

59. Huvos AG, Higinbotham NL, Miller TR. Bone sarcomas arising in fibrous dysplasia. *J Bone Joint Surg Am.* 1972;54:1047-1056.

60. Braddock GT, Hadlow VD. Osteosarcoma in enchondromatosis (Ollier's disease). Report of a case. *J Bone Joint Surg Br.* 1966;48:145-149.

61. Johnston RM, Miles JS. Sarcomas arising from chronic osteomyelitic sinuses. A report of two cases. *J Bone Joint Surg Am.* 1973;55:162-168.

62. Sim FH, Cupps RE, Dahlin DC, et al. Postradiation sarcoma of bone. *J Bone Joint Surg Am.* 1972;54:1479-1489.

63. Huvos A. *Bone Tumors: Diagnosis, Treatment, and Prognosis.* 2nd ed. Philadelphia, PA: Saunders; 1991.

64. Inskip PD, Ries LAG, Cohen RJ, et al. New malignancies following childhood cancer. In: Curtis RE, Freedman DM, Ron E, et al., eds. *New Malignancies Among Cancer Survivors: SEER Cancer Registries, 1973–2000 (NIH Publ. No. 05-5302).* Bethesda, MD: National Cancer Institute; 2006. Available at: http://seer.cancer.gov/publications/mpmono/Ch18_Childhood.pdf; Accessed August 2008.

65. Kalra S, Grimer RJ, Spooner D, et al. Radiation-induced sarcomas of bone: factors that affect outcome. *J Bone Joint Surg Br.* 2007;89:808-813.

66. Spiess H, Mays CW. Bone cancers induced by 224 Ra (Th X) in children and adults. *Health Phys.* 1970;19:713-729.

67. Shaheen M, Deheshi BM, Riad S, et al. Prognosis of radiation-induced bone sarcoma is similar to primary osteosarcoma. *Clin Orthop Relat Res.* 2006;450:76-81.

68. Loutit JF. Malignancy from radium. *Br J Cancer.* 1970;24:195-207.

69. Aub JC, Evans RD, Hempelmann LH, et al. The late effects of internally-deposited radioactive materials in man. *Medicine.* 1952;31:221-329.

70. Harrist TJ, Schiller AL, Trelstad RL, et al. Thorotrast-associated sarcoma of bone: a case report and review of the literature. *Cancer.* 1979;44:2049-2058.

71. Yamamoto T, Wakabayashi T. Bone tumors among the atomic bomb survivors of Hiroshima and Nagasaki. *Acta Pathol Jpn.* 1969;19:201-212.

72. Shigematsu I. Health effects of atomic bomb radiation. *Rinsho Byori.* 1994;42:313-319.

73. Harvey RT, Donald PJ, Weinstein GS. Osteogenic sarcoma of the maxillary alveolus occurring five years following the Chernobyl nuclear accident. *Am J Otolaryngol.* 1996;17:210-214.

74. Finkelstein MM, Kreiger N. Radium in drinking water and risk of bone cancer in Ontario youths: a second study and combined analysis. *Occup Environ Med.* 1996;53:305-311.

75. Newton WA Jr, Meadows AT, Shimada H, et al. Bone sarcomas as second malignant neoplasms following childhood cancer. *Cancer.* 1991;67:193-201.

76. Henderson TO, Whitton J, Stovall M, et al. Secondary sarcomas in childhood cancer survivors: a report from the Childhood Cancer Survivor Study. *J Natl Cancer Inst.* 2007;99:300-308.

77. Zilioli E, Ottaviani C. Osteosarcoma: concetti attuali di patologia e nuove prospettive terapeutiche. Nota I: aspetti bioimmulogici della neoplasia. *Chir Ital.* 1978;30:953-961.

78. Zilioli E, Ottaviani C. Osteosarcoma: concetti attuali di patologia e nuove prospettive terapeutiche. Nota II: criteri prognostici e terapia. *Chir Ital.* 1978;30:975-991.

79. Finkel MP, Jinkins PB, Tolle J, et al. Serial radiography of virus-induced osteosarcomas in mice. *Radiology.* 1966;87:333-339.

80. Finkel MP, Biskis BO, Farrell C. Pathogenic effects of extracts of human osteosarcomas in hamsters and mice. *Arch Pathol.* 1967;84:425-428.

81. Finkel MP, Biskis BO, Farrell C. Osteosarcomas appearing in Syrian hamsters after treatment with extracts of human osteosarcomas. *Proc Natl Acad Sci USA.* 1968;60:1223-1230.

82. Finkel MP, Biskis BO, Farrell C. Nonmalignant and malignant changes in hamsters inoculated with extracts of human osteosarcomas. *Radiology.* 1969;92:1546-1552.

83. Reilly CA Jr, Pritchard DJ, Biskis BO, et al. Immunologic evidence suggesting a viral etiology of human osteosarcoma. *Cancer*. 1972;30:603-609.
84. Finkel MP, Reilly CA Jr, Biskis BO. Pathogenesis of radiation and virus-induced bone tumors. *Recent Results Cancer Res*. 1976;54:92-103.
85. Eilber FR, Morton DL. Sarcoma-specific antigens: detection by complement fixation with serum from sarcoma patients. *J Natl Cancer Inst*. 1970;44:651-656.
86. Shah KV. SV40 and human cancer: a review of recent data. *Int J Cancer*. 2007;120:215-223.

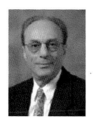

Imaging Assessment of Osteosarcoma in Childhood and Adolescence: Diagnosis, Staging, and Evaluating Response to Chemotherapy

Farzin Eftekhari

Abstract Osteosarcoma is an aggressive tumor of mesenchymal origin, capable of producing osteoid and immature bone. It is the most frequent primary malignant skeletal neoplasm in children and adolescents. Imaging studies play a major role in initial diagnosis, staging, and assessment of tumor response to chemotherapy. Conventional radiography is the prime imaging modality for diagnosis of bony tumors. Radionuclide bone scan is used in detection of metastatic lesions in the other bones. Computed tomography may be used as an adjunct to conventional radiography, but its main role is detection of pulmonary metastasis. The standard magnetic resonance imaging is the most specific modality for local staging and monitoring response to chemotherapy, and distinguishing postsurgical changes from residual tumor. Dynamic contrast-enhanced magnetic resonance imaging has been introduced to quantify the percentage of tumor necrosis, identify early responders, and thus predict survival. The role of ^{18}F fluorodeoxyglucose positron emission tomography (PET) in the staging and management of osteosarcoma is evolving. It has the advantage of total body imaging and may have an overall role in tumor staging and grading, detection of early response, and therefore, in the prognosis and detection of recurrence.

Introduction

Osteosarcoma is the most common primary malignant skeletal neoplasm in children and adolescents and is second only to plasma cell myeloma among all age groups. It is an aggressive tumor of mesenchymal origin that is capable of producing osteoid and immature bone, chondroid, and fibroblastic elements.[1–4] Advances in local and systemic control of the disease and limb salvage procedures have

---

F. Eftekhari (✉)
Department of Diagnostic Radiology, Division of Diagnostic Imaging, The University of Texas M.D. Anderson Cancer Center, Houston, TX, USA
e-mail: feftekhari@mdanderson.org

improved both the outcome and the quality of life for these generally young patients. Concurrent advances in imaging technology have not only allowed in-depth evaluation of the patient's tumor burden but have also played a major role in detecting early response to treatment and thus, in predicting the outcome.

Imaging studies are essential for diagnosing, staging, and grading the tumor; monitoring early response to chemotherapy; and detecting tumor recurrence. Additionally, imaging studies may be used to guide biopsies so that the most aggressive areas of large heterogeneous tumors are sampled; imaging studies may also be used to guide the administration of intra-arterial chemotherapy.

This chapter reviews both traditional and newer imaging techniques, highlighting their advantages, disadvantages, and pitfalls, and summarizing current imaging practices.

Classification

Osteosarcomas may be divided into two major categories: *primary* tumors that occur de novo in otherwise normal bone, and *secondary* tumors that develop in abnormal bone in the setting of a preexisting benign lesion, irradiated bone, retinoblastoma, or Paget disease of bone (Table 1). The majority of *primary* osteo-sarcomas occur in the metaphyseal portion of the long bones, with approximately 30% located in other parts of the skeleton.[1-4] Other morphological subtypes are intramedullary, intracortical, surface, extraskeletal, and gnathic osteosarcomas, and multicentric osteosarcoma or osteosarcomatosis.[1-4]

Fundamental Principles of Imaging

Conventional radiography, commonly referred to as "plain film," is the frontline and most important primary imaging modality used for the initial diagnosis of bone tumors. Radiographic findings also justify the consideration of a needle biopsy. The use of radiography is followed by the sequential application of other imaging modalities such as computed tomography (CT), magnetic resonance imaging (MRI), radionuclide scanning, and angiography. More recent modalities include ^{18}F-fluorodeoxyglucose (^{18}F-FDG) positron emission tomography (PET) and PET/CT.

Table 1 Locus in skeleton abstracted from refs. [1-4]

Locus in skeleton	%
Knee	50–75%
Femur	45–55%
Tibia	16–20%
Humerus	11–15%

Conventional Radiography

Primary Osteosarcomas

Primary conventional osteosarcomas (also called intramedullary or central) typically occur de novo in an otherwise normal bone during the second and third decades of life and are rare in patients younger than 6, or older than 60 years. Most osteosarcomas occur in the tubular bones of the appendicular skeleton. More than half of these tumors occur around the knee[1-4] (Table 1).

It is unusual for osteosarcomas to occur in the jaw, the spine, the pelvis, or the fibula, and they rarely occur in the cranium, the ribs, the scapula, the clavicle, the forearm, the hand, or the foot[1-4]; but the radiographic findings for these osteosarcomas will be similar to tumors found in the tubular bones. The metaphyseal region of the bone is the most common site for these tumors to occur, followed by the diaphyseal region. Tumors in the diaphyseal region tend to have a longer duration of symptoms compared to metaphyseal tumors. The metaphyseal lesions frequently extend into the diaphysis and open epiphysis, but primary epiphyseal tumors are quite rare[1-4] (Table 2).

Radiographic findings usually reflect the tumor's rate of growth, the status of bone destruction, and the extent of osteoid mineralization. A mixed pattern is most commonly seen, with areas of permeative destruction showing a wide zone of transition and a variable amount of mineralized osteoid (Fig. 1). When bone destruction is the dominant feature, or the tumor cannot produce enough osteoid/bone, the lesion appears osteolytic (Fig. 2). In contrast, when bone production is the dominant feature, the lesion will appear to be almost or totally osteoblastic (Figs. 3 and 4).

Outward tumor growth without bone expansion usually results in early destruction of the cortex and elevation of the periosteum. As a result, the ordinarily imperceptible periosteum forms thin layers of new bone. Various forms of periosteal reaction referred to as "Codman triangle" (Figs. 1 and 2), "paint-brush," "hair-on-end," and "sunburst", all point to the aggressive behavior of the tumor. An extraosseous soft tissue mass will be present in 80–90% of cases, and over 90% of those masses will contain clouds of mineralized osteoid[1-4] (Figs. 1 and 4).

Pathologic fractures are seen in 15–20% of cases of primary osteosarcoma, either at diagnosis or during chemotherapy.[1-4] In our experience, fractures have little, if any, impact on the outcome.[5] Discontinuous or skip metastases are seen in 25% of

Table 2 Locus in bone abstracted from refs. [1-4]

Locus in bone	%
Metaphyseal lesions	90–95%
Diaphyseal lesions	2–11%
Metaphyseal lesions extending to epiphysis	75–88%
Primary epiphyseal lesions	<1%

Fig. 1 Mixed osteolytic and osteoblastic osteosarcoma of distal femur in a 14-year-old female. Notice the typical metaphyseal location of the tumor with permeative destruction, "Codman triangle," and clouds of intraosseous and extraosseous mineralized osteoid (*arrows*)

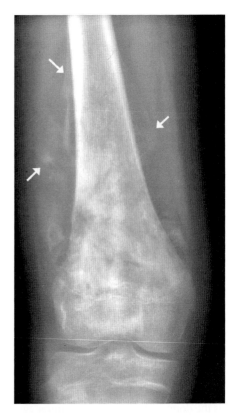

Fig. 2 Osteolysis-predominant osteosarcoma of distal femur in a 15-year-old female. Notice the typical metaphyseal location of the tumor and epiphyseal invasion (*arrowheads*), outward growth without expansion (*white arrow*), Codman triangle type of subperiosteal new bone formation (*black arrow*), cortical destruction and soft-tissue invasion (*white arrow*)

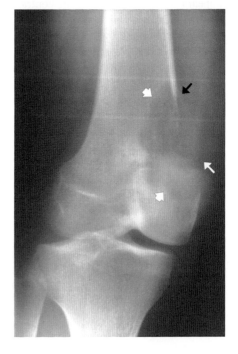

Fig. 3 Osteoid/bone-predominant osteosarcoma of distal femur in a 15-year-old male. Notice metaphyseal location, permeative destruction of the bone, and clouds of mineralized osteoid in the medullary bone (*arrows*)

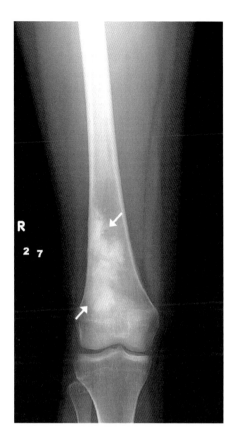

Fig. 4 Osteoblastic osteosarcoma of the fibula in a 12-year-old female. Notice the fluffy clouds of mineralized osteoid (*arrow*) engulfing the fibular head

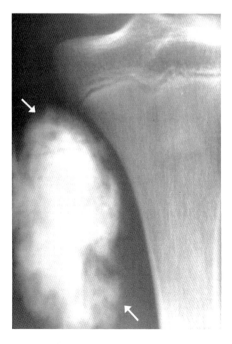

cases and appear proximal to the primary tumor, within the same bone.[1-4] The skip metastases may escape detection with conventional radiographic images and are best detected by MRI (Fig. 5). They may also be detected by ^{18}F-FDG PET.

Surface osteosarcomas arise from the juxtacortical regions of tubular bones; the parosteal type accounts for the majority (65%) and the periosteal type for 25% of these lesions.[1-4] The parosteal type tends to occur in females during the third and fourth decades of life, usually in the posterior aspect of the distal femur (Fig. 6) and the proximal tibia. Periosteal osteosarcomas tend to develop during the second and third decades of life, usually in the diaphyseal or the meta-diaphyseal regions (Fig. 7). Dedifferentiated parosteal osteosarcomas are high-grade tumors and are usually observed in older adults (Fig. 8).

Extraskeletal tumors constitute 1.2% of all osteosarcomas[1-4] (Fig. 9). They typically show more centrally condensed mineralized osteoid in contrast to myositis ossificans, where the mineralization starts in the periphery and matures concentrically (Fig. 10).

Gnathic osteosarcomas constitute 6–9% of all osteosarcomas[1-4] and are considered to be a distinct category of tumors with a predilection to occur in older children (Fig. 11).

Osteosarcomatosis (also known as multicentric osteosarcoma) is considered a morphological subtype, and it accounts for 3–4% of osteosarcomas.[1-4] Patients with this tumor type present with multiple synchronous osteoblastic lesions, usually in a mature skeleton (Fig. 12), or with a diffuse pattern (sclerosing osteosarcomatosis) (Fig. 13). Whether osteosarcomatosis represents a multicentric process or metastases from an often-seen dominant primary tumor is controversial.[1-4] A dominant and more aggressive lesion may be found in 93.3–100% of these cases, and the majority will exhibit pulmonary metastases at diagnosis.[6] The bone lesions appear either synchronously or within a few weeks of the symptomatic, radiographically diagnosed dominant osteosarcoma.[6]

Secondary Osteosarcomas

In contrast to primary (de novo) tumors, secondary osteosarcomas occur within an abnormal bone, for example, at the site of preexisting benign lesions such as fibrous dysplasia (Fig. 14), irradiated bone (Fig. 15), or Paget disease of bone (Fig. 16) and also in the setting of retinoblastoma. The prevalence of radiation-associated osteosarcomas is 0.02–4%. The latent period can vary from less than 3 years to 55 years.[7,8]

PEARL

Conventional radiography provides the fundamental basis for the primary diagnosis of osteosarcoma.

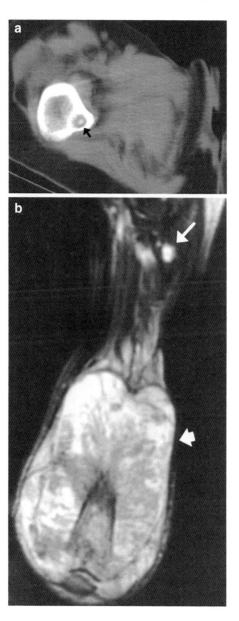

Fig. 5 Discontinuous (skip) metastasis from osteosarcoma of the distal femur in a 14-year-old male. Notice the lytic focus with central core of mineralized osteoid in the lesser trochanter of the femur seen on CT (*black arrow* in **a**) and as a hyperintense nodule on T2WI (*arrow* in **b**) proximal to the primary osteosarcoma (*arrowhead* in **b**). This was confirmed after amputation. MRI is superior to CT in detecting skip lesions

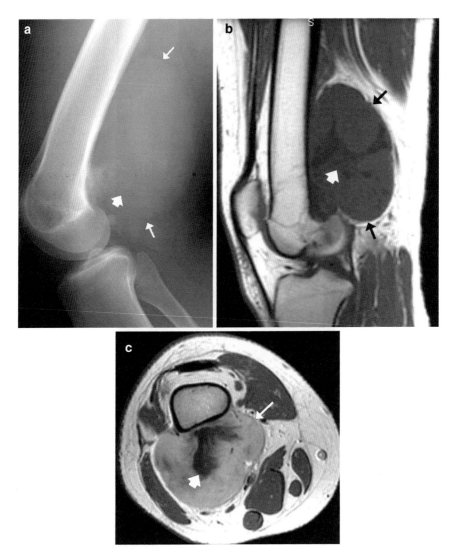

Fig. 6 Parosteal type of surface osteosarcoma of distal femur in a 20-year-old female. Notice the typical broad-based juxtacortical tumor arising from the posterior cortex of the distal femur (*arrows* in **a**). Notice the islands of mineralized osteoid within the mass (*arrowhead* in **a**). Notice the hypointense mass on T1WI (*arrows* in **b**) surrounding the hypointense mineralized matrix (*arrowheads* in **b**) and the large enhancing tumor on axial contrast-enhanced T1WI (*arrow* in **c**) that surrounds the hypointense mineralized osteoid (*arrowhead* in **c**)

Fig. 7 Periosteal type of surface osteosarcoma of tibia in an 11-year-old female. Notice the Codman type of periosteal new bone (*arrows*) and the absence of endosteal and medullary bone involvement in this case

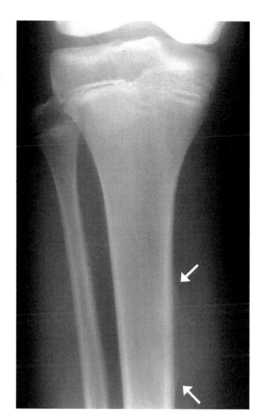

Fig. 8 Dedifferentiated parosteal osteosarcoma of distal femur in a 75-year-old female. Notice the aggressive periosteal new bone formation and the mineralized osteoid in the surrounding soft tissues (*arrows*)

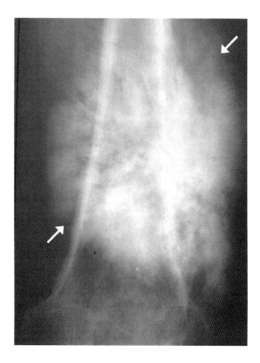

Extended Diagnostic and Therapeutic Imaging Modalities

Radionuclide Bone Scan

^{99m}Technitium (^{99m}Tc) is a radiotracer with an optimally short half-life that is taken up by the mineralized osteoid in both the primary tumor and the metastatic lesions. While moderately sensitive, the uptake is not specific and may also be seen in benign aggressive lesions such as aneurysmal bone cysts, complicated bone cysts, and other reparative processes such as myositis ossificans. Following a favorable response to effective chemotherapy, a decrease in tracer uptake may be seen.

> **PEARL**
>
> The principal role of a radionuclide bone scan is to detect the primary and additional tumor sites within the skeleton. It may occasionally demonstrate a response to therapy.

Angiography

Angiography was widely used in the 1980s, not only to guide the administration of intra-arterial chemotherapy but also for grading, local staging, and monitoring the tumor's response to chemotherapy (Fig. 17). The current role of angiography is to guide the administration of intra-arterial chemotherapy and provide ancillary monitoring of the tumor's response to chemotherapy. Table 3 outlines the degree of sensitivity and the specificity of angiography in assessing the effects achieved with intra-arterial chemotherapy (good necrosis), abstracted from a review of several publications.[9–15]

> **PEARL**
>
> The current role of angiography is to guide the administration of intra-arterial chemotherapy and provide ancillary monitoring of the tumor's response to chemotherapy.

Computed Tomography

CT is a good adjunct to conventional radiography in the diagnosis of osteosarcoma in tubular and specifically complex bones (i.e.,the pelvis, scapula, craniofacial regions), and small lesions adjacent to the endosteum. It is superior to conventional radiography in the detection of trace amounts of mineralized osteoid. CT can also

Table 3 Sensitivity and specificity of angiography in assessing the degree of response (necrosis) achieved with intra-arterial chemotherapy abstracted from a review of publications[9–15]

Investigator	Sensitivity	Specificity	Total patients
Kawai (1997)	5/5 (100%)	4/7 (57%)	12
Kunisada (1998)	7/8 (88%)	8/11 (73%)	19
Carrasco (1989)	43/47 (91%)	17/34 (50%)	81
Lang (1996) MRA (7 OS/2 Ewing)	5/5 (100%)	3/3 (100%)	8
Chuang (1982)	17/18 (94%)	21/24 (88%)	42
Kumpan (1986)	15/15 (100%)	7/7 (100%)	22
Wilkins (2003)	39/41 (95%)	5/6 (83%)	47

Good response: >90% necrosis. *MRA* = Magnetic resonance angiography in osteosarcoma (*OS*); Ewing sarcoma (Lang) (Courtesy: Norman Jaffe, MD)

depict the shell of the residual cortex, which helps distinguish benign expansile lesions, such as aneurysmal bone cysts, from osteosarcoma (Fig. 18). However, the primary role of CT is to detect pulmonary metastases.

PEARL

The primary role of CT is to detect pulmonary metastases.
CT is also used as an adjunct to conventional radiography in diagnosis.

Ultrasound

Because of its inherent physical limitations, gray-scale ultrasound typically has no role in the diagnosis or the staging of osteosarcoma. Because of its vascular kinetics, color Doppler ultrasound may help monitor a tumor's response to therapy.[16]

Standard Magnetic Resonance Imaging

MRI, with the aid of intravenous contrast material, has no particular role in the diagnosis of osteosarcoma. However, it is the most specific modality for local staging (Fig. 19). Because of its superb tissue contrast and multiplanar capability, MRI is superior to CT in the detection of discontinuous (skip) metastases (Fig. 6) and also of extension into the nearby joints. Non Mineralized osteoid is isointense to hypointense on T1WI and hyperintense on T2WI (Figs. 5, 6, and 19). Viable tumor should enhance when intravenous contrast is administered (Figs. 5 and 19). The hemorrhagic component of the tumor is generally hyperintense and necrosis is hypointense on T1WI; neither will enhance with contrast (Fig. 19). Necrotic tumor

Fig. 9 Extraskeletal osteosarcoma in the soft tissues adjacent to the fibula in an 11-year-old female. Notice the denser core of mineralized osteoid centrally (*arrow*). Contrast this with a case of myositis ossificans (see Fig. 10), wherein mineralization first appears in the periphery and progresses in a concentric fashion

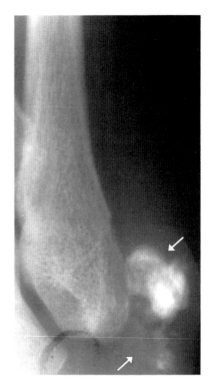

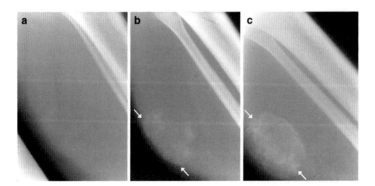

Fig. 10 An example of myositis ossificans in a 17-year-old female with painful swelling of her calf, clinically suspicious for sarcoma. She was referred for an ultrasound-guided needle biopsy. Ultrasound images (not shown) revealed diffuse edema of the gastrecnemius muscle containing a small amount of fluid in the center, but no calcifications. The patient denied any history of injury, but on direct questioning she admitted to being a long-distance jogger. Based on the history, the physical, and sonographic observations, a diagnosis of myositis ossificans was suggested and the needle biopsy was canceled by the radiologist. Nonetheless, the patient did get a biopsy done elsewhere that was not diagnostic. Conventional radiography (**a**) showed a swollen calf but no detectable calcifications. Serial follow-up radiograms 10 days (**b**) and 3 weeks later (**c**) showed concentric mineralization, confirming the diagnosis of myositis ossificans. Myositis ossificans may be a potential pitfall for extraskeletal osteosarcoma (Fig. 9). The clue to diagnosis is the development of peripheral and progressively concentric mineralization over a period of 30 days. The lack of a history of trauma should not dissuade physicians from accepting this diagnosis. Misdiagnosis is rampant, and the best strategy is a wait-and-watch attitude and follow-up by serial sonographic or radiographic examinations

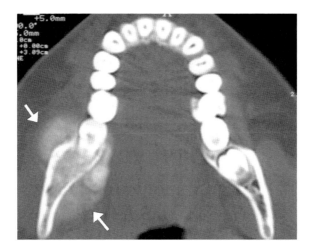

Fig. 11 Osteosarcoma of the mandible in a 16-year-old female. Notice an osteoid/bone-predominant osteosarcoma of the mandible with fluffy clouds of mineralized osteoid (*arrows*)

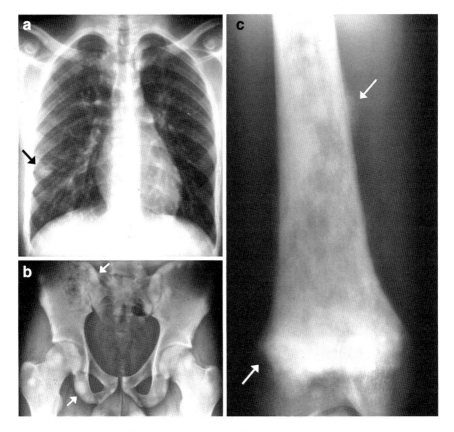

Fig. 12 Multifocal type of osteosarcomatosis in a 16-year-old male. Notice synchronous osteoblastic lesions of the left clavicle, ribs and pelvis in a mature skeleton (*arrows* in **a** and **b**), and a dominant aggressive lesion of the right femur (*arrows* in **c**), likely the primary site of osteosarcoma

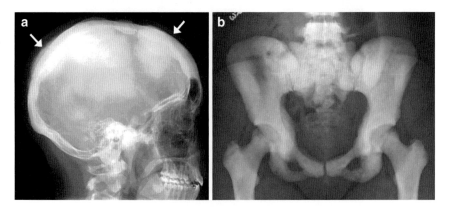

Fig. 13 Diffuse type of osteosarcomatosis (or sclerosing osteosarcomatosis) in a 19-year-old female. Notice the homogeneous sclerosis and thickening of the cranial vault (*arrows* **a**), and pelvic bones (**b**)

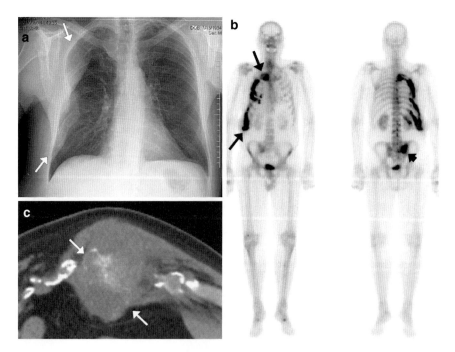

Fig. 14 Secondary osteosarcoma of the right ribs in a 73-year-old male with polyostotic fibrous dysplasia. Frontal chest radiogram (**a**) shows multiple expanded ribs with ground glass appearance representing fibrous dysplasia (*lower arrow* in **a**) and several destroyed ribs accompanied by a large soft tissue mass (*upper arrow* in **a**) representing the tumor. Anterior and posterior views of a nuclear bone scan showing tracer uptake by the abnormal ribs (*arrow* in **b**) and right sacral ala (*arrowhead* in **b**). CT scan obtained in decubitus position during biopsy (**c**) shows the tumor with scanty mineralized osteoid (*arrows* in **c**)

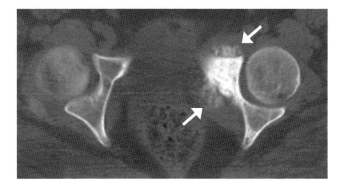

Fig. 15 Radiation-induced high-grade chondroblastic osteosarcoma of the left pubic bone in a 17-year-old female. The lesion (*arrows*) developed 13 years after partial resection and irradiation of an intraspinal/extraspinal ganglioneuroblastoma. Notice the osteoblastic lesion of the left pubic bone with aggressive periosteal new bone formation and soft tissue extension (*arrows*). The patient was treated by preoperative chemotherapy, surgical resection, and limb salvage procedure. She remains disease-free, as of February 2008

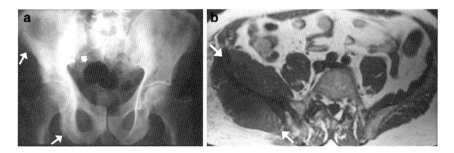

Fig. 16 Paget disease of the right hemipelvis complicated by osteosarcoma in a 74-year-old male. Conventional radiogram (**a**) showing thickened cortices and coarsened trabecular pattern of the right pubis, ischium, and ilium (*arrows* in **a**): classic findings for Paget disease. Also notice the shaggy outline and mixed lytic and sclerotic changes of the right ilium (*arrowhead* in **a**). T1WI MR showing an osteolytic tumor of the iliac bone and the associated mass involving the iliacus and gluteal muscles (*arrows* in **b**)

will be hyperintense on T2WI (Fig. 19), and the mineralized osteoid will be hypointense on all sequences. The use of contrast material is critical in monitoring the response to chemotherapy. In responsive tumors, the intraosseous component may not change in size, but the extraosseous component will decrease significantly. The use of contrast material should help differentiate viable tissue from nonviable tissue (Fig. 19). A decrease in tumor volume, peritumoral edema, and degree of enhancement are predictive of a good response,[17-19] but these decreases are observed in only two thirds of the cases.[18]

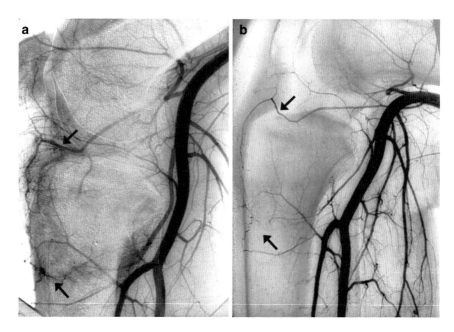

Fig. 17 Selective popliteal arteriogram in osteosarcoma of the proximal tibia shows the presence of a "tumor stain" caused by neovascularity before treatment (*arrows* in **a**) and its disappearance at the completion of chemotherapy (*arrow* in **b**)

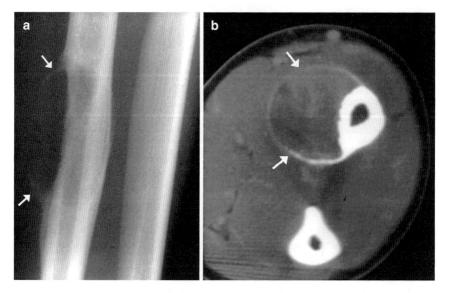

Fig. 18 Aneurysmal bone cyst of the tibia in a 12-year-old female. Notice the eccentric expansile mass with no mineralized matrix. The external "buttressing" (*arrow* in **a**) mimics the Codman triangle. The shell of the remaining cortex is not discernable on the conventional radiogram (**a**) but is detected on a CT scan (*arrows* in **b**)

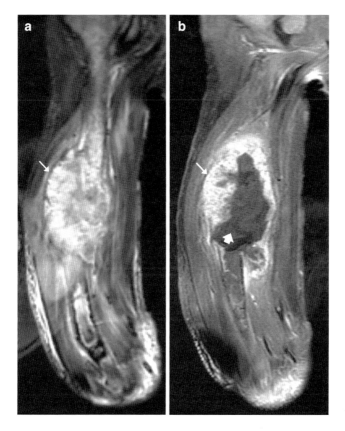

Fig. 19 Standard MRI of a telangiectatic osteosarcoma of the humerus in a 16-year-old female. Coronal fat-suppressed T2WI of the right humeral diaphysis showing a hyperintense mass invading the soft tissues (*arrows* in **a**), and fat-suppressed contrast-enhanced T1WI MR showing enhancement of the viable tumor (*arrows* in **b**) but not of the necrotic component (*arrowhead* in **b**)

PEARL

The role of standard contrast-enhanced MRI is in the local staging and the evaluation of response to chemotherapy. MR has no role in diagnosis.

Dynamic Contrast-Enhanced MRI

Dynamic contrast-enhanced MRI (DCE-MRI) is a functional imaging technique with a very high temporal resolution that is used to evaluate the status of tumor angiogenesis and the angiogenic parameters such as permeability or blood flow.[20-23] While the other imaging modalities indirectly indicate the effectiveness of therapy based on the anatomic information, they may also overestimate or underestimate the degree of response.[18–20] To overcome these shortcomings, DCE-MRI is being used to identify residual viable tissue within the tumor.[18–20,22] DCE-MRI is performed using an automated bolus injection of gadolinium at the rate of 3 mL/s or greater, with simultaneous acquisition of data at approximately 1 s/image; these data are used to generate a time-intensity curve. The technique can be performed easily during a standard MRI but requires special software for data analysis.[20–22]

The site of viable tissue can be identified primarily by the status of angiogenesis both directly (e.g., permeability or K_{trans}) and indirectly (e.g., the rate and amount of contrast enhancement). These angiogenic parameters can be quantified using the time-intensity curve. The data are useful for identifying residual viable tumor tissue and evaluating the treatment effects. Marcal and Choi studied the role of DCE-MRI in monitoring response to chemotherapy in sarcomas and correlated the change in tumor volume and ^{18}F-FDG PET activity and the percentage of tumor necrosis in the resected specimen.[20] They used the accepted criteria of ≥90% tumor necrosis in the resected specimen as a favorable response. The authors concluded that morphological changes using tumor *volume* were poor indicators of response. They also noted that area under the curve (AUC) from DCE-MRI and the maximum standardized uptake value (*SUV_{max}*) from ^{18}F-FDG PET were both highly sensitive and specific in predicting tumor response as well as outcome.[20–27] Other investigators have shown how quantitative response data from DCE-MRI can have a significant impact on the immediate surgical approach and the long-term survival of the patient .[21–25]

PEARL

DCE-MRI may be an early predictor of tumor response and final outcome. DCE-MRI is currently the most effective modality to identify and quantify residual viable tumor, but ^{18}F-FDG PET/CT may prove to be equally powerful.

---

^{18}F-FDG PET/CT

FDG is a marker of metabolic activity in tumors because most tumors have an increased rate of glycolysis and glucose transport.[25,26] ^{18}F-FDG is the most widely used PET tracer in oncology and specifically in osteosarcoma. However, there are insufficient data regarding its indications and benefits in oncology, in general, and in osteosarcoma, in particular.[25] The role of ^{18}F-FDG PET and ^{18}F-FDG PET/CT in the management of osteosarcoma is rapidly evolving.[25] While these modalities have

Imaging Assessment of Osteosarcoma in Childhood and Adolescence

no particular role in the initial diagnosis and local staging, they have the added advantage of whole-body imaging (Fig. 20). ^{18}F-FDG PET/CT can guide the interventional radiologists to sample the most biologically active regions of large heterogeneous tumors[21,22] and skip metastases. ^{18}F-FDG PET/CT can also be used for biologic grading of the tumor because the higher the uptake values, the higher the metabolic activity and, therefore, the grade.

PEARL

The Role of ^{18}F-FDG PET
Whole-body imaging capability to detect metastatic spread and skip lesions.
No role in diagnosis and local staging.
Potential role in tumor grading.
Guides biopsy to the most biologically active area of tumors.
Differentiates postoperative changes from residual viable tumor.
Monitors response to therapy and detects recurrence.

PEARL

^{18}F-FDG PET vs. Other Modalities
For primary diagnosis, conventional radiography and CT are superior to ^{18}F-FDG PET.
For local staging, MRI is superior to ^{18}F-FDG PET/CT.
For quantification of response and predicting prognosis, DCE-MRI is superior to PET.
For detection of pulmonary metastases, CT is superior to ^{18}F-FDG PET/CT.

---

^{18}F-FDG PET/CT also appears promising in its ability to monitor responses by depicting the change in tumor volume and SUV.[25,26] After chemotherapy and surgical resection are completed, ^{18}F-FDG PET/CT may help distinguish benign postoperative changes from the residual tumor. It can also help detect local recurrence and metastatic disease (Fig. 20). ^{18}F-FDG PET/CT is unable to differentiate low-grade and even high-grade *malignant* lesions from ^{18}F-FDG-avid *benign* lesions because their SUVs overlap; thus, it cannot be a substitute for a biopsy.[26]

Fig. 20 Metastatic small-cell osteosarcoma of right femur in a 15-year-old female (same patient as in Fig. 24). Coronal FDG PET shows metastatic lesions in the lungs, mediastinal nodes, right clavicle, spine, and left iliac crest (*arrows*)

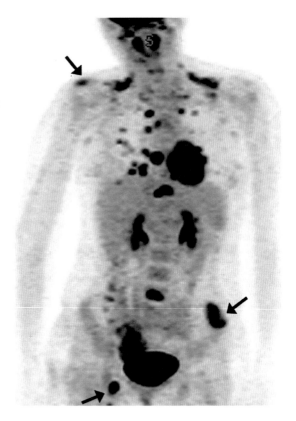

Monitoring Response to Chemotherapy

Patients with a favorable response to chemotherapy will show regression of the soft tissue mass, solidification of the periosteal reaction, mineralization of the osteolytic component, and containment of the fluffy osteoblastic component (Fig. 21). The apparent enlargement of the mineralized osteoid should not be mistaken for progression.

With a standard MRI, a favorable response will appear as a decrease in both tumor volume and tumor enhancement (Fig. 22) or near-complete necrosis (Fig. 23). In responsive tumors, the intraosseous component may not change in size, but the extraosseous component will decrease significantly. The use of contrast material should help differentiate viable tissue from nonviable tissue (Fig. 22). A decrease in tumor volume, peritumoral edema, and the degree of enhancement are predictive of a good response,[12,13] but these decreases are observed in only two thirds of the cases.[12] In one third of good responders whose

Imaging Assessment of Osteosarcoma in Childhood and Adolescence 53

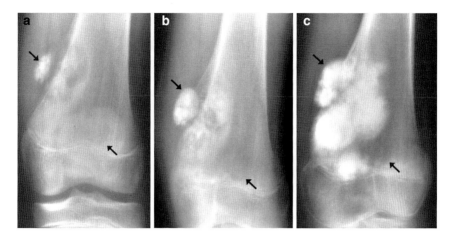

Fig. 21 Monitoring response to chemotherapy by conventional radiography in femoral osteosarcoma in a 13-year-old male. Notice progressive mineralization of the osteoid by bone (*arrows*) that should not be confused with disease progression

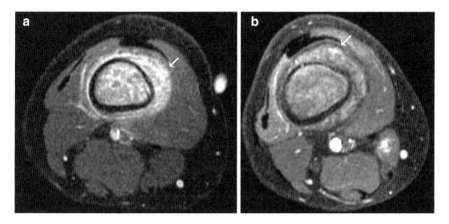

Fig. 22 Monitoring response to chemotherapy by standard MRI in a good responder. Osteosarcoma of distal femur in an 11-year-old female seen on a T1WI fat-suppressed contrast-enhanced MR (*arrow* in **a**) and post-therapy study showing the decrease in tumor volume and enhancement (*arrow* in **b**) corresponding to more than 99% necrosis seen on the resected specimen

tumor volume does not show a significant change, DCE-MRI will help document a favorable response.[18–22]

On ^{18}F-FDG PET/CT, favorable response appears as a visual decrease in metabolic activity and a sharp drop in SUV (Fig. 24), while poor response is indicated by little change or an increase in activity and SUV (Fig. 25).[26,27]

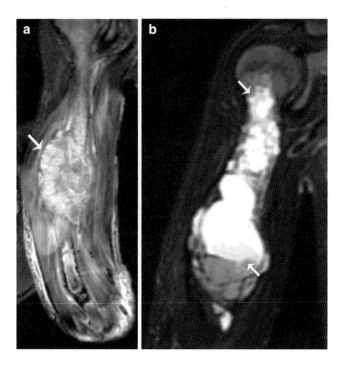

Fig. 23 Monitoring response to chemotherapy by standard MRI in a good responder. Telangiectatic osteosarcoma of the humerus in a 16-year-old female (same patient as in Fig. 19). Coronal T2WI fat-suppressed MR showing the tumor (*arrow* in **a**). Coronal T2WI fat-suppressed image after completion of therapy and before resection showing totally necrotic tumor (*arrows* in **b**), which correlated with >95% necrosis seen on the resected specimen

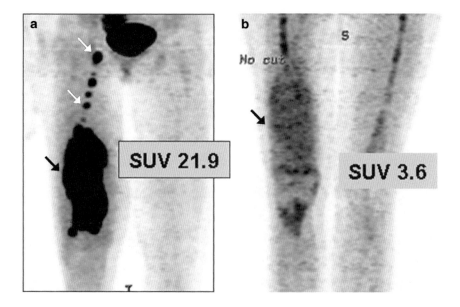

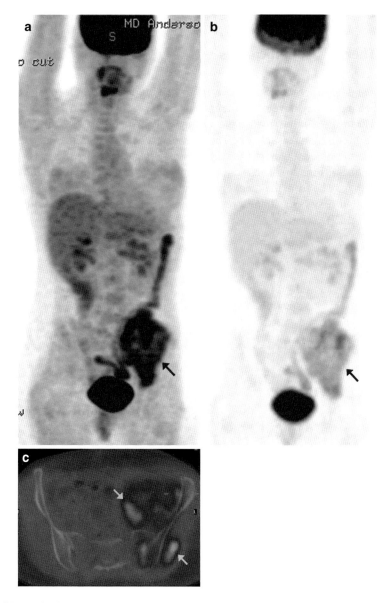

Fig. 25 Monitoring response to chemotherapy by FDG PET in a poor responder. A 41-year-old female with myxoid/chondroid osteosarcoma of the left ilium. Pretreatment FDG PET scan (**a**) showing a hypermetabolic tumor (*arrow* in **a**) with SUV of 8.6. On the post-treatment scan, SUV drops to only 6.3 (*arrow* in **b**), with significant residual viable tumor (*arrows* in **c**) correlating to only 79% necrosis seen on the resected specimen

◀──

Fig. 24 Monitoring response to chemotherapy by FDG PET in a good responder. Small-cell osteosarcoma of distal femur in a 15-year-old female metastatic to lymph nodes, bones, and lungs (same patient as in Fig. 20). Pretreatment FDG PET scan (**a**) showing the hypermetabolic tumor (*black arrow* in **a**) draining into the femoral lymph nodes (*white arrows* in **a**). Post-treatment scan showing a significant decrease in both volume and SUV, from 21.9 to 3.6

Post-Therapy Complications

During and after completion of intra-arterial and/or systemic chemotherapy, trophic changes may develop in the metaphyseal side of the cartilaginous growth plate. These are similar to trophic changes seen in other stressful conditions affecting the immature skeleton. These trophic changes manifest as alternating transverse radiolucent bands (growth-arrest lines) and radiodense bands (growth-recovery lines) (Fig. 26). These changes in both the infused limb and the contralateral limb may be from the local or systemic effect of cisplatin. The changes heal over time but may occasionally result in a wide nonossified defect in the metaphysis (Fig. 27).

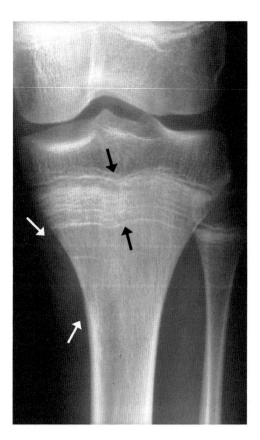

Fig. 26 Trophic changes of the contralateral knee due to the *systemic* effect of intra-arterial chemotherapy in a 14-year-old-male previously treated for osteosarcoma of the *right* femur. Notice the parallel bands of growth arrest and the growth recovery lines (*black arrows*). Also notice early metastasis to the *left* tibia (*white arrows*) concurrent with pulmonary metastases 2 years after initial diagnosis

Fig. 27 Trophic changes of the metaphysis after intra-arterial chemotherapy in an 11-year-old-female with osteosarcoma of the distal femur. Notice the parallel bands of growth arrest and the growth recovery lines in the femoral metaphysis (*black arrows*) and a wide defect of the tibial metaphysis (*white arrows*)

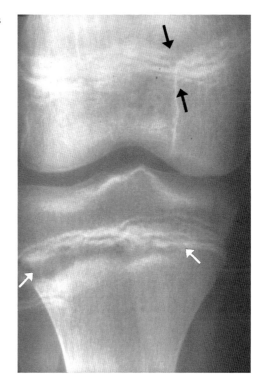

Local Recurrence of Osteosarcoma

A local recurrence may develop at the primary site (Fig. 28), the stump (Fig. 29), the resection site (Fig. 30), or near the prosthesis (Fig. 31). When the recurrent tumor is confined to the soft tissues and does not contain sufficient mineralized osteoid, it may escape detection by conventional radiography and even bone scan, but it will be detected by MRI or ^{18}F-FDG PET/CT.

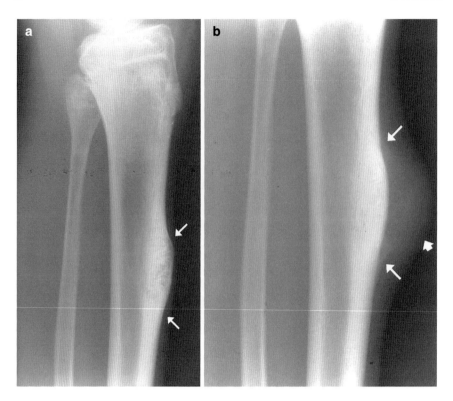

Fig. 28 Recurrent periosteal osteosarcoma of the tibia in a 14-year-old male. Notice the large soft tissue mass (*arrowhead* in **b**) and Codman triangle (*arrows* in **b**) that developed 7 months later at the site of the treated tumor (*arrows* in **a**)

Fig. 29 Recurrent osteosarcoma at the femoral stump in a 14-year-old male. Notice the recurrent tumor with homogeneously mineralized osteoid in the shaft of the stump (*arrow*). Those recurrent tumors that occur outside of the bony stump and do not produce, or are not capable of producing sufficient osteoid/bone may escape detection by conventional radiography

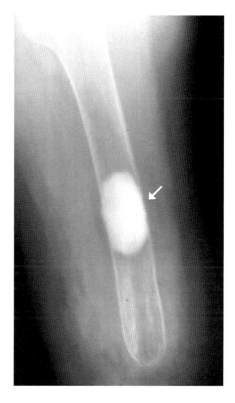

Fig. 30 Recurrent osteosarcoma of the fibula at the resection site in a 14-year-old male. Notice the fluffy clouds of mineralized osteoid at the resection site (*arrow*)

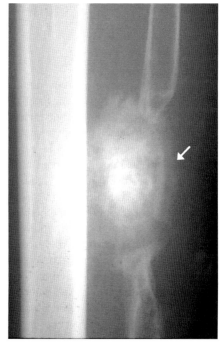

Fig. 31 Recurrent osteosarcoma of the femur in a 19-year-old male. Notice the fluffy clouds of mineralized osteoid (*arrows*) adjacent to the prosthesis

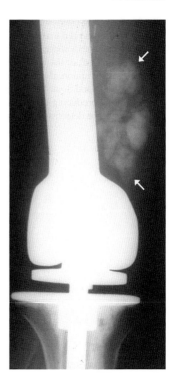

Conclusion

An accurate diagnosis of bone tumors requires both imaging and pathological evaluation. Imaging is used for local staging, grading, metastatic work-up, image-guided biopsy, and intra-arterial chemotherapy administration. Imaging also plays a critical role in detecting early response to chemotherapy and is a powerful tool in predicting a patient's outcome. It helps determine the effectiveness of preoperative chemotherapy, and the need for any additional postoperative chemotherapy. Among the currently available imaging modalities, conventional radiography remains the most reliable tool for initial diagnosis. MRI is the most reliable tool for local staging and quantifying response to chemotherapy. The major role for CT is to detect pulmonary metastasis and confirm radiographic diagnosis.

^{18}F-FDG PET/CT has no role in diagnosis, local staging, or detection of small lung metastases, but it may become a powerful competitor with MRI. Additionally, PET can perform whole-body imaging, depict the tumor's metabolic activity, and detect disease recurrence. The demonstration of early response to chemotherapy using imaging studies has been proclaimed a powerful predictor of 5-year patient survival,[20-22] but this role has not yet been confirmed in large-scale analysis.

Imaging Assessment of Osteosarcoma in Childhood and Adolescence 61

Acknowledgments The author wishes to thank Dr. Norman Jaffe for his continued support, Drs. Haesun Choi and Leonardo Marcal for sharing their research on DCE-MRI, Kristi Speights for editorial assistance, Mary Carr for secretarial assistance, and Juan Loya for assistance in illustration assistance.

References

1. Mira JM. Osseous tumors of intramedullary origin. In: Mira JM, ed. *Bone Tumors: Clinical, Radiologic, and Pathologic Correlations*. Philadelphia, Pa: Lea & Febriger; 1989:248-438.
2. Resnick D, Kyriakos M, Greenway GD. Tumor-like diseases of bone: imaging and pathology of specific lesions. In: Resnick D, ed. *Diagnosis of Bone and Joint Disorders*. 3rd ed. Philadelphia: Saunders; 1995:3662-3697.
3. Huvos AG. Osteogenic sarcoma. *Bone Tumors: Diagnosis, Treatment, and Prognosis*. Philadelphia, Pa: Saunders; 1991:85-156.
4. Dahlin DC, Coventy MB. Osteogenic sarcoma. A study of six hundred cases. *J Bone Joint Surg [Am]*. 1967;49:101-110.
5. Jaffe N, Spears R, Eftekhari F, et al. Pathologic Fracture in Osteosarcoma: Impact of chemotherapy on primary tumor and survival. *Cancer*. 1987;59:701-709.
6. Hopper KD, Moser RP, Haseman DB, et al. Osteosarcomatosis. *Radiology*. 1990;175:233-239.
7. Weatherby RP, Dahlin DC, Ivins JC. Postradiation sarcoma of bone: review of 78 Mayo Clinic cases. *Mayo Clin Proc*. 1981;56:294-306.
8. Lorigan JG, Libshitz HI, Peuchot M. Radiation-induced sarcoma of the bone: CT findings in 19 cases. *AJR*. 1989;153:791-794.
9. Kawai A, Sugihara S, Kunisada T, et al. Imaging assessment of the response of bone tumors to preoperative chemotherapy. *Clin Orthop Relat Res*. 1997;337:216-225.
10. Kunisada T, Ozaki T, Kawai A. Imaging assessment of the responses of osteosarcoma patients to preoperative chemotherapy: angiography compared with thallium-201 scintigraphy. *Cancer*. 1999;86(6):949-956.
11. Carrasco CH, Charnsangavej C, Raymond AK, et al. Osteosarcoma: angiographic assessment of response to preoperative chemotherapy. *Radiology*. 1989;170:839-842.
12. Lang P, Vahlensieck M, Matthay KK. Monitoring neovascularity as an indicator to response to chemotherapy in osteogenic and Ewing sarcoma using magnetic resonance angiography. *Med Pediatr Oncol*. 1996;26(5):329-333.
13. Chung VP, Benjamin R, Jaffe N, et al. Radiographic and angiographic changes in oseosarcoma after intraarterial chemotherapy. *AJR*. 1982;139:1065-1069.
14. Kumpan W, Lechner G, Wittich GR. The angiographic response of osteosarcoma following pre-operative chemotherapy. *Skeletal Radiol*. 1986;15(2):96-102.
15. Wilkins RM, Cullen JW, Odom L. Superior survival in treatment of primary nonmetastatic pediatric osteosarcoma of the extremity. *Ann Surg Oncol*. 2003;10(5):481-483.
16. Van der Woude HJ, Bloem JL, van Oostayen JA, et al. Treatment of high-grade bone sarcomas with neoadjuvant chemotherapy. The utility of sequential color Doppler sonography in predicting histopathologic response. *AJR*. 1995;165:125-133.
17. Abudu A, Davies AM, Pysent PB, et al. Tumour volume as a predictor of necrosis after chemotherapy in Ewing's sarcoma. *J Bone Joint Surg Br*. 1999;81:317-322.
18. Holscher HC, Bloem JL, Vanel D, et al. Osteosarcoma: chemotherapy-induced changes at MR imaging. *Radiology*. 1992;182:839-844.
19. Pan G, Raymond AK, Carrasco CH, et al. Osteosarcoma: MR imaging after preoperative chemotherapy. *Radiology*. 1990;174:517-526.
20. Marcal L, Choi H, Jackson E, et al. Use of Quantitative Dynamic Contrast MR Imaging to Monitor Musculoskeletal Sarcomas: Correlation with FDG PET and Pathology. E-poster. International Society for Magnetic Resonance in Medicine (ISMRM), Kyoto, Japan. 2004, May 15–21.

21. De Baere T, Vanel D, Shapeero LG, et al. Osteosarcoma after chemotherapy: evaluation with contrast material-enhanced subtraction MR imaging. *Radiology.* 1992;185:587-592.
22. Shapeero LG, Vanel D. Imaging evaluation of the response of high-grade osteosarcoma and Ewing sarcoma to chemotherapy with emphasis on dynamic contrast-enhanced magnetic resonance imaging. *Semin Musculoskelet Radiol.* 2000;4:137-146.
23. Vanel D, Verstraete KL, Shapeero LG. Primary tumors of the musculoskeletal system. *Radiol Clin North Am.* 1997;35:213-237.
24. Wunder JS, Paulian G, Huvos AG, et al. The histological response to chemotherapy as a predictor of the oncological outcome of operative treatment of Ewing sarcoma. *J Bone Joint Surg Am.* 1998;80:1020-1033.
25. Shankar LK, Hoffman JM, Bacharach S, et al. Consensus recommendations for the use of ^{18}F-FDG PET as an indicator of therapeutic response in patients in National Cancer Institute trials. *J Nucl Med.* 2006;47:1059-1066.
26. Brenner W, Bohuslavizki KH, Eary JF. PET imaging of osteosarcoma. *J Nucl Med.* 2003;44:930-942.
27. Eary JF, Conrad EU, Bruckner JD, et al. Quantitative [F-18] fluorodeoxyglucose positron emission tomography in pretreatment grading of sarcoma. *Clin Cancer Res.* 1998;4:1215-1220.

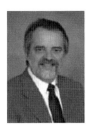

Osteosarcoma Multidisciplinary Approach to the Management from the Pathologist's Perspective

A. Kevin Raymond and Norman Jaffe

Abstract Osteosarcoma is a primary malignant tumor of the bone in which proliferating neoplastic cells produce osteoid and/or bone, if only in small amounts. This histological principle defines a tumor that usually affects young males more frequently than females, and disproportionately involves the long bones of the appendicular skeleton. These tumors are generally locally aggressive and tend to produce early, lethal systemic metastases. However, osteosarcoma is not a single disease but a family of neoplasms, sharing the single histological finding of osseous matrix production in association with malignant cells.

The majority (i.e., 75%) of cases are relatively stereotypical from the demographic, clinical, radiographic and histologic points of view. These tumors generally occur in the metaphyseal portion of the medullary cavity of the long bone and are referred to as "Conventional Osteosarcoma." The group is sub classified by the form of the dominant matrix present within the tumor, which may be bone, cartilage or fibrous tissue, and it is correspondingly referred to as osteoblastic, chondroblastic and fibroblastic osteosarcoma.

The remaining 25% of cases have unique parameters that allow reproducible identification of tumors which are biologically different from conventional osteosarcoma and are referred to as "Variants." The parameters identifying Variants fall into one of three major groups: (1) clinical factors, (2) histologic findings and (3) location of origin – within or on the cortex. Because of their inherent biological difference from Conventional Osteosarcoma, the Variants identify cases which must be excluded from analysis of data pertaining to the treatment of the majority of cases: Conventional Osteosarcoma.

The diagnostic parameters of osteosarcoma must be sufficiently inclusive to identify all the members of this potentially lethal tumor. Conversely, criteria for sub classification must be restricted to assure homogenous populations of tumors productively incorporating different biological behavior and the potential for development

---

A.K. Raymond (✉)
Department of Pathology, The University of Texas M.D. Anderson Cancer Center,
1515 Holcombe Blvd, Houston, TX, 77030-4009, USA
e-mail: kraymond@mdanderson.org

of unique treatment strategies which are different from those for Conventional Osteosarcoma. This can be designated "Classification Based Therapy" or "Therapy Based Osteosarcoma."

With this background, we will discuss the highly disciplined approach to the management of osteosarcoma from the pathologist's perspective. Factors governing the assessment of the response to preoperative chemotherapy will also be reviewed.

Introduction

Osteosarcoma is a primary malignant tumor of the bone in which proliferating neoplastic cells produce osteoid and/or bone, even if only in small amounts.[1,2] Osteoid is an extra cellular matrix and must be distinguished from type 1 collagen. The distinction, essentially, is between osseous collagen and nonosseous collagen. From a morphological perspective, osteoid can be defined as a pink (eosinophilic) material which is amorphous, homogeneous, refractile, occasionally curvilinear, and randomly oriented (Fig. 1). It can show varying degrees of calcification. Osteoid is intimately associated with the malignant cells that comprise osteosarcoma (Fig. 2).

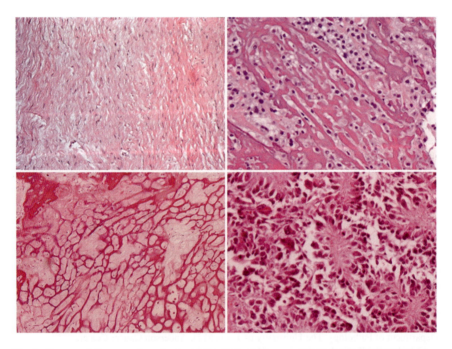

Fig. 1 Representative samples of osteoid. Sections appear as pink, (eosinophilic), amorphous, homogeneous, refractile material which is occasionally curvilinear and randomly oriented (Hematoxylin and eosin)

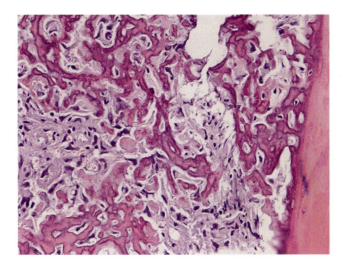

Fig. 2 Osteoid scaffolding with calcification (Hematoxylin and eosin)

Classification

Osteosarcoma may affect any bone, but it predominantly occurs in the metaphyseal regions of the appendicular skeleton. The distribution by age, sex, and site of the lesions in 962 patients seen at the M.D. Anderson Cancer Center is depicted in Fig. 3. Pain and swelling are the cardinal clinical symptoms, often accompanied by restriction in movement. The diagnosis and classification is made in conjunction with imaging studies, which are determined by the amount of ossification and calcification. The tumors may be purely lytic or sclerotic but usually have a combination of both features. Correlation with imaging is crucial for establishing the diagnosis.

From a pathological perspective, osteosarcoma may be classified as "Conventional Osteosarcoma" and "Osteosarcoma Variants." The osseous matrix (Fig. 4) is the single unifying feature, and classification is dependent on the predominant type. Classifications vary. A classification from Dahlin from the American Journal of Surgical Pathology is reproduced in Table 1[1] and suggested variants from 1977 to the present, from the M.D. Anderson Cancer Center, are depicted in Table 2.

Conventional Osteosarcoma

An algorithm can be formulated to help define the exact diagnosis. It commences with identification of the presence or absence of osteoid. If osteoid is present, the diagnosis is one of osteosarcoma. If osteoid is absent, another diagnosis must be considered. Here, it is important to correlate with radiologic features as core biopsies may not be representative of the lesion. A request for rebiopsy may sometimes

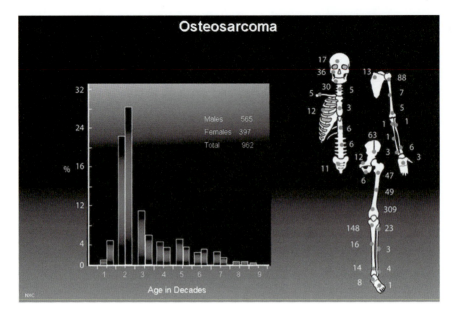

Fig. 3 Age, sex and anatomic distribution of osteosarcoma patients seen at the M.D. Anderson Cancer Center

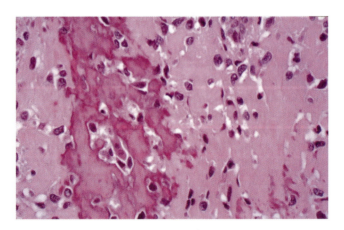

Fig. 4 Predominant osseous matrix in association with malignant cells, the single unifying feature of osteosarcoma (Hematoxylin and eosin)

be required, especially if the radiologic findings are highly suspicious for osteosarcoma, but the biopsy does not confirm the radiologic impression. The predominant matrix is then identified. This may comprise osteoid/bone, cartilage or fibrous tissue. If osteoid/bone is present, it is considered to be an osteoblastic osteosarcoma (Fig. 5). In imaging studies, it is identified as a bone producing tumor with sclerosis

Osteosarcoma Multidisciplinary Approach

Table 1 Dahlin's classification of osteosarcoma[1] Reproduced with permission from the Mayo Foundation

Osteosarcoma	
Conventional osteosarcoma	993
Others	281
Osteosarcoma in jaw	84
Osteosarcoma in Paget's disease	43
Postradiation osteosarcoma	52
Osteosarcoma in benign conditions	8
Telangiectatic osteosarcoma	44
Periosteal osteosarcoma	22
High-grade surface osteosarcoma	9
Low-grade osteosarcoma	16
Multicentric osteosarcoma	3
Parosteal osteosarcoma	56
Dedifferentiated chondrosarcoma	43
	1,274

Table 2 Osteosarcoma proposed M.D. Anderson Cancer Center Variants

Osteosarcoma: proposed variants (1977-present)	
Conventional osteosarcoma	Filigree osteosarcoma
Osteoblastic osteosarcoma	Osteosarcoma resembling osteoblastoma
Chondroblastic osteosarcoma	Chondroblastoma-like osteosarcoma
Low-grade central osteosarcoma	Chondromyxoid fibroma-like OS
Well-differentiated intraosseous OS	Periosteal-like osteosarcoma
Small cell osteosarcoma	Jaw osteosarcoma
Epithelioid osteosarcoma	Osteosarcoma of the skull
Plasmacytoid osteosarcoma	Intracortical osteosarcoma
Clear cell osteosarcoma	Parosteal osteosarcoma
Telangiectatic osteosarcoma	Parosteal osteogenic sarcoma
Paget's osteosarcoma	Juxta-cortical osteosarcoma
Postradiation osteosarcoma	Periosteal osteosarcoma
Radiation induced osteosarcoma	Periosteal osteogenic sarcoma
Osteosarcoma in fibrous dysplasia	Dedifferentiated parosteal osteosarcoma
Osteosarcoma in retinoblastoma	High-grade surface osteosarcoma
Osteosarcoma with rosatoid osteoid	Malignant fibrous histiocytoma
Sclerosing osteosarcoma	Dedifferentiated chondrosarcoma

infiltrating the cortex and fine ramifications into the soft tissue, often manifesting as an aggressive periosteal reaction (Fig. 6). The periosteal reaction may demonstrate a Codman's triangle, if the periosteum is elevated and sparse calcified tumor matrix is present at the junction. Alternatively, an exuberant calcified mass of bone matrix may produce a "sunburst" appearance of the periosteum and cortex. If the

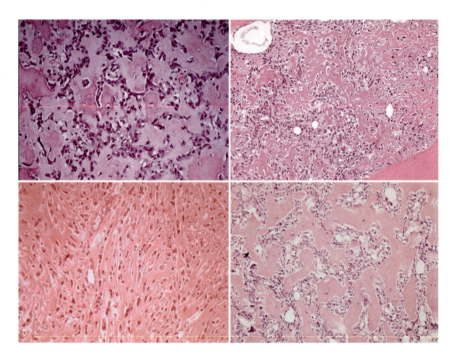

Fig. 5 Osteoblastic osteosarcoma. Pleomorphic spindle and polyhedral cells producing lace-like micro-trabeculae of osteoid and more mature bony trabeculae (Hematoxylin and eosin)

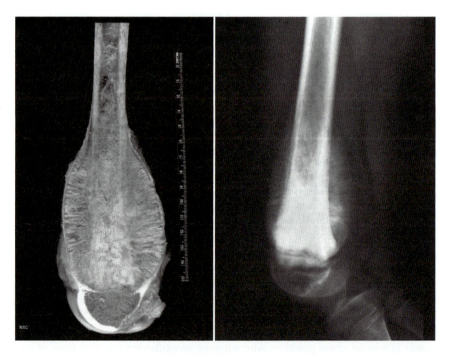

Fig. 6 Typical gross appearance of osteoblatic osteosarcoma involving the distal femoral metaphysis (L). The accompanying radiograph demonstrates a periosteal blastic reaction with invasion into the surrounding soft tissue (R)

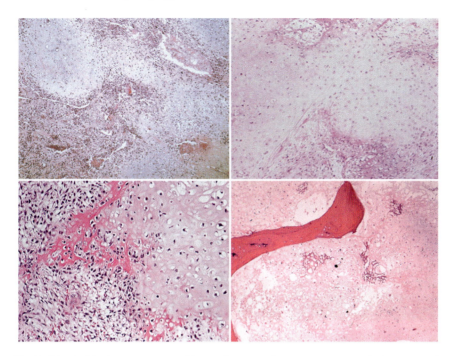

Fig. 7 Chondroblastic osteosarcoma. The cartilagenous elements are composed of pleomorphic cells that merge into sheets of malignant cells. Cartilage is present in several sections (Hematoxylin and eosin)

predominant matrix is cartilage, it is a chondroblastic osteosarcoma (Fig. 7) and on imaging, it may have a chondroid appearance with destructive infiltrative characteristics (Fig. 8). If the predominant matrix is scarce or absent, the diagnosis is fibroblastic osteosarcoma (Fig. 9). On gross pathologic examination, it has a sarcoma-like, soft and fleshy appearance, and the image is devoid of bone and cartilage (Fig. 10). Regardless of the degree of chondroid or fibrous tissue present, typical osteoid or bone production by tumor cells establishes a diagnosis of osteosarcoma.[1]

Osteoblastic, chondroblastic and fibroblastic osteosarcoma constitute 70% of the conventional types of osteosarcoma.

Osteosarcoma Variants

Variants can be subdivided into Clinical, Morphological and Surface entities. It is important to recognize this diagnostic and biologic diversity to ensure specific therapy and appropriate data analysis.

Clinical variants (~9%, overall) comprise jaw osteosarcoma (6%), Paget's Sarcoma (1%), postradiation osteosarcoma (1%), multicentric (multifocal) osteosarcoma (<1%)

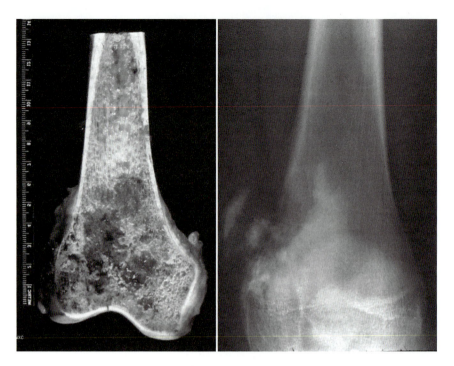

Fig. 8 Gross appearance of chondroblastic osteosarcoma (L) of the distal femur. In the accompanying radiograph there is a lytic lesion involving the medial half of the bone with invasion of the surrounding soft tissue (R)

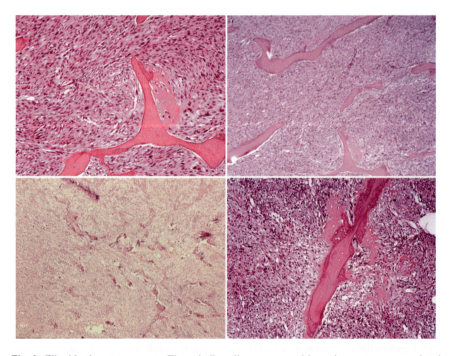

Fig. 9 Fibroblastic osteosarcoma. The spindle cells are arranged in various patterns associated with osteoid and more mature bone. (Hematoxylin and eosin)

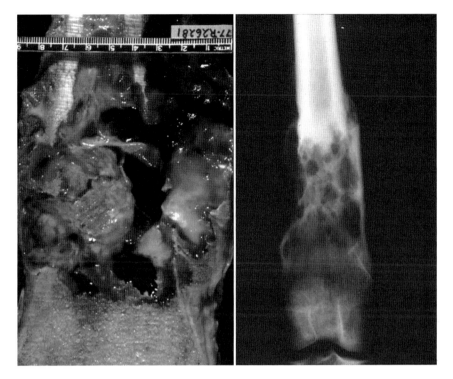

Fig. 10 Gross (fleshy) appearance of fibroblastic osteosarcoma of the distal tibia (L). The accompanying radiograph demonstrates a predominantly lytic lesion with a pathologic fracture (R)

and osteosarcoma in other categories (1%). Morphological variants (~7%, overall) comprise low-grade intraosseous osteosarcoma (1%), telangiectatic osteosarcoma (3%), small cell osteosarcoma (2%) and malignant fibrous histiocytoma (MFH) (2%). Cortical and surface variants (~7%, overall) comprise parosteal osteosarcoma (4%), dedifferentiated parosteal osteosarcoma (1%), periosteal osteosarcoma (1%) and high-grade surface osteosarcoma (1%).

The list of variants appears daunting (see also Chaps. 3 and 5). However, a comment on the "more frequently" encountered forms is appropriate.

Telangiectatic osteosacoma accounts for less than 5% of osteosarcomas.[3] The lesion is rapidly expansile and aggressive, and may simulate aneurysmal bone cyst. It is composed of loculated-blood filled spaces, partially lined by malignant cells producing sparse osteoid.[4-6] Small cell osteosarcoma is an uncommon variant which histologically resembles Ewing's sarcoma. Most of the tumors are composed of small round cells separated by collagenous bands of a fine eosinophilic matrix. The cells have ovoid nuclei and, unlike Ewing's Sarcoma, have a tendency to spindle.[7, 8] Modern molecular methods can help define Ewing's sarcoma and differentiate it from small cell osteosarcoma, but the specificity of this finding and the relationship of these two entities is questioned by some. Malignant fibrocytic histiocytoma tends to involve the ends of long bones; there may be less periosteal reaction. Pleomorphic spindle cells are noted, and multinucleated giant cells may be seen. An inflammatory background is not unusual, with a characteristic storiform or spiral nebular arrangement.[9-11] Low grade central osteosarcoma usually involves older patients, with the knee as a predilected site.[12] On imaging studies, the lesion may appear benign or may show dense sclerosis without massive destruction, as seen in conventional osteosarcoma. Spindle cells with variable amounts of bone and collagen are seen. The lesion may look more ominous on imaging. Histologically, it may resemble desmoplastic fibroma or fibrous dysplasia. Osteosarcoma developing in the setting of Paget's disease and in radiated bones is generally pleomorphic, as in conventional osteosarcoma, and the biological behavior is equally grave.

Osteosarcoma arising on the surfaces of bones is generally more indolent than those arising centrally. Four major subtypes may be recognized: parosteal osteosarcoma, periosteal osteosarcoma, high grade surface osteosarcoma and dedifferentiated parosteal osteosarcoma.

Parosteal osteosarcoma is a tumor usually seen in the third and fourth decades of life. Most tumours are situated on the surface of the posterior distal femur.[13, 14] The osteosarcoma usually presents as a dense mass adjacent to the cortex. Histologically, there is a mass of bone with varying stages of maturation, and fibrous stroma is present between the bone spicules. Computer tomography may assist in determining medullary invasion which must be distinguished from a benign potential mimic, myositis ossificans.

Dedifferentiated parosteal osteosarcoma commences as a low grade parosteal osteosarcoma and later develops a high-grade mesenchymal component which, on histological examination, is indistinguishable from conventional osteosarcoma. The tumor resembles parosteal osteosarcoma on imaging, but histologically, areas of high-grade and low-grade bone-forming sarcoma are present. Dedifferentiation has been cited to occur in 20% of low grade osteosarcomas.[15]

Periosteal osteosarcoma occurs most often in adolescence. It usually occurs on the surface of the shaft of a long bone. The characteristic histological feature is malignant cartilaginous tissue. It may be confused with chondrosarcoma.[14] The presence of osteoid, albeit minimally, and its occurrence in younger patients may assist in establishing the diagnosis and distinguishing it from chondrosarcoma.[16, 17]

High-grade surface osteosarcoma is a highly malignant surface tumor of bone. The imaging features may be similar to those of parosteal or periosteal osteosarcoma. It generally arises on the bone surface along the midshaft and usually does not invade the medullary cavity. The histological features are identical to those of high-grade conventional osteosarcoma. The matrix is not well-differentiated when contrasted with dedifferentiated parosteal osteosarcoma.[18]

Osteosarcomas of the jaw and skull are seen more often in an older age group compared to pediatric and adolescent patients.[19] Many osteosarcomas of the jaw show cartilaginous differentiation. They generally do not metastasize to distant sites.[20]

Osteosarcoma of the skull is extremely rare. It is highly malignant and, interestingly, does not exhibit chondroblastic differentiation.[15]

Radiation induced osteosarcoma develops in previously radiated bones. It is highly malignant and equivalent to conventional osteosarcoma. Multifocal sclerosing (multi-centric) osteosarcoma is highly malignant and affects multiple bones simultaneously.

The above classification lends itself to "Therapy Based Osteosarcoma." Standard primary chemotherapy is generally administered for osteoblastic, chondroblastic, fibroblastic and telangiectatic osteosarcoma. Intensification of chemotherapy may be recommended for postradiation osteosarcoma, Paget's disease, multicentric osteosarcoma, small-cell osteosarcoma (therapy integrated with that recommended for Ewing's sarcoma), dedifferentiated parosteal osteosarcoma and high-grade surface osteosarcoma. In contrast, surgical excision alone may be recommended for low grade central osteosarcoma, parosteal osteosarcoma, periosteal osteosarcoma and jaw osteosarcoma, provided there is no evidence of progression to high-grade mitotic activity.

Diagnostic Biopsy

Biopsy may be obtained by two different mechanisms: open and closed. Open biopsy is a surgical procedure performed under general anesthesia and may involve incision or excision of the tumor. It usually provides liberal amounts of tissue for diagnostic and investigational purposes. An open biopsy should preferably be performed by the surgeon who will perform the limb salvage procedure as the biopsy site and track must be completely excised in the subsequent definitive surgical procedure. Closed biopsy is obtained with a needle. This provides an aspirate and a core (Fig. 11). Several "passes" may have to be made to provide sufficient material for investigational purposes. The instruments employed for needle biopsy are illustrated in Fig. 12. A needle biopsy may be performed by an interventional radiologist. It is generally performed as an outpatient procedure under local anesthesia or conscious sedation. A rapid definitive strategy of treatment can be planned shortly upon receipt of the diagnosis.

The hazards of biopsy in patients with malignant primary bone and soft tissue tumors have been addressed.[21] An open biopsy may be fraught with complications, including tissue contamination, which may jeopardize the patient's candidacy for a limb salvage procedure. There is minimal contamination with needle biopsy (Fig. 13). The procedure was found to be accurate in 89% of 265 osteosarcoma patients in whom needle biopsy was performed at the M.D. Anderson Cancer Center.

Specimen Therapy Evaluation

The goals of therapy evaluation comprise confirmation of the diagnosis, status of the margin and extent of the disease, classification and subclassification of the neoplasm, imaging correlation and response to therapy. The response is both quali-

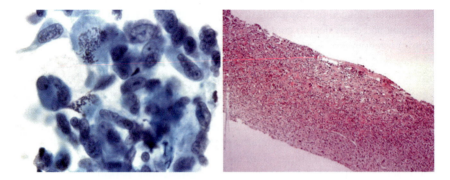

Fig. 11 Cellular aspirate (L) and core tissue (R) obtained by needle biopsy reveal malignant cytologic and architecture features, respectively

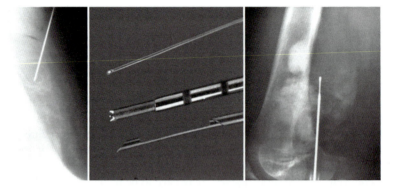

Fig. 12 Needles utilized for biopsy (*center panel*). The *left panel* demonstrates a cutting needle in bone. The *right panel* demonstrates a needle inserted into soft tissue. Upon withdrawal, the core of tissue along the spine of the needle will be evacuated

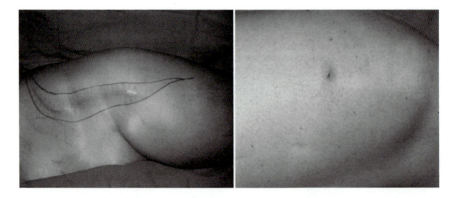

Fig. 13 Simple puncture wound (R) following a needle biopsy performed for a suspected case of osteosarcoma. Contrast the extensive scar (L) following an open biopsy to obtain a specimen in a patient with an osteosarcoma of the distal femur. The procedure was complicated by tumor contamination

tative and quantitative. To achieve these goals, representative sections of the tumor must be obtained. This is undertaken through a standardized work-up. One of the most important aspects of this workup is to identify the viable tumor, which is utilized as a guide for planning postoperative treatment.

Preparation of Gross Specimen

Specimens submitted from orthopedic oncologic surgical procedures range from resection to major ablative extirpation. The latter tends to be large, complex and somewhat intimidating. The goal of specimen examination is to reduce the specimen to the tumor and the parent bone. Details regarding the preparation of orthopedic specimens have been published.[22, 23] The pathologist should also review the clinical and imaging material before commencing preparation and examination.

External examination of the gross specimen of the skin is brief. The extent of contamination of the biopsy site by tumor and coexisting diseases are noted. Extensive vascular invasion can be grossly assessed by a cross-section of the significant draining vein or veins in the location where their paths are relatively consistent (e.g., popliteal or anticubital fossa). The specimen is dissected so that only the tumor and the parent bone remain (Fig. 14). After the soft tissues have been removed, the tumor-distorted bone is sectioned in one of the long axes in a plane that will maximally demonstrate the areas suspected for residual viable tumor. This results in a central "slab section" and two opposing "hemispheres" (Fig. 15). A Toledo Meat Saw (Toledo Scale, Toledo OH) or equivalent is utilized. The specimen should be photographed for permanent record.

A review of the preoperative angiogram in a patient treated with intra-arterial chemotherapy will assist in the above-mentioned process. More than 95% of osteosarcomas are hypervascular. Reduction and/or disappearance of tumor neovascularity and stain are sensitive but nonspecific indicators of a good response to therapy. Persistence of residual neovascularity after three courses of chemotherapy is almost always an indication of poor response to treatment, with significant amounts of residual viable tumor.[25–29] Response may also manifest with progressive mineralization (i.e., opacification) and reduction in tumor size.

The slab section is cut from end-to-end (for "mapping") and submitted for decalcification, processing and histologic analysis. An Isomet saw is used for this part of the dissection (Buechler, Lake Bluff, IL). This is a geologic saw with a diamond impregnated circular blade and water bath (Fig. 16).

Before decalcification of the cut slab, sections are reassembled into their prior anatomic configuration and a specimen radiograph is obtained. Each piece is assigned a section code that is recorded on the specimen radiograph (Figs. 17–20). The radiograph is labeled to match the numbering system (section code) of the processing cassettes. It also provides a permanent record of the submitted sections ("map"). Additional sections are taken from the unsampled hemispheres. These are referred to as "random" sections, as there is no corresponding radiographic record of their precise anatomic location.

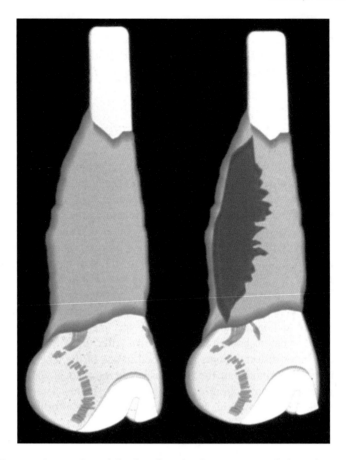

Fig. 14 Tumor and parent bone following dissection for assessment of chemotherapy response. The blue area represents the neoplasm and the red area, the site of suspected residual viable tumor. Reprinted with permission from Reprinted with permission from Raymond AK et al: Osteosarcoma chemotherapy effect: A prognostic factor: Semin Diag Pathol 4: 212–236. 1987

Histologic Analysis

A large number of morphological parameters are reviewed: classification and sub classification; the presence or absence of tumor; anatomic distribution, if tumor is present; qualitative and quantitative analysis of viable tumor; qualitative and quantitative analysis of tumor necrosis; and documentation of any reactive processes. Correlation with clinical and imaging findings and review of any additional investigational parameters are also noted.

Evaluation of chemotherapy effect requires not only the ability to detect tumor necrosis, but also makes the assumption that there has been adequate representation of the tumor. This can be tedious and time consuming. The single best prognostic factor following preoperative chemotherapy is tumor necrosis of above 90%.[29] It

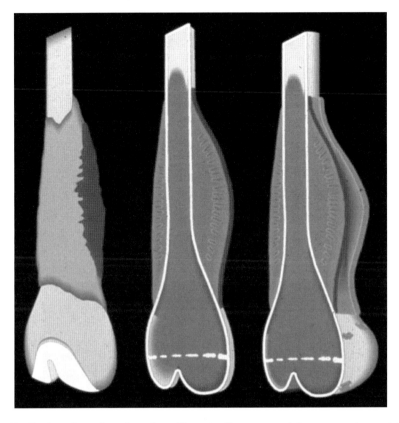

Fig. 15 The bone is cut in a plane that will maximally expose and demonstrate the suspicious area. This results in a slab section (*center*) and two opposing hemispheres. Reprinted with permission from Raymond AK et al: Osteosarcoma chemotherapy effect: A prognostic factor: Semin Diag Pathol 4: 212–236. 1987

has been advocated that postoperative chemotherapy be modified according to the histologic response of the effect of preoperative chemotherapy on the primary tumor.[29] However, this strategy is not universally accepted because of disparate histologic responses in simultaneously resected primary and metastatic tumors following treatment with neaoadjuvant therapy.[30]

The effects of chemotherapy are analyzed in terms of percent tumor necrosis. The hallmark of osteosarcoma necrosis is the dropout of neoplastic cells. Acellular tumor-produced matrix (i.e., osteoid, bone and cartilage) remains in areas previously occupied by viable tumor. Residual matrix is frequently accompanied by cellular debris and an ingrowth of rudimentary granulation tissue, hemosiderin deposition and/or fibrosis of varying density. An important criterion is the definitive absence of tumor cells. There may be scattered cells with significantly bizarre nuclear and/or cytoplasmic features or both; it can be difficult to assess whether these likely therapy-induced changes are malignant cells or atypical stromal cells. Questionable cellular changes in which there is no way to prove viability or identity

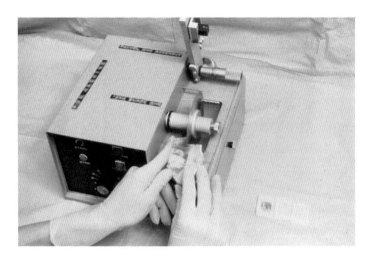

Fig. 16 Isomet geologic saw with diamond-impregnated circular blade and water bath Reprinted with permission from Raymond AK et al: Osteosarcoma chemotherapy effect: A prognostic factor: Semin Diag Pathol 4: 212–236. 1987

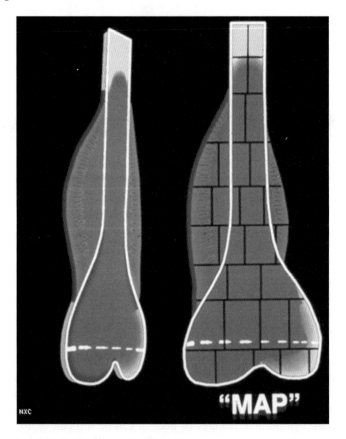

Fig. 17 Slab section is completely sectioned and will be entirely submitted for histologic analysis. Prior to decalcification and processing, the pieces are reassembled and used to prepare a specimen radiograph (Fig. 18). Reprinted with permission from Raymond AK et al: Osteosarcoma chemotherapy effect: A prognostic factor: Semin Diag Pathol 4: 212–236. 1987

Osteosarcoma Multidisciplinary Approach to the Management 79

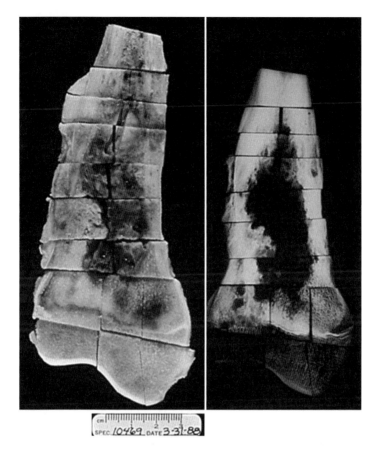

Fig. 18 Sections reassembled into their prior anatomic configuration (L) and a final specimen radiograph is obtained (R). Reprinted with permission from Raymond AK et al: Osteosarcoma chemotherapy effect: A prognostic factor: Semin Diag Pathol 4: 212–236. 1987

also create confusion, and these are, perhaps, best reported solely as "Present" or "Absent" (Fig. 21) in an accompanying note. Response to the treatment of the three major types of osteosarcoma is depicted in Figs. 22– 24.

Response to preoperative chemotherapy is a sensitive prognostic indicator that enables early identification of tumors in patients who have a high probability of surviving vs. those who potentially will not respond to treatment. The method is used to perform analyses of the effects of treatment and is not arbitrary. Reporting of the results must be clear, concise and accurate. This will also assist in planning the administration of optimum postoperative adjuvant chemotherapy.

Fig. 19 Osteosarcoma mapping. Specimen radiograph with mapping code. The specimen was cut, reassembled, coded, and submitted for specimen radiograph prior to decalcification. Cells demonstrating extensive therapeutic effect and indeterminate viability. Reprinted with permission from Raymond AK et al: Osteosarcoma chemotherapy effect: A prognostic factor: Semin Diag Pathol 4: 212–236. 1987

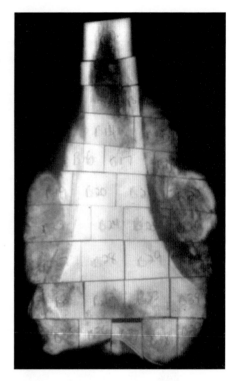

Fig. 20 "Map" created by using the specimen radiograph. Areas containing viable tumor indicated in white (periosteum, cortex, articular cartilage, epiphyseal plate and normal bone marrow). Reprinted with permission from Reprinted with permission from Raymond AK et al: Osteosarcoma chemotherapy effect: A prognostic factor: Semin Diag Pathol 4: 212–236. 1987[22]

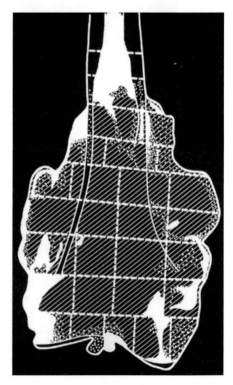

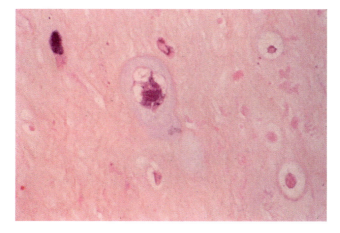

Fig. 21 Cells demonstrating extensive therapeutic effect and indeterminate viability. Best reported solely as "Present" or "Absent"

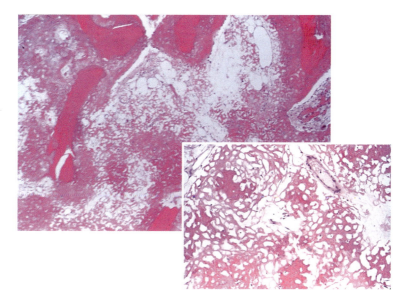

Fig. 22 Osteoblastic osteosarcoma with extensive response to preoperative chemotherapy. Residual acellular bone matrix remains. The lower panel demonstrates loss or dropout of many neoplastic cells (Hematoxylin and eosin)

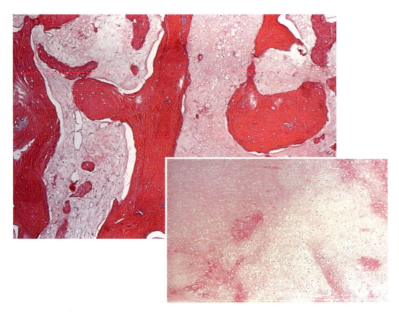

Fig. 23 Chondroblastic osteosarcoma following preoperative chemotherapy. Lobules of neoplastic cartilage with focal areas of osseous matrix. Many lacunae have undergone complete cell dropout and are empty (Hematoxylin and eosin)

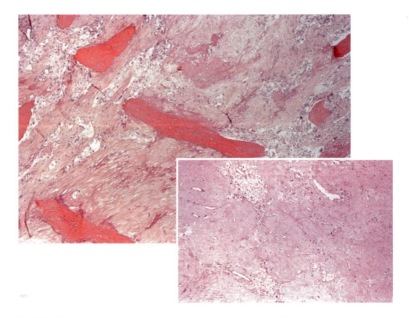

Fig. 24 Fibroblastic osteosarcoma response to preoperative chemotherapy showing loss of neoplastic cells. There is significant ingrowth of reactive stromal elements with appearance of edematous granulation tissue (Hematoxylin and eosin)

References

1. Dahlin DC, Unni KK. Osteosarcoma and its important recognizable variants. *Am J Surg Pathol*. 1977;1:61-72.
2. Lichtenstein L. *Bone Tumors*. 4th ed. St Louis: CV Mosby Company; 1972:215-243.
3. Unni KK. Osteosarcoma in bone. In: Unni KK, ed. *Bone Tumors*. New York: Churchill Livingston; 1988:107-133.
4. Matsuno T, Unni KK, Mc Cleod RA, et al. Telangiectatic osteosarcoma. *Cancer*. 1976;38:2538-2547.
5. Farr GH, Huvos SG, Marcove RC, et al. Telangiectatic osteogenic sarcoma: a review of twenty eight cases. *Cancer*. 1974;34:1150-1158.
6. Huvos AG, Rosen G, Bretsky SS, et al. Telangiectatic osteosarcoma; a clinicopathologic study of 124 cases. *Cancer*. 1982;49:1679-1689.
7. Eidekin J, Raymond AK, Ayala AC, et al. Small cell oseosarcoma. *Skeletal Radiol*. 1987;16:621-628.
8. Sim FH, Unni KK, Beabout JW, et al. Osteosarcoma with small cells simulating Ewing's tumor. *J Bone Joint Surg*. 1979;61A:207-215.
9. Dahlin DC, Unni KK, Matsumo T. Malignant (fibrous) histiocytoma of bone – fact or fancy? *Cancer*. 1977;39:1508-1516.
10. Wold LE. Fibrohistiocytic tumors of bone. In: Unni KK, ed. *Bone Tumors*. New York: Churchill Livingstone; 1988:183-197.
11. Balance WA, Mendelson G, Carter JA, et al. Osteogenic sarcoma. Malignant fibrous histiocytoma subtype. *Cancer*. 1988;62:763-771.
12. Unni KK, Dahlin DC, Mc Cleod RA. Intraosseous well differentiated osteosacoma. *Cancer*. 1977;40:1337-1347.
13. Ahuja SC, Villacin AB, Smith J, et al. Juxtacortical (parosteal) osteogenic sarcoma: histological grading and prognosis. *J Bone Joint Surg*. 1977;59:632-647.
14. Schajowicz F, Mc Guire MH, Araiyo ES, et al. Osteosarcomas arising on the surfaces of long bones. *J Bone Joint Surg*. 1988;70A:555-564.
15. Unni KK. Osteosarcoma of bone. In: Unni KK, ed. *Bone Tumors*. New York: Churchill Livingstone; 1988:107-133.
16. Hall RB, Robinson LH, Malawer MM, et al. Periosteal osteosarcoma. *Cancer*. 1985;55:165-171.
17. Unni KK, Dahlin DC, Beabout JW. Periosteal osteosarcoma. *Cancer*. 1976;37:2476-2485.
18. Wold LE, Unni KK, Beabout JW, et al. High-grade surface osteosarcoma. *Am J Surg Pathol*. 1984;8:181-186.
19. Unni KK. Osteosarcoma of bone. In: Unni KK, ed. *Bone Tumors*. New York: Churchill Livingstone; 1988:107-133.
20. Clark JL, Unni KK, Dahlin DC, et al. Osteosarcoma of the jaw. *Cancer*. 1983;51:2311-2316.
21. Mankin HJ, Lange TA, Spanier SS. The hazards of biopsy in patients with malignant primary bone and soft tissue tumors. *J Bone Joint Surg*. 1982;64:1121-1127.
22. Raymond AK, Ayala AG. Specimen management after chemotherapy. In: Unni KK, ed. *Bone Tumors*. New York: Churchill Livingstone; 1988:157-181.
23. Weatherby RP, Unni KK. Practical aspects of handling orthopedic specimens in the surgical pathology laboratory. *Pathol Annu*. 1982;17:1-31.
24. Raymond AK, Chawla SP, Carrasco HC, et al. Osteosarcoma chemotherapy effect: a prognostic factor. *Semin Diagn Pathol*. 1987;4:212-236.
25. Jaffe N, Knapp J, Chuang VP, et al. Osteosarcoma: Intra-arterial treatment of the primary tumor with *cis*-diamminedichloroplatinum-II (CDP) angiographic, pathologic, and pharmacologic studies. *Cancer*. 1983;51:402-407.
26. Carrasco CH, Chawla EP, Benjamin RS, et al. Arteriographic production of tumor necrosis after primary treatment of osteosarcoma in adults (abstract). *Proc Am Soc Clin Oncol*. 1987;6:126.
27. Carrasco CH, Charnasangavej C, Richli WR, et al. Angiographic response of assessment to preoperative chemotherapy in osteosarcoma. *Radiology*. 1989;170:839-843.

28. Kupman W, Lechner G, Wittich GR. The angiographic response of osteosarcoma following preoperative chemotherapy. *Skeletal Radiol*. 1985;15:96-102.
29. Benjamin RS. Chemotherapy for osteosarcoma. In: Unni KK, ed. *Bone Tumors*. New York: Churchill Livingstone; 1988:149-156.
30. Nachman J, Simon MA, Dean L, et al. Disparate histologic response in simultaneously resected primary and metastatic osteosarcoma. *J Clin Oncol*. 1987;5:1185-1190.

Conditions that Mimic Osteosarcoma

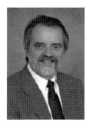

A. Kevin Raymond and Norman Jaffe

Abstract A variety of conditions may mimic osteosarcoma. The differential diagnosis includes benign and malignant tumors, infection and inflammatory processes arising from the musculoskeletal system. An accurate clinical history, imaging studies, and pathological evaluation are essential to establish the exact diagnosis. This chapter describes many of the conditions which may mimic the diagnosis of osteosarcoma. For convenience, the conditions are divided into several categories.

Introduction

The differential diagnosis of osteosarcoma is broad. Excluding the extremely unusual case, mimicking conditions can be divided into several well-defined groups.

The first group consists of malignant tumors that are the exception to the axiom that the production of osseous matrix defines osteosarcoma, i.e., osteosarcoma is a primary tumor of bone in which the neoplastic cells produce osteoid or bone, even if only small amounts.[1] These tumors are sarcomas that produce osseous matrix, yet are not considered osteosarcoma. This well-recognized but seldom-spoken-of phenomenon may occur in synovial sarcoma, dedifferentiated chondrosarcoma, clear cell chondrosarcoma, and mesenchymal chondrosarcoma and other tumors such as melanoma and a variety of carcinomas as well.

A second group of lesions that mimic osteosarcoma ranges from reactive matrix-producing lesions to benign neoplasia to highly malignant tumors. The distinction between these entities uses a more traditional approach to diagnosis that incorporates

---

A.K. Raymond (✉) and N. Jaffe
Department of Pathology, The University of Texas, M.D. Anderson Cancer Center,
1515 Holcombe Blvd, Houston, TX, 77030-4009, USA
e-mail: kraymond@mdanderson.org

the review of clinical information and imaging studies into the fabric of careful analysis of histologic detail. From a strategic and organizational point of view, it may be easiest to view this group by considering the specific forms of osteosarcoma that are mimicked by other pathologic processes.

Unequivocal distinction between conventional osteosarcoma and various manifestations of trauma (e.g., a stress fracture, true fracture, or hypertropic callus) can also be the source of significant diagnostic challenges.

Intraosseous lesions such as myxoma, fibromyoma, fibrous dysplasia, osteofibrous dysplasia and giant cell reparative granuloma of bone may cause significant diagnostic difficulty. At times, the distinction between a benign mixed tumor of the salivary (e.g., submandibular) gland and chondroblastic osteosarcoma can be surprisingly problematic.

Low-grade central, or intraosseous, osteosarcoma (well-differentiated intraosseous osteosaroma) can be difficult to segregate from other fibro-osseous processes such as fibrous dysplasia and osteofibrous dysplasia. Distinguishing telangiectactic osteosarcoma from other hemorrhagic cystic processes and giant cell-rich osteosarcoma from other giant cell-containing lesions can be vexing. Benign processes such as aneurysmal bone cysts and other lesions in which aneurysmal bone cyst-like features are encountered (e.g., giant cell tumor of bone, chondroblastoma, fibrous dysplasia, and osteoblastoma) may fuel this problem.

Although a rare problem, distinction between small-osteosarcoma and other small-cell processes can provide a diagnostic challenge. This distinction has become more bothersome with the recognition that the translocation t(11;22) can occur not only in Ewing sarcoma but also has now been reported, exceptionally, in a few cases of osteosarcoma. Further, larger studies to confirm these surprising findings are needed.

The separation of surface osteosarcoma from other surface processes can present unique challenges. However, there are very unique clinical, imaging, and histologic features that allow distinction between surface osteosarcoma and a variety of lesions grouped under the heading of "response to trauma," e.g., myositis ossificans, Nora's tumor, florid periostitis, fracture, and soft-tissue chondroma.

In essence, there are numerous conditions that must be differentiated from osteosarcoma. A partial list incorporating those described above and several others is given in Table 1. In all instances, the history, imaging studies, and histologic appearance must be taken into account to establish the diagnosis. Attention to strict diagnostic cytologic/histologic detail, while incorporating important clinical and imaging information as well as special studies (e.g., molecular testing), allows reproducible segregation between osteosarcoma and lesions with morphologic features that mimic osteosarcoma. This presentation will provide a brief discussion of some of these conditions. Described here are the traditional differential diagnosis, nontraditional entities (osteoid-producing entities that are not osteosarcoma), and other miscellaneous potentially confounding tumors and conditions

Table 1 Partial list of diagnoses in which patients may be referred with a diagnosis of "Osteosarcoma"

A partial list of tumors and conditions that may mimic Osteosarcoma
Chondrosarcoma
Chondrobalstoma (Codman's tumor)
Fibrous dysplasia and osteofibrous dysplasia (Ossifying fibroma)
Aneurysmal bone cyst
Telangiectatic osteosarcoma
Dediffereniated chondrosarcoma
Clear cell chondrosarcoma
Mesenchymal chondrosarcoma
Synovial sarcoma
Ewing sarcoma
Giant cell tumor of bone
Osteoid osteoma and osteoblastoma
Fracture
Osteomyelitis
Inflammatory metachronous hyperostosis
Myositis ossificans
Florid periostitis
Hypertrophic callus
Nora's disease

Traditional Differential Diagnosis

Chondrosarcoma

Chondrosarcoma is a malignant tumor characterized by the formation of cartilage by tumor cells.[2] It is seen more commonly in adults and is more prone to occur in the second to seventh decades of life. Males are more commonly affected than females (Fig. 1). It is frequently located in the pelvis and long bones, particularly the femur and humerus.

Chondrosarcoma may be subdivided into primary (conventional or medullary), dedifferentiated and secondary types. The tumor may be slow growing or highly malignant and metastasizing. Radiographically, the lesion is characterized by expansion of the medullary portion of the bone, thickening of the cortex, and endosteal scalloping. Annular, punctate or comma-shaped calcifications may be seen (Fig. 2).

Histologically, chondrosarcoma is typified by the formation of cartilage by tumor cells. Histologic distinction into types is based on the cellularity of the tumor, degree of pleomorphism of the cells and nuclei, and number of mitoses. High-grade

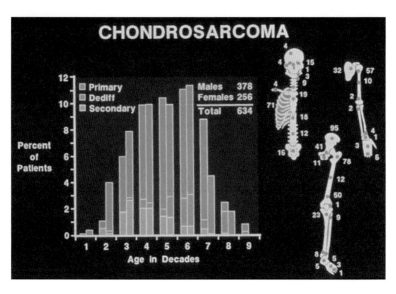

Fig. 1 Demographics of chondrosarcoma patients at the M. D. Anderson Cancer Center

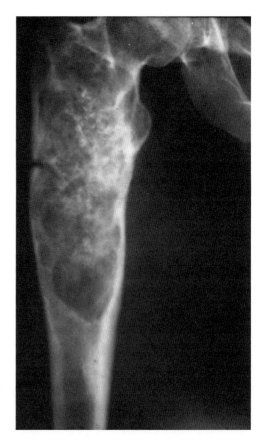

Fig. 2 Chondrosarcoma of the proximal femur. Plain films reveal an osteolytic lesion with "pop corn" appearance of intralesional mineralized content

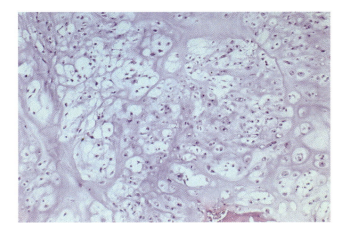

Fig. 3 Chondrosarcoma with large and vacuolated cells dispersed in intercellular cartilage (Hematoxylin & eosin)

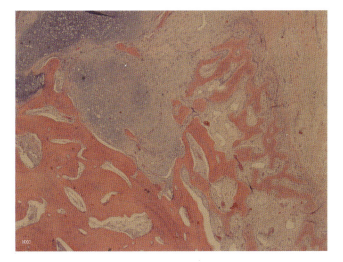

Fig. 4 Chondrosarcoma permeating between preexisting bony trabeculae (Hematoxylin eosin)

chondrosarcomas less closely resemble normal cartilage than do low-grade tumors. Figures 3–5 illustrate the histologic appearance of chondrosarcoma.

Chondroblastoma (Codman's Tumor)

Chondroblastoma represents less than 1% of all primary bone tumors. The lesion is seen primarily before skeletal maturity,[3] in the first and second decades of life.

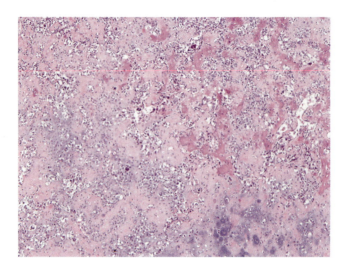

Fig. 5 Chondrosarcoma with modest hyperchromasia and increased pleomorphism of the nuclei (Hematoxylin & eosin)

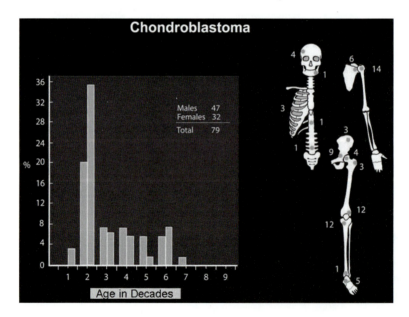

Fig. 6 Demographics of M.D. Anderson Cancer Center chondroblastoma patients

It is more common in males than in females. The demographics of patients with chondroblastoma treated at M.D. Anderson Cancer Center are depicted in Fig. 6. This benign tumor typically occurs in the epiphysis of long bones and usually is

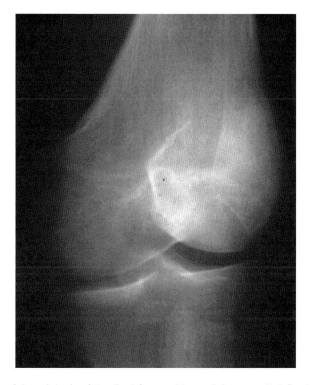

Fig. 7 Image of the epiphysis of the distal femur with a radiolucent well-defined, eccentrically located chondroblastoma

eccentrically located. It is radiolucent with a sclerotic border (Fig. 7). Periosteal new bone formation is rarely seen.

Histologically, the tumor is highly cellular, with relatively undifferentiated tissue comprising round and polygonal chondroblast-like cells. Multinucleated giant cells may be seen. Small amounts of more mature cartilaginous intercellular matrix and foci of intercellular calcifications are often present (Figs. 8–10). Pulmonary metastases have been reported in rare cases.[4]

The differential diagnosis for tumors located in the epiphysis also includes giant cell tumor of bone, clear cell chondrosarcoma, and cysts. These entities are described later in this chapter.

Fibrous Dysplasia and Osteofibrous Dysplasia (Ossifying Fibroma)

Fibrous dysplasia generally occurs in the first to fourth decades of life. Demographics of M.D. Anderson patients reveal a slightly greater number of females affected

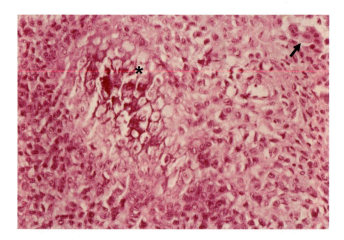

Fig. 8 Chondroblastoma with round chondroblasts and ovoid, often "grooved" nuclei and an occasional multinucleated giant cell (*arrow*). "Chicken wire" intercellular calcifications are seen toward the left center side (*asterisk*)

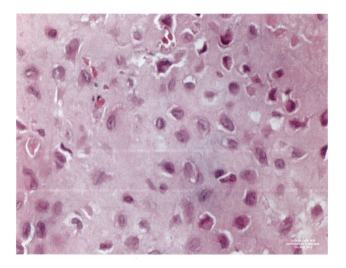

Fig. 9 Typical appearance of a chondroblastoma: chondroid differentiation with abundant matrix

than males (Fig. 11). The condition may occur in one or more sites.[5] The clinical spectrum varies from asymptomatic, monostotic lesions to extensive skeletal deformities. However, pain has been described in 70% of patients.[6] Patients with fibrous dysplasia also appear to have a slightly increased risk of developing sarcomas, usually osteosarcoma.[6-8]

Lesions in the long bones are located in the diaphyseal or metaphyseal region. They are centrally or eccentrically located and are described as areas of intramedullary

Conditions that Mimic Osteosarcoma 93

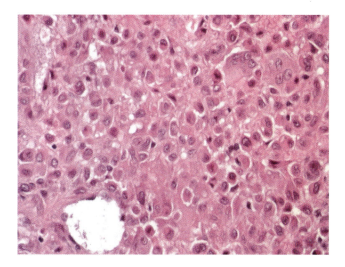

Fig. 10 Calcification in chondroblastoma

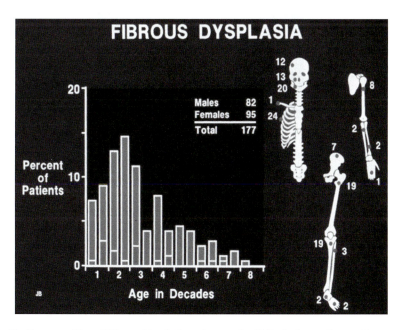

Fig. 11 Demographics of Fibrous Dysplasia patients at the M.D. Anderson Cancer Center

lucency with a hazy quality, a "ground glass" appearance (Fig. 12). There may be end-to-end scalloping with a zone of reactive sclerosis.

Histologic evaluation of fibrous dysplasia reveals swirling bland spindle cells. They are minimally atypical and monomorphic. The background is edematous and

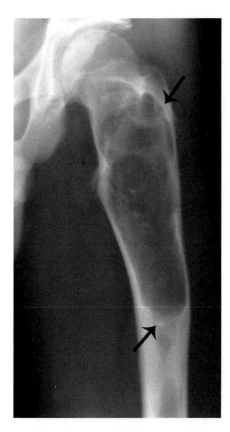

Fig. 12 Fibrous dysplasia of the femur in a 14-year-old male. Frontal radiogram of the proximal left femur showing a metadiaphyseal lesion that extends into the neck (upper arrow). Notice the thick internal septations in a "ground-glass" background, expansile nature and narrow zone of transition (lower arrow), features of long-standing benign process. This appearance has been likened to "shepherd's crook."

composed of randomly arranged trabeculae with a lack of osteoblastic rimming. The trabeculae are poorly oriented and tend to form irregular C- or S-shaped profiles (Figs. 13 and 14). Fibrous dysplasia frequently weakens the bone, causing secondary deformities. Lesions that have poorly defined areas of osteolysis, cortical destruction, and soft-tissue masses adjacent to the cortical destruction are suggestive of malignant transformation. Activating point mutations in the *GNAS1* gene, encoding a heterotrimeric G-protein regulatory the cAMP pathway, are associated with fibrous dysplasia.

Osteofibrous dysplasia – the term for ossifying fibroma preferred by Campanacci and Laus[9] generally occurs in the first decade of life, in the skeletally immature patient. It is more common in boys than in girls and is usually encountered

Conditions that Mimic Osteosarcoma 95

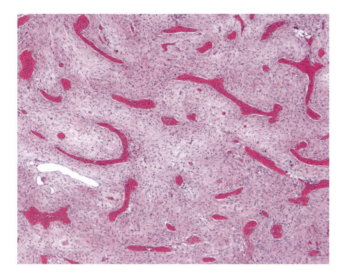

Fig. 13 Fibrous dysplasia. Swirling bland spindle cells, minimally atypical and monomorphic in an edematous background. Randomly arranged bone trabecula with lack of osteoblastic rimming (Hematoxilin & Eosin)

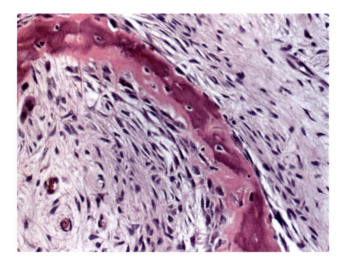

Fig. 14 High power view section of Fig. 13 highlighting the spindle cells and loose stroma

in the lower extremity below the knee (Fig. 15), most commonly the diaphysis of the tibia. Imaging studies reveal a "soap bubble" appearance within the medullary cavity (Fig. 16). Not infrequently, anterior tibial bowing may be observed. Histologically, the lesion is characterized by fibrous stroma with trabeculae of woven bone and osteoblastic rimming (Figs. 17 and 18).

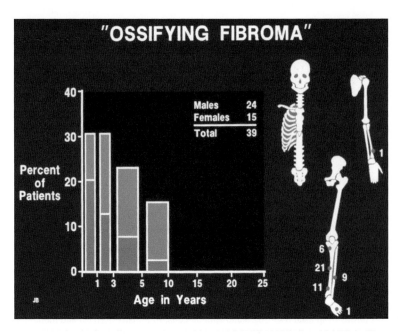

Fig. 15 Demographics of M.D. Anderson ossifying fibroma (osteofibrous dysplasia) patients

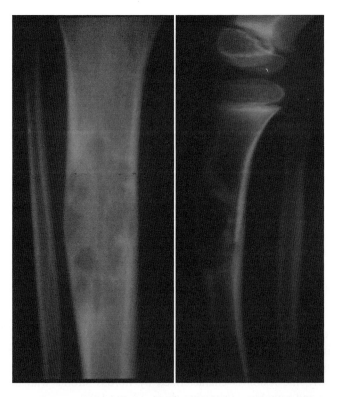

Fig. 16 Ossifying fibroma of diaphysis of tibia. Soap bubble appearance within the medullary (L) cavity with anterior bowing of the tibia (R)

Conditions that Mimic Osteosarcoma

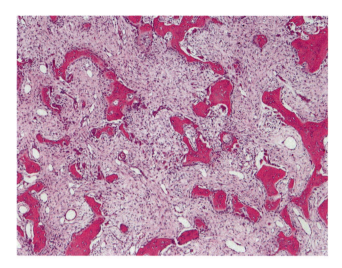

Fig. 17 Osteofibrous dysplasia. In contrast to fibrous dysplasia, the surfaces of the irregular trabecula tend to be conspicuously lined with osteoblasts

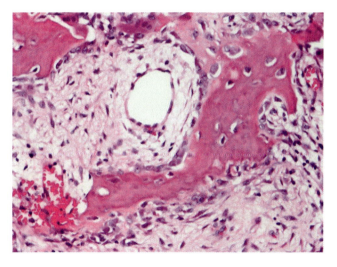

Fig. 18 High magnification view of Fig. 17 highlights the osteoblasts associated with the trabeculae

Fibrous dysplasia and osteofibrous dysplasia must be distinguished from low-grade central, or intraosseous, osteosarcoma (Well-differentiated osteosarcoma). The latter is extremely rare (1% of osteosarcomas) and has a survival rate of 80%. The demographics of patients with this tumor seen at M.D. Anderson are depicted in Fig. 19. It generally occurs in the second to fifth decades of life. An example in the distal femur is depicted in Fig. 20. It is large, destructive, and confined. The morbid anatomic appearance of the tumor is rock hard, gray white or ivory

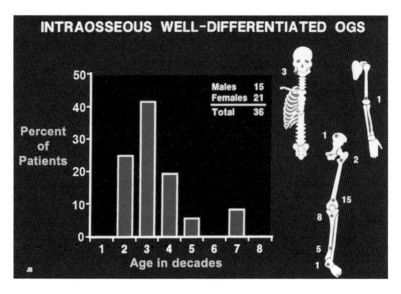

Fig. 19 Demographics of M.D. Anderson intraosseous well-differentiated osteosarcoma patients

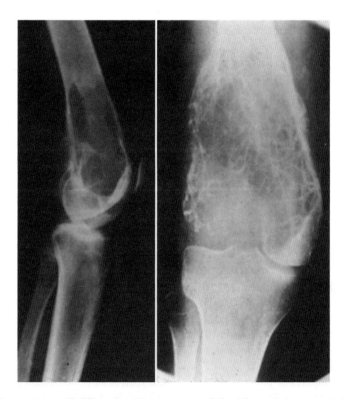

Fig. 20 Intraosseous well-differentiated osteosarcoma of distal femur. It is large and destructive, confined within the bone

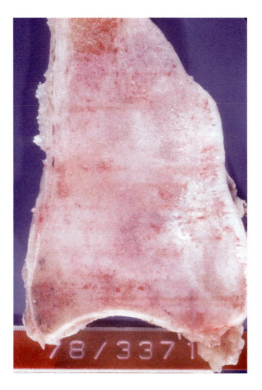

Fig. 21 Resected specimen of intraosseous well-differentiated osteosarcoma. It is rock hard, grey-white, homogenous, and confined

white, homogeneous, and confined (Fig. 21). The histologic appearance is depicted in Figs. 22 and 23. Extensive networks of well-formed lamellar bone trabeculae are typical.

The following factors distinguish fibrous dysplasia and osteofibrous dysplasia from conventional osteosarcoma. Fibrous dysplasia and osteofibrous dysplasia occur in the very young (Figs. 11 and 15). More than 60% are seen in patients younger than 5 years; more than 95% in patients younger than 10 years. These dysplasias generally involve the tibia, particularly in osteofibrous dysplasia. Imaging studies reveal fairly distinctive results. Fibrous dysplasia is characterized by a "ground glass" lesion and osteofibrous dysplasia by a "soap bubble" lesion with anterior bowing of the tibia. In contrast, osteosarcoma is overtly destructive, and a mass representing soft-tissue invasion is frequently seen. Histologic examination of fibrous dysplasia and osteofibrous dysplasia reveals an innocuous spindle-cell stroma background with angiocentric bone trabeculae. Woven bone is present in both. Osteoblastic rimming is present in osteofibrous dysplasia. As indicated earlier, mutations in the *GNAS1*

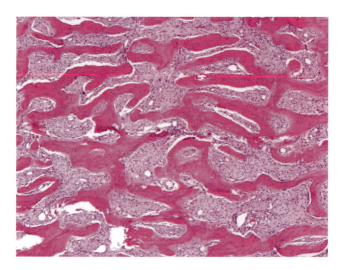

Fig. 22 Histological section of intraosseous well-differentiated osteosarcoma. The tissue section shows a moderately cellular fibrous stroma producing abundant matrix. (Hematoxilin Eosin)

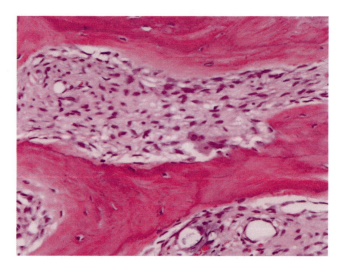

Fig. 23 High magnification view of Fig. 22 demonstrated that the osteosarcoma cells are spindled and only mild cytologically atypical. Such relatively banal histologic findings underscore the importance of correlation with the radiologic features

gene is associated with fibrous dysplasia. In contrast, conventional osteosarcoma is composed of highly anaplastic cells and randomly deposited matrix or mixed matrix with osteoid and cartilage.

Conditions that Mimic Osteosarcoma 101

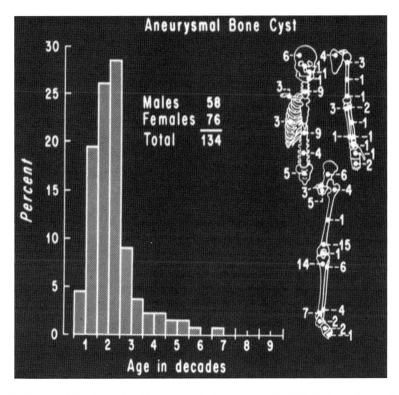

Fig. 24 Demographics of aneurismal bone cysts of patients seen at the M.D. Anderson Cancer Center

Aneurysmal Bone Cyst

Aneurysmal bone cysts arise de novo in bone and are prone to occur in the first to third decades of life.[10] Females are more commonly affected than males (Fig. 24). Pain and swelling are the most common complaints. Radiographically, a cyst is characterized by an area of lucency situated eccentrically in the medullary cavity in the metaphysis of a long bone, with well-defined margins, cortical thinning, and expansion. The interface is usually well defined (Fig. 25). Computed tomography and magnetic resonance may show internal septation and often multiple fluid–fluid levels. From a gross-anatomical perspective, the cyst presents as a hemorrhagic spongy mass. Histopathologic features include cavernous spaces, the walls of which lack the normal features of blood vessels. It is unusual for the spaces to have endothelial linings. The septa invariably contain giant cells. Almost all aneurysmal bone cysts also have solid areas (Figs. 26–28).

The differential diagnosis of the aneurysmal bone cyst includes telangiectatic osteosarcoma, as well as giant cell tumor and low-grade osteosarcoma, which are both described later in this chapter. Telangiectatic osteosarcoma is the most important.

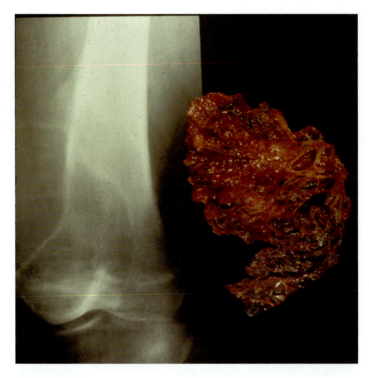

Fig. 25 Radiologic image and corresponding gross anatomic specimen of aneurysm bone cyst of the distal femur

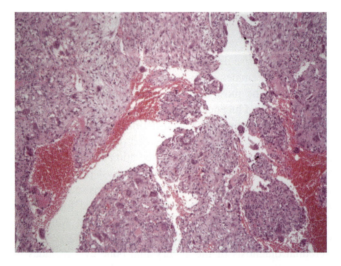

Fig. 26 Aneurysmal bone cyst with septa separating spaces containing loosely arranged spindle cells with accumulated blood and scattered multinucleated giant cells

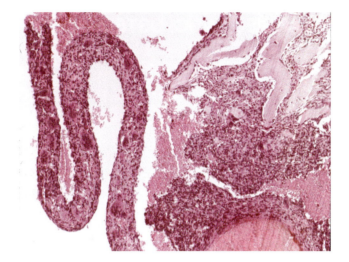

Fig. 27 Higher-power appearance of septa

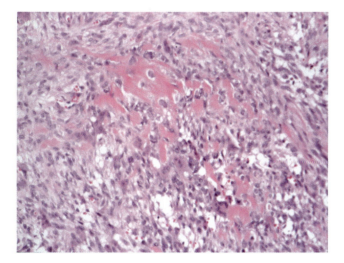

Fig. 28 Relatively solid aneurismal bone cyst. Loose arrangement of spindle cells. Osteoid is present

It accounts for 3% of all osteosarcomas. Observed demographic features are outlined in Fig. 29. It is prone to occur in the second decade of life and is more common in males than in females. Because of their overlap, the demographics are not very helpful when distinguishing an aneurysmal bone cyst from telangiectatic osteosarcoma. It is noted, however, that the spine is an unusual site for telangiectatic osteosarcoma.

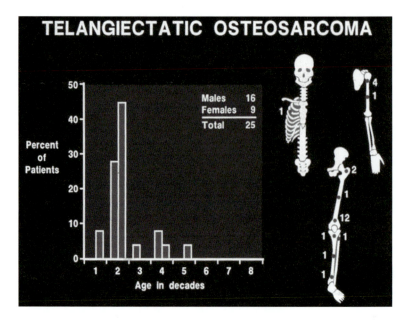

Fig. 29 Demographics of M.D. Anderson telangiectatic osteosarcoma patients

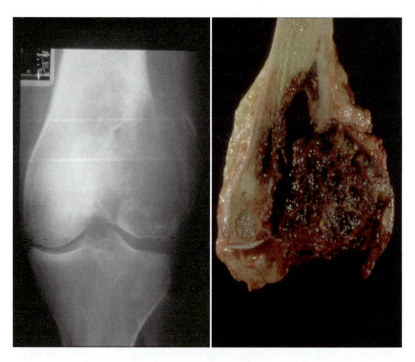

Fig. 30 Telangiectatic osteosarcoma of the distal femur. The image shows a destructive, eccentrically placed lytic lesion which is expansile, infiltrative, and ill defined (L). The gross specimen shows a hemorrhagic mass with blood filled cysts (R)

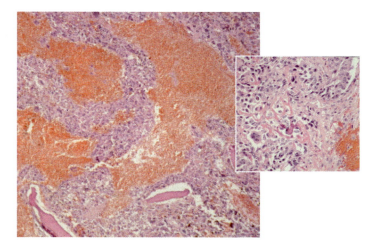

Fig. 31 Histologic features of telangiectatic osteosarcoma. The specimen shows blood-filled pseudocysts (no epithelial lining), membranes, malignant cells, and osteoid. Inset: high power field demonstrates the cytologic atypia

Telangiectatic Osteosarcoma

Telangiectatic osteosarcoma is a rapidly expansile, aggressive lesion composed of loculated blood-filled spaces, partially lined by malignant cells producing sparse osteoid. Radiographically, it appears as a purely lytic lesion with minimal, if any, sclerotic changes (Fig. 30). Histologic examination reveals a hemorrhagic mass with blood-filled cysts, septa, membranes, highly malignant anaplastic cells, and sparse, delicate osteoid (Fig. 31). By definition, it is a high-grade malignancy.

Nontraditional Osteoid-Producing Entities

In this section, exceptions to the rule that osteosarcoma is a primary malignancy of bone in which the neoplastic cells produce osteoid and/or bone, even if only in small amounts[1] are considered. Osteoid and/or bone may be noted in synovial sarcoma, dedifferentiated chondrosarcoma, clear cell chondrosarcoma, and mesenchymal chondrosarcoma.

Dedifferentiated Chondrosarcoma

Dedifferentiated chondrosarcoma is the most malignant of all chondrosarcomas. The condition occurs slightly more in men than in women and generally in older

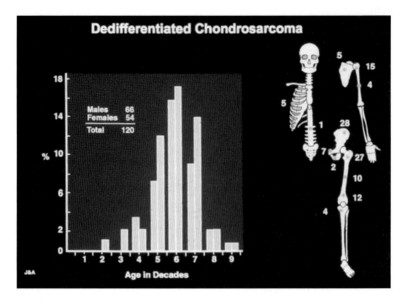

Fig. 32 Demographics of dedifferentiated chondrosarcoma

patients, in the fifth to seventh decade of life (Fig. 32). It presents with a skeletal distribution similar to that of chondrosarcoma. The patient typically reports pain of long duration followed by a more recent onset of rapid swelling and local tenderness. Imaging features vary, but the hallmark is a proliferative sarcoma engrafted on an aggressive indolent-appearing chondrosarcoma.[11] The lesion may resemble a conventional chondrosarcoma with areas of aggressive bone destruction and focal calcification (Fig. 33). Histologic analysis reveals a sharp interface between cartilage and a high-grade bone-producing sarcoma component,[12] with no transition (Fig. 34).

Clear Cell Chondrosarcoma

Clear cell chondrosarcoma is more prone to occur between the second and seventh decades of life and is more common in men than in women (Fig. 35). The tumor is most likely to occur in the epiphysis (Fig. 36). Histologic analysis reveals sheets of clear cells with osteoclast-like giant cells (Fig. 37). The tumor resembles a typical chondrosarcoma with bone production by osteoblasts. It is considered as a low-grade malignancy, and its clinical behavior is usually less aggressive than that of conventional chondrosarcoma.[13]

Conditions that Mimic Osteosarcoma

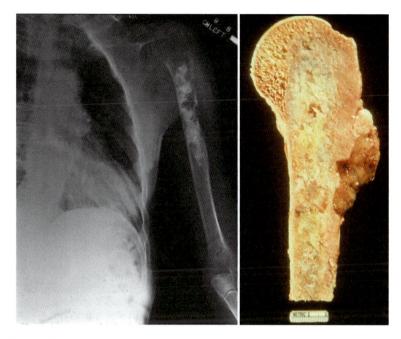

Fig. 33 Dedifferentiated chondrosarcoma of the proximal humerus (L). There is an osteolytic lesion with poorly defined margins. Punctate and annular calcifications present within the lesion. The gross specimen is on the right

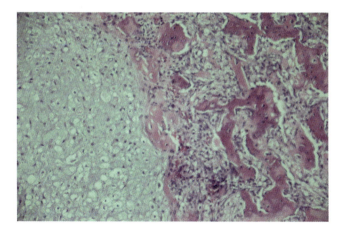

Fig. 34 Dedifferentiated chondrosarcoma. High power appearance between junction of chondrosarcoma and spindle cell sarcoma. The tumors do not merge but are juxtaposed. There is usually a sharp demarcation between the tumor and its dedifferentiated component

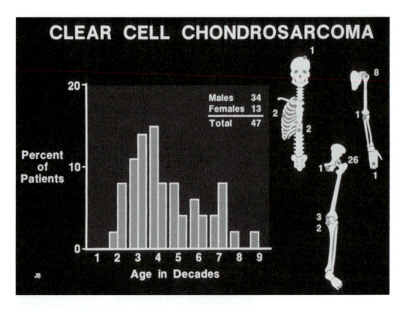

Fig. 35 Demographics of M.D. Anderson clear cell chondrosarcoma patients

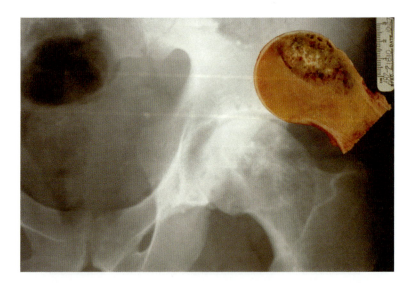

Fig. 36 Clear cell chondrosarcoma of the femoral head. The lesion is well demarcated and shows focal mineralization. Inset: Corresponding gross specimen

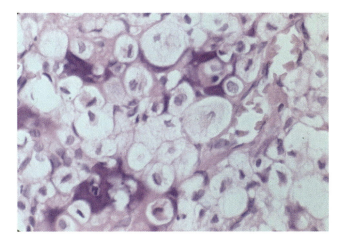

Fig. 37 High-power appearance of clear cell chondrosarcoma showing focal ossification intimately admixed with tumor cells. The tumor cells have centrally located round nuclei and abundant clear cytoplasm

Mesenchymal Chondrosarcoma

Mesenchymal chondrosarcoma is prone to occur in the second to third decades of life and is equally distributed between males and females (Fig. 38). It represents less than 1% of bone tumors. Its radiographic appearance is usually indistinguishable from that of conventional chondrosarcoma. The features are nonspecific but usually suggest a malignant tumor of cartilaginous derivation. Some tumors may exhibit a permeative growth pattern similar to that of round-cell tumors. Histologically, the tumor is typified by areas of differentiated cartilage with highly vascular spindle- or round-cell mesenchymal tissue.[14,15] Small cells in sheets with a "hemangiopericytoma-like" vascular pattern may be present (Fig. 39). The cartilage is non-mixing or transitional, and there is osteoid and/or bone production. Sox-9, a transcription factor involving in cartilage development, may be expressed in both mesenchymal chondrosarcoma and conventional chondrosarcoma (Fig. 40).

Synovial Sarcoma

This peculiar soft tissue sarcoma occurs in older children and young adults. It has the propensity to differentiate into two distinct elements: a spindle cell component and a distinct glandular component with epithelial differentiation comprise the biphasic form. A monophasic form consisting solely of spindle cells is the most common form. Characteristic cytogenetic abnormalities include a balanced

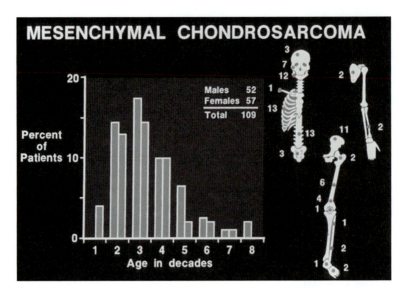

Fig. 38 Demographics of mesenchymal chondrosarcoma patients at the M.D. Anderson Cancer Center

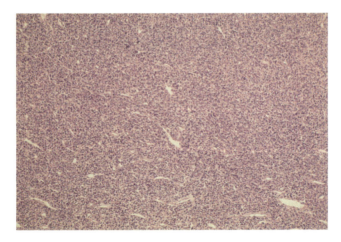

Fig. 39 Typical vascular pattern in mesenchymal chondrosarcoma. Vessels are surrounded by small malignant cells, which compress and deform them. Morphologically identifiable cartilage tissue is present in other areas of the specimen

translocation between chromosomes X and 18 resulting in one of several fusion transcripts (SYT/SSX1, SYT/SSX2 or very rarely SYT/SSX4). Cytogenetic or molecular demonstration of this event is diagnostically relevant

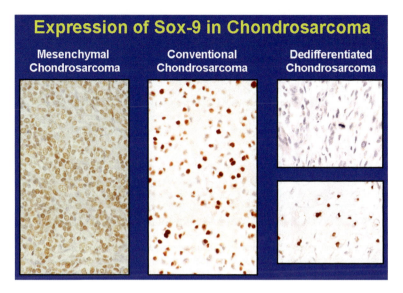

Fig. 40 Sox-9 expression in chondrosarcoma. *Left panel*: mesenchymal chondrosarcoma showing distinct nuclear expression of Sox-9, a transcription factor associated with cartilaginous development; *center panel*, conventional chondrosarcoma with intermediate quantity of Sox-9 and *right panel* dedifferentiated chondrosarcoma loss of Sox-9 in the dedifferentiated component with retention in the more well-differentiated component (*lower panel*). Courtesy of Czerniak B, M.D. Anderson Cancer Center

Miscellaneous Tumors and Conditions

Ewing Sarcoma

Ewing sarcoma is part of the Ewing family of tumors.[16] It accounts for approximately 6% of malignant bone tumors. The bones of the pelvis and extremities, particularly the lower extremities, are the most common sites involved.[17] In contrast to osteosarcoma, the diaphysis is more commonly affected than the metaphysis. Not infrequently, the entire bone may be involved. Imaging reveals multiple layers of subperiosteal new bone formation, referred to as an "onion skin" appearance (Fig. 41). (This appearance may also be seen in other conditions, e.g., osteomyelitis.) Lytic and blastic areas may be present. Occasionally, the radiographic appearance may be more characteristic of osteosarcoma with spicules radiating from the cortex. The tumor may also appear to arise on the surface of the bone, producing a saucer-like indentation of the surface. The radiographic findings should be distinguished from those of osteosarcoma, osteomyelitis, Langerhans cell histiocytosis (eosinophilic granuloma), and lymphoma of bone.

Microscopically, Ewing sarcoma is composed of sheets of round cells with round nuclei. The cells appear numerous and monotonous. They are separated into small compartments by bands of stroma, with very little stroma among the cells (Fig. 42).

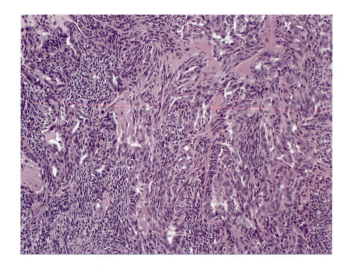

Fig. 41 Synovial sarcoma: This biphasic synovial sarcoma is composed of narrow spindle cells with scatted more epithelioid cell–forming glands with small lumens (original magnification, 100×). Monophasic (spindle cells only) is the more common morphologic forms of this disease and can be more challenging diagnostically. Patchy expression of epithelial membrane antigen (EMA) and cytokeratins is helpful and molecular techniques to demonstrate the characteristic SYT-SSX1 or SSX2 fusion event can aid in cases presenting a diagnostic challenge

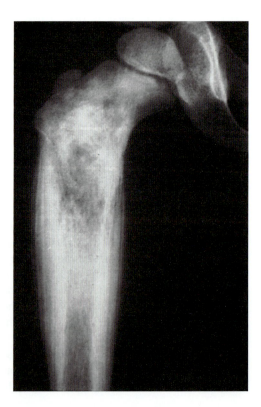

Fig. 42 Ewing's sarcoma of the femur. Lytic and blastic areas affecting the upper third of the femur with typical "onion skin" appearance arising from subperosteal new bone formation

Most Ewing sarcoma cells express CD99, a cell-membrane protein encoded by the MIC2 gene, which is located in the pseudoautosomal region at the end of the short arms of the X and Y chromosomes.[18] CD99 expression is not specific for Ewing sarcoma; it may be detected in lymphoblastic lymphoma, embryonal rhabdomyosarcoma, and other soft-tissue sarcomas. In Ewing sarcoma, CD99 often has a distinct membranous distribution.

The vast majority of cases of Ewing sarcoma are associated with translocation involving the *EWSR1* (22q12) locus. The most common translocation is between chromosome 11 containing FLI1 and EWSR1 on chromosome 22. Numerous variant translocations involving substitutes, most often for FLI1, but also EWSR1 are described. Molecular confirmation of a characteristic fusion event is an evolving standard of care in diagnosis of this tumor.

Giant Cell Tumor of Bone

Giant cell tumor constitutes 5% of skeletal tumors.[19] It usually presents with pain and a mass that has been present for several weeks to months. It most commonly occurs at the end of a long bone. Imaging demonstrates a lytic lesion centered in the epiphysis but involving the metaphysis and extending into the adjacent articular cortex (Fig. 43). Apart from a thin shell of subperiosteal new bone outlining the outer surface of the tumor, no periosteal reactions are present. There is no mineralized tumor matrix.

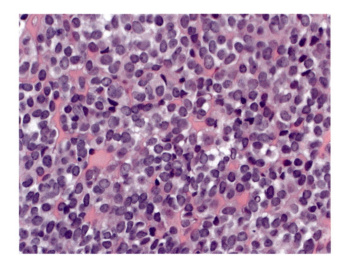

Fig. 43 Ewing sarcoma: Shown here at high magnification (original, 400×), Ewing sarcoma is a prototypical small round cell tumor with prominent nuclei and relatively small amounts of more subtle cytoplasm. While membranous expression of CD99 visualized with immunohistochemistry is helpful, demonstration of a characteristic rearrangement of EWSR1 is an evolving standard of care in diagnosis

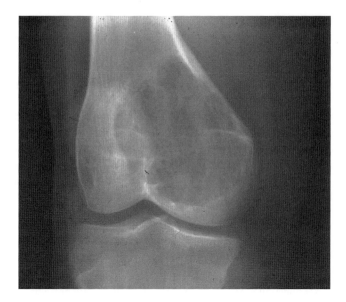

Fig. 44 Giant cell tumor of the distal femur. There is a geographic lytic lesion with irregular, but well-defined borders

Bony ridges at the periphery of a lobulated tumor will give the appearance of trabeculations within the tumor. The tumor is composed of a vascularized network of round, oval, or spindle-shaped stromal cells and multinucleated giant cells (Fig. 44). Osteoid production and ossification may be noted in small foci.[20,21]

Osteoid Osteoma and Osteoblastoma

Osteoblastoma and Osteoid osteoma typically occur during the first three decades of life. They are benign bone-forming tumors that are histologically similar but may have a different natural history. Osteoblastoma typically occurs in the spine, whereas osteoid osteoma frequently presents in the diaphysis of the femur and tibia.[22] The size of the tumor is an important determinant of whether the lesion is diagnosed as an osteoid osteoma or osteoblastoma. Schajowicz and Lemos[22,23] classified osteoid osteoma as possessing a nidus of 2 cm or less in greatest diameter. They designated such lesions as "circumscribed osteoblastomas." In their opinion, also, the term "benign osteoblastoma" should be dropped, and all these lesions should be considered potentially malignant. While somewhat controversial, this idea is reasonable as size is probably a continuous rather than discrete variable in relation to malignant potential. On the other hand, one does not want to overtreat small lesions. Malignant transformation of osteoblastoma with production of metastases has been documented.[23,24]

Conditions that Mimic Osteosarcoma   115

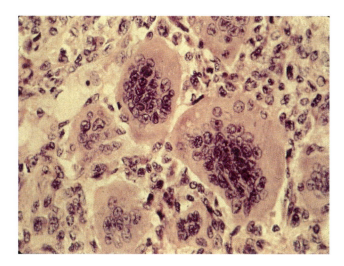

Fig. 45 Giant cell tumor with prominent multinucleated giant cells. The stromal cells contain a single large nucleus surrounded by a poorly defined cytoplasm that gives a syncticial appearance (Hematoxylin & eosin).

Imaging in osteoid osteoma and osteoblastoma reveals a well-circumscribed lesion; however, occasionally, cortical destruction with a soft-tissue mass may occur, especially if the tumor is of the more aggressive type. Bone destruction may be aggressive. Expansion and aneurysmal dilatation may occur (Fig. 45).

Histologically, the lesions contain osteoblasts with osteoid trabeculae (Fig. 46). The tumors behave unpredictably. The tumor depicted in Figs. 45 and 46 underwent malignant transformation into an osteosarcoma with metastases.

Fracture

Fracture, including a "stress" fracture, may occasionally be suspected to harbor an osteosarcoma (Fig. 47). In the early phases, a fracture may be characterized with abundant cellular activity with mitotic processes. The fracture may also exhibit exuberant callus, compounding the misdiagnosis. "Stress" fractures are often located in the tibial shaft and may occur after heavy marching or jogging. The history and imaging studies may be helpful in making the distinction.

Osteomyelitis

Osteomyelitis may present with a lytic and blastic reaction. One of the earliest signs is irregular rarefaction. In the acute phase, features suggest a permeative malignant

Fig. 46 Aggressive osteoblastoma in diaphysis of femur. The lesion appears as a lucent, expansile area with irregular sclerosis and no definite nidus. Ossification and calcification is present within the lytic area

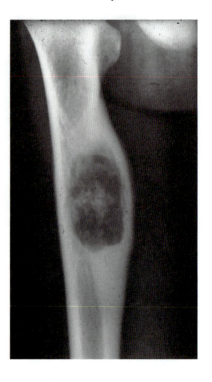

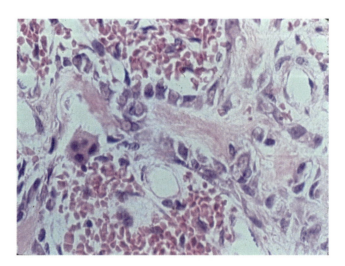

Fig. 47 Aggressive osteoblastoma. Rows of hypertrophic plump, so-called epithelioid osteoblasts surrounding osteoid or slightly calcified bone trabeculae

Conditions that Mimic Osteosarcoma 117

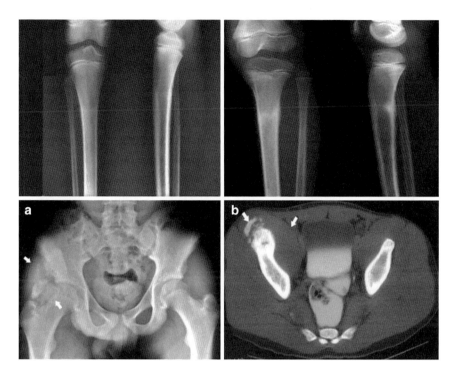

Fig. 48 Fracture proximal shaft of tibia. Patient referred with a diagnosis of osteosarcoma of proximal shaft of the tibia. He complained of pain and tenderness commencing 6 weeks earlier after jogging. *Upper panels*: A radiograph was obtained and dismissed as "normal." With persistence of the pain and increasing localized tenderness a repeat radiograph was obtained revealing a horizontal blastic area at the painful site. In comparing earlier (*left panel*) and later radiographs (*right panel*) a stress fracture was diagnosed and confirmed by computer tomography. *Lower panels*: Healing fracture of the iliac bone with callus formation, a potential pitfall for osteosarcoma. Frontal radiogram of the pelvis (**a**) showing fracture of the right ilium and an exuberant mineralized callus formation (*arrows*). Axial CT image at the corresponding level (**b**) showing an avulsion fracture of the right ilium, mineralized callus and a large hematoma of the iliopsoas muscles (*arrows*)

lesion similar to Ewing sarcoma. In the chronic phase, geographic areas of destruction may be seen (Fig. 48).

Inflammatory Metachronous Hyperostosis

Inflammatory metachronous hyperostosis. This is a chronic recurrent form of osteomyelitis which most commonly affects the clavicle, and later other bones (Fig. 49). Radiographic studies show a predominantly sclerotic process.

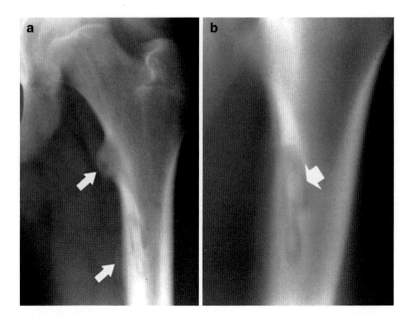

Fig. 49 Chronic active osteomyelitis in a 14-year-old male. Frontal conventional radiogram of the left femur (**a**) showing a sclerotic lesser trochanter (*upper arrow*), solid periosteal reaction and longitudinal sinus tracts within the thickened cortex (*lower arrow*). Frontal conventional tomogram of the left femur (**b**) showing a sequestrum (*arrow*) surrounded by serpiginous sinus tract

The condition is self-limited in that, with or without treatment, the bones eventually return to normal. Bacterial cultures were negative in two of the reported cases and a viral etiology could not be excluded.[25] The histology shows thickened bone spicules surrounded by reactive osteoblastic reactive bone and connective tissue. It is treated with analgesic medication.

Myositis Ossificans

In myositis ossificans, heterotopic calcification may occur in muscle or soft tissue. Fibroblastic proliferation is the dominant feature. The cells tend to be loosely arranged without organization. The osteoblasts form reactive new bone, and the osteoid undergoes mineralization to form parallel arrays of bone that appears almost normal. The imaging studies usually show a well-circumscribed lesion; computer tomography is usually helpful in demonstrating this feature (Fig. 50). The mass is not attached to the underlying cortex of the bone.

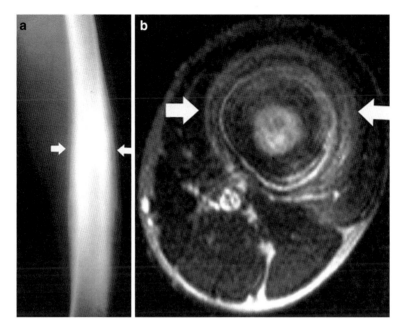

Fig. 50 Idiopathic hyperostosis of femur in a 14-year-old female with painful swelling. Lateral view of the femur (**a**) showing solid periosteal new bone formation and diffuse sclerotic reaction of both cortical and medullary bone (*arrows*). Axial T2WI, MR (**b**) showing multilayer periosteal new bone formation (*arrows*)

Bone Cysts

A variety of lesions that appear cystic may occur in bone. A unicameral bone cyst apparently results from a disturbance of growth at the epiphyseal line. It generally forms in the upper part of the diaphysis of the humerus, proximal femur, or proximal tibia. For example, a patient with a simple cyst in the proximal femur was referred to M.D. Anderson Cancer Center with a diagnosis of osteosarcoma. Three experienced pathologists supported the diagnosis, but it was refuted by a fourth. The cyst was treated by simple curettage. The patient has been well 5 years following the procedure.

Summary

A variety of benign and malignant conditions may mimic osteosarcoma. Some of the more common, a few less common, and several gleaned from the literature have been described in this chapter. These experiences would suggest that any condition – *anything* – affecting the musculoskeletal system could masquerade as osteosarcoma. To establish the correct diagnosis, a detailed history, imaging studies, and histologic findings must be obtained. Careful and conscientious correlation of findings with hallmarks of all three disciplines is essential. A high index of suspicion is important, and the possibility that non-tumorous conditions may mimic neoplastic conditions should constantly be borne in mind. The "burden of proof" that a condition is or is not osteosarcoma ultimately rests with the pathologist, but is informed by interactions with radiologic and clinical colleagues.

References

1. Dahlin DC, Unni KK. Osteosarcoma and its important recognizable variants. *Am J Surg Pathol.* 1977;1:61–72.
2. Sissons HA, Murray RO, Kemp HBS. *Orthopedic Diagnosis.* Berlin: Springer-Verlag; 1984: 102–107, 135–144, 214–215, 247–251.
3. Dahlin DC, Ivins JC. Benign chondroblastoma. *Cancer.* 1972;30:401–413.
4. Huvos AG. *Bone Tumors: Diagnosis, Treatment and Prognosis.* Philadelphia: WB Saunders; 1979.
5. Lichtenstein L, Jaffe HL. Fibrous dysplasia of bone. A condition affecting one, several or many bones, the graver cases of which may present abnormal pigmentation of skin, premature sexual development, hyperthyroidism or still other extra skeletal abnormalities. *Arch Pathol.* 1942; 33:777–816.
6. Harris WH, Dudley HR, Barray RJ. The natural history of fibrous dysplasia. *J Bone Joint Surg.* 1962; 44A:207–233.
7. Dorfman HD. Proceedings: malignant transformation of benign bone lesions. *Proc Natl Cancer Conf.* 1973; 7:901–913.
8. Huvos AG, Heilweil M, Bretsky SS. The pathology of malignant fibrous histiocytoma of bone. *Am J Surg Pathol.* 1985; 9:853–871.
9. Campanacci M, Laus M. Osteofibrous dysplasia of the tibia and fibula. *J Bone Joint Surg Am.* 1981; 63A:367–375.
10. Lichtenstein L. Aneurysmal bone cyst: observations in fifty cases. *J Bone Joint Surg Am.* 1957; 39A:873–882.
11. Dahlin DC, Beabout JW. Dedifferentiation of low grade chondrosarcomas. *Cancer.* 1971;28:461–466.
12. Mc Carty EF, Dorfman HD. Chondrosarcoma with dedifferentiation. A study of 18 cases. *Hum Pathol.* 1982;13:36–40.
13. Kumar R, David R, Cierney G. Clear cell chondrosarcoma. *Radiology.* 1985;154:45–48.
14. Dahlin DC, Henderson ED. Mesenchymal chondrosarcoma: further observations on a new entity. *Cancer.* 1962;15:410–417.
15. Salvador AH, Beabout JW, Dahlin DC. Mesenchymal chondrosarcoma – observations on 30 new cases. *Cancer.* 1971;28:605–615.
16. Gurney JG, Swensen AR, Bulterys M. Malignant bone tumors. In: Ries LAG, Smith MA, Gurney JG et al., eds. *Cancer Incidence and Survival Among Children and Adolescents: United States SEER Program 1975–1995 (NIH Pub. No. 99–4649).* Bethesda, MD: National Cancer Institute, SEER Program, 1999.
17. Cotterill SJ, Ahrens S, Paulussen M et al. Prognostic factors in Ewing's tumor of bone: analysis of 975 patients from the European Intergroup Cooperative Ewing's Sarcoma Study Group. *J Clin Oncol.* 2000;18:3108–3114.

18. Ambros IM, Ambros PF, Strehl S et al. MIC2 is a specific marker for Ewing's sarcoma and peripheral primitive neuroectodermal tumors. Evidence for a common histogenesis of Ewing's sarcoma and peripheral primitive neuroectiodermal tumors from MIC2 expression and specific chromosomal aberration. *Cancer*. 1991;67:1886–1893.
19. Goldenberg RR, Campbell CJ, Bonfiglio M. Giant cell tumor of bone: an analysis of two hundred and eighteen cases. *J Bone Joint Surg Am*. 1970;52:A619–A664.
20. Jaffe HL, Lichtenstein L, Portis RB. Giant cell tumor of bone: its pathologic appearance, grading, supposed variants and treatment. *Arch Pathol*. 1940;30:993–1031.
21. Cooper KL, Beabout JW, Dahlin DC. Giant cell tumor: ossification in soft-tissue implants. *Radiology*. 1984;153:597–602.
22. Schajowicz F, Lemos C. Osteoid osteoma and osteoblastoma: closely related entities of osteoblastic derivation. *Acta Orthop Scand*. 1970;41:272–291.
23. Schajowicz F, Lemos C. Malignant osteoblastoma. *J Bone Joint Surg Br*. 1976;58B:202–211.
24. Seki T, Fukada H, Ishi Y et al. Malignant transformation of benign osteoblastoma. *J Bone and Joint Surg Am*. 1975;57:424–426.
25. Eftekhari F, Jaffe N, Schwegal D et al. Inflammatory metachronous hyperostosis of the clavicle and femur in children. Report of two cases, one with long-term follow-up. *Skeletal Radiol*. 1989;18:9–14.

Treatment

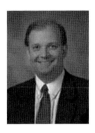

Surgical Management of Primary Osteosarcoma

Alan W. Yasko

Abstract Surgical strategies for the primary tumor for patients with extremity and pelvis osteosarcoma have evolved from the ablative to limb-sparing approaches over the past three decades. Favorable oncologic and functional outcomes with contemporary tissue-conserving techniques consistently observed in skeletally mature patients have prompted the application of similar approaches to a growing number of eligible skeletally immature patients.

In response to emerging long-term outcome data, current strategies have focused principally on refining the nature and scope of surgical resection to preserve uninvolved tissues, and on the adoption of novel biological and nonbiological skeletal and soft-tissue reconstruction methods to optimize function.

We focus on these clinical issues and discuss current efforts to advance the surgical management of the primary tumor and address the limitations of the definitive treatment of the primary tumor, including locally recurrent disease and complications of skeletal reconstructions.

Introduction

The definitive treatment of the primary tumor for patients with osteosarcoma is a bimodal approach that reflects the evolution of the understanding of the combined impact of chemotherapy and surgery. The migration from radical, limb ablation to conservative limb-sparing tumor resection for patients with extremity and pelvic osteosarcoma coincided with the emergence and refinement of effective multiagent chemotherapy regimens and markedly improved patient survival. The therapeutic paradigm shift from amputation alone, to amputation and adjuvant chemotherapy, and ultimately to contemporary induction chemotherapy followed by limb-sparing

A.W. Yasko (✉)
Department of Orthopaedic Surgery, Northwestern University, Feinberg School of Medicine, Orthopaedic Oncology, Chicago, IL, USA
e-mail: a-yasko@northwestern.edu

surgery and adjuvant chemotherapy has been supported by the long-term outcome data that reflects success in local tumor control with limb preservation and improved patient survival.[1]

Guided by the precise delineation of the primary tumor by MRI, the nature and scope of the definitive surgery has changed to adopt a more technically demanding, tissue-conserving approach that takes advantage of the advances made in prosthetic joint replacement design, allograft biology, and microvascular bone and soft tissue transfer techniques. The diagnosis, preoperative planning, surgery, and post treatment surveillance is a team effort within a disease-specific multidisciplinary care delivery model engaging orthopedic surgical oncologists, pediatric oncologists, musculoskeletal radiologists, and bone pathologists, which has resulted in greater precision and coordination of patient treatment and reproducible favorable patient outcomes. This cooperation is credited with the consistent achievement of function and cosmesis without compromise of local tumor control or patient survival.

Preoperative Assessment

Radiologic Imaging

Despite the many advances in diagnostic imaging, biplanar radiographs remain the foundation for the radiological diagnosis of osteosarcoma, determination of fracture risk, and assessment of tumor response to induction chemotherapy. The characteristics of osteosarcoma (i.e., the hallmark of biological aggressiveness, extent of bone involvement, and the degree of bone destruction) are described and defined by plain radiography.

The value of more complex imaging modalities, including MRI, CT, and more recently PET scanning, to the quality of oncologic care is undeniable, but their principal role currently is to delineate the local extent of tumor involvement for local tumor staging, and to identify the optimal site for biopsy.

Biopsy

Biopsy confirmation of the suspected diagnosis of osteosarcoma must be performed prior to proceeding with treatment. Surgical biopsies are still preferred by many orthopedic oncologists to obtain tissue for the diagnosis. The principles of a surgical biopsy must be followed to minimize the risk of contaminating uninvolved tissues. Small, longitudinally oriented incisions performed along the most direct track and targeting the soft tissue component of the osteosarcoma are most desirable to avoid complications. Despite compelling evidence regarding the hazards of poorly performed biopsies, prereferral procedures are still performed commonly by non-oncologic surgeons prior to evaluation by an orthopedic oncologist. This can pose a problem when the definitive surgery must be altered to accommodate excision of the biopsy track en bloc with the tumor specimen and can potentially compromise the definitive surgical resection procedure.[2,3]

Percutaneous biopsy techniques have been adopted slowly in most centers as the preferred method to obtain tissue for the diagnosis of osteosarcoma and other bone tumors.[4] The impact of this image-guided minimally invasive technique remains difficult to quantify, but with negligible procedure-related morbidity and minimal violation of the column of surrounding uninvolved tissue, the avoidance of an additional surgery for the biopsy is desirable.[5,6] Multiple needle passes, repeat procedures as necessary, and surgical biopsy are not precluded by this technique. Moreover, core needle and fine-needle aspirations have been effective methods to obtain sufficient sampling of pathologic tissue for an array of genetic and molecular studies.[7–12] The availability of musculoskeletal radiologists, interventional radiologists, cytologists and musculoskeletal pathologists expert in bone sarcomas improves the yield of a successful diagnosis. No delay in the initiation of chemotherapy is expected after a needle biopsy, but healing of the biopsy incision is necessary prior to starting the treatment.

A primary role of orthopedic oncologists at the initial assessment, even prior to the confirmation of the diagnosis of osteosarcoma, is to determine the structural integrity of the tumor-bearing segment of bone. External support through the application of an orthosis, immobilization by casting, and activity modification with protected weight-bearing or extremity use must be considered during the period of induction chemotherapy. In the presence of a fracture, immobilization by casting or rarely, limited internal fixation, should be used to reduce fracture motion, bleeding, soft tissue contamination and pain. If fracture fixation is performed injudiciously or prior to confirmation of the diagnosis, the definitive limb-sparing procedure can be compromised and the outcome adversely affected.[13]

Postinduction chemotherapy assessment of the bone and soft tissue extent of the primary disease is performed by plain radiography and MR imaging of the affected extremity. Consolidation of the periosteal reaction, ossification of the intra-osseous and extra-osseous components of the tumor, and healing of a pathologic fracture are radiologic indicators of tumor responsiveness to chemotherapy (Fig. 1).

Surgical Planning

Reassessment of the restaging studies precedes the completion of induction chemotherapy. Sufficient time is necessary prior to surgery to plan for the surgical procedure. The evaluation of joint involvement, the proximal and distal extent of the intraosseous tumor, the healing of a pathologic fracture, and proximity to the epiphyseal plate is necessary to finalize the oncologic and reconstruction plan. Skeletal reconstruction and soft tissue coverage procedures, if necessary, must be planned well in advance of the surgical date to permit adequate time to procure the implant for reconstruction.

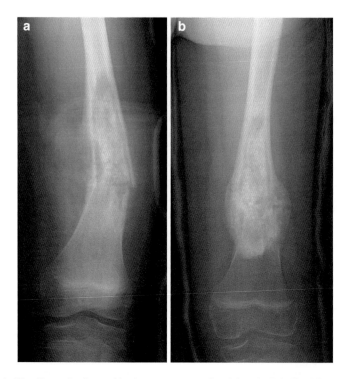

Fig. 1 (**a**) AP radiograph of osteoblastic osteosarcoma involving the left distal femur associated with pathologic fracture. (**b**) Following induction chemotherapy, the fracture healed and the soft tissue mass ossified indicative of a favorable response to chemotherapy

Surgery for the primary tumor is a two-step process that includes tumor extirpation and skeletal reconstruction that is completed in a single stage. Many factors influence the type of surgery that is recommended. Patient age, anatomic site of the tumor, cultural factors, surgeon bias, patient and family expectations, early and late surgical risks, and the inherent limitations of the reconstruction must be considered.

Several radiologic advances have contributed to the refinement of contemporary surgery. Digital imaging has emerged as a valuable assessment tool for more exact measurement of the dimensions of the bone segment and joint to be resected and reconstructed, to more precisely determine the margins of resection and match biologic implants or customize prosthetic devices to reconstruct a patient's anatomy.

Modular oncology prosthetic reconstruction systems provide almost real-time availability that was not achievable two decades ago. Bone bank inventories of large segment allografts also have increased to meet the demands of surgeons who desire a biologic reconstruction, rendering protracted wait times obsolete. Sophisticated orthopedic techniques in fracture management and joint arthroplasty are applied today to broaden the possibilities of surgeries that have a much greater probability of success. Microvascular surgical techniques have expanded the limb-sparing opportunities when advanced soft tissue transfers are necessary to avoid amputation.

The surgical planning must also consider the patient's chemotherapy schedule and coincide with bone marrow recovery following the last scheduled course of preoperative chemotherapy. Although the criteria for suitability for surgery vary, in general, adequate recovery or a trend toward recovery of the absolute neutrophil count is essential.

With careful preoperative planning, the medical condition of the patient can be optimized in preparation for surgery to minimize intra operative and postoperative risks. With proper coordination, the interruption of chemotherapy is brief, and re-initiation of therapy can commence usually within 2–3 weeks postoperatively.

Surgery

Limb-Sparing Tumor Resection

In general, three conditions must be met for limb-salvage surgery to be performed successfully: (1) evidence of clinical and radiographic response of the primary tumor to preoperative chemotherapy (for high-grade tumors); (2) ability to achieve a satisfactory surgical margin[14]; and (3) ability to reconstruct the extremity with reasonable likelihood of preserving or restoring meaningful function with minimal surgical morbidity, facilitating early resumption of chemotherapy.

The Musculoskeletal Tumor Society recognizes a wide local excision either by amputation or limb-salvage procedure as the recommended surgical approach. A wide excision removes the primary tumor en bloc along with its reactive zone and a cuff of normal tissue in all planes (Fig. 2). Conceptually, this strategy is applicable to all high-grade sarcomas. The single most powerful predictor of local tumor control is achieving satisfactory surgical margins. This type of resection successfully controls the local disease in greater than 95% of patients.[1] The challenge of achieving satisfactory margins when a pathologic fracture has developed can be overcome such that, in many series, fracture is not considered a major risk factor for local tumor recurrence if appropriate surgery is performed to account for the potential contamination of the soft tissues surrounding the fracture.[15–17]

One of the most controversial issues in the surgical management of osteosarcoma is the recommendation of limb-sparing surgery in patients who are skeletally very immature. Many surgeons maintain that limb conservation in patients younger than 8 years is a relative contraindication.[68] The survival of the construct, adjustments to accommodate skeletal growth, ability of the child to understand the need for activity restrictions, cooperation with physical therapy that may compromise the outcome must be considered in the decision-making process. Lower extremity reconstruction is associated with many more complications than the upper extremity. Site-specific risks and intrinsic limitations of each reconstruction method are in part dependent on the type of resection performed.

Bone resections fall into one of three types based on the anatomic site and extent of the involved bone to be excised. Because most osteosarcomas arise in the

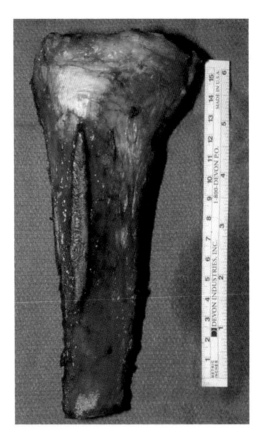

Fig. 2 En bloc resection of the proximal tibia osteosarcoma with in continuity excision of the biopsy track and a cuff of soft tissue surrounding the tumor

metaphysis of the long bone near the joint (>90%), the majority of the procedures that are performed for these tumors involve resection of both the segment of the tumor-bearing bone and the adjacent joint (osteoarticular resection). Historically, the majority of these resections were performed to include the entire joint. Concern for tracking of tumor into the joint arose from early observations of amputation specimens that exhibited tumor extension along the joint capsule and ligaments that stabilize the joint. The main advantage of the MRI is the precise identification of tumor involvement in the joint or along the ligament.

Presently, the majority of these osteoarticular resections are performed through the adjacent joint (intra-articular). If the tumor does extend along the joint capsule or ligamentous structures and/or invades the joint, the entire joint should be resected (extra-articular) to avoid violating areas involved with tumor.

Less frequently encountered is the clinical situation in which an osteosarcoma arises within the diaphysis or shaft region of the long bone (<10%). Confined to the diaphyseal portion of the long bones, the tumor-bearing segment of bone alone is resected (intercalary resection) with preservation of the adjacent proximal and distal joints. The sensitivity of the MRI to detect changes within the bone and soft tissues has allowed for a more precise surgical margin (within a few millimeters of the tumor) necessary to spare a joint, growth plate, or a tendon that, if sacrificed with the tumor, would have a major impact on limb function and patient outcome.

Even less frequently, there may be extensive involvement along the length of the bone that precludes adequate resection and reconstruction without sacrificing the entire bone. In this clinical situation, a whole bone resection involving both the proximal and distal joints is required.

For patients near or at skeletal maturity, the resultant bone defect can be reconstructed using the entire array of site-specific implants available, without concern for limb-length discrepancies resulting from resection or injury to one or both adjacent growth plates in the bone. In patients with appreciable skeletal growth remaining, both prosthetic and biological options for reconstruction are more limited.

Skeletal Reconstruction of the Extremity

Reconstruction alternatives have expanded parallelly with advances in biomechanical engineering, prosthesis design, metallurgy, allograft biology, and microvascular techniques. The reconstructive methods available should be discussed in the context of the clinical setting. Multiple factors influence the type of reconstruction selected, including the anatomic location, integrity of the surrounding structures, the extent of the resection, the risk and nature of potential early and late complications associated with a given type of reconstruction and the patient's age, the short and long-term expectations, and the anticipated functional demands.

Prosthetic Arthroplasty

This represents the most frequently used method by which the skeletal defect and the adjacent joint are reconstructed. It is used primarily about the knee, hip and shoulder (Fig. 3) when a mobile joint is desired.[18–23] Elbow arthroplasty is available for the uncommon occurrence of osteosarcoma arising in the distal humerus.[24] Anatomic and prosthetic design limitations restrict the routine use of prosthetic replacement for the wrist (distal radius) or ankle (distal tibia) joints for both adults and children.

The current generation of prostheses are available as modular systems to fit a particular anatomic size and length of the resected bone segment. Down-sized modular prostheses are available for the younger, skeletally immature patients, and custom-designed prostheses, if necessary, can be manufactured typically within 4 weeks.

All the prostheses for the knee are constrained (hinged) because of the obligatory resection of the ligamentous structures that support the joint. The epicenter of the tumor (distal femur or proximal tibia) dictates the type of prosthesis, the postoperative

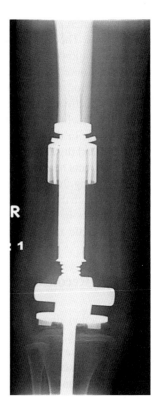

Fig. 3 AP radiograph of an expandable prosthetic reconstruction of the right knee in a skeletally immature patient following resection of a osteosarcoma in the distal femur

rehabilitation, and the time to full recovery. Prosthetic arthroplasties of the shoulders and hip are not constrained typically and require replacement only of the involved side of the joint, in the majority of cases.

Fixation of the prosthesis into the host bone is usually accomplished with polymethylmethacrylate cement. As of now, the experience with alternative methods of fixation, including cement-free fixation by bone ingrowth or alternative methods of fixation of the prosthesis stem, is encouraging, but remains investigational.[21,22]

The advantages of prosthetic arthroplasty include immediate joint stability without prolonged extremity immobilization and early restoration of function and ambulation with low early morbidity in both skeletally mature and immature patients. The incidence of early (within 1 year of surgery) prosthesis-related complications is consistently low, with an infection rate of less than 5% during the critical period when chemotherapy is administered postoperatively.[18-23] For this reason, prosthetic arthroplasty is desirable for the primary reconstruction of osteo-articular defects for patients who require adjuvant chemotherapy. Clearly, not all children are candidates for this method of reconstruction, even if wide surgical margins can be achieved without amputation. Anatomic limitations and prosthetic design and mechanical constraints restrict universal application, particularly in very young patients.

Tumors arising in the immature skeleton pose a unique problem for the orthopedic oncologist, particularly in patients with a substantial projected growth of the involved extremity. When the surgical resection includes sacrifice of a principal growth plate of a long bone, an appreciable limb-length discrepancy and functional deficit will result, if accommodations are not made within the construct. For more skeletally immature patients, the bones are small, and customized prostheses must be manufactured. The outcome success for any prosthetic limb-sparing reconstruction is predicated on the willingness to participate with rehabilitation,to cooperate with imposed activity restrictions, and to accept the certainty of multiple surgeries to maintain limb length and function, upon reaching skeletal maturity. The younger the patient, the greater the risk of prosthesis-specific complications that will require revision surgery and possibly, result in amputation.

The advent of the expandable prosthesis as a custom-manufactured device in 1983 in the United States, addressed the issue of skeletal growth and offered an alternative to amputation or rotationplasty for this patient population. The goal of surgical reconstruction was, and still remains, to maintain a mobile joint and provide a mechanism to accommodate for the loss of the growth center when the distal end of the bone is involved by tumor. The only prostheses available until recently were designed to be surgically lengthened periodically to achieve expansion. The need for multiple surgical procedures should be anticipated with this reconstructive approach during the period of the patient's skeletal growth. If revision is necessary. at skeletal maturity, the expandable prosthesis can be exchanged for a nonexpendable prosthetic arthroplasty. Mechanical failure of the expansion mechanism has been the principal limiting factor to the success of this method of reconstruction. In addition, although longitudinal bone growth is accommodated for by these implants, appositional growth is not, and this has been a cause of early loosening of both cemented and uncemented implants at the point of fixation to bone.

Over the past decade, prostheses that can be lengthened without surgery have been developed to obviate the need for repeated surgery. Two such devices are available on a custom-manufactured basis.[21,22,69] Lengthening of the prosthesis can be performed under sedation as an outpatient procedure frequently so small incremental expansions can recapitulate skeletal growth kinetics more physiologically (Fig. 4). The modifications in the design of newer-generation prostheses may also reduce the incidence of deep infection and prosthesis failure, but long-term follow-up is lacking. One such prosthesis can be used in patients who can have their joints preserved. The intercalary bone defect can be replaced with a prostheses using hydroxyapatite-coated extracortical plates that has been shown to be effective in preliminary studies.[21,22]

Clearly, any mechanical device has inherent limitations with respect to its durability. The primary shortcoming of this type of reconstruction is loosening of the prosthesis at the bone-cement interface owing to repetitive mechanical stresses and loads experienced during activities of daily life. This is a primary concern with lower extremity reconstructions. All implants will need to be replaced at some point in the

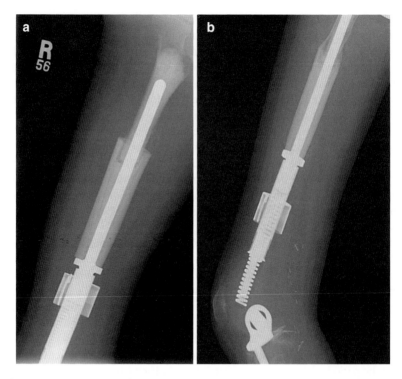

Fig. 4 (**a**) Lateral radiograph of a composite expandable prosthesis and intercalary allograft segment to restore bone stock in an effort to avoid loosening of the prosthesis. (**b**) Lateral radiograph shows expanded prosthesis and radiographic evidence of healing of the allograft segment to the host bone

long-term survivor's lifetime; however, most implants are revised long after active treatment for the primary disease has been completed.[19,23] The survivorship of prosthetic arthroplasty reconstructions varies and depends on multiple factors, including the site of reconstruction, and ranges from 60–90% estimated survival at 5 years to 50–80% at 10 years.[23,25–27,70] In general, given the young patient population for which these massive bone and joint resections are performed, it is anticipated that as patient survival improves, the rate of construct revisions will increase.

Biological Constructs

Although prosthetic devices may be expedient and provide many advantages in the short term, biological constructs are appealing for the prospects of long term durability. The major drawback of all biological solutions is the limited availability of patient-matched implants.

Surgical Management of Primary Osteosarcoma

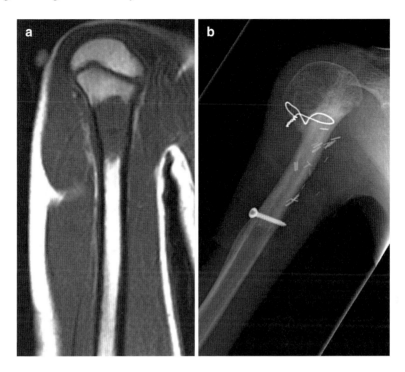

Fig. 5 (**a**) Coronal MRI of the proximal humerus reveals well delineated extent of the osteosarcoma in the right proximal humerus with a clear zone of uninvolved bone of the proximal epiphysis of the humerus. (**b**) Vascularized fibula graft reconstruction resulting in expedient healing with preservation of the humeral head resulting in full range of motion of the dominant right shoulder and unrestricted function

Autografts are ideal as host-derived implants, but are limited to the fibula as a donor bone. The vascularized fibular graft has broad utility, when long bone or pelvic defects require bridging and are the most predictably successful of the biological constructs.[28–32] Segmental defects in architecturally complex anatomic structures cannot be addressed using this method. Vascularized fibula grafts are used alone most frequently in the nonweight-bearing upper extremity to reconstruct the humerus and less commonly, the ulna or radius (Fig. 5). Vascularized fibula grafts are particularly useful in patients with compromised tissue beds (i.e., previous infection or multiple revisions) and can result in rapid healing. Because this type of reconstruction is used when the patient's native joint is spared, excellent long-term-function is anticipated. In a unique setting of resection of the proximal humerus in a very young patient, transfer of the proximal fibular epiphysis (and growth plate) can be used to address the limb-length discrepancy anticipated with excision of the growth plate of the humerus, as an alternative to an expandable prosthesis (Fig. 6).

Fig. 6 Vascularized fibula graft for the proximal humerus with preservation of the epiphysis to maintain a viable growth plate to allow for spontaneous growth of the affected left humerus

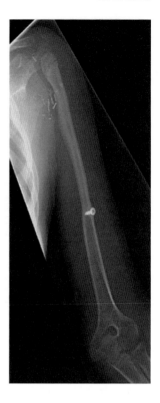

Allografts offer tremendous flexibility and utility to reconstruct almost any skeletal or osteoarticular defect. Maturation of tissue banking in the USA and in many other countries has increased the availability of anatomically matched tissue of low immunogenicity. Attractive as a biological solution with no patient harvest morbidity, allografts have increased the number of patients eligible for limb-sparing surgery with the hope of providing a durable reconstruction. Risks of allograft transplantation are not inconsequential and are divided equally among graft fracture, infection, and nonunion.[33–39]

The use of allografts in the pediatric population has been reported sporadically, especially for very immature patients. There are constraints, however, in the availability of appropriately small sized grafts; recent data in a series of patients younger than 10 years of age demonstrated their utility, when available, to exhibit similar healing patterns and, unfortunately, similar complications as noted in adults.[40]

As a biologic solution that restores bone stock and the adjacent joint surface, osteoarticular allografts are patient-matched constructs that have particular appeal for reconstruction.[36,37,40] Moreover, these allografts provide a site of attachment for host soft tissues in an effort to optimize active movement of the affected joint in anatomic locations where function is predicated on restoration of key muscle-tendon groups (hip abductor muscles through the gluteus tendon and quadriceps muscles through the patellar tendon for active extension of the knee).[41]

These grafts are readily available from regional bone banks. Current cryopreservation techniques can maintain viable, articular cartilage, thus affording the potential for a long-term, biologic reconstruction. This is particularly applicable about the knee, where the majority of prosthetic failures occur. Therefore, osteoarticular allografts are applied most frequently for reconstruction about the knee.

There are several significant disadvantages of large segmental allografts, however. The grafts must be fixed to the host bone and heal, to achieve the desired outcome. Prolonged limb immobilization, bracing or casting, and protected weight-bearing may be required for many months, even perhaps for up to a year. Moreover, there is a high complication rate associated with this method of reconstruction. Nonunions, fractures, and early infections are observed consistently in 15–20% of cases. A vascularized fibular graft can be used in combination with a large segment allograft to accelerate graft incorporation and reduce graft nonunion and fracture[42] (Fig. 7).

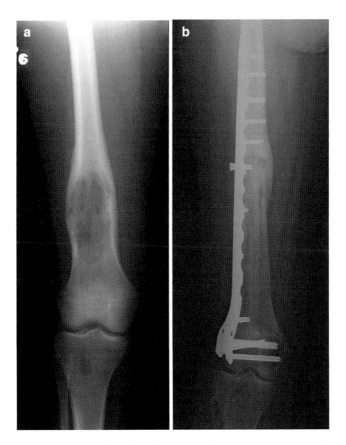

Fig. 7 (**a**) AP radiograph of the right distal femur revealing an osteosarcoma involving the distal diaphysis but without involvement of the epiphysis. (**b**) AP radiograph showing a composite segmental allograft and intramedullary placement of a vascularized fibula graft to expedite healing

The role of osteoarticular allografts as a method of primary reconstruction in adolescents is desirable, but is limited in skeletally immature patients (Figure 8). Growth considerations must be taken into account. If growth is anticipated, the resected bone and joint can be replaced with a longer construct at the time of implantation. If minimal growth is anticipated, no adjustment is necessary. Late complications, irrespective of the age of the patient and the precision of the anatomic match, include degenerative arthritis and joint instability.

The combination of a segmental allograft and prosthesis offers the advantages of both methods of reconstruction. The prosthesis is cemented into the allograft, which in turn must be fixed to the host bone to achieve incorporation. The allograft restores bone stock removed at the time of surgical resection, provides an attachment point for host soft tissues, and reduces the stresses on the prosthesis. The prosthesis provides a predictably stable joint articulation. This is useful particularly with expandable prostheses in which the additional length realized through the prostheses' adjustment effectively shortened the anchoring bone stock, thereby increasing the likelihood of long-term problems with bone stock deficiency. The experience with this approach has not been extensive.[43,44] As a primary mode of reconstruction, alloprosthesis composites possess risks similar to those of both osteoarticular allograft and prosthetic arthroplasty reconstructions. This method is used primarily in the proximal femur and proximal humerus when a mobile joint is the object of reconstruction. An interposition allograft may reduce the risk of aseptic loosening, the major limitation of any mechanical device in such a young patient population (Fig. 4).

Another use of the segmental graft methods is to achieve joint fusion. Although not as readily acceptable presently given the option of a mobile joint, no reconstruction that aims to preserve joint function will provide a lifelong solution in young patients who are long-term survivors of their disease. Although a nonmobile joint may be less desirable than a mobile joint to the majority of patients, in selected cases it may provide the best mode of reconstruction. Joint fusion is accomplished using either a large segment of allograft, autograft (fibula), or a combination of both. Plate fixation or intramedullary nail stabilization has been used to support the construct until healing at the host-graft junction has been achieved. Once the grafted bone has become incorporated by the host, the reconstruction is anticipated to last for the patient's lifetime. This method of reconstruction is the treatment of choice for the wrist (distal radius) and ankle (distal tibia) joints and is commonly used for the shoulder (proximal humerus) and knee (distal femur or proximal tibia). Arthrodesis of the hip (proximal femur) is usually reserved for the young patient and is difficult to achieve. For any allograft transplantation procedure, the risk of disease transmission of allogeneic tissue, albeit low, remains an inherent disadvantage.

Other Considerations

Extensive intraosseous tumor involvement may preclude adequate fixation of either a prosthesis or an allograft to a remnant of uninvolved host bone. Replacement of the entire bone is a viable alternative to limb disarticulation. Two options are available for reconstruction: whole bone (including adjacent proximal and distal joints) prosthetic arthroplasty, and whole bone allograft-prosthesis composite reconstruction. Too few of these types of reconstruction have been performed to comment on the incidence of complications or functional outcome anticipated. Expandable components would be necessary to accommodate skeletal growth deficiencies of both growth plates.

The application of bone transportation by distraction techniques (Ilizarov method) is an alternate approach to reconstruction of segmental bone defects that, at first glance has appeal, but mature data in a sufficient number of patients are lacking. Most data are from the European experience with few patients in each series.[45–50,53] Up to 10 cm mean length has been gained by this method at a slow rate of one centimeter per month. The major risk of this externally applied apparatus of trans-osseous pins and metal frames is infection of the pins protruding through the skin. This is problematic, particularly for patients anticipated to be episodically immunosuppressed during adjuvant chemotherapy. Meticulous pin care is necessary over a protracted period of time to prevent complications. Moreover, adjacent joint stiffness can develop and compromise functional outcome.

Pelvic resections represent a unique challenge. Fortunately, pelvic sarcomas in children and young adults are rare, with osteosarcoma arising in the innominate bones including patients of all ages of <10%.[51] Tumors in this site are associated with a poorer prognosis and a higher rate of local tumor recurrence (>20%).[48,52,53] In general, pelvic sarcomas present with locally advanced disease. Quality of life issues are paramount for these patients. The extent of the skeletal resection determines the functional deficit and influences the decision regarding the type of reconstruction, if any, to be offered to the patient to optimize function. Limb-sparing pelvic resections are achievable following the surgical principles for resection of tumors arising in the long bones of the extremity.[54]

If wide margins can be achieved without sacrificing both the femoral and sciatic nerves, an internal hemipelvectomy (with preservation of the limb) can be considered a viable alternative to hindquarter amputation. The pelvis can be left without reconstruction when a tumor confined to the pubis, ischium, or iliac wing is removed (hip joint preserved), without significant functional deficit. Resection of the hip joint without reconstruction results in suboptimal function, because the extremity remains flail, unstable, and weak, and is associated with significant limb shortening.

The reconstructive options for the pelvis vary and depend on the region resected. Periacetabular resections can be reconstructed with a large segment allograft pelvis/ hip prosthesis composite implant, pelvifemoral arthrodesis, or prosthetic spacer reconstruction (saddle prosthesis). A discussion of possible reconstructions summarized in recent reviews of the surgical management of pelvic sarcomas.[55,56] The method of reconstruction must be based on the clinical situation and the functional demands of the patient. In general, restoration of a disrupted pelvic ring or reconstruction of the hip joint may yield better function, but too few cases of any one type of reconstruction have been performed to demonstrate the superiority of one method over another.[42]

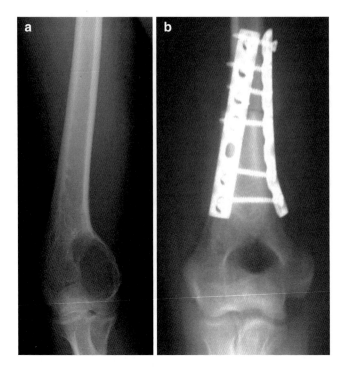

Fig. 8 (**a**) AP radiograph of a distal humerus osteosarcoma. (**b**) Osteoarticular allograft reconstruction after en bloc resection of the tumor

Judicious patient selection and careful preoperative counseling are important. Enthusiasm for maximizing function by pelvic and hip reconstruction must be tempered by the high complication rate (greater than 50%) reported to be associated with the various available reconstruction options. Deep infection is the most commonly observed complication of pelvic reconstructions and can be devastating to the patient. However, if complications are avoided, lower extremity function and ambulation may be facilitated, at least in the short term.

Too few patients have osteosarcoma of the mobile spine and sacrum. Techniques to achieve satisfactory surgical margins, as in patients with extremity tumors, have been examined, but too few reported data are available to assess the long-term oncologic impact.[57–59] Tumors in the expendable bones do not require reconstruction and therefore, preclude many of the early and late complications observed with skeletal reconstruction. These sites include the fibula, ribs, clavicle, scapular body, and portions of the pelvis as described above.

Soft Tissue Management

Adequate soft tissue coverage is critical to the success of any limb-salvage procedure. Multiple intra operative factors contribute to compromised wound healing, including surgical elevation of extensive soft tissue flaps, resection of large segments of bone and surrounding soft tissues, insertion of massive prosthesis or allograft, and long duration of the surgical procedure. These conditions, coupled with the deleterious effects of chemotherapy on soft tissue and bone healing, leave patients extremely vulnerable to wound-associated complications and deep infection. The risk is compounded during the period of adjuvant chemotherapy, when bone marrow suppression occurs. The development of these complications during this period can place the limb and the patient at risk and often prompts amputation.

Local transposition muscle flaps and free tissue transfers are extremely useful to provide a healthy, well-vascularized soft tissue envelope to cover the reconstruction. The liberal use of these methods has significantly reduced the incidence of infections associated with limb-salvage procedures, especially following resection and reconstruction of the proximal tibia.

Rotationplasty and Amputation

Rotationplasty (intercalary amputation) has been advocated for proximal tibial or distal femoral lesions. This procedure involves an intercalary resection of all structures within the region surrounding the tumor-bearing portion of the extremity, preserving only the neurovascular structures. The retained normal segment of the lower leg is rotated 180° and reattached to the proximal bone remnant. The intact ankle joint serves as the knee joint, thereby creating a functional below-knee amputation. The patient must wear a modified external limb prosthesis. The energy consumed with walking is less than that for above-knee amputees; however, the cosmetic result is undesirable for many patients. It is a durable alternative when a standard approach to limb salvage is not advisable. Acceptance in the United States is low because of social and emotional barriers.[60,61]

The present role of amputation in the treatment of the primary tumor in osteosarcoma is limited to patients with locally advanced disease that precludes the achievement of satisfactory surgical margins, tumors that progress on chemotherapy, or those that arise in anatomic sites that preclude a reconstructable limb. A greater percentage of very young patients with appreciable growth remaining at the time of diagnosis are considered for amputation because of the constraints of current methods to restore and preserve limb function. Vascular structures are infrequently involved by bone sarcomas, but can be resected and reconstructed if necessary. Likewise, major peripheral nerves vital to meaningful function of an extremity are rarely involved, and although cable grafting can be performed, these patients are usually not deemed candidates for limb-sparing surgery.

All patients with extremity osteosarcoma are candidates for amputation. Currently, it is incumbent on the orthopedic oncologist to determine the feasibility of performing a limb-sparing procedure based on clinical presentation, stage of the disease, local extent of tumor and involvement of vital structures, and tumor response to chemotherapy. The level of amputation is selected at the most distal site that will result in a wide surgical margin. The longer the limb stump, the greater ease of prosthetic fitting and improved function.[62–65]

Surveillance

Postoperative follow-up evaluations are critical to the success of the local treatment of osteosarcoma. Both oncologic and orthopedic issues must be addressed within the framework of a multidisciplinary treatment schema and the appropriate timeframe for the setting. Surgical surveillance mandates that the immediate postoperative assessment of the surgical site for incision healing be performed to clear the patient for resumption of chemotherapy. Near-term follow-up schedules are dependent on the nature of the reconstruction. During resumption of postoperative chemotherapy, surveillance is maintained to note progress in rehabilitation with joint range of motion and muscle strengthening.

Intermediate and long-term follow-up coincide with surveillance practices for high-grade osteosarcoma. Assessment for clinical and radiologic evidence of local tumor recurrence as well as for the status of the construct, for signs of wear or failure, is performed. At the time when the risk of local tumor recurrence diminishes, the construct-specific complications begin to appear.

Local Recurrence Management

Despite the improvements in chemotherapy, imaging, and surgical techniques, local recurrence in osteosarcoma has been reported at a rate of approximately 5%.[71] On multivariate analyses, independent prognostic factors for local tumor recurrence included poor response to chemotherapy and inadequate surgical margins. Median time to local recurrence is within the first 18 months. No statistical difference is observed among limb-sparing surgery, amputation and rotationplasty, assuming the indications for each are appropriate, and surgery is performed following accepted oncologic principles. The prognosis for patients after local recurrence of osteosarcoma is poor (5 year 19–29%), with survival predicated on the local recurrence-free interval and the presence of systemic recurrence at the time of diagnosis of the local recurrence. Complete removal of recurrent disease, by amputation or wide local excision, is essential to optimize the likelihood of survival.[66,67]

Summary

Effective chemotherapy regimens have changed the nature and scope of surgical management of primary sarcomas of the bone. Limb-sparing surgical procedures are performed in the majority of patients without a significantly increased risk of local tumor recurrence. Advances in technology have expanded the options available for skeletal reconstruction in the pediatric population. End-result analyses have helped refine the application of this technology to maximize function. Further advances are necessary to restore and maintain function in the long term.

References

1. Bacci G, et al. Influence of local recurrence on survival in patients with extremity osteosarcoma treated with neoadjuvant chemotherapy: the experience of a single institution with 44 patients. *Cancer.* 2006;106(12):2701-2706.
2. Mankin HJ, Mankin CJ, Simon MA. The hazards of the biopsy, revisited. Members of the musculoskeletal tumor society. *J Bone Joint Surg Am.* 1996;78(5):656-663.
3. Iemsawatdikul K, et al. Seeding of osteosarcoma in the biopsy tract of a patient with multifocal osteosarcoma. *Pediatr Radiol.* 2005;35(7):717-721.
4. White VA, et al. Osteosarcoma and the role of fine-needle aspiration: a study of 51 cases. *Cancer.* 1988;62(6):1238-1246.
5. Ahrar K, et al. Percutaneous ultrasound-guided biopsy in the definitive diagnosis of osteosarcoma. *J Vasc Interv Radiol.* 2004;15(11):1329-1333.
6. Puri A, et al. CT-guided percutaneous core needle biopsy in deep seated musculoskeletal lesions: a prospective study of 128 cases. *Skeletal Radiol.* 2006;35(3):138-143.
7. Kilpatrick SE, et al. The role of fine needle aspiration biopsy in the diagnosis and management of osteosarcoma. *Pediatr Pathol Mol Med.* 2001;20(3):175-187.
8. Dodd LG, et al. Utility of fine-needle aspiration in the diagnosis of primary osteosarcoma. *Diagn Cytopathol.* 2002;27(6):350-353.
9. Domanski HA, Akerman M. Fine-needle aspiration of primary osteosarcoma: a cytological-histological study. *Diagn Cytopathol.* 2005;32(5):269-275.
10. Jelinek JS, et al. Diagnosis of primary bone tumors with image-guided percutaneous biopsy: experience with 110 tumors. *Radiology.* 2002;223(3):731-737.
11. Mitsuyoshi G, et al. Accurate diagnosis of musculoskeletal lesions by core needle biopsy. *J Surg Oncol.* 2006;94(1):21-27.
12. Carrino JA, et al. Magnetic resonance imaging-guided percutaneous biopsy of musculoskeletal lesions. *J Bone Joint Surg Am.* 2007;89(10):2179-2187.
13. Adams SC, et al. Consequences and prevention of inadvertent internal fixation of primary osseous sarcomas. *Clin Orthop Relat Res.* 2008;467:519-525.
14. Bacci G, et al. Predictive factors for local recurrence in osteosarcoma: 540 patients with extremity tumors followed for minimum 2.5 years after neoadjuvant chemotherapy. *Acta Orthop Scand.* 1998;69(3):230-236.
15. Bramer JA, et al. Do pathological fractures influence survival and local recurrence rate in bony sarcomas? *Eur J Cancer.* 2007;43(13):1944-1951.
16. Scully SP, et al. Pathologic fracture in osteosarcoma: prognostic importance and treatment implications. *J Bone Joint Surg Am.* 2002;84-A(1):49-57.
17. Bacci G, et al. Nonmetastatic osteosarcoma of the extremity with pathologic fracture at presentation: local and systemic control by amputation or limb salvage after preoperative chemotherapy. *Acta Orthop Scand.* 2003;74(4):449-454.
18. van Kampen M, et al. Replacement of the hip in children with a tumor in the proximal part of the femur. *J Bone Joint Surg Am.* 2008;90(4):785-795.
19. Frink SJ, et al. Favorable long-term results of prosthetic arthroplasty of the knee for distal femur neoplasms. *Clin Orthop Relat Res.* 2005;438:65-70.
20. Belthur MV, et al. Extensible endoprostheses for bone tumors of the proximal femur in children. *J Pediatr Orthop.* 2003;23(2):230-235.
21. Gupta A, et al. Non-invasive distal femoral expandable endoprosthesis for limb-salvage surgery in paediatric tumours. *J Bone Joint Surg Br.* 2006;88(5):649-654.
22. Gupta A, et al. A knee-sparing distal femoral endoprosthesis using hydroxyapatite-coated extracortical plates. Preliminary results. *J Bone Joint Surg Br.* 2006;88(10):1367-1372.
23. Jeys LM, et al. Endoprosthetic reconstruction for the treatment of musculoskeletal tumors of the appendicular skeleton and pelvis. *J Bone Joint Surg Am.* 2008;90(6):1265-1271.
24. Weber KL, Lin PP, Yasko AW. Complex segmental elbow reconstruction after tumor resection. *Clin Orthop Relat Res.* 2003;415:31-44.

25. Biau D, et al. Survival of total knee replacement with a megaprosthesis after bone tumor resection. *J Bone Joint Surg Am*. 2006;88(6):1285-1293.
26. Myers GJ, et al. The long-term results of endoprosthetic replacement of the proximal tibia for bone tumours. *J Bone Joint Surg Br*. 2007;89(12):1632-1637.
27. Myers GJ, et al. Endoprosthetic replacement of the distal femur for bone tumours: long-term results. *J Bone Joint Surg Br*. 2007;89(4):521-526.
28. Chen, C.M., et al., Reconstruction of extremity long bone defects after sarcoma resection with vascularized fibula flaps: a 10-year review. *Plast Reconstr Surg*. 2007;119(3):915-924; discussion 925-926.
29. Friedrich JB, et al. Free vascularized fibular graft salvage of complications of long-bone allograft after tumor reconstruction. *J Bone Joint Surg Am*. 2008;90(1):93-100.
30. Moran SL, Shin AY, Bishop AT. The use of massive bone allograft with intramedullary free fibular flap for limb salvage in a pediatric and adolescent population. *Plast Reconstr Surg*. 2006;118(2):413-419.
31. Zaretski A, et al. Free fibula long bone reconstruction in orthopedic oncology: a surgical algorithm for reconstructive options. *Plast Reconstr Surg*. 2004;113(7):1989-2000.
32. Bae DS, Waters PM, Gebhardt MC. Results of free vascularized fibula grafting for allograft nonunion after limb salvage surgery for malignant bone tumors. *J Pediatr Orthop*. 2006;26(6):809-814.
33. Alman BA, De Bari A, Krajbich JI. Massive allografts in the treatment of osteosarcoma and Ewing sarcoma in children and adolescents. *J Bone Joint Surg Am*. 1995;77(1):54-64.
34. Brigman BE, et al. Allografts about the knee in young patients with high-grade sarcoma. *Clin Orthop Relat Res*. 2004;421:232-239.
35. Kohler R, et al. Massive bone allografts in children. *Int Orthop*. 1990;14(3):249-253.
36. Muscolo DL, et al. Intercalary femur and tibia segmental allografts provide an acceptable alternative in reconstructing tumor resections. *Clin Orthop Relat Res*. 2004;426:97-102.
37. Muscolo DL, et al. Partial epiphyseal preservation and intercalary allograft reconstruction in high-grade metaphyseal osteosarcoma of the knee. *J Bone Joint Surg Am*. 2004;86-A(12):2686-2693.
38. Deijkers RL, et al. Epidiaphyseal versus other intercalary allografts for tumors of the lower limb. *Clin Orthop Relat Res*. 2005;439:151-160.
39. Manfrini M, et al. Intraepiphyseal resection of the proximal tibia and its impact on lower limb growth. *Clin Orthop Relat Res*. 1999;358:111-119.
40. Muscolo DL, et al. Allograft reconstruction after sarcoma resection in children younger than 10 years old. *Clin Orthop Relat Res*. 2008;466(8):1856-1862.
41. Ramseier LE, et al. Allograft reconstruction for bone sarcoma of the tibia in the growing child. *J Bone Joint Surg Br*. 2006;88(1):95-99.
42. Chang DW, Weber KL. Use of a vascularized fibula bone flap and intercalary allograft for diaphyseal reconstruction after resection of primary extremity bone sarcomas. *Plast Reconstr Surg*. 2005;116(7):1918-1925.
43. Farid Y, et al. Endoprosthetic and allograft-prosthetic composite reconstruction of the proximal femur for bone neoplasms. *Clin Orthop Relat Res*. 2006;442:223-229.
44. Biau DJ, et al. Allograft-prosthesis composites after bone tumor resection at the proximal tibia. *Clin Orthop Relat Res*. 2007;456:211-217.
45. Erler K, et al. Reconstruction of defects following bone tumor resections by distraction osteogenesis. *Arch Orthop Trauma Surg*. 2005;125(3):177-183.
46. Dragan S, et al. The application of Ilizarov's "bone segment transport" method in the treatment of tumors and tumor-like changes in bone. *Ortop Traumatol Rehabil*. 2002;4(4):441-451.
47. Catagani MA, Ottaviani G. Ilizarov method to correct limb length discrepancy after limb-sparing hemipelvectomy. *J Pediatr Orthop B*. 2008;17(6):293-298.
48. Ozaki T, Hillmann A, Winkelmann W. Treatment outcome of pelvic sarcomas in young children: orthopaedic and oncologic analysis. *J Pediatr Orthop*. 1998;18(3):350-355.

49. Canadell J, Forriol F, Cara JA. Removal of metaphyseal bone tumours with preservation of the epiphysis. Physeal distraction before excision. *J Bone Joint Surg Br*. 1994;76(1):127-132.
50. Tsuchiya H, et al. Osteosarcoma around the knee. Intraepiphyseal excision and biological reconstruction with distraction osteogenesis. *J Bone Joint Surg Br*. 2002;84(8):1162-1166.
51. Fuchs B, et al. Osteosarcoma of the pelvis: outcome analysis of surgical treatment. *Clin Orthop Relat Res*. 2009;467(2):510-518.
52. Saab R, et al. Osteosarcoma of the pelvis in children and young adults: the St. Jude Children's Research Hospital experience. *Cancer*. 2005;103(7):1468-1474.
53. Ozaki T, et al. High complication rate of reconstruction using Ilizarov bone transport method in patients with bone sarcomas. *Arch Orthop Trauma Surg*. 1998;118(3):136-139.
54. Kollender Y, et al. Internal hemipelvectomy for bone sarcomas in children and young adults: surgical considerations. *Eur J Surg Oncol*. 2000;26(4):398-404.
55. Hosalkar HS, Dormans JP. Surgical management of pelvic sarcoma in children. *J Am Acad Orthop Surg*. 2007;15(7):408-424.
56. Hugate R Jr, Sim FH. Pelvic reconstruction techniques. *Orthop Clin North Am*. 2006;37(1):85-97.
57. Boriani S, et al. En bloc resections of bone tumors of the thoracolumbar spine. A preliminary report on 29 patients. *Spine*. 1996;21(16):1927-1931.
58. Liljenqvist U, et al. En bloc spondylectomy in malignant tumors of the spine. *Eur Spine J*. 2008;17(4):600-609.
59. Melcher I, et al. Primary malignant bone tumors and solitary metastases of the thoracolumbar spine: results by management with total en bloc spondylectomy. *Eur Spine J*. 2007;16(8):1193-1202.
60. Agarwal M, et al. Rotationplasty for bone tumors: is there still a role? *Clin Orthop Relat Res*. 2007;459:76-81.
61. Sawamura C, Hornicek FJ, Gebhardt MC. Complications and risk factors for failure of rotationplasty: review of 25 patients. *Clin Orthop Relat Res*. 2008;466(6):1302-1308.
62. Refaat Y, et al. Comparison of quality of life after amputation or limb salvage. *Clin Orthop Relat Res*. 2002;397:298-305.
63. Eiser C, et al. Quality of life implications as a consequence of surgery: limb salvage, primary and secondary amputation. *Sarcoma*. 2001;5(4):189-195.
64. Aksnes LH, et al. Limb-sparing surgery preserves more function than amputation: a Scandinavian sarcoma group study of 118 patients. *J Bone Joint Surg Br*. 2008;90(6):786-794.
65. Ginsberg JP, et al. A comparative analysis of functional outcomes in adolescents and young adults with lower-extremity bone sarcoma. *Pediatr Blood Cancer*. 2007;49(7):964-969.
66. Rodriguez-Galindo C, et al. Outcome after local recurrence of osteosarcoma: the St. Jude Children's Research Hospital experience (1970–2000). *Cancer*. 2004;100(9):1928-1935.
67. Nathan SS, et al. Treatment algorithm for locally recurrent osteosarcoma based on local disease-free interval and the presence of lung metastasis. *Cancer*. 2006;107(7):1607-1616.
68. Weisstein, J.S., R.E. Goldsby, and R.J. O'Donnell, *Oncologic approaches to pediatric limb preservation*. J Am Acad Orthop Surg, 2005. 13(8): p. 544–54.
69. Neel, M.D., et al., *Early multicenter experience with a noninvasive expandable prosthesis*. Clin Orthop Relat Res, 2003(415): p. 72–81.
70. Futani, H., et al., *Long-term follow-up after limb salvage in skeletally immature children with a primary malignant tumor of the distal end of the femur*. J Bone Joint Surg Am, 2006. 88(3): p. 595–603.
70. Bacci G, et al., *Local recurrence and local control of non-metastatic osteosarcoma of the extremities: a 27-year experience in a single institution*. J Surg Oncol, 2007. 96(2): p. 118–23.

The Role of Radiotherapy in Oseosarcoma

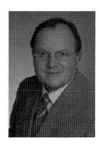

Rudolf Schwarz, Oyvind Bruland, Anna Cassoni, Paula Schomberg, and Stefan Bielack

Abstract A survey of the literature shows that the experience with radiotherapy (RT) in the local treatment of osteosarcoma (OS) is limited. This is due to various reasons: OS is a rare tumor and surgery is the treatment of choice with high local control rate, and uncertainty exists in regard to the efficacy and tolerance of radiotherapy. Publications on this topic were analyzed and will be reviewed. Furthermore, experience from the Cooperative Osteosarkomstudiengruppe (COSS)-Registry, including 100 patients (pts) treated using radiotherapy for OS, was analyzed.

The COSS-registry includes a total of 175 pts (5% of all pts) with histologically proven OS irradiated over the period of 1980–2007. 100 pts were eligible for analysis. The median age was 18 (3–66) years. Indication for RT was a primary tumor in 66, a local recurrence in 11, and metastases in 23 pts. 94 pts got external photontherapy; 2 pts, proton therapy; 2 pts, neutron therapy; and 2 pts, intraoperative RT. In addition, a group of 17 pts received bone-targeted radionuclide therapy by samarium-153-EDTMP-therapy alone or in combination with external RT. The median dose for external RT was 55.8 Gy (30–120). All the pts received chemotherapy in accordance with different COSS-protocols.

The median follow-up was 1.5 (0.2–23) years. Survival and local control rates at 5 years were calculated, and univariate and multivariate analyses performed. 41 pts are alive, 59 pts died. The overall survival rate after biopsy was 41% at 5 years, while the overall survival rates after RT for the whole group, for treatment of primary tumors, local recurrence, and metastases were 36%, 55%, 15%, and 0% respectively.

In 41 cases, local control was achieved, whereas local progression or local recurrence occurred in 59 cases, with a median time to local recurrence of 0.5 (0.1–4) years after RT. 15 pts were nonresponders to radiotherapy. Local control for the whole group was 30%. Local control rates for combined surgery and RT were significantly better than those for RT alone (48% vs. 22%, $p=0.002$). Local control for treatment of primary tumors, local recurrence, and metastases were 40%, 17%,

---

R. Schwarz (✉)
Radiation Oncologist, Department of Radiation Oncology, Medical Center Hamburg-Eppendorf, Martinistr. 52, Hamburg, D-20246, Germany
e-mail: rschwarz@uke.uni-hamburg.de

and 0% respectively. Local control for pts given an addition of samarium-153-EDTMP was poor, though not statistically significant . A dose of over 60 Gy had no significant effect on local control. Prognostic factors for survival were indication for RT, RT plus surgery vs. RT alone and tumor location. Prognostic factors for local control were indication for RT, and RT plus surgery vs. RT alone.

For the majority of pts, surgery remains the local treatment of choice. Radiotherapy is an important option as local treatment of unresectable tumors, following intralesional resection, or as palliation of symptomatic metastases. Survival prognosis of such pts, however, is poor. Despite the fact that many of these pts will eventually die, they may benefit in terms of prolonged survival and prolonged local control. The combination of surgery, radiotherapy, and chemotherapy can be curative. The consistent use of full-dose chemotherapy is of importance for the response to radiotherapy. Prognostic factors for survival are indication for RT, RT plus surgery vs. RT alone and tumor location. Prognostic factors for local control are indication for RT, and RT plus surgery vs. RT alone.

Introduction

A combination of neoadjuvant chemotherapy, surgery and postoperative chemotherapy is the standard treatment for pts with OS. Complete resection with clear margins is the gold standard in the local therapy.[1-4] The majority of pts are currently treated using limb salvage procedures.[1,2,5,6] However, limb salvage is not feasible in OS-pts with advanced extremity or axial tumors. In such cases, gross tumor resection may not be possible, and when achievable, the resection margins are close or positive.

The COSS group performed a multivariate analysis of 1,702 pts with OS. Histological response to neoadjuvant chemotherapy (>90% necrosis) and surgical remission were the main prognostic factors.[7] Picci et al.[8] reported that local recurrence after limb-salvage surgery is associated with less than wide surgical margins, a suboptimal response to chemotherapy , and complications from the biopsy procedure . Ozaki et al.[9] reported a local recurrence rate of 70% for 67 pts with pelvic OS. They also reported that a recurrence developed in 31 of 50 pts (62%) who underwent resection, and 16 (94%) of 17, who did not. Pts with spinal lesions also have a poor prognosis. Of 22 pts with spinal lesions treated by COSS, 15 pts (68%) experienced a local failure.[10] In head and neck OS, a local recurrence rate of approximately 50% has been reported, with the mandible as the most favorable site, followed by the maxilla, and then the extragnathic sites.[11] Single modality, nonoperative options have not been reliably effective in controlling the primary tumor.[12-14]

Historically, in the prechemotherapy era, Cade[15] used a strategy of high-dose radiotherapy and delayed amputation. Gaitan-Yanguas[16] showed a dose-response relationship with no lesions controlled at doses of 30 Gy, and all lesions controlled with doses of >90 Gy. Machak et al.[17] reported on a series of pts with extremity lesions who refused amputation and received neoadjuvant chemotherapy and radiotherapy. Local control was related to response after induction chemotherapy. All the 11 pts with

The Role of Radiotherapy in Oseosarcoma 149

a good response to neoadjuvant chemotherapy achieved local control after radiotherapy. The calculated local progression-free survival among nonresponders was 31% at 3 years, and 0% at 5 years. DeLaney et al.[18] reported on 41 pts with OS who were either not resected or were excised with close or positive margins and who underwent RT with external beam photons and/or protons at the Massachusetts General Hospital. Local control rates, according to the extent of resection, were 78.4% for gross total resection, 77.8% for subtotal resection, and 40% for biopsy only. The use of a bone-seeking radioisotope, samarium153ethylene diamine tetramethylene phosphonate (EDTMP), can provide additional radiation to osteoblastic OS.[19–22]

Publications reporting on the experience with radiation for local treatment of OS were analyzed and will be discussed. In addition, data from the COSS-Registry of 100 pts with radiotherapy for OS were analyzed.

Material/Methods

Since 1980, most OS pts from Germany, Austria, and Switzerland have been treated on protocols of the Cooperative Osteosarcoma Study Group (COSS). A uniform concept of preoperative and postoperative chemotherapy in combination with aggressive surgery has formed the basis of all consecutive neoadjuvant study protocols since 1980.[7] Registration was never limited to the typical young pts with localized limb tumors; rather, all pts with osteosarcoma were eligible. In addition to the pediatric population, many adults with OS were also registered.

The COSS-registry includes over 3,500 pts with histologically proven OS. A total of 175 pts (5%) were identified to have been externally irradiated over the period of 1980 – 2007. Inadequate follow-up concerning survival and/or local control, missing radiotherapy details or histologies other than OS were exclusion criteria for the analysis. After exclusion based on these criteria, 100 pts (2.9%) were eligible. Table 1 lists the patient characteristics. The median age was 18 (3–66) years, 57 pts were below 20 years and 43 pts, above 20 years of age. Indication for RT was a primary tumor in 66, a local recurrence in 11, and metastases in 23 pts. A total 65 pts were irradiated with curative, and 35 pts with palliative, intent. The anatomical sites of irradiated tumors or metastases were as follows : pelvis, 33; lower extremity, 29; spine, 13; head and neck, 13; thoracic sites, 10; and upper extremity, 2. The median follow-up was 1.5 (0.2–23) years after radiotherapy. Survival and local control rates at 5 years were calculated, and univariate and multivariate analyses performed.

Radiotherapy

Early COSS-Protocols did not include recommendations regarding radiotherapy; EURO.B.O.S.S. and EURAMOS-1 were the first protocols to do so.

Table 1 Patient characteristics

Indications for radiotherapy	
Primary tumor	66
Local recurrence	11
Metastasis	23
Age	
Median age	18 (3–66) years
<20 years	57
≥20 years	43
<40 years	86
≥40 years	14
Localisation of the treated tumors	
Pelvis	33
Spine	13
Thoracic sites	10
Head and neck	13
Lower extremity	29
Upper extremity	2

Radiotherapy was performed in 35 pts as preoperative (9), postoperative (24), or intraoperative (2) radiotherapy. The majority of pts (65) were treated with radiotherapy after biopsy, or for unresectable tumors or metastases in combination with chemotherapy.

Table 2 shows details of the RT. Ninety-four pts received linear accelerator-based external photon therapy. Special techniques were used in 6 pts (2 pts, Proton therapy; 2 pts, neutron therapy; and 2 pts, intraoperative RT). A group of 17 pts received high-dose samarium-153-EDTMP therapy for large and unresectable primary or recurrent tumors and/or metastases, alone or in combination with external RT,[23,24] some of them with high doses and stem cell rescue. Eight pts had bone metastases and nine pts, an advanced OS of the pelvis. For the treatment of hematopoetic toxicity, cryopreserved hematopoetic progenitor cells were used. The median dose for external RT was 55.8 Gy (30–120); for preoperative RT, 50 Gy (30–68) ; postoperative RT, 54 Gy (36–72); for RT without surgery, 56 Gy (30–75,6); for primary RT, 59.7 Gy (20–120); for local recurrence, 50.4 Gy (30–70); and for metastases, 45 Gy (30–66). Complications were not analyzed.

Chemotherapy

Chemotherapy was given to all pts according to the COSS protocol active at the time of enrollment. All protocols included high-dose methotrexate at 12 g/m^2 per course with leucovorin rescue. In addition, doxorubicin 60–90 mg/m^2 per course, cisplatin 90–150 mg/m^2 per course, ifosfamide 6–10 g/m^2 per course, and bleomycin, cyclophosphamide, and dactinomycin were used in varying combinations. For the

The Role of Radiotherapy in Oseosarcoma

Table 2 Radiotherapy (RT) characteristics

Treatment modalities	Patients
Preop RT	9
Postop RT	24
Intraop RT	2
RT/RCHTH	65
Radiotherapy	
External RT with photons	94
IMRT	3
Stereotactic RT	1
Neutrontherapy	2
Protontherapy	2
Intraoperative RT	2
Additionally Hyperthermia	2
Dose of radiotherapy	Gy
Median dose for external RT	55.8 (30–75.6)
Median dose for primary RT	59.7 (20–120)
Median dose for local recurrence	50.4 (30–70)
Median dose for metastases	45 (30–66)
Median dose preoperative RT	50 (30–68)
Median dose postoperative RT	54 (36–72)
Intraoperative RT	20
Extra corporal RT	120
Neutrons	12, 16
Total dose of irradiation	
<60 Gy	59 patients
≥60 Gy	41 patients

treatment of primary tumors, the duration of chemotherapy ranged from 24 to 38 weeks.[7] Therapy of relapse was not standardized; however, most protocols included general recommendations.[25] Surgical removal of all detectable tumor foci was recommended whenever feasible. The decision to use second-line chemotherapy and the choice of drugs were left to the discretion of the treating physician. Since 1990, COSS has suggested carboplatin and etoposide, if chemotherapy is considered.

Assessment of Response

For pts with assessable, unresected or partially resected disease, local control was defined as durable stabilization or regression of tumor demonstrable on cross-sectional imaging with CT or MRI. Local failure in these pts was defined as tumor growth on cross-sectional imaging and was invariably accompanied by progression of local symptoms. For pts whose disease had been grossly resected, local control was defined as the absence of tumor regrowth demonstrable on cross-sectional imaging with CT or MRI.

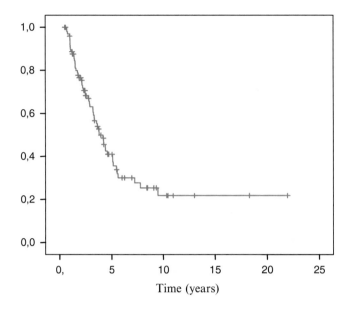

Fig. 1 Cumulative overall survival for all patients ($n = 100$)

Statistical Analysis

An analysis of the overall survival and local control rates was performed using the Kaplan–Meier method.[26] The log-rank test was used to compare the survival curves.[27] Multivariate analyses of overall survival and local control were completed using the Cox proportional hazards model.[28] The overall survival rate was calculated for all the pts from the time of biopsy (Fig. 1). All other overall survival and local control rates were calculated from the end of radiotherapy. Only four variables (dose <60 Gy vs. ≥60 Gy, RT plus surgery vs. RT alone as local treatment, tumor location extremity vs. axial tumors, and indication for RT primary tumor and local recurrence vs. metastases) that resulted in a significant value in univariate analysis were included in the multivariate models.

Results

Survival

The overall survival rate after biopsy was 41% at 5 years (Fig. 1). At the last follow-up, 41 pts were alive, 59 pts had died. The overall survival rate after RT for the whole group was 36% at 5 years (Fig. 2). The results for the overall survival rates are demonstrated in Table 3. There is a highly significant difference in survival between treatment with RT plus surgery and that with RT alone (62%

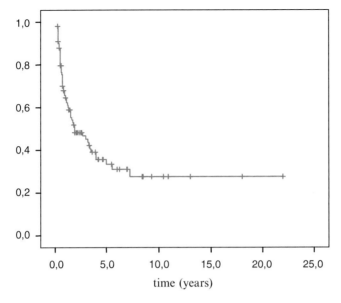

Fig. 2 Cumulative survival for all patients after RT

Table 3 Results for overall survival (OS)

Group	Patients n	OS at 5 years (%)	OS at 10 years (%)	p
Localization				
Extremity tumors	31	43	37	0.057
Axial tumors	69	28	–	
Indication				
Primary	66	48	39	<0.0001
Local recurrence	11	13	–	
Metastasis	23	–	–	
Local treatment				
RT plus surgery	35	63	–	<0.0001
RT alone	65	22	18	
Modality				
Only external RT	83	38	30	0.191
Additional 153-Sam	17	15	–	
RT dose				
<60 Gy	59	27	22	0.145
≥60 Gy	41	41	35	
Age				
<20 years	57	41	41	0.761
≥20 years	43	31	22	

vs. 26%, $p<0,0001$, Fig. 3). The overall survival rates for the treatment of primary tumors, local recurrences, and metastases were 55%, 15%, and 0% (Fig. 4) respectively. Pts with extremity tumors had a better chance of survival

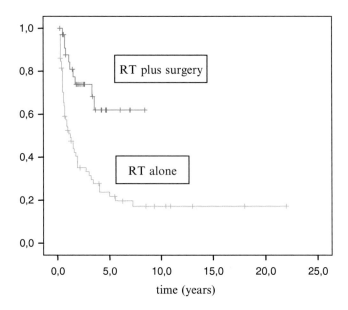

Fig. 3 Cumulative survival for patients after RT plus surgery vs. RT alone ($p<0.0001$)

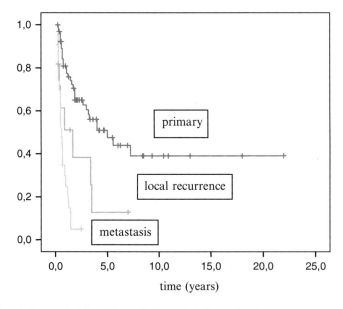

Fig. 4 Cumulative survival for different indications (primary, local recurrence, metastasis)

than pts with axial tumors (55% vs. 29%, $p=0.016$). The survival rate for pts with additionally administered samarium-153-EDTMP in comparison to that of other pts was not significantly different (42% vs. 15%, $p=0.137$). Age had no significant influence on survival.

Table 4 Results for local control (LC)

Group	Patients n	LC at 5 years (%)	LC at 10 years (%)	p
Localization				
Extremity tumors	31	35	35	0.156
Axial tumors	69	27	–	
Indication				
Primary	66	39	39	<0.0001
Local recurrence	11	18	–	
Metastasis	23	–	–	
Local treatment				
RT plus surgery	35	48	–	0.002
RT alone	65	22	22	
Modality				
Only external RT	83	34	34	0.127
Additional ^{153}Sam	17	10	–	
RT dose				
<60 Gy	59	30	30	0.790
≥60 Gy	41	32	32	
Age				
<20 years	57	33	33	0.516
≥20 years	43	28	28	

Local Control

The results for the local control rates are shown in Table 4. In 41 cases, local control could be achieved; in 59 cases, a local progression or local recurrence occurred with a median time to local failure of 0.5 (0.1–4) years after RT. Fifteen pts were nonresponders to radiotherapy. The local control rate for the whole group was 30% at 5 years (Fig. 5). The local control rate for combined surgery and RT was significantly superior to that of RT alone (48% vs. 22%, $p=0.002$, Fig. 6). The local control rates for treatment of primary tumors, local recurrence, and metastases were 40%, 17%, and 0% respectively (Fig. 7). Local control for pts who received additional samarium-153-EDTMP-therapy was worse than for those with only external RT; however, the difference was not significant. A dose of over 60 Gy had no significant effect on local control.

Prognostic Factors

The prognostic factors for survival were indication for RT, RT plus surgery vs. RT alone and tumor location of the irradiated tumor site (Table 5).The prognostic factors for local control were indication for RT, and RT plus surgery vs. RT alone (Table 6).

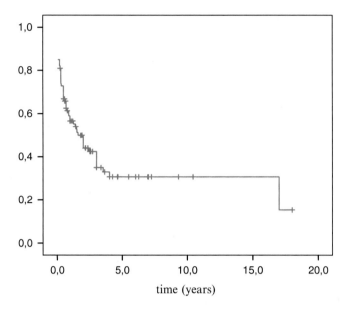

Fig. 5 Cumulative local control for all patients ($n=100$)

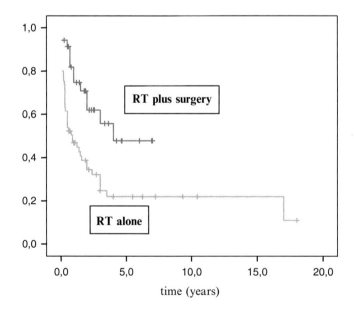

Fig. 6 Cumulative local control for patients after RT plus surgery vs. RT alone ($p=0.002$)

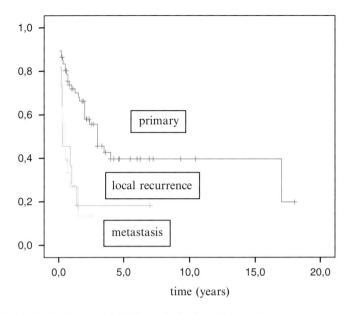

Fig. 7 Cumulative local control for different indications (primary, local recurrence, metastasis)

Table 5 Multivariate analysis of prognostic factors for overall survival

Factor		Hazard ratio(95% confidence intervall)	p-value
RT modality	RT + surgery	1	
	RT alone	5.149 (2.4–10.8)	<0.0001
RT indication	Primary	1	
	Local recurrence	3.738 (1.6–8.5)	0.002
	Metastasis	5.252 (2.6–10.3)	<0.0001
Tumor location	Axial	1	
	Extremity	0.542 (0.28–1.0)	0.058
Dose	<60 Gy	1	
	≥60 Gy	0.708 (0.4–1.2)	0.231

Discussion

The combination of neoadjuvant and adjuvant chemotherapy with complete resection of the primary tumor with clear margins is the standard treatment for pts with OS.[1–4,8] A high percentage of pts are currently being treated using limb salvage

Table 6 Multivariate analysis of prognostic factors for local control

Factor		Hazard ratio(95% confidence intervall)	p-value
RT modality	RT + surgery	1	
	RT alone	2.743 (1.4–5.28)	<0.003
RT indication	Primary	1	
	Local recurrence	3.353 (1.5–7.3)	0.003
	Metastasis	2.98 (1.4–5.9)	0.002
Tumor location	Axial	1	
	Extremity	0.628 (0.3–1.1)	0.139
Dose	<60 Gy	1	
	≥60 Gy	1.12 (0.6–1.9)	0.686

procedures.[1,2,5,6] Local control of the primary or recurrent tumor is of great importance for cure.[7,25] Although limb salvage surgery can be done in many pts with OS, some pts have extremely challenging extremity or axial tumors, and complete resection is difficult to achieve. In these cases, gross tumor resection may not be possible, and when achievable, the resection margins are close or positive.

In pts with surgery as local treatment, the definition of histopathological remission is possible. In radiotherapy for gross tumor after biopsy or partial resection of the tumor, an alternative definition is necessary. Local control has to be defined as durable stabilization or regression of tumor demonstrable on cross-sectional imaging with CT or MRI (see above). Because of the osteoblastic stroma in OS, tumors may not necessarily shrink, even if a response occurs. Local failure in these pts has to be defined as tumor growth on cross-sectional imaging. It was invariably accompanied by progression of local symptoms. For pts whose disease had been grossly resected, local control has to be defined as the absence of tumor regrowth demonstrable on cross-sectional imaging with CT or MRI.

The limited success of radiotherapy in the past has been attributed to a suggested low cellular radiosensitivity of OS tumor cells. However, Larsen et al.[29] had demonstrated that the parameters of the radiation cell survival curves (α and β) of three OS cell lines, are in the same order as those of most nonsarcoma cell lines derived from tumors known to be clinically radiocurable. Another paper showed that the doses required by these OS cell lines to achieve 50% survival (D50%) were much lower than the D50% of a human melanoma line, known to be radioresistant.[30] However, tumor radiocurability is determined by various radiobiological factors such as cellular radiosensitivity, tumor hypoxia, reoxygenation, tumor size, repair, and proliferation rate. In clinical reality, the efficacy of radiotherapy is often limited by large tumor size and a significant proportion of hypoxic cells.[31] In addition, tumor location may prohibit the safe delivery of adequate radiation doses.

Radiotherapy as single modality has not been reliably effective in controlling the primary tumor.[12–14] Cade[15] advocated a strategy – "a holding action"; giving high-dose radiotherapy to relieve local pain. He then restricted delayed amputation to pts without evidence of lung metastases during subsequent follow-up.

Ozaki et al.[9] reported for the COSS, a local recurrence rate of 70% for 67 pts with pelvic OS. Recurrence developed in 31 out of 50 (62%) pts who underwent resection, and 16 (94%) out of 17 pts who did not. Out of 30 pts with intralesional surgery, or no surgery, 11 pts took radiotherapy and had better overall survival compared with 19 pts who went without radiotherapy ($p = 0.0033$). The Cox proportional hazard model revealed that existence of primary metastasis, intralesional surgery, or no surgery, and no local radiotherapy were by themselves poor prognostic factors. Pts with spinal lesions also have a poor prognosis. Of 22 pts treated by the Cooperative Osteosarcoma Study Group, 15 (68%) experienced a local failure.[10] Sundaresan et al.[32] described that some OS of the spine respond to radiotherapy.

The publication by Machak et al.[17] reported a local control rate at 5 years of 56% in 31 extremity OS pts who were treated with external beam radiotherapy to a median dose of 60 Gy, and neoadjuvant chemotherapy. Among pts with a good imaging and good biochemical (as assessed by normalization of alkaline phosphatase) response, no local failure was observed. Caceres et al.[33] noted a high response rate among pts with limb OS treated by chemotherapy and 60 Gy of RT. In 80% of those pts, biopsies after treatment were negative. DeLaney et al.[18] reported on 41 pts with OS that were either not resected or were excised with close or positive margins and who underwent RT with external beam photons and/or protons at the Massachusetts General Hospital. The survival rates in DeLaney's series and in ours are similar. In the Boston Series, the actuarial survival at 5 years according to the extent of surgery was 74.4% for gross total resection; 74.1% for subtotal resection; and 25% for biopsy only. The local control rate at 5 years according to the extent of resection was 78.4% for gross total resection; 77.8% for subtotal resection; and 40% for biopsy only, compared with 48% for pts with surgery and radiotherapy and 22% for those with radiotherapy alone in our series. Both, the poor overall survival and local control rates support the need for multidisciplinary local treatment for further improvement in treatment results.

A clear dose-response relationship could not be demonstrated in the analysis of DeLaney or in ours This might have been an effect of limited size and heterogeneity of the populations. In the series of Machak et al.[17] and our own series, long-term local control after RT doses of 60 Gy and chemotherapy could be demonstrated. Gaitan-Yanguas[16] showed a dose-response relationship with no lesions controlled at doses of 30 Gy, and all lesions controlled with doses of >90 Gy. Lombardi et al.[34] used hypofractionated, accelerated radiotherapy to overcome the intrinsic radioresistance of OS.

New techniques allowing local dose escalation are emerging. Several series utilized intraoperative radiotherapy to increase the dose and spare later reactions.[35–38] Hong et al.[36] described extracorporeal irradiation (ECI) in the management of 16 pts with primary malignant bone tumors, four of them with OS. After en bloc resection, a single dose of 50 Gy was delivered to the bone segment extra corporeally. At a median follow-up of 19.5 months, there were no cases of local recurrence or graft failure. One patient required amputation due to chronic osteomyelitis. Oya et al.[37] reported 39 pts with OS of the extremities, who were treated with high-dose intraoperative radiotherapy. The irradiation field included the tumor plus an adequately wide margin, and excluded the major vessels and nerves. A dose of 45–80 Gy was delivered with electrons or X-rays. The cause-specific and relapse-free 5-year survival rate was 50% and 43%, respectively. Distant metastases developed in 23 pts; 19 died and 4 were alive for >10 years. Nine local recurrences were found 4–29 months after IORT. Functional status was examined in 21 pts; four of them needed nonnarcotic analgesics, and 17 (81%) were free of pain. Five pts had a minor to moderate functional deficit, and 16 had only cosmetic alterations without a functional deficit. Hence, IORT may be a treatment option in specialized centers.

With modern radiation techniques, higher radiation doses can be delivered with fewer side effects. Highly conformal RT techniques such as intensity modulated RT (IMRT), image-guided radiotherapy (IGRT), proton therapy, and heavy ion therapy are suitable techniques.[18,39–42] The availability of these techniques has encouraged radiation oncologists to treat OS with doses of ≥ 70 Gy. In a Japanese series of 15 pts with unresectable OS treated with carbon ion therapy the actuarial survival rate was 45%.[42] However, because of limited experience and follow-up, no definite conclusions can be drawn about these high radiation doses.

A local recurrence has a worse prognosis in comparison to primary tumors. The overall survival and local control at 5 years in DeLaney's[18] series (overall survival 78,8% vs. 54%; $p < 0.05$, and local control 73.8% vs. 48%; $p < 0.05$) and our series (overall survival 55% vs. 15%, $p < 0.0001$, and local local control 40% vs. 17%, $p < 0.0001$) were better for patients with radiotherapy for primary tumor.

Preoperative radiotherapy was reported by several groups.[43–45] Chambers et al.[43] reported on 33 pts with preoperative RT and resection for craniofacial OS. They reported an overall survival rate of 73% at 5 years.[43] Dincsbas et al.[45] analyzed 64 pts with neoadjuvant and adjuvant chemotherapy, preoperative RT in 44 cases, and limb sparing surgery. The median follow-up was 44 months. at which the tumor necrosis rate was $\geq 90\%$ in 87% of the pts. The 5-year local control and overall survival rates were 97.5% and 48.4% respectively. The authors concluded that preoperative RT, when combined with chemotherapy, may facilitate the chance of extremity-sparing surgery with good local control .

Neutron therapy was used in some centers on the basis of an assumedly improved radiobiological effectiveness of neutrons. Two pts were treated with neutrons in the COSS-series. Other small series have been reported,[46] but on their basis alone, no definitive conclusions can be made. Neutrons are available only in a very limited number of centers worldwide.

Prophylactic lung irradiation (PLI) without effective adjuvant and neoadjuvant chemotherapy was used three decades ago.[47] Currently there is no indication for PLI, because effective chemotherapeutic agents are used nowadays in the treatment protocols.[47,48]

The use of a bone-seeking radioisotope, samarium-153-EDTMP, can provide additional radiation to disseminated skeletal metastases and osteoblastic OS.[19–23,49–53] Several series have shown that provision of high-dose samarium-153-EDTMP and peripheral blood stem cells to pts with favorable imaging results can deliver an additional 40 to 200 Gy of radiation to lesions of osteoblastic OS.[22,52] In our series The overall survival and local control rates for pts with external beam radiotherapy and samarium-153-EDTMP were worse than those for pts with external beam radiotherapy only. This can be explained by the fact that all the pts receiving samarium-153-EDTMP-therapy had advanced local tumors and/or multiple metastases. Over and above that, the differences in overall survival and local control were not significant. Further studies aiming to define the exact role of this multimodal concept are warranted.

Chemotherapy is of great importance for the efficacy of radiation as local treatment.[54] Intra-arterial chemotherapy for OS was introduced in the Eighties.[55–57] Estrada-Aguilar et al.[57] reported on five pts treated with intra-arterial cisplatin and concurrent radiotherapy for nonresectable OS. Long-term local control was achieved in all the pts. Two pts were long-term survivors with no evidence of local or systemic relapse 56 and 77 months after therapy.[57] Radiosensitizers have also been used. Martinez et al.[58] reported on intra-arterial infusion of the radiosensitizer 5′-bromodesoxyuridine (BUdR) combined with hypofractionated irradiation and chemotherapy for primary treatment of OS. Nine pts were treated; local control was achieved in seven cases, and four pts survived 6–10.5 years after irradiation.

Chemotherapy was given to 85% of the pts in DeLaney's series and to all the pts in Machak's and our own series.[17,18] Local control was related to response after induction chemotherapy. All 11 pts with a good response to neoadjuvant chemotherapy achieved local control after radiotherapy. The calculated local progression-free survival among nonresponders was 31% at 3 years and 0% at 5 years.[17]

DeLaney et al.[18] analyzed 14 pts for chemotherapy response. Six pts had a good histological or imaging response, and 8 pts had either moderate or poor response. Of those with a good response, none developed local failure, but for those with a moderate or poor response, the local control rate was only 35.7% ($p < 0,05$). Mahajan et al.[53] analyzed 39 high risk, metastatic, and/or recurrent pts treated with a combination of external beam radiotherapy to 119 sites in combination with different chemotherapeutic drugs, most commonly ifosfamide or methotrexate; 11 pts also received samarium-153-EDTMP-therapy. Objective and potentially durable responses were documented using PET-CT and bone scans. Improvement was demonstrated in 72%, of the pts, stable disease in 25% and progression in 3%.

In most cases chemotherapy can be continued during radiotherapy, but enhancement of radiation toxicity is likely to occur with several agents, and the combination of chemotherapy and radiation may result in severely acute and late side effects. This is of particular concern when the spinal cord is within the treatment volume. High-dose methotrexate should be avoided during radiotherapy. Adriamycin (doxorubicin) should be avoided because of enhanced intestinal toxicity and increased skin toxicity. Concurrent ifosfamide should be avoided if a significant volume of the bladder is in the radiation field. The nucleoside analog gemcitabine can be used as a radiation enhancer in OS.[53,59,60] Given as a radiation enhancer one day after samarium-153-EDTMP infusion, additional efficacy has been observed in some pts.[53,59,60]

Conclusions

For the majority of osteosarcomas, surgery remains the local treatment of choice. Radiotherapy is an important option as local treatment of unresectable tumors, following intralesional resection, or as palliation of symptomatic metastases. The probability of long-term survival, however, is low. Despite the fact that many of the pts will eventually die of their disease, they may benefit in terms of prolonged survival and prolonged local control. The combination of surgery, radiotherapy, and chemotherapy can be curative. The consistent use of full-dose chemotherapy is of importance for the response to radiotherapy. In the COSS series, prognostic factors for survival are an indication for RT, RT plus surgery vs. RT alone and tumor location. Prognostic factors for local control are an indication for RT, and RT plus surgery vs. RT alone.

We thank Matthias Kevric from COSS-registry for his support in this analysis, and Christoph IntVeen, for the statistical analysis.

References

1. Bacci G, Ferrari S, Bertoni F, et al. Long-term outcome for patients with nonmetastatic osteosarcoma of the extremity treated at the Istituto Ortopedico Rizzoli according to the Istituto Ortopedico/osteosarcoma-2 protocol: an updated report. *J Clin Oncol*. 2000;18:4016-4027.
2. Bielack S, Kempf-Bielack B, Schwenzer D, et al. Neoadjuvante Therapie des lokalisierten Osteosarkoms der Extremitäten. Erfahrungen der Cooperativen Osteosarkomstudiengruppe COSS an 925 Patienten. *Klin Paediatr*. 1999;211:260-270.
3. Ferguson WS, Goorin AM. Current treatment of osteosarcoma. *Cancer Invest*. 2001;19:292-315.
4. Provisor AJ, Ettinger LJ, Nachman JB, et al. Treatment of nonmetastatic osteosarcoma of the extremity with preoperative and postoperative chemotherapy: a report from the Children's Cancer Group. *J Clin Oncol*. 1997;15:76-84.
5. Weis LD. The success of limb-salvage surgery in the adolescent patient with osteogenic sarcoma. *Adolesc Med*. 1999;10:451-458.
6. Lindner NJ, Ramm O, Hillmann A, et al. Limb salvage and outcome of osteosarcoma: the University of Muenster experience. *Clin Orthop*. 1999;358:83-89.
7. Bielack SS, Kempf-Bielack B, Delling G, et al. Prognostic factors in high-grade osteosarcoma of the extremities or trunk: an analysis of 1, 702 patients treated on neoadjuvant cooperative oseosarcoma study group protocols. *J Clin Oncol*. 2002;20:776-790.
8. Picci P, Sangiorgi L, Bahamonde L, et al. Risk factors for local recurrences after limb-salvage surgery for high-grade osteosarcomas of the extremities. *Ann Oncol*. 1997;8:899-903.
9. Ozaki T, Flege S, Kevric M, et al. Osteosarcoma of the pelvis: experience of the cooperative osteosarcoma study group. *J Clin Oncol*. 2003;21:334-341.
10. Ozaki T, Flege S, Liljenqvist U, et al. Osteosarcoma of the spine: experience of the cooperative osteosarcoma study group. *Cancer*. 2002;94:1069-1077.
11. Kassir RR, Rassekh CH, Kinsella JB, et al. Osteosarcoma of the head and neck: meta-analysis of nonrandomized studies. *Laryngoscope*. 1997;107:56-61.
12. Jenkin RD, Allt W, Fitzpatrick PJ. Osteosarcoma: an assessment of management with particular reference to primary irradiation and selective delayed amputation. *Cancer*. 1972;2:393-400.
13. De Moor NG. Osteosarcoma: a review of 72 cases treated by megavoltage radiation therapy, with or without surgery. *S Afr J Surg*. 1975;13:137-146.

The Role of Radiotherapy in Oseosarcoma 163

14. Beck JC, Wara WM, Bovill EG Jr, et al. The role of radiation therapy in the treatment of osteosarcoma. *Radiology*. 1976;120:163-165.
15. Cade S. Osteogenic sarcoma: a study based on 133 patients. *J R Coll Surg Edinb*. 1955;1:79-111.
16. Gaitan-Yanguas M. A study of the response of osteogenic sarcoma and adjacent normal tissues to radiation. *Int J Radiat Oncol Biol Phys*. 1981;7:593-595.
17. Machak GN, Tkachev SI, Solovyev YN, et al. Neoadjuvant chemotherapy and local radiotherapy for high-grade osteosarcoma of the extremities. *Mayo Clin Proc*. 2003;78:147-155.
18. DeLaney TF, Park L, Goldberg SI, et al. Radiotherapy for local control of osteosarcoma. *Int J Rad Oncol Biol Phys*. 2005;61:492-498.
19. Bruland ØS, Skretting A, Solheim ØP, et al. Targeted radiotherapy of osteosarcoma using 153 Sm-EDTMP. A new promising approach. *Acta Oncologica*. 1996;35:381-384.
20. Bruland ØS, Skretting A, Saeter G, et al. Targeted internal radiotherapy in osteosarcoma patients using 153Sm-EDTMP. *Med Ped Oncol*. 1996;27:215.
21. Bruland ØS, Phil A. On the current management of osteosarcoma: a critical evaluation and proposal for a modified treatment strategy. *Eur J Cancer*. 1997;33:1725-1731.
22. Anderson PM, Wisemann GA, Dispenzieri A, et al. High-dose samarium-153 ethylene diamnine tetramethylene phosphonate phosphonate: low toxicity of skeletal irradiation in patients with osteosarcoma and bone metastases. *J Clin Oncol*. 2002;20:189-196.
23. Franzius C, Bielack S, Sciuk J, et al. High-activity samarium-153-EDTMP therapy in unresectable osteosarcoma. *Nuklearmedizin*. 1999;38:337-340.
24. Franzius C, Schuck A, Bielack SS. High-dose Samarium-153 ethylene diamine tetramethylene phosphonate: low toxicity of skeletal irradiation in patients with osteosarcoma and bone metastases. *J Clin Oncol*. 2002;20:1953-1954.
25. Kempf-Bielack B, Bielack SS, Jürgens H, et al. Osteosarcoma Relapse after combined modality therapy: an analysis of unselected patients in the cooperative osteosarcoma study group (COSS). *J Clin Oncol*. 2005;23:559-568.
26. Kaplan EL, Meier P. Nonparametric estimation from incomplete observations. *J Am Stat Assoc*. 1958;53:457-481.
27. Mantel M. Evaluation of survival data and two new rank order statistics arising in its consideration. *Cancer Chemother Rep*. 1996;50:163-170.
28. Cox DR. Regression models and life-tables (with discussion). *J R Stat Soc (B)*. 1972;34:187-220.
29. Larsen RH, Bruland ØS, Hoff Å, et al. Inactivation of human osteosarcoma cells in vitro by 211At-TP-3 monoclonal antibody; comparison with Astatine-21-labelled bovine serum albumon, free Astatine-211 and external-beam X rays. *Rad Res*. 1994;139:178-184.
30. Larsen RH, Bruland ØS, Hoff P, et al. Analysis of the therapeutic gain in the treatment of human osteosarcoma microcolonies in vitro with 211At-labelled monoclonal antibodies. *Br J Cancer*. 1994;69:1000-1005.
31. Olsen DR, Bruland ØS. Is osteosarcoma a radioresistant tumor? *Towards the Eradication of Osteosarcoma Metastases – An Odyssey*. The Norwegian Radium Hospital; 1998:73–76.
32. Sundaresan N, Rosen G, Ag H, et al. Combined treatment of osteosarcoma of the spine. *Neurosurgery*. 1988;23:714-719.
33. Caceres E, Zaharia M, Valdivia S, et al. Local control of osteogenic sarcoma by radiation and chemotherapy. *Int J Radiat Oncol Biol Phys*. 1984;10:35-39.
34. Lombardi F, Gandola L, Fossati-Belani F, et al. Hypofractionated accelerated radiotherapy in osteogenic sarcoma. *Int J Rad Oncol Biol Phys*. 1992;24:761-765.
35. Calvo FA, Ortiz de Urbina D, Sierrasesumaga L, et al. Intraoperative radiotherapy in the multidisciplinary treatment of bone sarcomas in children and adolescents. *Med Pediatr Oncol*. 1991;19:478-485.
36. Hong A, Stevens G, Stalley P, et al. Extracorporeal irradiation for malignant bone tumors. *Int J Radiat Oncol Biol Phys*. 2001;50:441-447.
37. Oya N, Kokubo M, Mizowaki T, et al. Definitive intraoperative very high-dose radiotherapy for localized osteosarcoma in the extremities. *Int J Radiat Oncol Biol Phys*. 2001;51:87-93.
38. Sabo D, Bernd L, Buchner M, et al. Intraoperative extracorporeal irradiation and replantation in local treatment of primary malignant bone tumors. *Orthopäde*. 2003;32:1103-1112.

39. Uhl V, Castro JR, Knopf K, et al. Preliminary results in heavy charged particle irradiation of bone sarcoma. *Int J Radiat Oncol Biol Phys.* 1992;24:755-759.
40. Castro JR, Linstadt DE, Bhary JP, et al. Experience in charged particle irradiation of tumors of the skull base: 1977–1992. *Int J Radiat Oncol Biol Phys.* 1994;29:647-655.
41. Hug EB, Munzenrieder JE. Charged particle therapy for base of skull tumors: Past accomplishments and future challenges. *Int J Radiat Oncol Biol Phys.* 1994;29:911-919.
42. Kamada T, Tsujii H, Tsuji H, et al. Efficacy and safety of carbon ion radiotherapy in bone and soft tissue sarcomas. *J Clin Oncol.* 2002;20:4466-4471.
43. Chambers RG, Mahoney WD. Osteogenic sarcoma of the mandible, current management. *Am Surg.* 1970;36:463-471.
44. Eilber FR, Morton DL, Eckhardt J, et al. Limb salvage for skeletal and soft tissue sarcomas: multidisciplinary preoperative therapy. *Cancer.* 1984;53:2579-2584.
45. Dincbas FO, Koca S, Mandel NM, et al. The role of preoperative radiotherapy in nonmetastatic high-grade osteosarcoma of the extremities for limb-sparing surgery. *Int J Radiat Oncol Biol Phys.* 2005;62:820-828.
46. Carrie C, Breteau N, Negrier S, et al. The role of fast neutron therapy in unresectable pelvic osteosarcoma: preliminary report. *Med Pediatr Onco.* 1994;22:355-357.
47. Burgers JM, van Glabbeke M, Busson A, et al. Osteosarcoma of the limbs. Report of the EORTC-SIOP03 trial 20781 investigating the value of adjuvant treatment with chemotherapy and/or prophylactic lung irradiation. *Cancer.* 1988;61:1024-1031.
48. Whelan JS, Burcombe RJ, Janinis J, et al. A systematic review of the role of pulmonary irradiation in the management of primary bone tumours. *Ann Oncol.* 2002;13:23-30.
49. Appelbaum FR, Sandmaier B, Brown PA, et al. Myelosuppression and mechanism of recovery following administration of 153Samarium-EDTMP. *Antibody Imunoconjug Radiopharm.* 1988;1:263-270.
50. Turner JH, Claringbold PG, Heytherington EL. A phase I study of samarium 153 ethylene diamine tetramethylene phosphonate therapy for dissiminated skeletal metastases. *J Clin Oncol.* 1989;7:1926-1931.
51. Turner JH, Martindale AA, Sorby P. Samarium [153]EDTMP therapy of dissiminated skeletal metastasis. *Eur J Nucl Med.* 1989;15:784-795.
52. Franzius C, Bielack S, Sciuk J, et al. High-activity samarium-EDTMP therapy followed by autologues peripheral blood stem cell support in unresectable osteosarcoma. *Nuklearmedizin.* 2001;40:215-220.
53. Mahajan A, Woo SY, Kornguth DG, et al. Multimodality treatment of Osteosarcoma: radiation in a high-risk cohort. *Pediatr Blood Cancer.* 2007;. doi:10.1002/pbc.21451.
54. Anderson PM. Effectiveness of radiotherapy for osteosarcoma that responds to chemotherapy. *Mayo Clin Proc.* 2003;78:145-146.
55. Jaffe N, Knapp J, Chuang VP, et al. Osteosarcomas: Intra-arterial treatment of the primary tumor with Cis-diammine-dichloroplatinum II (CDP). Angiographic, pathologic, and pharmacologic studies. *Cancer.* 1983;51:402-407.
56. Kinsella TJ, Glatstein E. Clinical experience with intravenous radiosensitizers in unresectable sarcomas. *Cancer.* 1987;59:908-915.
57. Estrada-Aguilar J, Greenberg H, Walling A, et al. Primary treatment of pelvic osteosarcoma. *Cancer.* 1992;69:1137-1145.
58. Martinez A, Goffinet DR, Donaldson SS, et al. Intra-arterial infusion of radiosensitizer (BUdR) combined with hypofractionated irradiation and chemotherapy for primary treatment of osteogenic sarcoma. *Int J Radiat Oncol Biol Phys.* 1985;11:123-128.
59. Anderson PM (2002) Samarium + gemcitabine concept. Presented at: Children's Oncology Group meeting; October 26, St. Louis, Mo.
60. Anderson P, Aguilera D, Pearson M, et al. Outpatient chemotherapy plus radiotherapy in sarcomas: improving cancer control with radiosensitizing agents. *Cancer Control.* 2008;15:38-46.

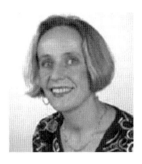

Osteosarcoma Lung Metastases Detection and Principles of Multimodal Therapy

Dorothe Carrle and Stefan Bielack

Abstract The management of pulmonary metastases poses a challenge to the multidisciplinary team involved in the treatment of osteosarcoma. A postal survey on the management of pulmonary metastases in osteosarcoma involving 17 representatives from international study groups and selected institutions was performed in which a response rate of 94% was achieved. The results showed uniform approaches in areas like the imaging methods used for initial staging and the use of manual exploration with thoracotomy. However, it demonstrated diverse practices regarding exploration of the unaffected site in unilateral pulmonary disease, and the approach to lesions disappearing under chemotherapy. Furthermore, agreement on the size of a lesion considered to distinguish between benign and of metastatic origin, varied. Based on the survey and a review of the current literature, detection methods and principles of multimodal therapy will be discussed. Prognostic factors in synchronous and metachronous pulmonary metastases and their implications for a multimodal therapy is also presented.

Introduction

Osteosarcoma, like other malignant bone tumors, metastasizes mainly by hematogenous spread resulting in lung metastases, with a major impact on patients' prognosis. The management of pulmonary metastases poses a challenge to the multidisciplinary team involved in the treatment of osteosarcoma. Key aspects to be considered include the choice and interpretation of imaging modalities, the appropriate surgical approaches, and optimal systemic therapy. For the purpose of the Pediatric and Adolescent Osteosarcoma Symposium in Houston, March 2008, a postal survey was carried out to ascertain current practices regarding the diagnostic and therapeutic aspects in the management of osteosarcoma lung metastases.

D. Carrle (✉)
Pediatrics 5 (Oncology, Haematology, Immunology), Klinikum Stuttgart, Olgahospital, Bismarckstr. 8, D-70176, Stuttgart, Germany
e-mail: coss@olgahospital-stuttgart.de

Postal Survey

Seventeen representatives from international study groups and selected institutions who have published major clinical series on metastatic osteosarcoma in recent years were approached. A 94% response rate was achieved, with 16 out of 17 representatives submitting a completed questionnaire. The results of the survey are shown in Table 1a–1f.

As for the imaging methods used to detect lung metastases, thoracic Computed Tomography (CT) was uniformly applied at initial staging (Table 1a) Its use during routine follow-up varied, however, with CT-scanning being applied by 10 of 16 respondents, while others relied on conventional chest X-ray (with some indicating the use of both methods) (Table 1a). Regarding the size of a lesion considered sufficient to distinguish between benign and of metastatic origin, uniformity was achieved in that lesions of less than 5 mm cannot be reliably classified by imaging. The majority of respondents regarded a lesion size >5 cm as sufficient to be certain of its metastatic origin. One respondent refused to draw any definite conclusion from CT-imaging, regardless of size, as resection of the lesion would always be performed (Table 1c).

Table 1a Survey on the management of pulmonary metastases in osteosarcoma. The number of responses (*n*) amongst the 16 participants in the survey varied with each item questioned. At initial staging which imaging method do you use as part of staging for pulmonary metastases in a patient who presents with osteosarcoma for the first time?

Imaging method	*N*
Chest X-ray	12/15[a]
CT-scan	16/16
FDG-PET	3/12[a]

[a]Reasons for use of FDG-PET were specified: only as part of additional investigation if suspicious findings; within a protocol to evaluate usefulness, not for staging but for response assessment

Table 1b Survey on the management of pulmonary metastases in osteosarcoma. The number of responses (*n*) amongst the 16 participants in the survey varied with each item questioned. At routine follow-up (after completion of therapy for localized osteosarcoma) which imaging methods do you use?

Imaging method	*N*
Chest X-ray	12/15[a]
CT-scan	10/16[a, b]
FDG-PET	1/12[c]

[a]1/16 CT only if chest X-ray abnormal
[b]1/16 baseline CT, further follow-up with CXR
[c]Reasons for use of FDG-PET were specified: only as part of additional investigation if suspicious findings; only if patient has postoperative changes in the chest

Osteosarcoma Lung Metastases Detection and Principles of Multimodal Therapy

Table 1c Survey on the management of pulmonary metastases in osteosarcoma. The number of responses (*n*) amongst the 16 participants in the survey varied with each item questioned. Is CT sufficient to distinguish between a metastases and a benign lesion, depending on the size of the lesion?

Size of lesion	N
>5 cm	12/15[a]
1–4.9 cm	11/15[a]
0.5–0.9 cm	5/16
<0.5 cm	0/15

[a]One respondent added comments like generally or possibly

Table 1d1 Survey on the management of pulmonary metastases in osteosarcoma. The number of responses (*n*) amongst the 16 participants in the survey varied with each item questioned. Imaging findings in situation Tables 1a or 1b are suspicious for lung metastases
Which is the first surgical procedure you recommend?

Method	N
CT-guided biopsy	1/16
Thoracoscopy	2/16
Open Thoracotomy	13/16

Table 1d2 Survey on the management of pulmonary metastases in osteosarcoma. The number of responses (*n*) amongst the 16 participants in the survey varied with each item questioned. Imaging findings in situation Tables 1a or 1b are suspicious for lung metastases. Is manual exploration routinely recommended at thoracotomy?

	N
Yes, Manual exploration	16/16

The vast majority of respondents (81%) would proceed directly to open thoracotomy as the initial therapeutic approach, without performing further diagnostic procedures complementary to the CT-scan (Table 1d1). Manual exploration during thoracotomy was uniformly accepted as standard (Table 1d2). In contrast, the need for exploration of the contralateral side in seemingly unilateral pulmonary disease was not uniformly accepted; approximately one third of the respondents considered unilateral exploration as sufficient (Table 1e).

The approach towards pulmonary metastases, which seemingly disappear during induction chemotherapy, was the most heterogeneous, with half of the respondents preferring surgical exploration and the others supporting a watch and see strategy.

The answers to our survey underlined uniformity in some areas and demonstrated strikingly diverse practices in others. Heterogenous approaches even amongst experts in the field reflect the current lack of evidence regarding practical aspects of management in a rare disease and call for longitudinal research on the clinical efficacy of diagnostic and therapeutic procedures. The results of the survey will be discussed throughout this chapter in their respective contexts.

Table 1e Survey on the management of pulmonary metastases in osteosarcoma. The number of responses (*n*) amongst the 16 participants in the survey varied with each item questioned. A patient with osteosarcoma without prior history of metastatic disease is found to have findings characteristic of lung metastases. If imaging suggests only unilateral involvement, would you routinely recommend surgical exploration of the unaffected side?

	N
Unilateral exploration	6/16[a]
Bilateral exploration	11/16[a]

[a]One respondent indicated both methods, choice of method would depend on duration of relapse-free interval (RFI)

Table 1f Survey on the management of pulmonary metastases in osteosarcoma. The number of responses (*n*) amongst the 16 participants in the survey varied with each item questioned. In case of primary (=synchronous) lung metastases that "disappear" during chemotherapy would you still recommend surgical exploration?

	N
Surgical exploration	8/16[a]
Observation	8/16[a]

[a]One respondent indicated discrepant opinion between oncologist and surgeon: oncologist recommends surgery but surgeons disagree

Table 2a Site of involvement of primary metastases

	COSS[1]	Rizzoli[2]
Sites of involvement	No of patients	No of patients
All metastatic sites	202 (100%)	57 (100%)
Isolated lung mets	124 (61%)	43 (75%)
Combined lung and extrapulmonary mets	40 (20%)	9 (16%)
Isolated extrapulmonary mets	36 (18%)	5 (9%)
Multiple extrapulmonary organs involved	2 (1%)	0 (0%)

Mets Metastases

Location and Frequency of Metastases

Metastatic disease, which is detectable with current imaging methods is present in less than 20% of high-grade osteosarcoma at initial diagnosis. The most frequent site of metastases is the lung, both in case of synchronous (Table 2a)[1,2] and in case of metachronous metastases[3,4] (see Table 2b). However, extrapulmonary involvement is increasingly observed as a second or subsequent recurrence.[5,6]

Table 2b Sites of involvement of recurrent metastases in the COSS-cohort[3]

Sites of involvement	No of patients	% of total no of patients with relapse	% of total no of patients with metastases	% of total no of patients with pulmonary metastases
All recurrences	576	100	–	–
Mets + local relapse	31	5.3	–	–
Local relapse only	44	7.6	–	–
Mets only	501	87.0	100	–
Lung mets	469	81.4	93.6	100
Isolated lung mets	373	64.8	74.4	79.5
Combined lung and extrapulmonary sites	96	16.7	16.7	20.5
Isolated distant bone mets	45	7.8	9.0	–
Distant bone mets	90	15.6	–	–
Other isolated extrapulmonary mets	12	2.1	2.3	–
Extrapulmonary/extraosseous mets	54	9.4	10.7	–
Unilateral lung mets	227	–	–	52.1[a]
Bilateral lung mets	209	–	–	47.9
Laterality unknown	33	–	–	–
Pleural disruption by lung mets	66	–	–	14.1

Mets Metastases

[a] of Patients with known laterality of pulmonary involvement

Role of Imaging in Pulmonary Metastases

CT-Scanning: Possibilities and Limitations

Computed tomography has been the standard imaging modality used to diagnose pulmonary metastases from sarcoma since the 1980s. This is also reflected by the uniform practice of using CT-scanning in the initial staging of osteosarcoma, revealed by our survey. However, limitations of both sensitivity and specifity are well established.[7-10]

While still being the most exact imaging method available, CT does not reliably allow the determination of the number of metastatic lesions: Under- and to a lesser extent, overestimation of their true number compared to intra-operative findings has been reported in several series.[10-13] Poor correlation between CT-findings and histologically confirmed pulmonary metastatic disease continues to be an issue of concern, even in the area of modern CT scanning. This is proven by a recent retrospective study from the Memorial Sloan-Kettering Cancer Center (MSKCC)[14] in which CT-findings in 28 young patients with metastatic osteosarcoma undergoing a total of 54 thoracotomies were compared with findings at thoracotomy. In 19/54 (35%), more histologically proven (viable or non-viable) metastatic lesions were detected than predicted by preoperative CT-scanning. There was concordance with preoperative CT-findings in 15/54 (28%), and, fewer metastases than predicted were found in 20/54 (37%). Of particular concern, is the fact that preoperative CT scanning missed a total of 146 out of 329 (44%) lesions with a possible malignant potential, of which almost two thirds (209) turned out to be osteosarcoma, histologically.[14]

Unfortunately, CT imaging is also not sufficient to distinguish benign from malignant lesions. In a retrospective analysis of 43 children and young adults with presumed unilateral osteosarcoma metastases treated at MSKCC between 1980 and 2002, histology of resected nodules revealed benign lesions in 15 patients.[15] The proportion of patients with benign lesions was even higher in a cooperative Italian/Scandinavian series, with 22 out of 51 patients demonstrated to have a benign histology of all resected lesions. Among some of the other 29 patients of this series who had metastatic nodules, coexistence of malignant and benign lesions was observed.[13] The previously mentioned study from MSKCC performed on osteosarcoma patients treated between 1996 and 2004 showed that, even in the area of modern CT scanning, there continues to be a poor correlation between CT-findings and histologically proven metastatic disease.[14] Histology of benign lung lesions most commonly showed fibrosis, followed by intrapulmonary lymph nodes, normal lung, congestion/hemorrhage, benign calcification, pneumonia/consolidation, abscess, granuloma, and rare findings like old suture material.[14]

The aforementioned retrospective cooperative Italian/Scandinavian series of 119 thoracic CT-scans in 51 patients treated between 1988 and 1997 could not define the safe criteria for distinguishing between metastatic and benign lesions, but demonstrated some tendencies[13]: Benign lesions tended to be smaller (<5 mm) than metastatic nodules; however, there was no size small enough to guarantee a benign histology as 10/25 nodules <5 mm turned out to be metastatic. There was also a tendency for a decreased likelihood of metastases with smaller numbers of nodules, but no number was small enough to rule them out. Four out of 13 patients, who had only a solitary nodule radiologically, had histologically confirmed metastatic disease, whereas all patients with more than seven nodules had metastases.

Changes in CT-morphologic features during chemotherapy are often assumed to predict or exclude metastatic origin (Fig. 1). However, this may be an erroneous assumption. Picci et al[13] analyzed follow-up CTs under chemotherapy in patients who had had abnormal initial scans. Benign nodules had a tendency to retain a constant size and also a stable number. In contrast, change (either increase or decrease) in number or in size of suspicious lesions was more often observed with metastases. However, once again, neither criterion was sensitive or specific enough to allow discrimination between benign and malignant origin.

Therefore, CT provides us with some clues, but not with definitive criteria which would allow for the prediction of the nature of radiomorphologic abnormalities with a reasonable level of certainty.

Nuclear Imaging of Pulmonary Metastases

Bone scintigraphy (with phosphorus compounds labeled with Technetium) is primarily used to detect osseous metastases, but radionuclide uptake may be seen in large osteoblastic pulmonary metastases.[16] However, the technique will not detect small metastases or those that do not produce sufficient amounts of osteoid matrix.

PET-imaging has gained increasing acceptance in tumor imaging, and, with increasing availability of this modality, its clinical value in pulmonary metastatic osteosarcoma needs to be critically assessed. According to our survey, FDG-PET-scanning is still not regarded as a routine method in either staging or follow-up of osteosarcoma.

Published data on the role of FDG-PET scans to detect primary lung metastases is limited. Most series on FDG-PET in sarcoma, due to their wide histological inclusion criteria and the lack of subgroup analyses, do not allow conclusions specific to osteosarcoma.[17–19] To our knowledge, the largest series on pulmonary metastases of osteosarcoma included 32 patients with both synchronous and metachronous lesions from the University Hospital Muenster[20]: Franzius et al retrospectively compared the results of 49 F-18-FDG-PET scans with thoracic spiral CT scans. The sensitivity, specifity, and overall accuracy of F-18-FDG-PET scans for lung metastases were 0.50, 1.00 and 0.92, respectively (on an examination-based analysis). Comparable values for spiral CT were 0.75, 1.00 and 0.96. CT therefore turned out to be superior compared to F-18-FDG-PET. The sensitivity of F-18-FDG-PET was inferior, especially in small lung lesions of ≤9 mm.[20]

Similarly, a lower sensitivity for PET detection of lung metastases compared to chest CT scan was recently described by Völker et al[21] for pediatric sarcoma in general. However, their prospective study of 46 pediatric sarcoma patients included only three patients with pulmonary metastatic osteosarcoma.

Data regarding the role of FDG-PET in the pulmonary follow-up of osteosarcoma is even more scarce. A study, again from Muenster, which compared the ability of FDG-PET to detect recurrances from malignant primary bone tumors, with conventional imaging, included 13 patients with pulmonary/pleural metastases in recurrent Ewing tumors or osteosarcoma. An inferior sensitivity of FDG-PET to detect pulmonary recurrances (0.85) was observed compared to CT-scans (0.1).[22]

Iaguru et al[19] compared the detection rate of pulmonary metastases by F-18-FDG-PET with that of thoracic CT-scans in 40 patients with bone resp. soft tissue sarcoma at initial staging and during routine follow-up. Sensitivity and specifity were 0.68 and 0.98 for PET and 0.95 and 0.92 for CT. The inferior performance of PET compared with chest CT for detection of sub-centrimetric pulmonary nodules, as noticed in this study and others, should be expected in view of the physical limitations of spatial resolution inherent to most current PET-scanners. However, the inferiority of PET for lesions sized >1 cm was somewhat unexpected, and differences in biological behavior between metastases and PET-avid primary tumors were discussed. Potential explanations for the limited sensitivity of FDG-PET include partial volume effects because of the small size of metastases,[23] blurring of lesions caused by breathing, different expressions of glucose transporter proteins in metastases and primary tumors, and a location close to the myocardium with its physiologically high glucose metabolism.[19,20]

In summary, there is no optimal imaging method available which reliably detects or excludes pulmonary metastases from osteosarcoma. Despite technological advances and despite the introduction of new imaging modalities, thoracic CT-scanning remains the most reliable imaging tool. Awareness of the limitations of imaging in general, and of CT in particular, has major implications for surgical strategies.

Implications of Imaging on Therapy

Manual Exploration Mandatory

Patients with metastatic osteosarcoma will only be cured if all metastases are removed during surgery.[1,3,24–26] As imaging is not sensitive enough to detect all lesions, careful and thorough manual palpation of the lungs has become the standard intraoperative approach in pulmonary metastasectomy for various underlying histologies[27,28] and particularly for osteosarcoma,[27,29,30] where the presence of osteoid resulting in a "grain of salt"-like consistency facilitates the palpation even of very small nodules. According to our survey, this method is uniformly recommended by international study groups and specialized centers (Table 1d2).

No Role for Thoracoscopy

According to our survey, there is little if any role for thoracoscopic interventions when it comes to removing pulmonary osteosarcoma metastases. Only two institutions indicated that thoracoscopy might be the first surgical procedure in suspicious lesions, whereas thoracotomy with manual exploration was advocated by all the remaining participants except for one (Table 1d1).

McCormack et al[31] have prospectively evaluated the role of video-assisted thoracoscopy (VATS) in the resection of pulmonary metastases. Due to a 56% failure rate of the VATS-intervention compared with thoracotomy, their study was terminated early. In 14 of the 18 patients studied, additional lesions (proving to be malignant in ten patients) were detected when VATS was followed by thoracotomy. The major downside of this technique was that metastases escaping detection by preoperative CT-scan were subsequently not visualized even during thoracoscopy, consequently not offering the option of manual lung palpation. Hence complete resection, though of utmost prognostic importance, was impeded. Similarly, Castagnetti et al[32] described a low detection rate of pulmonary metastases by thoracoscopy in ten patients undergoing thoracoscopy for metastatic osteosarcoma. Non-visualization of lesions which had been clearly detected on CT-scans was again reported.

Thoracoscopy does not allow to visualize deep seated metastases. As evidenced by Kayton et al's[14] CT analysis of 183 lesions, only one third are pleural-based or abutting the pleura, while almost half of all lesions are located at least 5 mm away from the closest pleural surface, thereby evading detection by thoracoscopy.

Another concern in the use of VATS-procedures for metastasectomy is the risk of port-site seeding.[33] Several mechanisms have been implicated, including direct contact of the chest wall with tumor during extraction, disruption of tumor and contamination of instruments, transtumoral dissection, and leaving contaminated fluid inside the chest cavity at the end of the procedure.

Approach to Unilateral Disease

About 1/3 of the institutions and study groups represented in our survey reported withholding from exploration of the contralateral side in patients with radiographic evidence of unilateral pulmonary involvement only (Table 1e). Different approaches towards unilateral lung disease are also manifest from published series on metastastic osteosarcoma from different groups and institutions, either favoring unilateral[10,11,34,35] or bilateral exploration.[2,7,15] Information on the side of subsequent relapse after unilateral thoracotomy is available from several reports: In a series from the Mayo Clinic and Seattle,[10] only 2 of 23 patients with antecedent unilateral thoracotomy relapsed on the contralateral and 11 on the ipsilateral side. In the Rizzoli series[35] of 94 patients, a unilateral surgical approach was pursued. The side of subsequent relapse was contralateral in half of all patients.

In the other half, the lungs were either affected ipsi- or bilaterally. Since the exact proportion of patients with ipsilateral relapse was not reported, an estimation on how many relapses might have been prevented by contralateral exploration is not possible.

In contrast to the publications discussed above, which would favor unilateral surgery, others point towards potential benefits of bilateral approaches even in seemingly unilateral disease. For example, eight of ten patients who relapsed after unilateral lung surgery in a series reported by Saeter et al[11] developed their recurrences in the contralateral lung. Also, at MSKCC,[15] seven of nine patients with seemingly unilateral early metastatic recurrences (i.e., occurring within 2 years of diagnosis of osteosarcoma) were later proven to have bilateral involvement: Bilateral exploration led to the detection in six patients, whereas contralateral involvement became evident by a subsequent relapse occurring within a year, in one patient. In contrast, only one of five patients with unilateral late metastases subsequently developed a contralateral relapse.[15]

Two recent studies reported non-detection of contralateral pulmonary metastases by CT-imaging: Among three thoracotomies performed at the MSKCC in patients with unilateral involvement, one revealed osteosarcoma on the contralateral lung despite negative CT-imaging.[14] In a larger, though more unselected cohort with a wide spectrum of malignant diseases, 23% of a total of 13 patients with unilateral metastases as determined by helical CT-scan were found to have contralateral metastases upon palpation during thoracotomy.[28]

In summary, the rationale for bilateral exploration in seemingly unilateral disease stems from the limited sensitivity of imaging methods and from follow-up data of patients developing contralateral disease after unilateral thoracotomy.

Approach to Lesions "Disappearing" During Chemotherapy

In our survey, the approach towards synchronous pulmonary metastases which seemed to disappear during induction chemotherapy was anything but uniform and opinions were equally divided between a surgical and a watch and wait strategy (Table 1f). In several studies, surgical resection was not performed in such situations[8,26,36,37] In contrast, a more aggressive surgical approach has been advocated by others.[12,30,38] In an Italian report of 26 patients undergoing complete metastasectomy, the number of lesions detected by CT had decreased by 73 during preoperative chemotherapy. However, the amount of resected lesions ($n=191$) outranged both the number detected on the preoperative scans ($n=93$) and the amount suggested by the initial scans ($n=169$). Even the number of histologically proven metastases among the 191 resected lesions ($n=140$) was higher than the estimate from the preoperative scan.[2] In the recent series from MSKCC, three of three patients who underwent thoracotomy despite seemingly complete disappearance of lung lesions on preoperative CT-scans had histological evidence of osteosarcoma in the resected specimens.[14]

Treatment and Outcome of Primary Pulmonary Metastases

Survival Probability with Multimodal Therapy

Some reports have specifically addressed treatment and outcome of primary pulmonary metastatic disease. Table 3a summarizes the survival rates obtained in some recent studies.[1,25,26,39–41] In most series, survival data was given for isolated lung disease; survival data for combined lung metastases (i.e., lung plus extrapulmonary metastases) was rarely available. To our knowledge, the largest series on patients with primary pulmonary metastases (isolated or combined) is the one of 164 consecutive Cooperative Osteosarcoma Study Group (COSS) patients.[1] In this study, the 5-year overall survival expectancy for 124 patients whose metastases were limited to the lungs and for 40 patients with combined lung metastases were 33% and 20%, respectively. Reported survival probabilities in other series have ranged widely,[25,41] probably due to low patient numbers, differences in the length of follow-up, and heterogeneous selection criteria.

Tumor-Related Prognostic Factors in Primary Pulmonary Metastases

It is important to understand the impact of various tumor characteristics on prognosis, particularly those which will influence the therapeutic approach. For one, a strong correlation between the type of lung involvement as well as the number of metastases and prognosis is evident. Unilateral disease is associated with a better prognosis than bilateral involvement both when metastatic disease is confined to the lung[1,12,24,26] and also when additional extrapulmonary metastases are present.[1] A low number of metastases was associated with superior outcomes in several studies[1,8,12,25,26,41] even though different cut-offs for the number of nodules were applied.

Table 3a Survival in patients with primary pulmonary dissemination as only metastatic site

Author	N	N (isolated lung metastases)	Survival			
			EFS		OAS	
Bacci et al, 2000[41]	28	28	2 years	36%	2 years	53%
Daw et al, 2006[26]	25	23	NA		5 years	26%
Goorin et al, 2002[39]	35	28	NA		2 years	52%
Kager et al, 2003[1]	164	124	5 years	19%	5 years	33%
Marina et al, 1992[40]	31	18	NA		3 years	50%
					4 years	30%
Tsuchiya, 2002[25]	46	46	NA		5 years	18%

The best prognostic subgroup seems to consist of patients with solitary lung metastases,[1] who may enjoy survival expectancies very similar to those of patients with seemingly localized disease.

Rationale for Surgery in Primary Pulmonary Metastases

Complete surgical resection of all malignant lesions has consistently been shown to be of paramount prognostic importance in osteosarcoma; consequently, an aggressive surgical approach must also be pursued in primary metastatic disease. In our COSS series, patients with residual (macroscopic) tumor burden had a fivefold increased risk of dying compared to those in whom a complete surgical resection was achieved. In that series, no patient was alive beyond 5 years without complete surgery.[1] Other series of primary osteosarcoma metastases to the lung[24–26] confirm the outstanding prognostic importance of complete surgical resection also evident from series on primary metastatic osteosarcoma in general[1,2,24,37] For instance, Daw et al[26] analyzed the impact of surgical remission in a group of 21 patients with pulmonary metastases only and found a significant survival benefit for the ten patients in whom surgical remission was achieved (5-year survival 40.0 vs. 0%; $p=0.005$). Aggressive thoracotomy thus plays a critical role in any curative approach for primary pulmonary metastatic osteosarcoma and should be attempted whenever complete resection seems at least a remote possibility. Such an approach should not be limited by sheer number or by a large size of pulmonary lesions.

Role of Chemotherapy in Primary Metastases

Introduction of chemotherapy into the therapeutic concept of localized osteosarcoma has dramatically improved long-term outcome and, today, chemotherapy is an essential component of multimodal treatment. Based on an observed association of metastatic disease with shorter pre-diagnostic symptom duration, Bacci et al[42] have speculated that different biologic behavior of primary metastatic osteosarcoma rather than the extent of disease might account for a decreased susceptibility to treatment and hence, poor prognosis. This hypothesis was not substantiated by data from a large cohort from our COSS-group,[43] where primary metastatic disease was associated with prolonged symptom duration before diagnosis, as well as with large size of the primary tumor, both indicators of advanced disease.[43] Identical age and sex distribution as well as identical response rates to induction chemotherapy again argued against basic biological differences between primary metastatic and seemingly localized osteosarcoma.[43] Histologic response is a key prognostic factor distinguishing itself in a long-term survival difference of approximately 25%.[43]

Osteosarcoma Lung Metastases Detection and Principles of Multimodal Therapy 177

Interestingly, a good histological response of the primary tumor predicts better outcomes not only in localized disease, but also in primary metastatic osteosarcoma, as evidenced by data both from the MSKCC[24] and from COSS.[1] The fact that patients with synchronous metastases obviously benefit from a good response to chemotherapy is a strong argument for the up-front use of first line chemotherapeutic agents with proven efficacy against osteosarcoma. If this holds true, the use of upfront-window experimental treatment with unproven efficacy in patients with resectable metastatic osteosarcoma, as suggested by some investigators[24,25] might not be beneficial.

In summary, approximately half of those patients with primary metastatic osteosarcoma in whom an aggressive surgical approach results in successful removal of all tumor deposits and who also receive state-of-the-art chemotherapy can become long-term survivors. The inferior cure rate of primary metastatic compared to localized disease cannot be attributed to ineffective chemotherapy alone, but relates to the technical challenges of complete surgical resection of all disease manifestations.

Pulmonary Metastases at Recurrence

Survival

Combined modality therapy in osteosarcoma results in disease-free survival rates of 65–70%.[44] Distant recurrence of osteosarcoma remains the primary cause of treatment failure, with the lung being the most frequent site of relapse. Reported survival rates in relapsed osteosarcoma as reported in series including all sites of relapse have varied widely – probably because of variations in inclusion criteria – from 20%[45] to 36% after 3 years[46] (see Table 3b[3,6,10,34,45–49,58]). In a selected cohort of 36 patients who did not receive chemotherapy for primary disease, the 2-year survival probability was even 65%.[49] Most series dedicated to pulmonary recurrences originate from the surgical literature and – with few exceptions – suffer from an inherent selection bias in that only patients advancing to the surgical department were included and poor-risk patients with extensive disease were thus underrepresented.[50–57] Survival data of large cohorts of unselected patients with recurrent osteosarcoma might give a more balanced view on the outlook of patients with pulmonary relapse: Overall survival rates at 5 and at 10 years were 23% and 18%, respectively, in the COSS series including 576 first recurrences.[3] In the subgroup of 373 patients with metastases limited to the lungs, 2 and 5-year survival rates were 38% and 28%, respectively. Several publications report on patients who achieved surgical remissions and survived several re-recurrences.[5,6,10,11,35,46,47,59] In an unselected cohort of 249 affected COSS-patients, the 5-year overall survival after the second and subsequent (up to the fifth) relapse ranged from 13% to 18%.[5]

Table 3b Survival in patients recurrent osteosarcoma

Authors	N	All recurrences Outcome EFS		OAS		N	Pulmonary metastases only Outcome EFS		OAS	
Bacci et al, 2005[6]	235	5 y	28%	5 y	29%	202[a]	5 y	30%	NA	
Chou et al, 2005[48]	43	3 y	14%	3 y	35%	22	NA		NA	
Crompton et al, 2006[47]	37[b]	10 y	15%			25	NA		NA	
Duffaud et al, 2003[59]	33	NA		3 y	32%	24	NA		3 y	38%
				5 y	24%				5 y	28%
Fagioli et al, 2002[45]	32	3 y	12%	3 y	20%	26	NA		NA	
Ferrari et al, 2003[58]	162	5 y	16%	3 y	33%	125	5 y	18%	5 y	33%
				5 y	28%					
Goorin et al, 1984[34]	41	NA		NA		32	NA		5 y	32%
Goorin et al, 1991[49]	52	NA		NA		43	NA		NA	
	26[c]	NA		2 y	25%	NA	NA		NA	
	26[d]	NA		2 y	65%					
Hawkins and Arndt, 2003[10]	59	4 y	6%	4 y	23%	36	4 y	7%	4 y	28%
Kempf-Bielack et al, 2005[3]	576	NA		5 y	23%	373	NA		2 y	38%
				10 y	18%				5 y	28%
Saeter et al, 1995[11]	60[e]	NA		5 y	24%	NA				
Tabone et al, 1994[46]	42	2 y	38%	2 y	43%	20	NA		2 y	48%
		3 y	27%	3 y	36%				3 y	40%

Data of oncology series of recent years
[a]Lung combined with extra-pulmonary metastases
[b]Localized disease at initial presentation
[c]With primary chemotherapy
[d]No primary chemotherapy
[e]Metastases only

Prognostic Factors in Pulmonary Recurrence

In the COSS-series, risk factors predicting outcome of recurrent osteosarcoma included the interval from diagnosis of primary disease to relapse (time to relapse), the number of metastatic lesions, bilateral pulmonary involvement and the presence of pleural disruption, e.g., lung metastases extending by contiguous growth into the pleural cavity, the chest wall, diaphragm or mediastinum, or causing malignant pleural effusion.[3] Prognostic significance of the number of metastatic pulmonary nodules with different cutoffs[6,10,25,57,58] – and a significantly inferior outcome with bilateral pulmonary metastases compared to unilateral involvement[10,57,58] have also been reported by others. The interval to relapse was shown to correlate with prognosis in several other studies[6,10,25,48,52,58,59] while yet others were not able to detect such a correlation.[11,46,49,51,57]

In case of multiple relapse, the interval to the subsequent relapse again seems to correlate with outcome.[5] A high number of metastases in second relapse was a negative prognostic factor detected by multivariate analysis in the COSS-cohort.[5] The location and number of lesions cannot be viewed independently from resectability, which, like in primary metastatic disease is the most important treatment related risk factor as evidenced below.

Treatment and Prognosis of Metachronous Pulmonary Metastases

Surgery in Relapsed Osteosarcoma

In the COSS-experience, long-term survival was exclusively seen among patients who achieved a second surgical remission.[3] Upon multivariate analysis, failure to operate was the strongest negative prognostic factor for the entire cohort (with a relative risk (RR) of 4.97 for OAS (overall survival) in patients not undergoing surgery) and retained significance even in patients who did not achieve a second surgical complete remission (RR 1.81 for OAS). Surgical remission also correlated with survival in multiple smaller series and the inability to achieve second complete remission (CR) was associated with exceptionally poor outcomes, with OAS of maximally 5–8[25] but mostly 0%.[6,10,11,46,48,58,59] Surgical remission continues to be a prognostic factor of striking importance in subsequent relapses.[5,6]

Aggressive surgery therefore, is once again unanimously accepted as an essential component of curative treatment.

Second Line Chemotherapy in Relapsed Osteosarcoma

The benefit of second line chemotherapy in relapsed osteosarcoma is far less well established than the role of surgery. Hawkins and Arndt[10] analyzed the outcome of

30 patients with isolated pulmonary metastases who achieved a second complete surgical remission. In univariate analysis, a trend towards improved survival was shown for 15 patients treated with surgery alone compared to 15 patients receiving a combination of surgery and chemotherapy (45% vs. 13% $p=0.008$). In their study, chemotherapy had generally been reserved for patients with unresectable recurrent tumors or – at the discretion of the treating physician – for patients with early or multifocal disease recurrences, a strong selection bias in allocation of chemotherapy for patients with unfavorable prognostic factors. Ferrari et al[58] observed a significant correlation between the use of second line chemotherapy and prolonged survival in a subgroup of 48 patients who had unresectable relapsed osteosarcomas, OAS for 14 patients receiving chemotherapy was 53% at 1 year, compared to 12% for those 34 not treated with chemotherapy. However, no patient was alive at 2 years in either cohort. Interestingly, the authors could not demonstrate a correlation between the use of chemotherapy and outcome in patients who had achieved a second CR. Caution in the interpretation of this finding will take into account a bias to use chemotherapy more frequently in patients with unfavorable disease characteristics, including short relapse free interval, higher number of metastatic lesions, or involvement of extrapulmonary sites.

Saeter et al[11] from the Norwegian Radium Hospital reported improved survival with the use of "adequate" (i.e., based on drugs not used in first line therapy) second line chemotherapy irrespective of surgical treatment. Upon univariate analysis, the 5-year OAS of 60 patients differed significantly between 25 undergoing such chemotherapy and 35 receiving inadequate or no systemic treatment. However, again, in the subgroup of 30 patients who achieved a second complete surgical remission no effect of chemotherapy was evident.[11] Multivariate analysis of the COSS data showed an association with improved survival and the use of second line chemotherapy in all patients with relapse (5-year OAS 25% vs. 22%) (multivariate analysis relative risk (RR) for OAS 1.40; $p=0.007$) as well as in the subgroup not achieving a second CR (1-year OAS 28% vs. 16%; 2-year OAS 4% vs. 2%) (RR 1.53 for OAS; $p=0.025$). Somewhat in contrast to the smaller series described above, better event-free (EFS) survival with chemotherapy was also observed in the subgroup achieving a second surgical CR (2-year EFS 34% vs. 30%, 5-year EFS 22% vs. 20%) (RR for EFS 1.50; $p=0.007$). These findings would suggest an adjuvant – albeit (admittedly) rather limited – adjuvant effect of second line chemotherapy, even in heavily pretreated patients.

In the search for useful therapeutic strategies, high-dose chemotherapy with stem cell rescue was investigated in osteosarcoma with adverse prognostic features. However, several series have failed to detect any beneficial effect on survival in relapsed and in primary metastatic disease.[45,60,61] Hence, this practice has been largely abandoned.

In summary, there is agreement that the efficacy of current second line chemotherapy is, at best, very limited. Patients who fail to achieve a second surgical remission seem to live a few months longer with chemotherapy. Those who receive chemotherapy in conjunction with complete surgical removal of the recurrence may or may not benefit.

Summary and Perspectives for the Future

Computed tomography of the chest remains the method of choice to detect pulmonary metastases from osteosarcoma, even though it is far from being perfectly suited to meet the challenge. Thoracic surgery must include manual exploration, and we would recommend operation even in cases of questionable lesions, and to reoperate, if necessary several times, if there was any doubt about having left, even a single questionable nodule behind.

Efforts to improve outcomes should focus on optimizing imaging methods, on further refinements in surgical strategies and on the improvement of chemotherapeutic regimens. There is a dire need for additional effective agents. Due to the rarity of the disease large scale multinational trials will be required to determine their true value for patients with metastatic osteosarcoma.

Participants of the Survey Agreed to their Names Being Published

Mark Bernstein; Children's Oncology Group; Halifax, Canada
Stefan Bielack; Cooperative Osteosarcoma Study Group, Stuttgart, Germany
Laurence Brugieres; Société Française de lutte contre les Cancers de l'Enfant et de l'adolescent, Villejuif, France
Najat Daw; St. Jude's Hospital; Memphis, USA
Stefano Ferrari; Instituto Ortopedico Rizzoli, Bologna, Italy

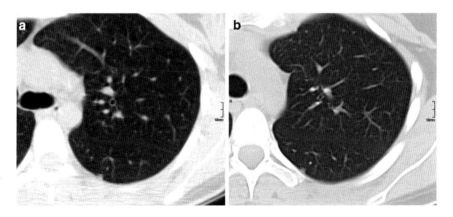

Fig. 1 (courtesy of Prof. P. Winkler, Olgahospital Stuttgart, Prof. I. Arlat Katharinenthospital Stuttgart and Dr. M. Schilling Radiologische Praxis, Stuttgart-Bad Canstatt): Computed tomographic image of the chest showing a small lung lesion (a) at initial staging and (b) 9 1/2 months later, after completion of chemotherapy in a 17 year old female patient with osteosarcoma of the right proximal tibia. The small lesion remained unchanged during chemotherapy. Histology confirmed its metastatic origin.

Allen Goorin; Dana-Faber Cancer Institut, Boston, MA, USA
Norman Jaffe; Divison of Pediatrics, M.D. Anderson Cancer Center, Houston, USA
Neyssa Marina; Children's Oncology Group; Stanford,USA
Paul Meyers; Memorial Sloan-Kettering Cancer Center, New York USA
Shreyaskumar Patel; The Sarcoma Center, M.D. Anderson Cancer Center, Houston,USA
Luis Sierrasesumaga Ariznavarreta; Department of Pediatrics, University Clinic of Navarra, Pamplona, Spain
Sigbjorn Smeland/Kirsten S. Hall; Scandinavian Sarcoma Group; Oslo, Norway
Hiroyuki Tsuchiya, H. Kanazawa; Japan
Jeremy Whelan; University College of London, London; UK

References

1. Kager L, Zoubek A, Pötschger U, et al. Primary metastatic osteosarcoma: Presentation and outcome of patients treated on neoadjuvant Cooperative Osteosarcoma Study Group protocols. *J Clin Oncol.* 2003;21:2011-2018.
2. Bacci G, Briccoli A, Rocca M, et al. Neoadjuvant chemotherapy for osteosarcoma of the extremities with metastases at presentation: Recent experience at the Rizzoli Institute in 57 patients treated with cisplatin, doxorubicin, and a high dose of methotrexate and ifosfamide. *Ann Oncol.* 2003;14:1126-1134.
3. Kempf-Bielack B, Bielack SS, Jürgens H, et al. Osteosarcoma relapse after combined modality therapy: An analysis of unselected patients in the Cooperative Osteosarcoma Study Group (COSS). *J Clin Oncol.* 2005;23:559-568.
4. Chi SN, Conklin LS, Qin J, et al. The patterns of relapse in osteosarcoma: The Memorial Sloan-Kettering experience. *Pediatr Blood Cancer.* 2004;42:46-51.
5. Bielack SS Kempf-Bielack B, Branscheid D, et al. Second and subsequent recurrences of osteosarcoma: Presentation, treatment, and outcomes of 249 consecutive Cooperative Osteosarcoma Study Group (COSS) patients. J Clin Oncol 2009; 27:557-65.
6. Bacci G, Briccoli A, Longhi A, et al. Treatment and outcome of recurrent osteosarcoma: Experience at Rizzoli in 235 patients initially treated with neoadjuvant chemotherapy. *Acta Oncol.* 2005;44:748-755.
7. Pastorino U, Gasparini M, Tavecchio L, et al. The contribution of salvage surgery to the management of childhood osteosarcoma. *J Clin Oncol.* 1991;9:1357-1362.
8. Kaste SC, Pratt CB, Cain AM, et al. Metastases detected at the time of diagnosis of primary pediatric extremity osteosarcoma at diagnosis: Imaging features. *Cancer.* 1999;86(8):1602-1608.
9. McCarville MB, Kaste SC, Cain AM, et al. Prognostic factors and imaging patterns of recurrent pulmonary nodules after thoracotomy in children with osteosarcoma. *Cancer.* 2001;91(6):1170-1176.
10. Hawkins DS, Arndt CA. Pattern of disease recurrence and prognostic factors in patients with osteosarcoma treated with contemporary chemotherapy. *Cancer.* 2003;98:2447-2456.
11. Saeter G, Høie J, Stenwig AE, et al. Systemic relapse of patients with osteogenic sarcoma. Prognostic factors for long term survival. *Cancer.* 1995;75:1084-1093.
12. Harris MB, Gieser P, Goorin AM, et al. Treatment of metastatic osteosarcoma at diagnosis: A Pediatric Oncology Group Study. *J Clin Oncol.* 1998;16:3641-3648.
13. Picci P, Vanel D, Briccoli A, et al. Computed tomography of pulmonary metastases from osteosarcoma: the less poor technique. A study of 51 patients with histological correlation. *Ann Oncol.* 2001;12:1601-1604.
14. Kayton ML, Huvos AG, Casher J, et al. Computer tomographic scan of chest underestimates the number of metastatic lesions in osteosarcoma. *J Ped Surg.* 2006;41:200-206.

Osteosarcoma Lung Metastases Detection and Principles of Multimodal Therapy 183

15. Su WT, Chewning J, Abramson S, et al. Surgical management and outcome of osteosarcoma patients with unilateral pulmonary metastases. *J Pediatr Surg.* 2004;39:418-423.
16. Brady AP, Ennis JT. The scintigraphic detection of ossific mediastinal and pulmonary metastases in osteosarcoma. *Br J Radiol.* 1990;63:978-980.
17. Garcia J, Kim E, Wong F, et al. Comparison of Fluorine – 18-FDG PET and Technetium-99 m-MIBI SPECT in Evaluation of Musculoskeletal Sarcomas. *J Nucl Med.* 1996;37:1476-1479.
18. Arush M, Israel O, Postovsky S, et al. PET/CT with 18FDG in the dectection of local recurrence and distant metastases in Pediatric Saracoma. *Ped Blood Cancer.* 2007;49:901-905.
19. Iagaru A, Chawla S, Menendez L, et al. 18-FDG-PET and PET/CT for detection of pulmonary metastases from musculoskeletal sarcomas. *Nucl Med Commun.* 2006;27:795-802.
20. Franzius C, Daldrup-Link HE, Sciuk J, et al. FDG-PET for pulmonary metastases from malignant primary bone tumors: Comparison with spiral CT. *Ann Onc.* 2001;12:479-486.
21. Völker T, Denecke T, Steffen I, et al. Positron emission tomography for staging of pediatric sarcoma patients: Results of a prospective multicenter trial. *J Clin Oncol.* 2007;25:5435-5441.
22. Franzius C, Daldrup-Link HE, Wagner-Bohn A, Sciuk J, et al. FDG-PET for detection of recurrences from malignant primary bone tumors: Comparison with conventional imaging. *Ann Oncol.* 2002;13(1):157-160.
23. Soret M, Bacharach S, Buvat I. Partial volume effect in PET tumor imaging. *J Nucl Med.* 2007;48:932-945.
24. Meyers PA, Heller G, Healey JH, et al. Osteogenic sarcoma with clinically detectable metastasis at initial presentation. *J Clin Oncol.* 1993;11:449-453.
25. Tsuchiya H, Kanazawa Y, Abdel-Wanis ME, et al. Effect of timing of pulmonary metastases identification on prognosis of patients with osteosarcoma: The Japanese Musculoskeletal Oncology Group study. *J Clin Oncol.* 2002;20:3470-3477.
26. Daw NC, Billups CA, Rodriguez-Galindo C, et al. Metastatic osteosarcoma. *Cancer.* 2006;106:403-412.
27. Rusch VW. Surgical techniques for pulmonary metastasectomy. *Sem Thoracic Cardiovasc Surg.* 2002;14:4-9.
28. Parsons AM, Ennis EK, Yankaskas BC, Parker LA Jr, Hyslop WB, Detterbeck FC. Helical computed tomography inaccuracy in the detection of pulmonary metastases: Can it be improved. *Ann Thorac Surg.* 2007;84(6):1830-1836.
29. La Quaglia MP. Osteosarcoma. Specific tumor management and results. *Chest Surg Clin N Am.* 1998;8:77-95.
30. Picci P. Osteosarcoma (osteogenic sarcoma). *Orphanet J Rare Dis.* 2007;2:6.
31. McCormack PM, Bains MS, Begg CB, et al. Role of video-assisted thoracic surgery in the treatment of pulmonary metastases: Results of a prospective trial. *Ann Thorac Surg.* 1996;62(1):213-216.
32. Castagnetti M, Delarue A, Gentet JC. Optimizing the surgical management of lung nodules in children with osteosarcoma: Thoracoscopy for biopsies, thoracotomy for resections. *Surg Endosc.* 2004;18:1668-1671.
33. Sartorelli KH, Partrick D, Meagher DP. Port-site recurrence after thoracoscopic resection of pulmonary metastasis owing to osteogenic sarcoma. *J Pediatr Surg.* 1996;31:1443-1444.
34. Goorin AM, Delorey MJ, Lack EE, et al. Prognostic significance of complete surgical resection of pulmonary metastases in patients with osteogenic sarcoma: Analysis of 32 patients. *J Clin Oncol.* 1984;2(5):425-431.
35. Briccoli A, Rocca M, Salone M, et al. Resection of recurrent pulmonary metastases in patients with osteosarcoma. *Cancer.* 2005;104:1721-1725.
36. Bacci G, Mercuri M, Briccoli A, et al. Osteogenic sarcoma of the extremity with detectable lung metastases at presentation. Results of treatment of 23 patients with chemotherapy followed by simultaneous resection of primary and metastatic lesions. *Cancer.* 1997;79:245-254.
37. Mialou V, Philip T, Kalifa C, et al. Metastatic osteosarcoma at diagnosis: Prognostic factors and long-term outcome – the French pediatric experience. *Cancer.* 2005;104:1100-1109.
38. Ward WG, Mikaelian K, Dorey F, et al. Pulmonary metastases of stage IIB extremity osteosarcoma and subsequent pulmonary metastases. *J Clin Oncol.* 1994;12:1849-1858.

39. Goorin AM, Harris MB, Bernstein M, et al. Phase II/III trial of etoposide and high-dose ifosfamide in newly diagnosed metastatic osteosarcoma: A pediatric oncology group trial. *J Clin Oncol*. 2002;20:426-433.
40. Marina NM, Pratt CB, Rao BN, et al. Improved prognosis of children with osteosarcoma metastatic to the lung(s) at the time of diagnosis. *Cancer*. 1992;70:2722-2727.
41. Bacci G, Ruggieri P, Bertoni F, et al. Local and systemic control for osteosarcoma of the extremity treated with neoadjuvant chemotherapy and limb salvage surgery: The Rizzoli experience. *Oncol Rep*. 2000;7:1129-1133.
42. Bacci G, Ferrari S, Longhi A, et al. High-grade osteosarcoma of the extremity: Differences between localized and metastatic tumors at presentation. *J Pediatr Hematol Oncol*. 2002;24:27-30.
43. Bielack SS, Kempf-Bielack B, Delling G, et al. Prognostic factors in high-grade osteosarcoma of the extremities or trunk: An analysis of 1,702 patients treated on neoadjuvant cooperative osteosarcoma study group protocols. *J Clin Oncol*. 2002;20:776-790.
44. Bielack SS, Machatschek JN, Flege S, et al. Delaying surgery with chemotherapy for osteosarcoma of the extremities. *Expert Opin Pharmacother*. 2004;5:1243-1256.
45. Fagioli F, Aglietta M, Tienghi A, et al. High-dose chemotherapy in the treatment of relapsed osteosarcoma: An Italian Sarcoma Group Study. *J Clin Oncol*. 2002;20:2150-2156.
46. Tabone MD, Kalifa C, Rodary C, et al. Osteosarcoma recurrences in pediatric patients previously treated with intensive chemotherapy. *J Clin Oncol*. 1994;12:2614-2620.
47. Crompton BD, Goldsby RE, Weinberg VK, et al. Survival after recurrence of osteosarcoma: A 20-year experience at a single institution. *Pediatr Blood Cancer*. 2006;47:255-259.
48. Chou AJ, Merola PR, Wexler LH, et al. Treatment of osteosarcoma at first recurrence after contemporary therapy: The Memorial Sloan-Kettering Cancer Center experience. *Cancer*. 2005;104:2214-2221.
49. Goorin AM, Shuster JJ, Baker A, et al. Changing pattern of pulmonary metastases with adjuvant chemotherapy in patients with osteosarcoma: Results from the multiinstitutional osteosarcoma study. *J Clin Oncol*. 1991;9:600-605.
50. Antunes M, Bernardo J, Salete M, et al. Excision of pulmonary metastases of osteogenic sarcoma of the limbs. *Eur J Cardiothorac Surg*. 1999;15:592-596.
51. Roth JA, Putnam JB Jr, Wesley MN, et al. Differing determinants of prognosis following resection of pulmonary metastases from osteogenic and soft tissue sarcoma patients. *Cancer*. 1985;55:1361-1366.
52. Han MT, Telander RL, Pairolero PC, et al. Aggressive thoracotomy for pulmonary metastatic osteogenic sarcoma in children and young adolescents. *J Pediatr Surg*. 1981;16:928-933.
53. Al-Jilaihawi AN, Bullimore J, Mott M, et al. Combined chemotherapy and surgery for pulmonary metastases from osteogenic sarcoma. Results of 10 years experience. *Eur J Cardiothorac Surg*. 1988;2:37-42.
54. Snyder CL, Saltzman DA, Ferrell KL, et al. A new approach to the resection of pulmonary osteosarcoma metastases. Results of aggressive metastasectomy. *Clin Orthop Relat Res*. 1991;270:247-253.
55. Heij HA, Vos A, de Kraker J, et al. Prognostic factors in surgery for pulmonary metastases in children. *Surgery*. 1994;115:687-693.
56. Temeck BK, Wexler LH, Steinberg SM, et al. Metastasectomy for sarcomatous pediatric histologies: Results and prognostic factors. *Ann Thorac Surg*. 1995;59:1385-1389.
57. Meyer WH, Schell MJ, Kumar AP, et al. Thoracotomy for pulmonary metastatic osteosarcoma. An analysis of prognostic indicators of survival. *Cancer*. 1987;59:374-379.
58. Ferrari S, Briccoli A, Mercuri M, et al. Postrelapse survival in osteosarcoma of the extremities: Prognostic factors for long-term survival. *J Clin Oncol*. 2003;21:710-715.
59. Duffaud F, Digue L, Mercier C, et al. Recurrences following primary osteosarcoma in adolescents and adults previously treated with chemotherapy. *Eur J Cancer*. 2003;39:2050-2057.
60. Sauerbrey A, Bielack S, Kempf-Bielack B, et al. High-dose chemotherapy (HDC) and autologous hematopoietic stem cell transplantation (ASCT) as salvage therapy for relapsed osteosarcoma. *Bone Marrow Transplant*. 2001;27:933-937.
61. Janinis J, McTiernan A, Driver D, et al. A pilot study of short-course intensive multiagent chemotherapy in metastatic and axial skeletal osteosarcoma. *Ann Onc*. 2002;13:1935-1944.

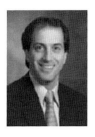

Surgical Treatment of Pulmonary Metastases from Osteosarcoma in Pediatric and Adolescent Patients

Matthew Steliga and Ara Vaporciyan

Osteosarcoma is the most common primary bone malignancy in the United States, comprising approximately 56% of the primary bone tumors.[1,2] Most patients present with local disease; their treatment is outlined in greater detail elsewhere in this book. However, 10–20% of patients diagnosed with osteosarcoma will have radiographic evidence of synchronous isolated pulmonary metastases at the time of initial presentation. Of the patients without synchronous pulmonary metastases, 40–55% will develop metachronous pulmonary metastases.[3–5]

Resection of isolated pulmonary metastases from osteosarcoma is a treatment option which has been shown to correlate with survival benefit and cure in select individuals. These patients are best addressed in a multidisciplinary fashion, with the involvement of a thoracic surgeon with experience in pulmonary metastasectomy. A proper evaluation and thorough preoperative testing is crucial to select those who may derive benefit from surgical resection.

This chapter will discuss the historical background of pulmonary metastasectomy, the indications for operative management, the preoperative assessment, the surgical intervention, and postoperative surveillance, as well as review of the outcomes for pulmonary metastasectomy, with a focus on application to osteosarcoma in the pediatric and adolescent population.

Historical Background

Resection of metastatic disease has never been evaluated in a randomized controlled trial. Completion of such a trial would be difficult because resection of limited pulmonary metastases has become standard practice. Randomization to a nonsurgical

---

M. Steliga (✉)
4301 W. Markham Street, Little Rock AR 72205
e-mail: masteliga@uams.edu

arm would be unacceptable based on multiple case series and comparisons to historical controls suggesting long term benefits of resection.

One of the first English publications on pulmonary metastasectomy was the report by Barney and Churchill in 1939.[6] The authors reported the resection of a lung mass which was found to be a metastasis from a previously resected renal cell carcinoma. The patient survived 23 years and died of unrelated causes, showing no sign of recurrence on autopsy. This demonstrated the feasibility of metastasectomy and the potential benefit in what was historically deemed incurable. A study of a series of 25 patients published by Ochsner and colleagues in 1963 suggested that a longer disease-free interval was associated with better survival after resection of pulmonary metastases. Four of their twenty-five patients with various primary tumors had survived for more than 5 years without recurrence.[7] A review of the Mayo Clinic experience from 1941 through 1962 analyzed the outcomes of 205 patients who had undergone a total of 221 operations for resection of pulmonary metastases. They demonstrated that patients had a 30% 5 year survival following pulmonary metastasectomy.[8] Many reports of pulmonary metastasectomy over the years included collections of cases with different tissue types. The limited numbers of patients who are candidates for resection has led to relatively limited numbers in the reports; nevertheless, the observation of long term survivors after surgical resection of metastases lends strong support to this potentially curative procedure.

The aforementioned studies reviewed populations which were mostly comprised of adults. There is limited information about the pediatric and adolescent population, but similar benefits have been demonstrated in this age range as well. In 1961, Richardson presented the results of a survey of pediatric and thoracic surgeons. The combined experience of this unknown number of physicians included eight children who were 5 year survivors out of a total of 35 who had undergone pulmonary metastasectomy for various histologies of tumors.[9] The first paper that specifically addressed pediatric osteosarcoma pulmonary metastasectomy was published in 1971 by Martini and colleagues. Historically, patients with metastatic disease to the lung from osteosarcoma had less than 5% survival at 3 years from initial diagnosis. Their cohort of patients who had undergone resection of pulmonary metastases had significantly improved the outcome compared to the historical control: 9 of 22 (41%) surviving beyond 3 years, compared to a 5% 3 year survival for historical controls.[10] Several of their patients had undergone bilateral and multiple thoracotomies over time. In 1991, data was republished on these same patients indicating that four of the patients had gone on to survive over 20 years after resection of osteosarcoma metastases.[11]

Presentation and Evaluation

Most metastatic lesions in the lung tend to be peripheral, and since the pulmonary parenchyma itself lacks sensory innervation, most pulmonary metastases are asymptomatic. Sometimes, albeit rarely, more central metastases may involve airways leading to cough, hemoptysis, pain, postobstructive pneumonia, or wheezing. Peripheral metastases have presented as pneumothorax, but this is not common. Pain or discomfort in the chest wall usually indicates involvement of parietal pleura, the chest wall, or distinct metastases to the chest wall itself, not the lung tissue. These patients present a significant challenge, as by definition they have extra-pulmonary disease. In isolated, carefully selected settings, they are still approached surgically. Those patients who do present with symptoms, often have advanced unresectable metastatic disease, but this is not an absolute contraindication to resection. Most resectable pulmonary metastases, therefore, are discovered on imaging studies obtained for metastatic workup or surveillance after resection of the primary tumor.

For decades, detection of pulmonary metastases relied on plain film radiographs which are still part of standard patient evaluation today. However, Computed Tomography is now the standard radiographic test for the detection and evaluation of pulmonary metastases.[12] Current high speed multislice scanners can provide accurate anatomic details of metastases, their location, number, and relation to pulmonary vasculature and airways. Reconstructions can be computer generated in different planes and in three dimensions, aiding surgical planning and intraoperative localization. One limitation of CT scans is the possibility of motion artifact from patient movement or respiration, which reduces the resolution. The few seconds of breath holding required can pose some difficulty in younger children who may require sedation for successful imaging.

Pulmonary metastases most often appear as well circumscribed nodules which may be single or multiple. Unfortunately, this appearance is not uniform, and metastatic disease may be represented as diffuse opacities, miliary nodules or other nonspecific findings which may be difficult to distinguish from infectious etiologies, atelectasis, scar, or benign granulomas. These nonspecific findings demonstrate the importance of comparison to previous films when evaluating patients with possible metastases. Fortunately, in patients with osteosarcoma metastasis, nodules are, frequently, discreet and, not infrequently, calcified, especially after response to systemic therapy.

PET and integrated CT/PET scans are currently used extensively in patients to evaluate the possibility of extra-pulmonary metastatic disease. Evaluation of lung parenchyma with PET does not show much benefit over chest CT.[13] A high resolution CT will detect nodules as small as 2–3 mm in size, whereas FDG labeled PET images usually require an area of increased uptake to be greater than or equal to 5–8 mm, to be detectable. In addition, the CT component of a PET-CT is obtained without contrast and is not commonly a high resolution scan. The benefit of PET scans may be in the evaluation of treatment response after systemic therapy. Reduction or loss of FDG avidity is indicative of a response to chemotherapy. Additional studies will help elucidate the role of PET scanning in the management of metastatic osteosarcoma. Since routine PET scanning does not effectively evaluate all the long bones and the calvarium, bone scans are routinely done to complete the evaluation for extra-pulmonary metastasis.

Preoperatively, patients should also undergo a physiologic evaluation in conjunction with the above mentioned anatomic evaluation. Patients who are to undergo pulmonary resection should, at the very least, have a complete pulmonary function testing done. Most children have normal lung parenchyma and normal pulmonary function, and most metastasectomies are limited to small wedge resections. However, for children who may have underlying pulmonary disease, those who may need to undergo resection of significant lung volume such as lobectomy, bilobectomy, or pneumonectomy, or those undergoing repeat resection for recurrence, assessment of their pulmonary function is crucial. For these patients, additional testing will be necessary and is beyond the scope of this chapter. The estimation of post-resection pulmonary function is one of the more challenging aspects of determining if a patient is a candidate for resection, andthe latter should be done by a surgeon with expertise in this field.

Many adults undergoing lung resection often have significant risk for concomitant cardiac disease, necessitating a thorough preoperative cardiac evaluation. Most children and adolescents on the other hand, have normal cardiovascular physiology and preoperative cardiac evaluation is not necessary. However, previous treatment with doxorubicin, a known cardiotoxic agent, may be associated with decreased cardiac function. This decreased cardiac function may not be clinically evident, but significant pulmonary resection may not be tolerated in these patients. In these cases, preoperative echocardiography provides important information regarding ventricular function and pulmonary arterial pressures which may be limitations to surgical resection.

Indications for Surgical Resection

The reviews of pulmonary metastasectomy, which demonstrated increased survival rates, have consistently shown that the most significant predictor of survival is achieving a complete resection.[14–16] Therefore, the goal of surgical resection of pulmonary metastases from osteosarcoma is to render the patient completely disease free. "Tumor debulking" or "cytoreductive surgery" with incomplete resection has not demonstrated any survival benefit for patients with pulmonary metastases.

If nodules seen on imaging studies are clinically and radiographically consistent with metastases, then the decision to offer surgery is based on the presence of four criteria (see Table 1). The primary site must be controlled without evidence of recurrence, or a completed resection of the primary is planned. Additionally, all the

Table 1 Criteria for resection of pulmonary metastases

Primary tumor must be resected or resectable
All nodules must be anatomically resectable
Predicted postoperative pulmonary reserve must be adequate
No extra-pulmonary sites of metastases

pulmonary nodules must be anatomically resectable, the patient's predicted postoperative pulmonary reserve must be adequate, and there must be no extra-pulmonary sites of metastatic spread.

These criteria have been reaffirmed by numerous authors.[12,17–19] Preoperative biopsy is not always indicated if there are multiple lesions that are clinically and radiographically consistent with metastatic nodules. Although solitary pulmonary nodule in adults may infrequently represent a new primary lung tumor rather than a metastasis, this is less common in the pediatric population, especially in those with a history of osteosarcoma.

A number of prognostic variables have been reported as factors which correlate with survival after pulmonary metastasectomy and will be discussed later in this chapter. While these variables may be correlated with decreased survival, none are absolute contraindications, assuming that the patient can potentially be rendered free of disease.

Surgical Resection

There are several considerations to the pre and peri-operative management when planning a resection of pulmonary metastases. Placement of epidural catheters is beneficial for pain management after thoracotomy in the perioperative period; however, this may not always be technically possible in the pediatric population. Other methods of pain control, including systemic narcotic, local anesthetics delivered at surgery or with indwelling catheters, are also options for post operative pain management.

General anesthesia with one lung ventilation is necessary for visualization in the chest and palpation of the nodules. Placement of double lumen endotracheal tubes or bronchial blockers, the two methods of achieving one-lung ventilation, can pose significant challenges in the younger patient. An experienced anesthesiologist is a crucial part of the operative team.

Nodules may be resected from the lungs using a variety of incisions, the most common of which is the posterolateral thoracotomy (see Fig. 1). This incision usually divides the latissimus muscle but preserves the serratus anterior muscle and provides excellent exposure of the entire ipsilateral hemithorax. A muscle-sparing thoracotomy utilizes a similar skin incision but mobilizes rather than divides the latissimus dorsi and serratus anterior muscles. This modification can limit operative exposure, but the preserved integrity of the chest muscles has been thought to improve postoperative recovery. In patients with lower extremity amputations, common in osteosarcoma patients, preservation of the latissimus can be significant. An obvious drawback to any thoracotomy is the limitation to one hemithorax. Contralateral nodules would necessitate a staged approach with exploration and resection on the contralateral side after adequate recovery from the first procedure (usually 3–6 weeks). In the absence of radiographic evidence of contralateral nodules, contralateral exploration is not routinely advocated. While there is no data to support this approach in children, there is some data in adults which demonstrates

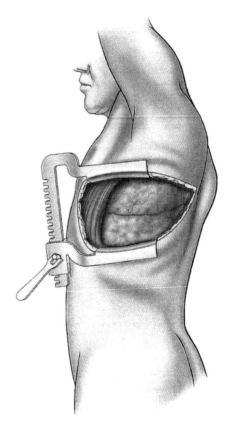

Fig. 1 A posterolateral thoracotomy provides wide access to the ipsilateral hemithorax

equivalent outcomes for patients with unilateral disease and ipsilateral exploration only.[20]

For patients presenting with bilateral disease, bilateral exploration is possible with either a median sternotomy or a transverse thoracosternotomy. The median sternotomy provides access to both pleural spaces simultaneously, and the postoperative pain is usually less than that in a thoracotomy. Although both lungs can be palpated and exposed in this fashion, exposure is more limited especially for lesions at the bases of the lungs and posteriorly (see Fig. 2). This is most difficult for nodules in the left lower lobe; the approach is better suited for bilateral upper lobe disease.

Another approach to bilateral exploration is the transverse thoracosternotomy also referred to as the "clamshell" approach. A transverse incision in the submammary crease is used to open both pleural spaces, and the sternum is divided horizontally, providing bilateral access. Although this incision does afford better access to the lower lobes, it has been associated with more postoperative pain than

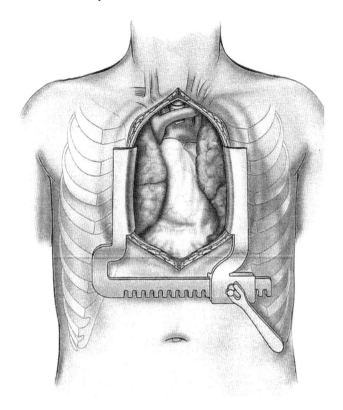

Fig. 2 A median sternotomy provides simultaneous bilateral access; however, operative access is limited

that in a median sternotomy (see Fig. 3). For this reason, it has not been commonly utilized.

Minimally invasive techniques have become more commonplace in all surgical diseases. Thoracoscopy has several significant advantages compared to open thoracic surgery. The incisions are significantly smaller and, coupled with the lack of any rib spreading, the postoperative pain is less. Some series have even demonstrated shorter hospital stays. Unfortunately, the major limitation to thoracoscopy is the lack of intraoperative tactile sensation. Most pulmonary metastases are not visible on the visceral pleural surface. Palpation is the standard technique for location of the nodules, prior to resection.[21–23] Thoracoscopy severely limits the ability to identify these nodules. Other drawbacks to thoracoscopic resection include the concern over poor margins of resection and even port site recurrences after removing tumors through small access incisions.[24,25]

Several different approaches have been used to assist with the intraoperative thoracoscopic location of nodules for resection. Percutaneously placed guidewires have been introduced into the lesions using CT guided positioning.[26] Blue dye can

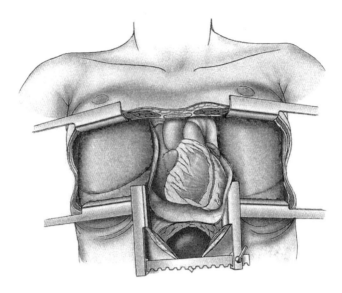

Fig. 3 A transverse thoracosternotomy or "clamshell" approach provides simultaneous bilateral access; however, it is associated with greater postoperative pain

be injected subpleurally overlying the nodule to assist with location.[26] One author has reported injection of radioisotopes into the lesion; the nodule is then identified intraoperatively with the use of a gamma probe to facilitate location of the lesion.[27] Dilute barium has also been used to mark the lung tissue, so that it may be localized with the aid of fluoroscopy.[28] Unfortunately, all of the aforementioned techniques require an additional interventional procedure based on CT imaging. More importantly, all of these techniques rely on the ability of high resolution CT imaging to identify all the metastases. If they are not seen on the CT scan, they cannot be localized.

Despite the high resolution of modern CT imaging, tiny nodules unseen on CT are routinely found during open thoracotomy. A 2007 publication by Parsons et al. validated this when two different radiologists' interpretations were compared to intraoperative findings.[29] The two radiologists' interpretations of the spiral CT images were completely accurate in only 19% of the cases. Missed metastases were found intraoperatively in 46% of the cases that were based on spiral CT imaging. A prospective trial was carried out in which patients underwent thoracoscopic metastasectomy, with conversion to thoracotomy during the same operation. Over half of the patients (56%) were found to have additional metastatic nodules that were only found at thoracotomy.[30] The study had planned on enrolling 50 patients prospectively. This difference was found to be statistically significant with the evaluation of the first 18 patients, and the study was closed. Other authors have revealed similar limitations to the sensitivity of thoracoscopy and CT imaging.[21,22,29]

One solution is an approach combining thoracoscopy and a subxiphoid "hand-port" incision that allows a hand to be introduced into each pleural space without thoracotomy.[31] This approach is reported to have the benefit of bilateral intraoperative palpation without large thoracic incision or rib spreading. The concept has appeal; however, its application in a pediatric and adolescent patient population is limited by the size of the patient. Therefore, an open approach remains the standard method of resection and complete evaluation of the lung tissue, especially in this younger patient population.

Despite the limitations of thoracoscopy, it is an important approach used by surgeons in several clinical scenarios relevant to metastatic disease. Thoracoscopy is very useful for obtaining tissue for diagnosis. Patients with a single nodule can be approached with a thoracoscopic wedge resection.[23] This is particularly appealing, if there is suspicion that the nodule may be of benign etiology, and that diagnosis is not possible with less invasive methods such as CT guided needle biopsy. In some cases, the imaging studies may suggest pleural studding, malignant effusion or multiple small nodules not amenable to resection. These patients may require a tissue biopsy for confirmation of this form of unresectable intrapleural disease. In these settings, thoracoscopy and biopsy are often possible through a single 5–10 mm port site incision. Finally, an isolated >1 cm nodule with a disease free interval of many years may be approached thoracoscopically, as the likelihood of additional nodules, in this scenario, is low.

The actual technique of resection most commonly employed is a wedge resection. Less common resections include anatomic resections, such segmentectomy, lobectomy, bilobectomy, and pneumonectomy.

Wedge resection refers to excision of lung parenchyma in a nonanatomic fashion, whereas anatomic resections such as segmentectomy, lobectomy and pneumonectomy follow the bronchial anatomy and pulmonary vasculature. Anatomic resections are the standard for primary lung malignancies because of the propensity for lymphatic invasion and central nodal involvement. Pulmonary metastases, on the other hand, are most often resected as wedge resections, preferably with 1 cm margins. The possibility of developing further metastatic disease in the future supports the resection of the least amount of lung tissue for negative margin. Most often wedge resections are performed with surgical staplers, allowing efficient excision with good hemostasis and pneumostasis. Nodules can also be focally excised with electrocautery and/or laser. These modalities may be useful for deeper lesions, which are difficult to excise with staplers without damaging large sections of lung. Anatomic resections may occasionally be necessary for nodules in close proximity to bronchial and/or vascular structures, and these are not contraindicated as long as the patient's pulmonary function permits the planned resection. Despite the greater loss of lung parenchyma that accompanies these operations, carefully selected patients who have undergone extensive resections, including lobectomy, sleeve lobectomy and even pneumonectomy, have demonstrated long term survival. In 1992, Putnam and colleagues reported on 19 patients who had undergone pneumonectomy for metastatic disease and another 19 with aggressive resections, including en bloc resection of chest wall, diaphragm, pericardium, or vena cava. This high risk group demonstrated 25% 5 year survival with an operative mortality of 5%.[32]

The involvement of mediastinal lymph nodes from pulmonary metastases is not common. The data that exists is retrospective and based on selected node dissection.

In these reviews, patients with sarcoma have fewer nodal metastases than carcinoma patients.[33,34] In one review, only 10% of the highly selected patients with osteosarcoma who received nodal dissection actually had nodal involvement.[35] The impact of nodal metastasis on survival was examined by Veronesi and associates. In their retrospective review, patients without nodal metastasis had a 60% 5 year survival, while those with hilar and mediastinal metastasis had a 17% and 0% 5 year survival respectively.[33] Further prospective data is needed to verify the importance of nodal metastasis.

In summary, resection of the least amount of lung necessary to obtain negative margins is the goal of pulmonary metastasectomy. More extensive resections can be performed if necessary, but this may limit the potential for re-resection should the disease recur in the remaining lung tissue. Decisions regarding these more aggressive resections should take into account the prognostic factors discussed earlier in the chapter.

Nonresectional, ablative techniques such as percutaneous radiofrequency ablation (RFA)[36] and stereotactic external beam radioablation have become popular lately. Their application in metastasectomy has been mostly for unresectable disease, to control a single nodule or multiple rapidly growing nodules for palliation. For potentially resectable metastatic disease, ablative techniques have several significant limitations. The first is their dependence on imaging studies rather than palpation, similar to the limitation of thoracoscopy. Peripheral air embolization has been a reported consequence of pulmonary RFA, and in the case of either technique, the possibility of damage to bronchial, vascular, and/or cardiac tissues may be significant, especially in centrally placed lesions.

Outcomes

Historical reviews have demonstrated the viability of pulmonary metastasectomy as a treatment option. Frequently, these consisted of little more than case reports or small cohort reviews. The data for pediatric populations are even more limited. The largest modern review was performed by Pastorino and colleagues as part of The International Registry of Lung Metastases (IRLM). They analyzed the data from the resection of lung metastases in 5,206 patients at 18 centers throughout Europe, Canada, and the United States.[14] Eighty-eight percent of the patients underwent complete resection. The patient population was of mixed tumor types with epithelial malignancies (43%) as the most common, followed closely by sarcoma (42%), and significantly fewer with germ cell (7%) melanoma (6%). The remaining 2% of malignancies included several types including Wilms' tumor and teratoma. Osteosarcoma accounted for 734 cases, the largest sarcoma histology subgroup (38% of all sarcomas). Prognostic factors such as: complete resectability, disease free intervals (DFI) greater than 36 months, solitary metastases, and histology of Wilms' or germ cell tumors were found to have a more favorable outcome. Overall actuarial survival was reported as 36% at 5 years compared to 13% at 5 years for those who were not completely resected (see Fig. 4).

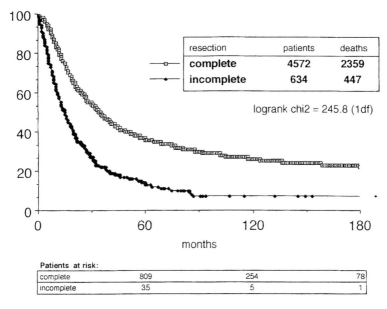

Fig. 4 Overall actuarial survival up to 15 years for complete vs. incomplete metastasectomy in the IRLM database. (From ref. [14])

A DFI of 0–11 months was associated with a 5 year survival of 33%, whereas patients with a DFI greater than 36 months, exhibited a 45% five year survival. Patients with single metastases had a 5 year survival of 43%, whereas those with 2 to 3 metastases had a 5 year survival of 34%. Those with 4 or more metastases had a 27% five year survival. Patients with germ cell tumors clearly had the best survival with a 68% five year survival. The 5 year survival for epithelial tumors (37%) and sarcomas (31%) did not differ statistically, but melanoma was clearly the worst with only a 21% five year survival (Table 2).

Operative mortality was cited as 1% overall, with 2.4% mortality for the subgroup of patients unable to be completely resected. The strengths of this analysis lie in the large number of patients included from multiple institutions; a limitation, however, is the combination of different tumor types which may have different biologic behavior. Subgroup analysis was not reported for the different age ranges or tumor types.

More germane to the topic of this chapter was a retrospective review of 137 patients under 21 years of age, with metastatic osteosarcoma identified over a 20 year period. Patients who had undergone metastasectomy ($n=93$) had significantly improved mean survival (33.6 months) compared to those who did not undergo resection ($n=38$, mean survival 10.1 months). The 5 year overall survival for those who underwent thoracotomy was 29%; this included patients who went to thoracotomy, but were found unresectable (6% in their series). Among the patients who did not undergo thoracotomy, the 5 year survival was 2.6%. The number of pulmonary lesions, extension to the pleura, unilateral vs. bilateral metastasis, or resection margins did not influence survival. However, response to preoperative chemotherapy,

Table 2 Median survival, 5 year survival and 10 year survival from the IRLM data for 5,206 patients broken down by completeness of resection, disease free interval, number of metastases, and tumor histology

	Median survival	5 year survival	10 year survival
Complete resection	35 months	36%	26%
Incomplete resection	15 months	13%	7%
DFI 0–11 months	29 months	33%	27%
DFI 12–35 months	30 months	31%	22%
DFI >36 months	49 months	45%	29%
1 metastasis	43 months	45%	31%
2–3 metastases	31 months	34%	21%
4 or more metastases	27 months	27%	19%
Germ cell tumors	NR	68%	63%
Epithelial tumors	40 months	37%	21%
Sarcomas	29 months	31%	26%
Melanomas	19 months	21%	14%

measured by tumor necrosis percentage, and a DFI greater than 1 year were associated with better survival following resection. (5 year survival 55.6% vs. 12.3%).[4] The authors supported resection and even repeat resection for pulmonary metastasis, especially when patients demonstrated a favorable response to chemotherapy.

Similar modern findings were reported by a smaller retrospective review from Japan. Although the study included metastasectomy for osteosarcoma and soft tissue sarcoma, the osteosarcoma subgroup (44 patients comprising adults as well as children) were noted to have a 5 year survival of 42.7% and a 10 year survival of 38.5%.[16] The ability for complete resection was the only significant variable associated with prolonged survival that was noted on multivariate analysis.

Although not conclusive, the wealth of retrospective data supports surgical resection of pulmonary metastasis from osteosarcoma in carefully selected patients. It would appear that the primary selection criteria that should be considered is the ability to achieve a complete resection (with the attendant physiologic issues addressed earlier in this chapter). The number of lesions is a lesser consideration and should only have an impact in the decision to operate if it precludes a complete resection. Response to chemotherapy and the DFI are important when considering resection, but long term survival even after a failed response to chemotherapy and short DFI have been reported. Therefore, surgical resection should not be withheld in an otherwise resectable patient, solely based on a poor response to chemotherapy or a short DFI. Careful assessment of these patients should include the morbidity of the operation, especially if an extended resection is required, and its impact on quality of life.

Extended resection of metastases includes large parenchymal resection (pneumonectomy or bilobectomy) or en bloc resection with chest wall or other major structures (vascular, cardiac, vertebral etc.). The data supporting this form of aggressive therapy is even more limited than the literature on metastasectomy, but some small retrospective studies from mixed tumor populations do exist. A retrospective review of adult patients with various tumor histologies reported on 19 patients with a pneumonectomy and an additional 19 patients with en bloc resection of metastatic disease in continuity with chest wall, diaphragm, pericardium or vena cava.[32] Thirty three of the 38 patients were able to have complete resection. The operative mortality for the entire group was 5%, with both the deaths occurring after right pneumonectomy (10.5% mortality after pneumonectomy).[37] This is similar to the operative risk for pneumonectomy for primary lung cancer. The five year actuarial survival was 25%. Although this review analyzed outcomes on adults, it is reasonable to apply these principles to similarly selected younger patients.

Additional support for selective application of aggressive surgery was found in the IRLM data. A subgroup analysis was performed of the patients in the registry who had received a pneumonectomy. The 5 year survival of this group was 20%, again supporting an aggressive approach in highly selected patients.

Finally, even cardiopulmonary bypass has been explored for highly selected cases. These reports are anecdotal, consisting of a case report or a very heterogeneous case series, but they demonstrate that even aggressive central lesions involving cardiac structure can be resected with long term benefit.[38,39]

Surveillance and Recurrence

Following resection of pulmonary metastases, patients should be examined with regularly scheduled chest x-rays, CT scans of the chest, history and physical exam. There seems to be no standard consensus in the follow-up interval. What is clear is that immediate postoperative chest CT scans and PET scans can be difficult to interpret, secondary to altered anatomy and postoperative inflammation. A chest CT taken 1 to 3 months after surgery should be obtained as a baseline study. All future CT scans will be compared to this study and recurrence determined by the development of a persistent growing nodule. The subsequent scans should be obtained frequently during the first 2 years, and annually for life. The absolute frequency of scanning is impacted by the length of the DFI, the number of metastasis resected, and the tumors doubling time. However, all patients, regardless of favorable prognostic factors should be followed annually for life.

Recurrent metastatic disease may be reevaluated for repeat thoracotomy and resection. Prior metastasectomy is not a contraindication to surgery, provided that the aforementioned principles are still met. The patients' pulmonary function may be diminished from baseline because of prior loss of lung parenchyma. This mandates evaluation with repeat pulmonary function tests. Reoperative surgery has the additional challenge of adhesions which often obliterate the pleural space, leading to longer operations and a higher incidence of postoperative airleak. Despite the challenges of reoperative cases, these patients can demonstrate cure and increased survival rates.

Pastorino and colleagues discussed recurrences and repeat resection in their review of the IRLM data. Overall, 53% of all the patients who underwent complete resection developed recurrence with a median time of 10 months after resection. Sarcoma patients who had recurrences were limited to intrathoracic recurrence 66% of the time, and 53% of those who relapsed, underwent a second metastasectomy. Overall, patients who underwent a second metastasectomy had a 44% five year survival, and 29% had a 10 year survival, supporting repeat metastasectomy in this highly selected group of patients.[14]

Repeated surgical resection of pulmonary metastases was evaluated by Kandolier and colleagues who reviewed 35 patients over a 20 year span; these patients had been free of disease after initial metastasectomy and went on to develop further pulmonary metastases.over a 20 year span This group of patients had mixed histologic tumor types. Their 5 year survival rates were 48%, and they had a 10 year survival of 28%. Grouping patients by tumor type did not reveal a significant difference in survival. A disease free interval of over 40 months between the first and second metastasectomies was associated with significantly longer survival.[40]

Temeck et al. reviewed reoperative metastasectomy for sarcoma metastases in a pediatric population.[41] Seventy patients were reviewed who had undergone a second ($n=70$), a third ($n=27$), or a fourth operation ($n=10$) were reviewed. CT had underestimated the overall number of nodules by 39%. A complete resection was possible in 73% of the second thoracotomies, 87% of the third thoracotomies, and 70% of the fourth thoracotomies. One operative mortality (1%) was reported in a patient who had undergone attempted resection which was found to be unresectable. Complications involved air leak (5.6%), wound infection in one patient and pneumonia in two patientsThe second time thoracotomy patients had a 5.6 year median survival if resectable compared to the 0.7 years ,if unresectable. There was a similar advantage of resectable over unresectable tumors among the third time thoracotomy patients The fourth time thoracotomy patients had less benefit, but it was still statistically significant (2.2 year median survival compared to 0.2 years if unresectable). Neither sex, age, histology, location of primary tumor, chemotherapy before second thoracotomy, nor size of the nodules had any impact on survival.

Similar conclusions were reached by Briccoli and colleagues who reviewed 94 patients with metastatic ostesarcoma.[42] At their institution, 570 patients underwent treatment for osteosarcoma of the limbs. Two hundred and sixty seven of these patients had metastases isolated to the lung and underwent resection. After metastasectomy, 40% of those patients ($n = 94$) represented with isolated lung metastases and underwent repeat resection. Thirty-one of the 94 (32.9%) who underwent a second operation survived without evidence of disease. Their 3- and 5-year event free actuarial survival from the first metastasectomy was 45% and 38% respectively, while it was 33% and 32% after the second metastasectomy. Smaller groups of patients went on to have third, fourth, and fifth thoracotomies for resection; these groups did contain patients who went on to survive disease free.

These data clearly show that prior resection, as a prognostic factor, should not deter resection of pulmonary metastasis. If the previously prescribed indications are present and a complete resection can be achieved, then surgical resection should be offered.

Future Directions

Refinements in technology related to CT imaging resolution may improve the sensitivity of CT for locating pulmonary nodules. Previous reports highlighting the limitations of CT imaging relied on older generation scanners with 5–10 mm slice thickness.[21,22,29] It remains to be seen whether the sensitivity of higher resolution scanners can approach the sensitivity of intraoperative palpation. If so, this may lend more support to image guided local therapy, such as radiofrequency ablation, cryoablation, or external beam radiation. Additionally, if CT scanning improves detection, thoracoscopic resection after CT localization may become appropriate initial therapy as well.

Summary

In summary, patients with metastatic osteosarcoma due to isolated pulmonary metastases comprise a population which may derive survival benefits and a potential long term cure with surgical resection. These patients have historically demonstrated poor outcome, and resection can usually be performed with acceptable operative morbidity and mortality. Despite the lack of randomized controlled trials, comparison of multiple reviews consistently demonstrates improved survival and a potential cure for patients who would otherwise have only palliative options. Even aggressive resections, in carefully chosen patients, can offer a chance for long term survival. All patients with even remotely resectable disease should be evaluated by a thoracic surgeon with experience in complex intrathoracic resections.

References

1. Wang, LL, Chintagumpala, M, and Gebhardt, MC. Osteosarcoma: epidemiology, pathogenesis, clinical presentation, diagnosis, and histology. *Uptodate*. 2007.
2. National Cancer Institute. Cancer Incidence and Survival among Children and Adolscents: United States SEER Program 1975–1995. 1995;89-110.
3. Ward WG, Mikaelian K, Dorey F, et al. Pulmonary metastases of stage IIB extremity osteosarcoma and subsequent pulmonary metastases. *J Clin Oncol*. 1994;12:1849-1858.
4. Harting MT, Blakely ML, Jaffe N, et al. Long-term survival after aggressive resection of pulmonary metastases among children and adolescents with osteosarcoma. *J Pediatr Surg*. 2006;41:194-199.
5. Tsuchiya H, Kanazawa Y, Abdel-Wanis M, et al. Effect of timing of pulmonary metastases identification on prognosis of pateints with osteosarcoma: the Japanese musculoskeletal oncology group study. *J Clin Oncol*. 2002;20:3470-3477.
6. Barney JD, Churchill EJ. Adenocarcinoma of the kidney with metastasis to the lung cured by nephrectomy and lobectomy. *J Urol*. 1939;42:269-276.
7. Ochsner A, Clemmons E, Mitchell W. Treatment of metastatic pulmonary malignant lesions. *J Lancet*. 1963;83:16-24.

8. Thomford N, Woolner L, Clagett O. The surgical treatment of metastatic tumors in lungs. *J Thorac Cardiovasc Surg*. 1963;49:357-363.
9. Richardson WR. Progress in pediatric cancer surgery. *Arch Surg*. 1961;82:641-655.
10. Martini N, Huvos AG, Mike V, et al. Multiple pulmonary resections in the treatment of osteogenic sarcoma. *Ann Thorac Surg*. 1971;12:271-280.
11. Beattie EJ, Harvey JC, Marcove R, et al. Results of multiple pulmonary resections for metastatic osteogenic sarcoma after two decades. *J Surg Oncol*. 1991;46:154-155.
12. Virgo KS, Naunheim KS, Johnson FE. Preoperative workup and postoperative surveillance for patients undergoing pulmonary metastasectomy. *Thorac Surg Clin*. 2006;16:125-131.
13. Aquino SL, Kuester LB, Muse VV, et al. Accuracy of transmission CT and FDG-PET in the detection of small pulmonary nodules with integrated PET/CT. *Eur J Nucl Med Mol Imaging*. 2006;33:692-696.
14. Pastorino U, Buyse M, Friedel G, et al. Long-term results of lung metastasectomy: prognostic analyses based on 5206 cases. *J Thorac Cardiovasc Surg*. 1997;113:37-49.
15. Temeck BK, Wexler LH, Steinberg SM, et al. Metastasectomy for sarcomatous pediatric histologies – results and prognostic factors. *Ann Thorac Surg*. 1995;59:1385-1390.
16. Suzuki M, Iwata T, Ando S, et al. Predictors of long-term survival with pulmonary metastasectomy for osteosarcomas and soft tissue sarcomas. *J Cardiovasc Surg*. 2006;47:603-608.
17. Rusch VW. Pulmonary metastasectomy. Current indications (Review). *Chest*. 1995;107:322s-331s.
18. Lanza LA, Putnam JB Jr. Resection of pulmonary metastases. In: Roth JA, Ruckdeschel JR, Weisenberger TH, eds. *Thoracic Oncology*. 2nd ed. Philadelphia: W.B. Saunders; 1996:569-589.
19. Putnam JB Jr, Roth JA. Secondary tumors in the lungs. In: Shields TW, ed. *General Thoracic Surgery*. 4th ed. Philadelphia: Williams & Wilkins; 1994:1334-1352.
20. Younes RN, Gross JL, Deheinzelin D. Surgical resection of unilateral lung metastases: is bilateral thoracotomy necessary? *World J Surg*. 2002;26:1112-1116.
21. Kayton ML, Huvos AG, Casher J, et al. Computed tomographic scan of the chest underestimates the number of metastatic lesions in osteosarcoma. *J Pediatr Surg*. 2006;41:200-204.
22. Parsons AM, Detterbeck FC, Parker LA. Accuracy of helical CT in the detection of pulmonary metastases: is intraoperative palpation still necessary? *Ann of Thorac Surg*. 2004;78:1910-1916.
23. Castagnetti M, Delarue A, Gentet JC. Optimizing the surgical management of lung nodules in children with osteosarcoma – thoracoscopy for biopsies, thoracotomy for resections. *Surg Endosc*. 2004;18:1668-1671.
24. Sartorelli KH, Partrick D, Meagher DP. Port-site recurrence after thoracoscopic resection of pulmonary metastasis owing to osteogenic sarcoma. *J Pediatr Surg*. 1996;31:1443-1444.
25. Walsh GL, Nesbitt JC. Tumor implants after thoracoscopic resection of a metastatic sarcoma. *Ann Thorac Surg*. 1995;59:215-216.
26. Mack MJ, Gordon MJ, Postma TW, et al. Percutaneous localization of pulmonary nodules for thoracoscopic lung resection. *Ann Thorac Surg*. 1992;53:1123-1124.
27. Chella A, Lucchi M, Ambrogi MC, et al. A pilot study of the role of TC-99 radionuclide in localization of pulmonary nodular lesions for thoracoscopic resection. *Eur J Cardiothorac Surg*. 2000;18:17-21.
28. Moon SW, Wang YP, Jo KH, et al. Fluoroscopy-aided thoracoscopic resection of pulmonary nodule localized with contrast media. *Ann Thorac Surg*. 1999;68:1815-1820.
29. Parsons AM, Ennis EK, Yankaskas BC, et al. Helical computed tomography inaccuracy in the detection of pulmonary metastases: can it be improved? *Ann Thorac Surg*. 2007;84:1830-1837.
30. McCormack PM, Bains MS, Begg CB, et al. Role of video-assisted thoracic surgery in the treatment of pulmonary metastases: results of a prospective trial. *Ann Thorac Surg*. 1996;62:213-216.
31. Mineo TC, Ambrogi V, Paci M, et al. Transxiphoid bilateral palpation in video-assisted thoracoscopic lung metastasectomy. *Arch Surg*. 2001;136:783-788.
32. Putnam JB, Suell DM, Natarajan G, et al. Extended resection of pulmonary metastases – is the risk justified. *Ann Thorac Surg*. 1993;55:1440-1446.
33. Veronesi G, Petrella F, Leo F, et al. Prognostic role of lymph node involvement in lung metastasectomy. *J Thorac Cardiovasc Surg*. 2007;133:967-972.

34. Dominguez-Ventura A, Nichols F. Lymphadenectomy in metastasectomy. *Thorac Surg Clin.* 2006;16:139-143.
35. Pfannschmidt J, Mode J, Muley T, et al. Nodal involvement at the time of pulmonary metastasectomy: experiences in 245 patients. *Ann Thorac Surg.* 2006;81:448-454.
36. Ghaye B, Bruyere PJ, Dondelinger RF. Nonfatal systemic air embolism during percutaneous radiofrequency ablation of a pulmonary metastasis. *AJR Am J Roentgenol.* 2006;187:W327-W328.
37. Koong HN, Pastorino U, Ginsberg RJ. Is there a role for pneumonectomy in pulmonary metastases? *Ann Thorac Surg.* 1999;68:2039-2043.
38. Vaporciyan AA, Rice D, Correa AM, et al. Resection of advanced thoracic malignancies requiring cardiopulmonary bypass. *Eur J Cardiothorac Surg.* 2002;22:47-52.
39. Ying C, Gang S. Successful resection of osteosarcoma pulmonary metastasis extending into left side of heart under cardiopulmonary bypass: a case report. *Chin Med J.* 2002;115(11):1743-1744.
40. Kandioler D, Kromer E, Tuchler H, et al. Long-term results after repeated surgical removal of pulmonary metastases. *Ann Thorac Surg.* 1998;65:909-912.
41. Temeck BK, Wexler LH, Steinberg SM, et al. Reoperative pulmonary metastasectomy for sarcomatous pediatric histologies. *Ann Thorac Surg.* 1998;66:908-912.
42. Briccoli A, Rocca M, Salone M, et al. Resection of recurrent pulmonary metastases in patients with osteosarcoma. *Cancer.* 2005;104:1721-1725.

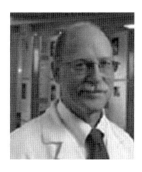

Non-Surgical Treatment of Pulmonary and Extra-pulmonary Metastases

Pete Anderson

Abstract Studies have demonstrated that chemotherapy alone is usually unsuccessful as exclusive therapy for osteosarcoma (Cancer 95:2202–2201, 2002). Information will be presented for situations where non-surgical alternatives could be considered as useful, if not necessary, adjuncts to chemotherapy. In the thorax these include treatment of pleural effusions, chest wall lesions, central lung or mediastinal osteosarcoma, as well as recurrences in patients with limited pulmonary reserve. Other situations include too many metastases to easily resect, axial osteosarcomas, bone metastases, liver and brain metastases.

Non-surgical local control measures include radiation with chemotherapy for radiosensitization, bone-seeking radioisotopes (e.g., ^{153}Sm-EDTMP, ^{223}Ra), bisphosphonates, heat (radiofrequency ablation), freezing and thawing (cryoablation), and intracavitary or regional (aerosol) therapy. Because of the predictable and common pattern of pulmonary metastases in osteosarcoma, aerosol therapy also offers an attractive regional treatment strategy. Principles and use of aerosol cytokines (e.g., GM-CSF, IL-2), and aerosol chemotherapy with gemcitabin will be discussed. Individual cases illustrating strategy and techniques will be presented.

Introduction

In recurrent osteosarcoma, surgery always best if possible and disease is localized.[2] Chemotherapy can be thought of as reduction of disease to make local control measures possible or more effective. In the absence of local control, chemotherapy is usually palliative. Jaffe showed that chemotherapy alone was of temporary benefit and that surgery was required in the vast majority.[1] This chapter details non-surgical approaches and strategies for both definitive and palliative treatment of pulmonary

P. Anderson (✉)
Children's Cancer Hospital, University of Texas MD Anderson Cancer Center, Unit 87, Pediatrics, 1515 Holcombe Blvd., Houston, TX, 77030-4009, USA
e-mail: pmanders@mdanderson.org

and extra-pulmonary metastases. Use of these strategies may allow families and providers that "expect the worst to hope for the best" (ETWBHFTB).[3] Figure 1 illustrates the schema of osteosarcoma metastasis treatment. In this group of patients, therapy must balance indications, risks, and alternatives. Individualized therapy is necessary.

Patients with osteosarcoma may see relapse as part of just part of their life narrative that is very rich in detail.[4-6] When discussing this with Lynn Harter, we decided that not only was the life narrative a very poignant summary of what they have been through, but also that it was universal that patients wanted the chance to write a few more chapters in this rich, life narrative. Interruption and delay of normal life tasks for young people with osteosarcoma metastases is expected. A therapeutic alliance to help provide quality time and/or durable response to therapy is what is sought. Although it is the natural tendency of health care providers to feel that the odds are just too high to justify attempts at "cure," effective palliation and extension of good quality life is now possible for many with relapsed or recurrent osteosarcoma.[7] It would seem that for some, an attitude of being grateful for function and the opportunity to enjoy life facilitates health care providers to coordinate complex care issues.[8] On the other hand, an attitude of feeling that "things are being done to me, not for me" will result in withdrawal of care and attempts at palliation.

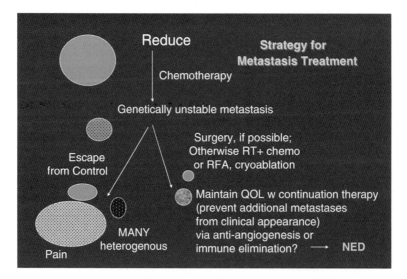

Fig. 1 Strategy for osteosarcoma metastasis treatment. Chemotherapy with drugs is useful for reduction of disease burden. Local control of measurable disease with surgery or other measures is done to further reduce potential for escape from cancer control. Durable responses often require continuation chemotherapy

Reduction of Recurrent or Metastatic Osteosarcoma with Drugs (Chemotherapy)

Because of the side effects and many hospitalizations associated with prior standard therapy cisplatin+doxorubicin and high dose methotrexate, young people with recurrent or metastatic osteosarcoma may refuse additional chemotherapy. Most teenagers and young adults with osteosarcoma, however, are willing to try outpatient chemotherapy if toxicity and hospitalization are less than their initial encounter with cancer chemotherapy. Table 1 compares inpatient osteosarcoma regimens with some that have modifications for outpatient use for recurrent and metastatic osteosarcoma.

Use of agents that inhibit VEGF may promote entry of chemotherapy into tumors as well as increase effectiveness of systemic control during radiation by reducing effect of compensatory VEGF production.[37–39] Shor et al. have summarized pre-clinical effects and action of tyrosine kinase inhibitors on sarcomas including osteosarcoma.[40] Aerosol GM-CSF seems well tolerated and is currently a slowly accruing COG clinical trial.[25,26] Aerosol gemcitabine is another approach that has good biologic rationale.[41,42] Canine studies are currently underway at UC Davis *Carlos Rodriguez, PI). Inhibition of mTOR (e.g., Rapamycin) and IGF-1 production and/or IGF-R1 signaling may be additional molecular means to inhibit the malignant phenotype of osteosarcoma.[43–49]

Zoledronate is perhaps the most potent bisphosphonate currently commercially available.[36] Zoledronate has been shown not only to be helpful for metastatic bone pain, but also to be directly toxic to osteosarcoma cells.[34,35] Bone seeking isotopes target similarly to bone surfaces but have the advantage of also targeting to osteoblastic metastases.[31–33,50] However, heterogeneity of areas of tumor making bone may limit distribution within osteosarcoma. Thus, zoledronate and bone-seeking isotopes may be useful adjuncts to chemotherapy and radiations but probably cannot adequately "sterilize" areas within metastases that are not actively making bone.

Use of any of these outpatient chemotherapy regimens should be balanced by weighing of indications, risks, and alternatives for a patients' particular situation. Alopecia is a common and not entirely irrevelant quality-of-life (QOL) consideration, particularly in young women.[13,51,52] Chemotherapy for radiosensitization seems to better control lesions than radiotherapy alone in osteosarcoma.[7,13,18,53–55] Choice of regimen for radiosensitization is often a function of what has been effective previously as well as need for systemic control.[7]

Reduction of Osteosarcoma with "Physical" Means: Using Physics!

Local control measures (e.g., surgery) are "site specific" and do not per se control disease at other, remote locations. Since local control surgery to remove a source of potential future recurrence as well as metastastic spread, such efforts seem to be

Table 1 Inpatient vs. outpatient osteosarcoma chemotherapy

Agent/Class I	Inpatient	Outpatient/Comment	Reference
Anthracycline	Doxorubicin CI[a]	Dexrazoxane/doxorubicin[b]	9,10
		Doxorubicin liposomes[b]	
Cisplatin	120 mg/M2 IA[c]	60 mg/M2/day CI x 2 days or 20–30 mg/M2/day x 4	11,12
	60 mg/M2/day iv	with hydration	
	24 h x 3 days hydration		13
	60 mg/M2 intrapleural		14
Carboplatin (CBDCA)	With ifos + etop ("ICE")	CBDCA less effective than cisplatin in osteosarcoma	15,16
Ifosfamide with MESNA	Bolus + hydration substitute CPM if hypophosphatemia before a cycle 1.8–3 g/M2/day x 3–5 days	Mix Ifos + Mesna 1:1No hydration; CI well tolerated. 2.8 g/M2 daily x 5. MESNA only day 6. polonesetron + aprepitant for anti-emetics	17,18
Cyclophosphamide (CPM) ± Vinorelbine	1.2 g iv q 3 weeksAlopecia	CPM 50 mg po dailyNo alopecia 25 mg/M2 iv	19,20
Methotrexate	12 g/M2 (max 20) Leucovorin iv until[MTX] < 0.1 µM	Oral NaHCO$_3$, po hydration then HDMTX 3 liter iv fluidBack pack/pump replaced qd po leucovorin until[MTX] < 0.1 µM polonesetron qd x 2	21
Gemcitabine + Docetaxel	Not an inpatient	d1,8 600–975 mg/M2 iv over 30–90 min	
	Regimen	d8 40–100 mg/M2 iv over 1 h	22,23
Bevacizumab (Avastin)	Usually outpatient	5 mg/kg iv q 2 weeks	24
		20–30 min infusion possible	
Temozolomide (Temodar)	Usually outpatient	75 mg/M2 daily (for radiosensitization)	
		Daily	18
Aerosol GM-CSF		250 mcg in 2 cc NS BID	25,26
		1 week on/1 week off	
L-MTP-PE	Usually outpatient	2 mg/M2 iv over 1 h	27,28
		2x/weeks x 12 weeks, then weekly x 24 weeks	
		Total weeks: 36; total doses: 48	
[153]Sm-EDTMP (Quadramet)	High dose with stem cells 14 days later	1–2 mCi/kg iv over 5 min	29,3031–33
Zoledronate (Zometa)	Usually outpatient	4 mg iv over 1 h	32,34–36
		Fewer side effects if 1 h	

IGF-R1 inhibition[d] (investigational)	Usually outpatient	Instead of 15 min infusion	
		9 mg/kg iv over 1 h q1 week	R1504
		10 mg/kg iv q 2 weeks	SCH717454
		To be determined (oral)	OSI-906

[a]CI- continuous infusion (usually 75–90 mg/M2 iv over 2–3 days; e.g., AOST 0331)

[b]Dexrazoxane (Zinecard) 750 mg/M2 iv over 15 min, then doxorubicin 75 mg/M2 iv over 15 min. Doxil 40 mg/M2 iv over 2–3 h with hands/feet on ice and observation for anaphylactoid reactions

[c]Intra-arterial

[d]IGFR agents are currently investigational. R1507 (Roche) clinical trial is SARC011; see wwwsarctrials.com for information about participating centers; Dr Dejka Araujo is PI of SARC 011 at MD Anderson (2007-0515). P04720 is the multi-site clinical trial of SC717454. Dr. Pete Anderson is PI of this study at MD Anderson (2007-0881); Dr Ed Kim is PI of clinical trial of OSI 906 (MDACC 2007-0075)

important for durable success in osteosarcoma.[1,2] Nevertheless, surgery is not possible nor practical for patients with some locations or multiple sites of recurrence and/or osteosarcoma metastases.

Radiation Therapy

Radiotherapy in combination with chemotherapy can have some benefit in local control of osteosarcoma tumors and lesions.[13,53–56] Preoperative radiation can also be considered as a means to facilitate surgery in sarcoma or a means to finish the task of local control when surgical margins are positive.[56–59] PET-CT is excellent for following durability of response of radiotherapy for a lesion.[55] PET-CT has 90% sensitivity for detection of bone involvement compared to 57% for CT or MRI for pediatric sarcoma bone lesions.[60] Areas that contain hardware are hard to image using CT and MRI; PET-CT can be particularly helpful these situations, too.

Although proximal tibia, femur, and distal femur limb salvage is now considered routine, for some other locations of osteosarcoma, local control can be particularly challenging and close or + margins are a problem. These include chest wall, central lung lesions, head and neck locations, and the pelvis, especially the sacrum. Figure 2 shows how PET-CT can facilitate radiotherapy treatment planning and follow-up of osteosarcoma involving the sacrum. Figure 3 shows details of maxillary metastases successfully treated with radiation and chemotherapy. Figure 4 shows a case in which RT seemed effective in 1 small pleural based and 2 chest wall lesions. L-MTP-PE was used to attempt to reduce chance of additional lung and pleural metastases. Once off therapy, 1 lesion recurred requiring surgery to be done. Figure 5 shows some images of a patient with osteosarcoma brain metastases recurring in brain 5 years s/p initial therapy and 2 years after removal of a solitary lung metastasis. She had response to doxorubicin liposomes and bevacizumab for 8 months then had progression. She had surgery for 2 major lesions and sterotactic RT for a remaining supraorbital lesion. Six weeks later she had whole brain radiotherapy for osteosarcoma. Recovery has been complete.

Thermal Ablation

After imaging and placing probes to deliver heat (radiofrequency ablation; RFA) or freezing and thawing cycles (cryoablation) thermal ablation is another means of local control of tumors.[61–66] Lesions must be observable using CT or ultrasound (>1 cm) and not so large that heating or freezing becomes difficult (<5 cm). Locations near blood vessels cannot be adequately ablated because of removal of heat or cold by the blood leaves a Cuff of viable tumor surrounding the vessel. RFA requires anesthesia, but recovery times are generally very short (1–2 days), but

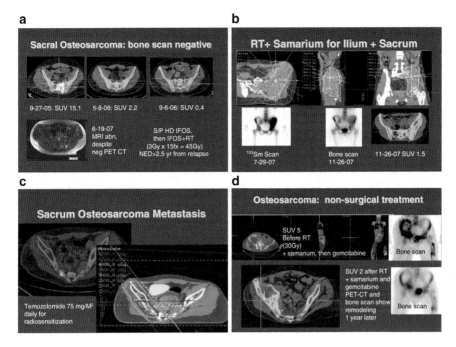

Fig. 2 Imaging of osteosarcomas involving the sacrum before and after local control with radiation in combination with samarium and/or chemotherapy. (a) This patient is now NED s/p removal of 1 lung metastasis with good function >2.5 years from relapse. Patients in panels (b) and (c) had no symptoms during radiotherapy and continue to have normal function. Patient in (d) also had lung and liver metastases and was given oral continuation chemotherapy with oral cyclophosphamide, Rapamycin and valproate. Lung metastases removed at 1 year had 100% necrosis and he is now off chemotherapy therapy >2 years s/p relapse. Bone scan shows response despite bone remodeling of ilium + sacral relapse

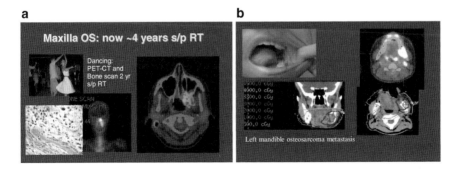

Fig. 3 Maxillary Osteosarcoma. (a) Primary disease responded to standard therapy, then ifosfamide with reduction in SUV on PET-CT and marked elevation of Alkaline phosphastase becoming normal. Bone scan remained avid. 55Gy RT was given in 5 weeks with cycles of ifosfamide at beginning and end of RT. Mucositis resolved in 4 weeks and patient is now 5 years from diagnosis. (b) Maxillary osteosarcoma metastasis (biopsy proven) treated with RT and temozolomide. Pain improved and oral lesion resolved in about 6 weeks

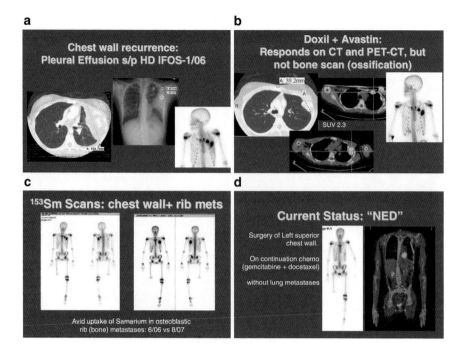

Fig. 4 Images of a teenager with osteosarcoma chest wall and pleural fluid osteosarcoma. After progression s/p high dose ifosfamide (**a**), she was treated with both non-surgical and surgical means. Initial chemotherapy to reduce disease burden and effusion was doxorubicin liposomes and bevacizumab (**b**). Local control was radiotherapy and samarium gemcitabine (**c**). Following completion of L-MTP-PE, relapse in 1 of the 2 chest wall nodules occurred. She received samarium again (**c**). Local control was surgery was done; she is now "NED" on continuation chemotherapy with good quality of life on the outpatient regimen gemcitabine + docetaxel (**d**)

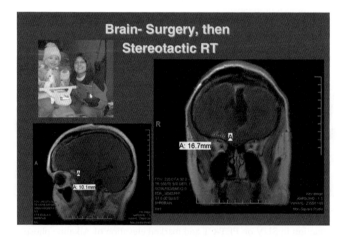

Fig. 5 Brain metastases of osteosarcoma. This patient was treated with chemotherapy to reduce disease then surgery. After removal of 2 lesions, sterotactic RT and then whole brain radiotherapy using temozolomide as radiation sensitizer was done. She has regained good health and is able to care for her active 3 year old daughter without difficulty

some patients may have symptoms for 1–2 weeks.[67] If tumors are near the skin, there is a greater chance for a burn and/or future wound problem. Temperature sensors can be placed in adjacent areas during the procedure (e.g., spine, skin) to make sure areas that do not need thermal ablation do not get too much heat during the procedure.

RFA has been best studied for tumors in the liver. Hepatic location, size, and number of lesions will determine feasibility. Administration of doxorubicin liposomes following the procedure may increase the zone of surrounding necrosis.[68,69] Bone lesions are also possible to destroy using RFA.[70] If metal is present, heat transfer makes thermal ablation procedures relatively contraindicated.

Lung and chest wall lesions are more difficult to destroy because of potential for pneumothorax.[71–74] However, in patients with prior thoracotomies, incidence of pneumothorax seems reduced, probably because of pre-existing pleural adhesions from prior surgery. In patients with low pulmonary reserve (e.g., FVC 45% or less), or a location that would require a large wedge resection that would reduce pulmonary reserve, RFA or cryoablation may actually provide good balance of local control and preservation of lung function. Cryoabation is another option for lung tumors.[64,65] Figure 6 illustrates versatility of RFA to treat both lung and bone-forming osteosarcoma lesions. Sometimes just providing local control to some lesions with non-surgical means will then allow a surgeon to plan for definitive surgical procedure for the remaining osteosarcoma metastasis.

Summary and Conclusion

Unfortunately, there is no recipe for control of osteosarcoma metastases; it is more like cooking. To achieve best results, experienced sarcoma specialists employ the guiding principles of (a) reduction of disease is better than allowing it to grow and cause worse problems, (b) interventions should be done in the spirit of improving

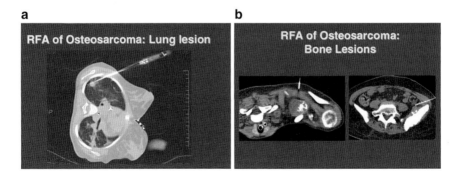

Fig. 6 Thermal ablation of osteosarcoma lesions. Radiofrequency ablation (RFA) is a technique to destroy tumor nodules using heat. A probe is placed into the lesion using CT guidance, then energy is delivered to kill tumor cells. (**a**) lung lesion, (**b**) bone lesions treated with RFA

quality of life and reducing or eliminating sources of pain and loss of function, and (c) even when health care teams and families expect the worst, active intervention and treatment may also allow some hope for additional meaningful time to write future chapters in the life narratives of these special patients.

Acknowledgments The author thanks the many members of the MD Anderson Cancer Center that make multidisciplinary care for metastases possible including Dr. Kamran Ahrar (interventional radiology), Dr. Andrea Hayes-Jordan (Pediatric Surgery), Dr. Ara Vaporciyan (thoracic Surgery), Dr. Rudolfo Nunez (Nuclear Medicine), Dr. Nancy Fitzgerald (Pediatric Radiology), Maritza Salazar-Abshire, RN, Margaret Pearson , CNP, and Kathy Cornelius.

References

1. Jaffe N, Carrasco H, Raymond K, et al. Can cure in patients with osteosarcoma be achieved exclusively with chemotherapy and abrogation of surgery? *Cancer.* 2002;95:2202-2210.
2. Kempf-Bielack B, Bielack SS, Jurgens H, et al. Osteosarcoma relapse after combined modality therapy: an analysis of unselected patients in the Cooperative Osteosarcoma Study Group (COSS). *J Clin Oncol.* 2005;23:559-568.
3. Anderson P. Osteosarcoma relapse: expect the worst, but hope for the best. *Pediatr Blood Cancer.* 2006;47:231-238.
4. Charon R. Narrative and medicine. *N Engl J Med.* 2004;350:862-864.
5. Harter LM, Japp PM. Technology as the representative anecdote in popular discourses of health and medicine. *Health Commun.* 2001;13:409-425.
6. Harter LM, Japp PM, Beck CS. *Narratives, Health, and Healing.* Mahwah, NJ: Lawrence Erlbaum Associates; 2005. 516 pp.
7. Anderson P, Salazar-Abshire M. Improving outcomes in difficult bone cancers using multi-modality therapy, including radiation: physician and nursing perspectives. *Curr Oncol Rep.* 2006;8:415-422.
8. Norville D. *Thank You Power: Making the Science of Gratitude Work for You.* Nashville: Thomas Nelson; 2007.
9. Anderson PM, Pearson M. Novel therapeutic approaches in pediatric and young adult sarcomas. *Curr Oncol Rep.* 2006;8:310-315.
10. Skubitz KM. Phase II trial of pegylated-liposomal doxorubicin (Doxil) in sarcoma. *Cancer Invest.* 2003;21:167-176.
11. Wilkins RM, Cullen JW, Odom L, et al. Superior survival in treatment of primary nonmeta-static pediatric osteosarcoma of the extremity. *Ann Surg Oncol.* 2003;10:498-507.
12. Wilkins RM, Cullen JW, Camozzi AB, et al. Improved survival in primary nonmetastatic pediatric osteosarcoma of the extremity. *Clin Orthop Relat Res.* 2005;438:128-136.
13. Anderson P, Kornguth D, Ahrar K, et al. Non-surgical treatments for young people with high-grade sarcoma metastases. *Pediatr Health.* 2008;2 (in press).
14. Boyer MW, Moertel CL, Priest JR, Woods WG. Use of intracavitary cisplatin for the treatment of childhood solid tumors in the chest or abdominal cavity. *J Clin Oncol.* 1995;13:631-636.
15. Ferguson WS, Harris MB, Goorin AM, et al. Presurgical window of carboplatin and surgery and multidrug chemotherapy for the treatment of newly diagnosed metastatic or unresectable osteosarcoma: pediatric Oncology Group Trial. *J Pediatr Hematol Oncol.* 2001;23:340-348.
16. Daw NC, Billups CA, Rodriguez-Galindo C, et al. Metastatic osteosarcoma. *Cancer.* 2006;106:403-412.
17. Skubitz KM, Hamdan H, Thompson RC Jr. Ambulatory continuous infusion ifosfamide with oral etoposide in advanced sarcomas. *Cancer.* 1993;72:2963-2969.
18. Anderson P, Aguilera D, Pearson M, Woo S. Outpatient chemotherapy + radiotherapy in sarcomas: improving cancer control with radiosensitizing agents. *Cancer Control.* 2008;15:38-46.

Non-Surgical Treatment of Pulmonary and Extra-pulmonary Metastases   213

19. Ferrari A, Grosso F, Stacchiotti S, et al. Response to vinorelbine and low-dose cyclophosphamide chemotherapy in two patients with desmoplastic small round cell tumor. *Pediatr Blood Cancer*. 2007;49:864-866.
20. Casanova M, Ferrari A, Bisogno G, et al. Vinorelbine and low-dose cyclophosphamide in the treatment of pediatric sarcomas: pilot study for the upcoming European Rhabdomyosarcoma Protocol. *Cancer*. 2004;101:1664-1671.
21. Anderson P. Chemotherapy for osteosarcoma with high-dose methotrexate is effective and outpatient therapy is now possible. *Nat Clin Pract Oncol*. 2007;4:624-625.
22. Leu KM, Ostruszka LJ, Shewach D, et al. Laboratory and clinical evidence of synergistic cytotoxicity of sequential treatment with gemcitabine followed by docetaxel in the treatment of sarcoma. *J Clin Oncol*. 2004;22:1706-1712.
23. Maki RG. Gemcitabine and docetaxel in metastatic sarcoma: past, present, and future. *Oncologist*. 2007;12:999-1006.
24. Reidy DL, Chung KY, Timoney JP, et al. Bevacizumab 5 mg/kg can be infused safely over 10 minutes. *J Clin Oncol*. 2007;25:2691-2695.
25. Anderson PM, Markovic SN, Sloan JA, et al. Aerosol granulocyte macrophage-colony stimulating factor: a low toxicity, lung-specific biological therapy in patients with lung metastases. *Clin Cancer Res*. 1999;5:2316-2323.
26. Wylam ME, Ten R, Prakash UB, et al. Aerosol granulocyte-macrophage colony-stimulating factor for pulmonary alveolar proteinosis. *Eur Respir J*. 2006;27:585-593.
27. Anderson P. Liposomal muramyl tripeptide phosphatidylehtanolamine (L-MTP-PE):ifosfamide containing chemotherapy in osteosarcoma. *Future Oncol*. 2006;2 (in press).
28. Meyers PA, Schwartz CL, Krailo MD, et al. Osteosarcoma: the addition of muramyl tripeptide to chemotherapy improves overall survival – a report from the Children's Oncology Group. *J Clin Oncol*. 2008;26:633-638.
29. Anderson PM, Wiseman GA, Erlandson L, et al. Gemcitabine radiosensitization after high-dose samarium for osteoblastic osteosarcoma. *Clin Cancer Res*. 2005;11:6895-6900.
30. Anderson PM, Wiseman GA, Dispenzieri A, et al. High-dose samarium-153 ethylene diamine tetramethylene phosphonate: low toxicity of skeletal irradiation in patients with osteosarcoma and bone metastases. *J Clin Oncol*. 2002;20:189-196.
31. Anderson P. Samarium for osteoblastic bone metastases and osteosarcoma. *Expert Opin Pharmacother*. 2006;7:1475-1486.
32. Anderson P, Nunez R. Samarium lexidronam (153Sm-EDTMP): skeletal radiation for osteoblastic bone metastases and osteosarcoma. *Expert Rev Anticancer Ther*. 2007;7:1517-1527.
33. Bruland OS, Skretting A, Solheim OP, Aas M. Targeted radiotherapy of osteosarcoma using 153 Sm-EDTMP. A new promising approach. *Acta Oncol*. 1996;35:381-384.
34. Ory B, Blanchard F, Battaglia S, et al. Zoledronic acid activates the DNA S-phase checkpoint and induces osteosarcoma cell death characterized by apoptosis-inducing factor and endonuclease-G translocation independently of p53 and retinoblastoma status. *Mol Pharmacol*. 2007;71:333-343.
35. Gralow J, Tripathy D. Managing metastatic bone pain: the role of bisphosphonates. *J Pain Symptom Manage*. 2007;33:462-472.
36. Russell RG. Bisphosphonates: mode of action and pharmacology. *Pediatrics*. 2007;119(Suppl 2):S150-S162.
37. Willett CG, Boucher Y, di Tomaso E, et al. Direct evidence that the VEGF-specific antibody bevacizumab has antivascular effects in human rectal cancer. *Nat Med*. 2004;10:145-147.
38. Winkler F, Kozin SV, Tong RT, et al. Kinetics of vascular normalization by VEGFR2 blockade governs brain tumor response to radiation: role of oxygenation, angiopoietin-1, and matrix metalloproteinases. *Cancer Cell*. 2004;6:553-563.
39. Tong RT, Boucher Y, Kozin SV, et al. Vascular normalization by vascular endothelial growth factor receptor 2 blockade induces a pressure gradient across the vasculature and improves drug penetration in tumors. *Cancer Res*. 2004;64:3731-3736.
40. Shor AC, Agresta SV, D'Amato GZ, Sondak VK. Therapeutic potential of directed tyrosine kinase inhibitor therapy in sarcomas. *Cancer Control*. 2008;15:47-54.

41. Gordon N, Koshkina NV, Jia SF, et al. Corruption of the Fas pathway delays the pulmonary clearance of murine osteosarcoma cells, enhances their metastatic potential, and reduces the effect of aerosol gemcitabine. *Clin Cancer Res.* 2007;13:4503-4510.
42. Koshkina NV, Kleinerman ES. Aerosol gemcitabine inhibits the growth of primary osteosarcoma and osteosarcoma lung metastases. *Int J Cancer.* 2005;116:458-463.
43. Khanna C, Helman LJ. Molecular approaches in pediatric oncology. *Annu Rev Med.* 2006;57: 83-97.
44. Krishnan K, Khanna C, Helman LJ. The biology of metastases in pediatric sarcomas. *Cancer J.* 2005;11:306-313.
45. Wan X, Mendoza A, Khanna C, Helman LJ. Rapamycin inhibits ezrin-mediated metastatic behavior in a murine model of osteosarcoma. *Cancer Res.* 2005;65:2406-2411.
46. Savage SA, Woodson K, Walk E, et al. Analysis of genes critical for growth regulation identifies insulin-like growth factor 2 receptor variations with possible functional significance as risk factors for osteosarcoma. *Cancer Epidemiol Biomarkers Prev.* 2007;16:1667-1674.
47. Shevah O, Laron Z. Patients with congenital deficiency of IGF-I seem protected from the development of malignancies: a preliminary report. *Growth Horm IGF Res.* 2007;17:54-57.
48. Mochizuki S, Yoshida S, Yamanaka Y, et al. Effects of estriol on proliferative activity and expression of insulin-like growth factor-I (IGF-I) and IGF-I receptor mRNA in cultured human osteoblast-like osteosarcoma cells. *Gynecol Endocrinol.* 2005;20:6-12.
49. MacEwen EG, Pastor J, Kutzke J, et al. IGF-1 receptor contributes to the malignant phenotype in human and canine osteosarcoma. *J Cell Biochem.* 2004;92:77-91.
50. Bruland OS, Nilsson S, Fisher DR, Larsen RH. High-linear energy transfer irradiation targeted to skeletal metastases by the alpha-emitter 223Ra: adjuvant or alternative to conventional modalities? *Clin Cancer Res.* 2006;12:6250s-6257s.
51. Lemieux J, Maunsell E, Provencher L. Chemotherapy-induced alopecia and effects on quality of life among women with breast cancer: a literature review. *Psychooncology.* 2007;17:317-328.
52. Batchelor D. Hair and cancer chemotherapy: consequences and nursing care – a literature study. *Eur J Cancer Care (Engl).* 2001;10:147-163.
53. Machak GN, Tkachev SI, Solovyev YN, et al. Neoadjuvant chemotherapy and local radiotherapy for high-grade osteosarcoma of the extremities. *Mayo Clin Proc.* 2003;78:147-155.
54. Anderson PM. Effectiveness of radiotherapy for osteosarcoma that responds to chemotherapy. *Mayo Clin Proc.* 2003;78:145-146.
55. Mahajan A, Woo SY, Kornguth DG, et al. Multimodality treatment of osteosarcoma: radiation in a high-risk cohort. *Pediatr Blood Cancer.* 2008;50:976-982.
56. Dincbas FO, Koca S, Mandel NM, et al. The role of preoperative radiotherapy in nonmetastatic high-grade osteosarcoma of the extremities for limb-sparing surgery. *Int J Radiat Oncol Biol Phys.* 2005;62:820-828.
57. DeLaney TF, Trofimov AV, Engelsman M, Suit HD. Advanced-technology radiation therapy in the management of bone and soft tissue sarcomas. *Cancer Control.* 2005;12:27-35.
58. DeLaney TF, Park L, Goldberg SI, et al. Radiotherapy for local control of osteosarcoma. *Int J Radiat Oncol Biol Phys.* 2005;61:492-498.
59. Patel S, Delaney TF. Advanced-technology radiation therapy for bone sarcomas. *Cancer Control.* 2008;15:21-37.
60. Volker T, Denecke T, Steffen I, et al. Positron emission tomography for staging of pediatric sarcoma patients: results of a prospective multicenter trial. *J Clin Oncol.* 2007;25:5435-5441.
61. Ahrar K. The role and limitations of radiofrequency ablation in treatment of bone and soft tissue tumors. *Curr Oncol Rep.* 2004;6:315-320.
62. Ahrar K, Wallace MJ, Matin SF. Percutaneous radiofrequency ablation: minimally invasive therapy for renal tumors. *Expert Rev Anticancer Ther.* 2006;6:1735-1744.
63. Allaf ME, Varkarakis IM, Bhayani SB, et al. Pain control requirements for percutaneous ablation of renal tumors: cryoablation versus radiofrequency ablation – initial observations. *Radiology.* 2005;237:366-370.
64. Ahmed A, Littrup P. Percutaneous cryotherapy of the thorax: safety considerations for complex cases. *AJR Am J Roentgenol.* 2006;186:1703-1706.

65. Wang H, Littrup PJ, Duan Y, et al. Thoracic masses treated with percutaneous cryotherapy: initial experience with more than 200 procedures. *Radiology*. 2005;235:289-298.
66. Simon CJ, Dupuy DE. Percutaneous minimally invasive therapies in the treatment of bone tumors: thermal ablation. *Semin Musculoskelet Radiol*. 2006;10:137-144.
67. Carrafiello G, Lagana D, Ianniello A, et al. Post-radiofrequency ablation syndrome after percutaneous radiofrequency of abdominal tumours: one centre experience and review of published works. *Australas Radiol*. 2007;51:550-554.
68. Ahmed M, Goldberg SN. Combination radiofrequency thermal ablation and adjuvant IV liposomal doxorubicin increases tissue coagulation and intratumoural drug accumulation. *Int J Hyperthermia*. 2004;20:781-802.
69. Goldberg SN, Kamel IR, Kruskal JB, et al. Radiofrequency ablation of hepatic tumors: increased tumor destruction with adjuvant liposomal doxorubicin therapy. *AJR Am J Roentgenol*. 2002;179:93-101.
70. Goetz MP, Callstrom MR, Charboneau JW, et al. Percutaneous image-guided radiofrequency ablation of painful metastases involving bone: a multicenter study. *J Clin Oncol*. 2004;22:300-306.
71. Nguyen CL, Scott WJ, Goldberg M. Radiofrequency ablation of lung malignancies. *Ann Thorac Surg*. 2006;82:365-371.
72. Kybosh M, Yamakado K, Nakatsuka A, et al. Percutaneous radiofrequency ablation of lung neoplasms: initial therapeutic response. *J Vasc Interv Radiol*. 2004;15:463-470.
73. Suh RD, Wallace AB, Sheehan RE, et al. Unresectable pulmonary malignancies: CT-guided percutaneous radiofrequency ablation – preliminary results. *Radiology*. 2003;229:821-829.
74. Grieco CA, Simon CJ, Mayo-Smith WW, et al. Image-guided percutaneous thermal ablation for the palliative treatment of chest wall masses. *Am J Clin Oncol*. 2007;30:361-367.

Review of the Past, Impact on the Future

Adjuvant Chemotherapy in Osteosarcoma

An Odyssey of Rejection and Vindication

Norman Jaffe

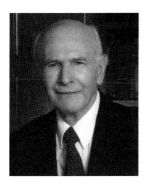

Osteosarcoma is the most common malignant bone tumor affecting children and adolescents. The biological behavior is consistent with the premise that pulmonary micrometastases are present at diagnosis in the majority of patients. These are silent and undetected on imaging studies. They usually surface six to twelve months following amputation of the primary tumor and if untreated are responsible for the patients demise. Until the 1970s the tumor was generally considered to be chemoresistant. However, in the early 1970's, two chemotherapeutic agents were found to be active in osteosarcoma. These comprised Adriamycin (doxorubicin) and high-dose Methotrexate with Citrovorin factor rescue (Leucovorin rescue). The administration of high-dose Methotrexate following amputation alone or in combination with other agents yielded a cure rate of 40-65 percent. This was attributed to the destruction of the pulmonary micrometastases. The improved survival due chemotherapy did not go unchallenged. The Mayo Clinic adduced data to suggest that there had been a "natural improvement" in the cure rate over several years and that it should not necessarily be assumed that chemotherapy, particularly high-dose Methotrexate, was responsible for the improvement. The veracity of historical controls and the efficacy of high dose Methotrexate were also disputed by additional claims from the Mayo Clinic. Principal among these was recent advances in diagnostic techniques i.e. CT lung and radionuclide bone scans.

To resolve the problem a multi-institutional randomized osteosarcoma trial (MIOS) was launched. A series of patients was treated by amputation and postoperatively with multiagent chemotherapy comprising high-dose Methotrexate Adriamycin, Cisplatin, Bleomycin, Cyclophosphamide and Dactinomycin. A second series of patients was treated with amputation only (concurrent controls). Treatment by amputation and postoperative adjuvant chemotherapy achieved a 66 percent two-year disease-free survival. In contrast, patients treated by amputation alone garnered a significantly worse outcome: less than 20 percent survival. The latter was comparable

---

N. Jaffe (✉)
Children's Cancer Hospital, University of Texas M.D. Anderson Cancer Center, 1515 Holcombe Boulevard, Unit #87, Houston, TX, 77030-4009, USA
e-mail: njaffe@mdanderson.org

to survival in the historical control series. Chemotherapy was thus found to be effective and comparison of the results with historical controls was validated.

The above experience was further substantiated by an additional concurrent randomized trial. An editorial by James Holland in the Journal of Clinical Oncology commented on the results of the randomized trial(s) and offered suggestions for the conduct of future trials. The acceptance of chemotherapy as an integral and essential component for the treatment of osteosarcoma launched a new era in the conquest of this disease.

Introduction

Those who do not remember the past are condemned to repeat it.[1]

Osteosarcoma is the most common malignant bone tumor in the pediatric age. A higher incidence occurs in adolescents and young adults, but it is not uncommon in the pre-teenage individual. The biological behavior of osteosarcoma is consistent with the premise that silent pulmonary micrometastases are present in at least 80–90 of patients at the time of diagnosis. These metastases are not detectable using conventional imaging or computerized tomography (CT). However, their presence is

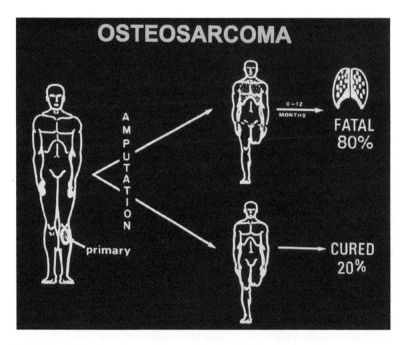

Fig. 1 Biological behavior of osteosarcoma. Silent pulmonary micro-metastases are present in 80–90% of patients at diagnosis. Following amputation, in the absence of effective postoperative therapy, overt metastases appear within 1 year. In optimum circumstances only 20% of patients in whom metastases are absent survive

inferred from prior experiences in which the majority of patients were treated by amputation. At the time of amputation, imaging studies demonstrated that the lungs were free of tumor. However, 6 to 12 months following amputation, 80–90% of patients usually developed overt pulmonary metastases (Fig. 1). Effective therapy to eradicate these metastases was not available, and patients invariably died of disease within 12 months of ablation of the primary tumor. This consistent outcome was documented by Friedman and Carter in a 1972 review of 1,337 patients. They reported a survival rate of 19.7% in patients treated with amputation.[2]

The poor prognosis following surgical ablation of primary tumors prompted Sir Stanford Cade, a surgeon/radiotherapist, to advocate a program of preoperative radiation therapy followed by elective amputation, if pulmonary metastases were absent.[3] The intent was to avoid unnecessary mutilation in patients destined to die of pulmonary metastases. Radiation therapy comprised 7,000–8,000 rad administered by supra-voltage technique over 6 to 8 weeks. After an interval of 6 to 8 months, in the absence of pulmonary metastases, ablative surgery was performed. Amputation was not performed, however, if pulmonary metastases had developed or if control of the primary tumor was exceptionally good (absence of local relapse). Consequently, a minority of patients could escape amputation altogether. Nonetheless, the outlook for patient survival remained dire, prompting Cade to quote the remarks of a celebrated surgeon of international repute in summarizing a scientific meeting on "bone sarcoma": "If you do not operate, they die; if you do operate, they die just the same– gentlemen, this meeting should be completed with prayers."[3]

With the consistent development of pulmonary metastases, osteosarcoma was considered a systemic disease that would require systemic therapy for its eradication and cure. A variety of systemic therapeutic measures for destroying the pulmonary micrometastases were thus investigated. These measures included immunotherapy and chemotherapeutic agents extant at that time. However, until the 1970s, none proved successful, and osteosarcoma came to be considered a chemo-resistant tumor.

The Promise of Chemotherapy

Comparison of Results with Historical Controls

In 1948, Farber et al. reported that the folic-acid antagonist 4-aminopteroyl-glutamic acid (aminopterin) produced temporary remissions in acute childhood leukemia.[4] The agent was subsequently synthesized for clinical application as methotrexate. In 1954, Golden et al.[5] demonstrated that in mice with leukemia, large doses of methotrexate, followed by citrovorin factor (later designated leucovorin) after a delayed interval, destroyed the leukemic cells and simultaneously afforded protection of normal host tissues; citrovorin factor is the antidote to methotrexate and supplies the product surceased by methotrexate.[5] The therapeutic strategy, designated "high-dose methotrexate with citrovorin factor rescue" (later, "leucovorin rescue"), was investigated by Burchenal[6] in adults and Djerassi et al[7] in children. In the clinical arena, the strategy was found to be valid, safe, and effective for the treatment of leukemia

In view of the grave prognosis for patients with osteosarcoma and the absence of an effective therapeutic mechanism for destroying the pulmonary metastases, the strategy was investigated in patients with osteosarcoma and overt pulmonary disease. Treatment was implemented in 1970 at the Children's Hospital Medical Center in Boston (currently the Boston Children's Hospital) and the adjacent Children's Cancer Research Foundation ("Jimmy Fund"), a component of the current Dana-Farber Cancer Institute. Permission to undertake the investigation required sole approval from Dr Sidney Farber, director of the foundation; institutional review boards had not been established at that time.

The first patient selected for therapy had undergone a hemipelvectomy for osteosarcoma of the ileum and had developed pulmonary metastases 9 months later. All potential putative side effects of the new therapeutic approach that were known at that time were outlined to the patient and her mother. Both consented to the treatment. It included an initial dose of vincristine based upon experimental evidence that the drug, in concentrations achievable in vivo, increased the uptake of methotrexate in vitro.[8] (Vincristine was subsequently discarded because it was not considered clinically effective and may have contributed to toxicity.)

Treatment commenced with a continuous infusion of 5% dextrose water, which was maintained for 72 h. Methotrexate was administered at an initial dose of 50 mg/kg. It was dissolved in 500 mL of 5% dextrose water for intravenous infusion over 6 h. Citrovorin factor ($6–15$ mg/m^2) was initiated 2 h after the completion of the methotrexate infusion, and 12 doses were administered at 6 h intervals, with the dose adjusted according to the surface area of the patient and the quantity of methotrexate administered. With experience and compelling evidence that high-dose methotrexate could be delivered safely and effectively, the dose was escalated at 3-week intervals.[9]

The patient had begun the treatment with bilateral pulmonary metastases. A durable complete response was attained with 200 mg/kg methotrexate (Fig. 2). To ensure adequate tumoricidal concentrations, a dose of 250 mg/kg (12.5 g/m^2) was adopted for future therapeutic administration. This dose was arbitrarily chosen since facilities to test serum methotrexate concentrations in the blood were not available. With the discovery that this therapeutic strategy was effective, treatment was offered to 12 additional patients with pulmonary and/or bone metastases. Responses were attained in four.[9]

A practice was then implemented of administering high-dose methotrexate with leucovorin rescue as postoperative adjuvant therapy after ablation of patients' primary tumors.[10] The objective was to destroy the putative silent pulmonary micrometastases. The rationale underlying this strategy was derived from experiments published by Skipper et al., Laster et al., and Schabel.[11–13] The strategy proved effective. Subsequently, as postoperative adjuvant therapy, high-dose methotrexate was administered alone or in combination with doxorubicin (Adriamycin) in three studies. Over the ensuing 15 years, survival rates of 40–65% were achieved: 40% with methotrexate alone and up to 65% with methotrexate and doxorubicin.[14,15] In comparison with the historical controls reported in the literature, with a maximal survival rate of less than 20%, the results were significant. Other investigators who utilized high-dose methotrexate in combination with doxorubicin, cisplatin, and cyclophosphamide recorded similar experiences.[16–18]

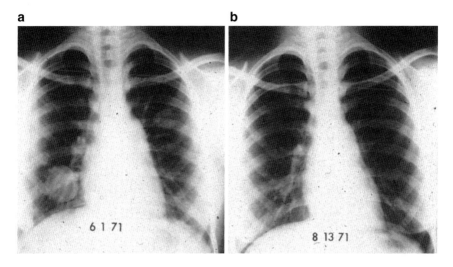

Fig. 2 (**a**) (*left*). Chest radiograph of patient with metastases in the right lower lobe and left upper lobe. (**b**) (*right*). Two months later following high dose Methotrexate therapy complete regression of both lesions had occurred. This material is reproduced with permission of Wiley–Liss, Inc., a subsidiary of John Wiley & Sons Inc. (Jaffe N et al. Cancer, 31: 1367–1373, 1973)

Controversy: Are Historical Controls Valid?

However, the claim that improved survival rates could be attributed to chemotherapy, particularly high-dose methotrexate, was refuted. Muggia and Louie asserted that there was "wide disparity on the fate of adjuvant treatment in osteosarcoma" and that "assessment of data from adjuvant trials ranges from unbridled optimism to cautious noncommittal reporting to outright pessimism."[19]

The skepticism by Muggia and Louie was bolstered by data from the Mayo Clinic. The investigators there reported a disease-free survival rate of 40% in patients treated by amputation and prophylactic whole-lung radiotherapy.[20] A later communication noted a steady progression toward improved survival over several years (from 1963–1965 to 1972–1974). Prior to 1969, the survival rate had been constant, around 20% (in keeping with the historical controls summarized by Friedman and Carter)[2]; however, after 1969, the rate "spontaneously" increased to 40–50% without the apparent benefit of postoperative adjuvant treatment[21] (Fig. 3). A follow-up report further confirmed that the period during which patients were treated had a strong influence on survival and that there were no significant differences in survival rates between patients treated solely by amputation and those treated by amputation supplemented with chemotherapy and pulmonary radiation.[22]

A number of factors were suggested by the Mayo Clinic investigators and others as possible contributors to the discrepancy between the Mayo Clinic's higher survival rates in the absence of chemotherapy and the survival rates reported by the Freidman and Carter report and others (see later). These factors, none of which were

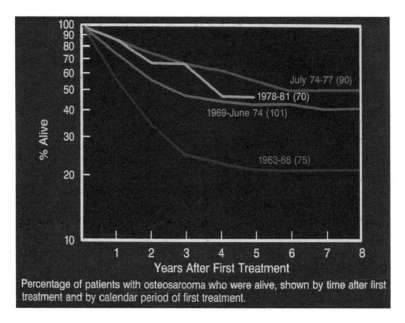

Fig. 3 Historical survival rates over several sequential periods at the Mayo clinic demonstrating improvement in osteosarcoma patients treated by amputation without effective chemotherapy. Reprinted with permission from Taylor WF, Ivins J, Prichard D, et al. Trends and variability in survival among patients with osteosarcoma: a 7-year update. Mayo Mayo Clin Proc 1985; 60(2): 91–104

shown to be definitive, were as follows: (1) Historical and contemporary controls were not truly comparable. (2) New diagnostic techniques (e.g., CT for detecting pulmonary metastases) had altered the staging of the patients. (3) A change in the biology and the "natural history" of the disease had occurred. (4) Patients were being referred earlier for treatment. This possibility was inferred from the supposition that prior to the 1950s, medical attendants may have been reluctant to refer patients to a major medical center for immediate treatment once osteosarcoma was diagnosed or suspected. However, with improved surgical techniques, reticence had perhaps dissipated. Thus, in more recent years, patients with less advanced disease may have been referred earlier, which could have affected survival rates because earlier diagnosis and treatment are usually associated with a more favorable outcome. (5) A tourniquet in conjunction with frozen-section biopsy, followed by immediate amputation, had been practiced at the Mayo Clinic. For inexplicable reason(s), patients so treated in 1969–1974 did significantly better than those treated in 1963–1968.[21,22]

The reports on historical survival rates from the Mayo Clinic differed sharply from those published by the Dana-Farber Cancer Center, M. D. Anderson Cancer Center, and Memorial Sloan-Kettering Cancer Center[8,18,23–26] (Figs. 4–6). These institutions confirmed the Friedman and Carter report.[2] In their publications, survival rates varied from 5 to 20%, and in contrast to the results at the Mayo Clinic, at the Dana-Farber Cancer Center, the worst survival rates had occurred during the most recent calendar years.[10] Communications from the Rizzoli Orthopaedic

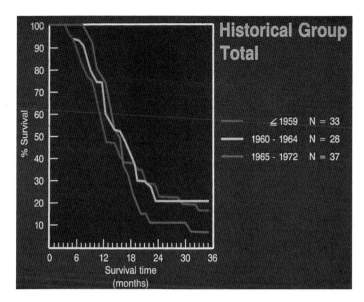

Fig. 4 Historical control survival rates over several sequential periods of osteosarcoma patients at the Dana Farber Cancer Institute demonstrating survivals less than 20% following treatment with amputation. Reprinted with permission from Jaffe N, et al. Adjuvant Methotrexate and Citrovorum–Factor Treatment of Osteogenic Sarcoma. New J Med 291: 994–97, 1974

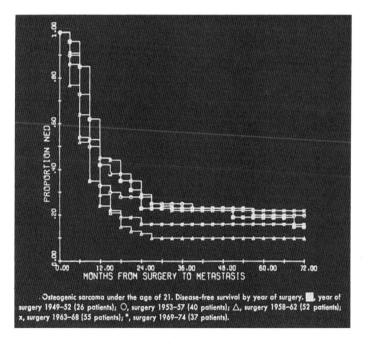

Fig. 5 Historical control survival rates over several sequential periods at the Memorial Sloan Kettering Cancer Center demonstrating survival of 25% or less following amputation. Reprinted with permission from Mike V and Marcove RC: Osteogenic sarcoma under the age of 21. Experiences at Memorial Sloan Kettering Cancer Centre. In: Immunotherapy of cancer. Present status of trials in man. In: Terry WD and Windhorst D (eds.) Raven Press, New York, pp 271–82, 1978 Progress in Cancer Research, Vol VI

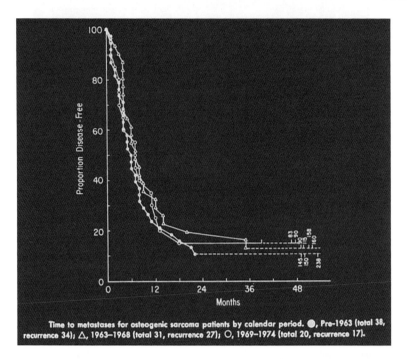

Fig. 6 Historical control survival rates over several sequential periods at the MD Anderson Cancer Center demonstrating survival of 20% or less in osteosarcoma patients treated by amputation. Reprinted with permission from Gehan EA et al: Osteosarcoma. The MD Anderson Experience 1850–1974. In: Immunotherapy of cancer. Preset status of trials in man. In: Terry WD and WIndhorst D (eds.) Raven Press, New York, pp 271–82, 1978 Progress in Cancer Research, Vol Vi

Institute in Bologna, Italy, described similar historical survival curves (and similar improvements with chemotherapy).[27,28]

The contention that CT scans (which had only recently been introduced) had altered the staging status of patients could not be substantiated. The absence of pulmonary metastases and the pristine status of the lungs in patients treated at the Children's Hospital Medical Center in Boston had been confirmed by pulmonary laminograms, a practice extant at that time. Further, CT scans did not appear to be vastly superior to conventional chest radiographs for detecting pulmonary metastases. According to several contemporary published reports, the differences between rates of CT detection of lesions and rates of detection with conventional radiographs and pulmonary laminograms varied from 1.9 to 9.3%.[29–33] Nevertheless, skepticism in regard to the benefit of postoperative adjuvant chemotherapy persisted.

Additional reports demonstrating responses to methotrexate and attesting further to its efficacy in osteosarcoma were published.[34–44] The responses provided evidence that methotrexate augmented the therapeutic effects of radiation therapy in destroying overt pulmonary metastases (Figs. 7–10 depict a representative case) and enhanced the opportunity for performing safer surgical procedures in limb salvage operations (Figs. 11 and 12 depict a representative case). When the primary tumor was treated with methotrexate, it not only induced necrosis but also the

Adjuvant Chemotherapy in Osteosarcoma

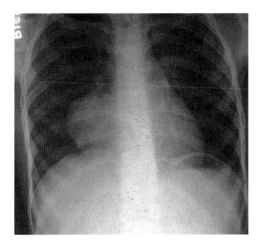

Fig. 7 Pulmonary metastasis in the paracardiac region of the right lower lobe of a patient following amputation for an osteosarcoma of the distal femur. Radiation (1,500 rad) was delivered to avert possible bronchial invasion or obstruction

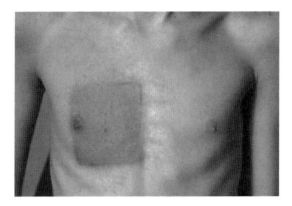

Fig. 8 Radiation reaction confined to the portal of radiation. High dose methotrexate was administered after completion of radiation therapy and the vesicular erythematous eruption developed concurrently with the administration of methotrexate. Reprinted with permission Jaffe N et al. Favorable response of metastatic osteogenic sarcoma to pulse high dose methotrexate with citrovorin rescue and radiation therapy. Cancer 31: 1367–73, 1973

formation of a pseudo-capsule, and when administered postoperatively, it eliminated residual viable microscopic cells at the resection site. This result improved the opportunity for local control. The potential for methotrexate to eradicate "skip" metastases was also noted. These strategies were implemented in a multidisciplinary setting following the observation that "rescue" with leucovorin rendered methotrexate nonmyelosuppressive. Methotrexate could thus be administered on a weekly basis alone or at more prolonged intervals in combination with other agents, particularly doxorubicin.[36,43] Toxicity was minimal, although for unknown reasons, a fatality was occasionally encountered.[40,41]

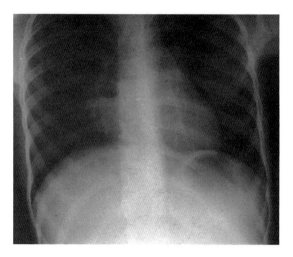

Fig. 9 A chest radiograph obtained concomitantly with the appearance of the skin eruption demonstrated cavitation in the superior portion of the para-cardiac lesion observed in Fig. 8 Reprinted with permission from Jaffe N et al: Favorable response of metastatic osteogenic sarcoma to pulse high dose methotrexate with citrovorin rescue and radiation therapy. Cancer 31: 1367–73, 1973

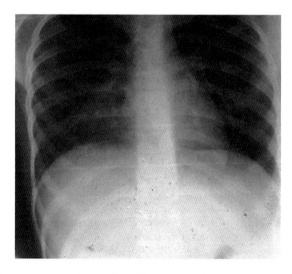

Fig. 10 Complete response attained in the radiation-chemotherapy treatment of the right paracardiac lesion in the patient depicted in Fig. 9. Streaks of residual fibrosis are present

These reports on methotrexate demonstrating improved survival, eradication of pulmonary metastases, enhancement of limb-salvage procedures, and reduction of potential toxicity were published over the ensuing decade. However, the efficacy of chemotherapy, and in particular of high-dose methotrexate, for the treatment of osteosarcoma remained controversial. The controversy centered particularly on the Mayo Clinic report that questioned the validity of historical controls as the basis of comparison for the newly reported studies in which

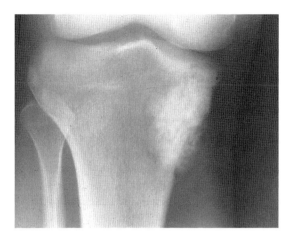

Fig. 11 Osteosarcoma of the proximal tibia. The typical features of an osteoblastic lesion extending into the subcutaneous tissues are present. Clinical signs and symptoms included pain, swelling, localized tenderness and warmth. Limitation of joint movement was present

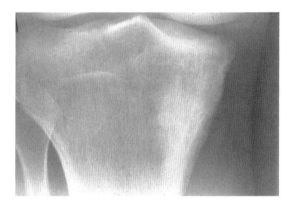

Fig. 12 Complete healing and reconstitution of bone achieved following seven courses of high dose Methotrexate was achieved. All clinical signs and symptoms of an active lesion disappeared. A limb salvage procedure was performed and pathological examination of the resected specimen demonstrated 100% tumor destruction

methotrexate treatment was considered successful. As a result, the Mayo Clinic launched a randomized trial that compared the incidence of pulmonary metastases in patients treated solely by amputation (concurrent controls) and in patients treated by amputation plus postoperative high-dose methotrexate. The study did not demonstrate an advantage with high-dose methotrexate. Survival rates in both arms were approximately 40%.[45]

The Mayo Clinic trial, published in 1984, was followed by an acerbic editorial by Carter "Adjuvant Chemotherapy in Osteosarcoma: The Triumph that Isn't."[46]

However, analysis of the conduct of the Mayo Clinic trial revealed that one quarter of the patients did not receive the recommended methotrexate treatment. There were also departures from the published dose, schedule, and duration of treatment. These discrepancies were emphasized in a letter to the *Journal of Clinical Oncology* and the validity of utilizing historical controls in osteosarcoma was again stated.[47] This letter prompted the following response from Carter: "…the debate about crucial importance of sticking to a regimen recipe with biblical fervor seems to occur only when negative data begin to be reported."[48]

Feinstein et al.,[49] in an effort to diffuse the controversy, suggested that stage migration and new diagnostic techniques may have produced misleading statistics for cancer survival and were possibly responsible for variations in the reported results. They labeled this idea "The Will Rogers Phenomenon," derived from Rogers' entertaining assertion that "When the Okies left Oklahoma and moved to California, they raised the average intelligence level in both states." However, the explanation had no effect in assuaging the controversy. Several investigators insisted that clinical trials utilizing concurrent controls (as opposed to historical controls) were essential to demonstrate the stated efficacy of chemotherapy in osteosarcoma.[50-52] Others inquired whether it was "ethical not to conduct a prospectively controlled trial of adjuvant chemotherapy in osteosarcoma."[53]

The Multi-Institutional Osteosarcoma Study

The call for a prospectively controlled trial of adjuvant chemotherapy did not go unchallenged.[54] It was again emphasized that until the beginning of the 1970s, patients with osteosarcoma had been treated with surgery, radiation, immunotherapy, and ineffective chemotherapy. Survival rates had been less than 20%. This population of patients provided a stable historical-control group that had been repeatedly confirmed by several institutions and investigators. Similar data for the period prior to the 1970s had been published by the Mayo Clinic. There was no explanation for the apparent "natural" improvement in survival over the subsequent defined period reported by the Mayo Clinic. It was also noted that some Mayo Clinic patients had received a variety of additional treatments, including adjuvant chemotherapy and radiation to the lungs. It was suggested that a discussion about, or confirmation of, historical controls was possibly moot in view of newly available effective chemotherapy (i.e., methotrexate). It was also emphasized that CT, tomography, and conventional imaging had no bearing on historical controls as it remained to be demonstrated whether these investigations would indeed render historical controls invalid.

Of major importance was the fact that the survival rates reported in the historical-control series had been gleaned from a large number of patients. It was conceded that histologic findings, tumor size, tumor location, patient age, patient sex, and other factors could influence the outcome of individual patients; however, these factors assumed less significance when similar or identical results were consistently reported among a large number of patients and by numerous independent investigators.

Further, statistical regression methods were available to compensate and adjust for differences when comparing the large volume of historical-control patients with those in current studies.[55]

It was again emphasized that with the administration of effective chemotherapy, pulmonary metastases had not developed in 12–24 months in more than 50% of patients, a significant difference in comparison with historical controls. The 5-year survival rate in patients who received chemotherapy had matured at 50–60%, as described above. Hence it appeared more ethical and fruitful to administer potentially effective (new) chemotherapy to *all* patients rather than to reconfirm (again) the bleak prognosis in concurrent, randomly assigned controls treated solely with surgery.

The additional advantages of the administration of chemotherapy were also emphasized. Thus, experience had revealed that many patients who were treated with seemingly partially effective chemotherapy developed pulmonary metastases that were reduced in number and delayed in their appearance compared with the historical controls.[56] This reduced burden of metastases had been a major factor in successfully treating patients with relapses by thoracotomy and other measures, thereby augmenting the number of long-term survivors.[36,43]

Effective chemotherapy also had had a major impact on the evolution of treatment of the primary tumor. Thus, in contrast to previous practices, transmedullary amputation as opposed to disarticulation had been adopted with increasing frequency, rotationplasty was being offered to more patients, and limb salvage was being considered wherever possible. Limb salvage was generally preceded by preoperative chemotherapy (later designated "neoadjuvant chemotherapy"), which, as indicated earlier, had been found to improve the safety of the surgical procedure.[57]

Finally, the suggestion that physicians in 1930–1950 were reluctant to refer patients to major medical centers was rejected. There was no evidence that lag time, onset of symptoms, and time to diagnosis had influenced the validity of historical controls.

Nevertheless, the role and efficacy of adjuvant chemotherapy in osteosarcoma were again questioned. Link and Vietti[58] asserted "that the role for chemotherapy improving the safety and local rate of limb-sparing procedures which provide clean surgical margins likewise remains conjectural." D'Angio and Evans[59] expressed uncertainty in regard to the role of methotrexate and other agents in osteosarcoma: "…it remains to be seen whether this extremely costly treatment – or any adjuvant drug or drugs – is actually of value when given in this fashion. Whatever the outcome, more than a decade has been lost in vacillation, uncertainty and indecision."

The oscillating dispute gained currency and could not be aborted. The criticisms coalesced, and it was elected to perform a concurrent controlled trial. Included in the list of investigators who would conduct the trial were physicians who had previously published articles attesting to the efficacy of high-dose methotrexate.[14,15,18] The trial was designated The Multi-institutional Osteosarcoma Study (MIOS). The stated rationale and intent were to confirm or refute the "dismal prognosis reported in historical controls" as compared with concurrent controls, which had not been employed in the recently reported "successful" studies. A chemotherapy regimen based principally on publications by Rosen et al.[60,61] was selected for investigation.

It comprised bleomycin, cyclophosphamide, dactinomycin, high-dose methotrexate, doxorubicin, and cisplatin and was to be administered for 45 weeks after amputation to a group of patients selected by randomization. As a comparative concurrent control, a newly diagnosed series of patients also selected by randomization were to be treated solely by amputation.

The MIOS, published in 1986[62] revealed a 65% disease-free survival rate in patients treated with amputation and postoperative adjuvant chemotherapy. Patients treated solely by amputation (concurrent controls) had a survival of less than 20%. The result in the concurrent-control series was thus similar to that of the historical controls. The result confirmed that there had been no change in the natural history of the disease. The report also stated that "the beneficial effects in relapse-free survival attributed to adjuvant chemotherapy in previous uncontrolled trials were *likely* to be real." (author emphasis). Postoperative chemotherapy was thus shown definitively to be effective.

The Ramifications of MIOS

The MIOS was later endorsed by a similar concurrent randomized trial conducted by Eilber et al. It was reported initially in an abstract at the American Society of Clinical Oncology (ASCO) in 1986 and formally in the *Journal of Clinical Oncology*.[63] Holland berated Eilber at the ASCO meeting for conducting the trial and, in an editorial accompanying the formal publication,[64] criticized the use of a "concurrent control arm" bereft of adjuvant chemotherapy when effective agents were available. He proposed criteria for randomized trials and emphasized the need to investigate the feasibility of pilot candidate regimens while assessing human and economic costs. He also stressed the necessity for a thorough literature review (cf. validity of historical controls) and an in-depth study of raw data in an assessment of one's own clinical setting.

The MIOS had been forged on the anvil of scientific rigor at tremendous sacrifice. Self-recrimination and grief developed in a number of parents whose children in the nonchemotherapy arm of the study had had relapses because they had not received potentially effective therapy in the first instance. The burden of proof documenting a bleak prognosis without effective chemotherapy had been secured originally with a large number of historical-control patients in whom identical results had been observed. The responses achieved with methotrexate had never previously been observed with any other chemotherapeutic agent and should have provided adequate incentive to proceed immediately with this potentially effective treatment.

Acceptance of Adjuvant Therapy for Osteosarcoma

Confirmation of the efficacy of high-dose methotrexate alone and in combination with other agents and recapitulation of the historical controls launched a new era in the treatment of osteosarcoma. The necessity of administering chemotherapy to all

Adjuvant Chemotherapy in Osteosarcoma 233

patients with osteosarcoma was confirmed by other investigators. Winkler and Bielack wrote in 1988, "Adjuvant chemotherapy has proven efficacy and is indicated in all cases of classic osteosarcoma."[65] Utilizing pre- and postoperative treatment, cure rates in the vicinity of 65–75% have since been attained, and limb salvage has became an established form of treatment.

Denouement

This odyssey has recorded the saga of controversies and difficulties encountered in the effort to forge optimum therapy for patients with osteosarcoma. The author recognizes that the differences and controversies were based upon the prevailing opinion and understanding of the disease extant at various times. Investigations were conducted and implemented in an effort to provide what was considered to be optimum treatment. Opinions and views were not always concordant. As a consequence, the author locked horns with many colleagues, former fellows, and investigators. Nonetheless, this discord did not compromise the association, the professional relationships and the friendship he was honored and privileged to enjoy with them over the course of many years. These relationships are keenly appreciated. Photographs of several investigators who contributed to the development of therapy for osteosarcoma are depicted in Figs. 13 and 14.

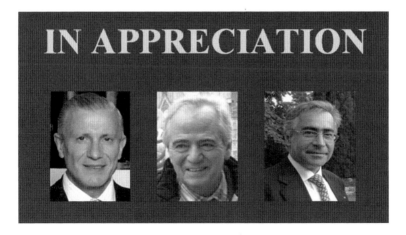

Fig. 13 Photographs of principal investigators from the Rizzoli Institute, Bologna, Italy who were the first to confirm the use of historical controls as a valid basis of comparison in investigating new agents for the treatment of Osteosarcoma (ref. 27). *Left*: Mario Campannaci; *Center*: Gaetano Bacci; *Right*: Piero Picci

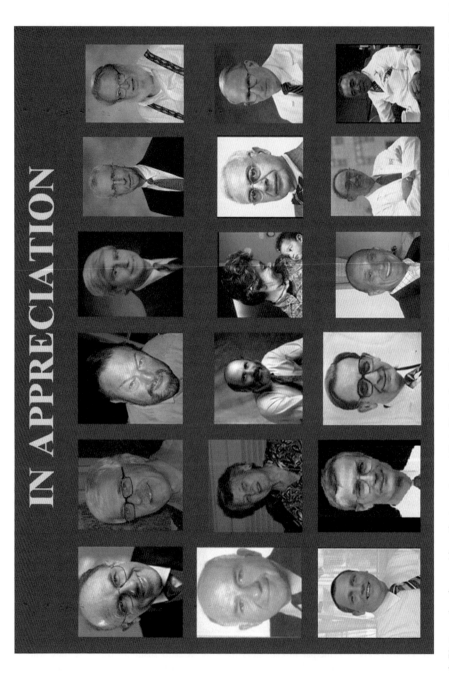

Fig. 14 Photographs of several investigators who contributed to the investigation and management of osteosarcoma. *Bottom row*: (*Left* to *right*): Stefan Bielack, Kurt Winkler, James F Holland, Gerald Rosen, Charles B Pratt, Wataru W Sutow. *Middle row*: Joseph V Simone, Teresa J Vietti, Michael P Link, Audrey E Evans, Giulio J D'Angio, Frederick R Eilber. *Top row*: Franco M Muggio, Alan M Goorin, Steven K Carter, Herbert Abelson, John H Edmonson, William F Taylor

References

1. Santayana G. *The Life of Reason, or The Phases of Human Progress.* 2nd ed. New York: Scribner; 1936.
2. Friedman M, Carter SK. The therapy of osteogenic sarcoma: current status and thoughts for the future. *J Surg Oncol.* 1972;45:482-510.
3. Cade S. Osteogenic sarcoma. A study based on 113 patients. *J R Coll Surg Edinb.* 1955;l:79-111.
4. Farber S, Diamond LK, Mercer RD, et al. Temporary remissions in children in acute leukemia produced by folic acid antagonist 4-aminopteroyl-glutanic acid (aminopterin). *New Engl J Med.* 1946;238:787-793.
5. Golden A, Mantel N, Greenhouse SW, et al. Effect of delayed administration of Citrovorin factor on the antileukemic effectiveness of aminopterin in mice. *Cancer Res.* 1954;14:43-48.
6. Burchenal JH. Human leukemias. *Bibl Hematol.* 1975;40:65-77.
7. Djerassi I, Abir E, Boyer GL, et al. Long term remissions in childhood acute leukemia: use of infrequent infusions of methotrexate: supportive roles of platelet transfusions and citrovorum factor. *Clin Pediatr.* 1966;5:502-509.
8. Zager RF, Frisby SA, Oliverio VT. The effects of antibiotics and cancer chemotherapeutic agents in the cellular transport and antitumor activity of methotrexate in L1210 murine leukemia. *Cancer Res.* 1973;33:1670-1676.
9. Jaffe N. Recent advances in the chemotherapy of osteogenic sarcoma. *Cancer.* 1972;30:1627-1631.
10. Jaffe N, Frei E III, Traggis D, Bishop Y. Adjuvant methotrexate treatment and citrovorum factor in osteogenic sarcoma. *New Engl J Med.* 1974;291:994-997.
11. Skipper HE, Schabel FM, Wilcox WS. Experimental evaluation of potential anticancer agents. XIV. Further study of certain basic concepts underlying chemotherapy of leukemia. *Cancer Chemother Rep:.* 1964;35:1-28.
12. Laster WR Jr, Mayo JG, Simpson-Herren L, et al. Success and failure in the treatment of solid tumors. II. Kinetic parameters and cell cure of moderately advanced carcinoma. *Cancer Chemother Rep.* 1969;53:169-188.
13. Schabel FM Jr. Concepts for systemic treatment of micro-metastases. *Cancer.* 1975;35:15-24.
14. Goorin AM, Delorey M, Gelber RD, et al. Dana-Farber Cancer Institute/The Children's Hospital adjuvant chemotherapy trials for osteosarcoma: three sequential studies. *Cancer Treat Symp* 1985;3:155-159.
15. Goorin AM, Perez-Atayde A, Gebhardt M, et al. Weekly high dose methotrexate and doxorubicin for osteosarcoma: The Dana Farber Cancer Institute/The Children's Hospital Study III. *J Clin Oncol.* 1987;5:1178-1184.
16. Rosen G, Nirenberg A, Caparros B, et al. Osteogenic sarcoma: eight-percent, three-year disease-free survival with combination chemotherapy (T-7). *Natl Cancer Inst Monogr.* 1981;56:213-220.
17. Sutow WW, Gehan EA, Vietti TG, et al. Multidrug chemotherapy in primary osteosarcoma. *J Bone Joint Surg Am.* 1976;58:629-633.
18. Pratt C, Shanks E, Hustu O, et al. Adjuvant multiple drug chemotherapy for osteosarcoma of the extremity. *Cancer.* 1979;39:51-57.
19. Muggia FM, Louie AC. Five years of adjuvant chemotherapy: more questions than answers. *Cancer Treat Rep.* 1978;62:30-36.
20. Rab CT, Ivins JC, Childs RE, et al. Elective whole lung irradiation in the treatment of osteogenic sarcoma. *Cancer.* 1976;38:939-942.
21. Taylor WF, Ivins JG, Dahlin D, et al. Osteogenic sarcoma experience at the Mayo Clinic, 1963–1974. In: Terry WD, Windhorst D, eds. *Immunotherapy of Cancer. Present Status of Trials in Man*, Progress in Cancer Research and Therapy, vol. VI. New York: Raven Press; 1978:257-269.

22. Taylor WF, Ivins JC, Prichard DJ, et al. Trends and variability in survival among patients with osteosarcoma: a 7-year update. *Mayo Clin Proc.* 1985;60(2):91-104.
23. Frei E III, Blum R, Jaffe N. Sarcoma: natural history and treatment. In: Terry WD, Windhorst D, eds. *Immunotherapy of Cancer. Present Status of Trials in Man*, Progress in Cancer Research and Therapy, vol. VI. New York: Raven Press; 1978:248-255.
24. Gehan EA, Sutow WW, Urube Botero T, et al. Osteosarcoma. The MD Anderson experience 1850–1974. In: Terry WD, Windhorst D, eds. *Immunotherapy of Cancer. Present Status of Trials in Man*, Progress in Cancer Research and Therapy, vol. VI. New York: Raven Press; 1978:271-282.
25. Miké V, Marcove RC. Osteogenic sarcoma under the age of 21. Experiences at Memorial Sloan Kettering Cancer Center. In: Terry WD, Windhorst D, eds. *Immunotherapy of Cancer. Present Status of Trials in Man*, Progress in Cancer Research and Therapy, vol. VI. New York: Raven Press; 1978:282-293.
26. Marcove RC, Mike V, Hajek JV, et al. Osteogenic sarcoma in childhood. *NY State J Med.* 1971;71:855-859.
27. Campanacci M, Bacci G, Bertoni F, et al. The treatment of osteosarcoma of the extremities: twenty years' experience at the Instituto Ortopedico Rizzoli. *Cancer.* 1981;48:1569-1581.
28. Bacci G, Gherlinzoni F, Picci P, et al. Adriamycin-methotrexate high dose versus Adriamycin-methotrexate moderate dose as adjuvant chemotherapy for osteosarcoma of the extremities: a randomized study. *Eur J Cancer Clin Oncol.* 1986;22:1337-1345.
29. Bacci G, Picci P, Calderoni P, et al. Full lung tomograms and bone scanning in the initial workup of patients with osteogenic sarcoma. A review of 126 cases. *Eur J Cancer Clin Oncol.* 1982;18:967-971.
30. Muhm JR, Prichard DJ. Computed tomography for detection of pulmonary metastases in patients with osteogenic sarcoma. *Proc Am Assoc Cancer Res.* 1980;21:593.
31. Cohen M, Provisor A, Smith WL, et al. Efficacy of whole lung tomography on diagnosing metastases from solid tumors in children. *Radiology.* 1981;141:375-378.
32. Gordon RE, Mettler FA Jr, Wicks J, et al. Chest x-rays and full lung tomograms in gynecologic malignancy. *Cancer.* 1983;52:559-562.
33. Wilimas J, Hammon E, Champion J, et al. The value of computerized tomography (CT) as a routine follow-up procedure for patients with Wilms tumor. *Am Soc Clin Oncol.* 1983;2:80 (Abstr 34).
34. Jaffe N, Farber S, Traggis D, et al. Favorable response of metastatic osteogenic sarcoma to pulse high dose methotrexate with citrovorin rescue and radiation therapy. *Cancer.* 1973;31:1367-1373.
35. Jaffe N, Watts H, Fellows K, et al. Local en bloc resection for limb preservation. *Cancer Treat Rep.* 1978;62:217-223.
36. Jaffe N, Frei E III, Traggis D, et al. Weekly high-dose methotrexate-citrovorum factor in osteogenic sarcoma pre-surgical treatment of primary tumor and of overt pulmonary metastases. *Cancer.* 1977;39:45-50.
37. Frei E, Jaffe N, Gero M, et al. Guest editorial. Adjuvant chemotherapy of osteogenic sarcoma: progress and perspectives. *J Natl Cancer Inst.* 1978; 60:3-10.
38. Jaffe N, Frei E III, Watts H, et al. High dose methotrexate in osteogenic sarcoma: a 5-year experience. *Cancer Treat Rep.* 1978;62:259-264.
39. Jaffe N. Progress report on high-dose methotrexate (NSC-740) with citrovorum rescue in the treatment of metastatic bone tumors. *Cancer Chemother Rep.* 1974;58:275-280.
40. Jaffe N, Traggis D. Toxicity of high-dose methotrexate (NSC-740) and citrovorum factor (NSC-3590) in osteogenic sarcoma. *Cancer Chemother Rep.* 1975;6:31-36.
41. Pitman SW, Parker M, Tattersall MH, et al. Clinical trial of high-dose methotrexate (NSC-740) with citrovorum factor (NSC-3590) – toxicologic and therapeutic observations. *Cancer Chemother Rep.* 1975;6:43-49.
42. Jaffe N, Frei E III, Traggis D, et al. High-dose methotrexate with citrovorum factor in osteogenic sarcoma. Progress report II. *Cancer Treat Rep.* 1977;61:675-679.

Adjuvant Chemotherapy in Osteosarcoma

43. Jaffe N, Traggis D, Cassady JR, et al. Multidisciplinary treatment for macrometastatic osteogenic sarcoma. *Br Med J.* 1976;2:1039-1041.
44. Jaffe N, Link M, Traggis D, et al. The role of high dose methotrexate in osteogenic sarcoma. Sarcomas of soft tissue and bone in childhood. *Natl Cancer Inst Monogr.* 1981;56:201-206.
45. Edmonson JH, Green SJ, Ivins JC, et al. A controlled pilot study of high-dose methotrexate as postsurgical adjuvant treatment for primary osteosarcoma. *J Clin Oncol.* 1984;2:152-156.
46. Carter SK. Adjuvant chemotherapy in osteogenic sarcoma.The triumph that isn't? *J Clin Oncol.* 1984;2:147-148.
47. Jaffe N. Adjuvant chemotherapy in osteogenic sarcoma. *J Clin Oncol.* 1984;2:1179-1181.
48. Carter SK. Reply: adjuvant chemotherapy in osteosarcoma. *J Clin Oncol.* 1984;2:1181.
49. Feinstein AR, Sosin DM, Wells CK. The Will Rogers phenomenon. Stage migration and new diagnostic techniques as a source of misleading statistics for survival in cancer. *N Engl J Med.* 1985;312:1604-1608.
50. Goorin AM, Frei E III, Abelson HT. Adjuvant chemotherapy for osteosarcoma: a decade of experience. *Surg Clin North Am.* 1981;61:1379-1389.
51. Kolate GB. Dilemma in cancer treatment. *Science.* 1980;209:792-794.
52. Brostrom LA, Apairsi T, Ingimarsson SN, et al. Can historical controls be used in current clinical trials in osteosarcoma? Metastasis and survival in a historical and concurrent group. *Int J Radiat Oncol Biol Phys.* 1980;6:1717-1721.
53. Lang EB, Levin AS. Is it ethical not to conduct a prospectively controlled trial of adjuvant chemotherapy in osteosarcoma? *Cancer Treat Rep.* 1982;66:1699-1704.
54. Jaffe N, van Eys J, Gehan E. Response to: "Is it ethical not to conduct a prospectively controlled trial of adjuvant chemotherapy in osteosarcoma?". *Cancer Treat Rep.* 1983;67:743-744.
55. Cox DR. Regression models and life tables (with discussion). *J R Stat B.* 1972;187-220.
56. Jaffe N, Smith E, Abelson HT, et al. Osteogenic sarcoma: alterations in the pattern of pulmonary metastases with adjuvant chemotherapy. *J Clin Oncol.* 1983;1:251-254.
57. Jaffe N, Traggis D, Cohen DG. The impact of high dose methotrexate in the management of osteogenic sarcoma. In: *Proceedings of the Twelfth International Cancer Congress*, vol. 10. Oxford: Pergamon Press; 1979:175-179.
58. Link MP, Vietti TJ. Reply: Role of adjuvant chemotherapy in the treatment of osteosarcoma. *Cancer Treat Rep.* 1983;67:744-745.
59. D'Angio GJ, Evans AE. Bone tumors – a commentary. In: D'Angio GJ, Evans AE, eds. *Bone Tumours and Soft-Tissue Sarcomas*, Progress in Cancer Research and Therapy, vol. VI. Baltimore, MD: Edward Arnold; 1985:121-124.
60. Rosen G, Murphy ML, Huvos AG, et al. Chemotherapy en bloc resection and prosthetic bone replacement in the treatment of osteogenic sarcoma. *Cancer.* 1976;37:1-11.
61. Rosen G, Marcove RC, Huvos AG, et al. Primary osteogenic sarcoma: eight year experience with adjuvant chemotherapy. *J Cancer Res Clin Oncol.* 1983;106(Suppl):55-67.
62. Link MP, Goorin AM, Miser A, et al. The effect of adjuvant chemotherapy on relapse-free survival in patients with osteosarcoma of the extremity. *New Engl J Med.* 1986;314:1600-1606.
63. Eilber FR, Dauglass HI Jr, Mendel ER, et al. Adjuvant Adriamycin and cisplatin in newly-diagnosed nonmetastatic osteosarcoma of the extremity. *J Clin Oncol.* 1986;4:353-362.
64. Holland JF. Adjuvant chemotherapy of osteosarcoma: no runs, no hits, two men left on base. *J Clin Oncol.* 1987;5:4-6.
65. Winkler K, Bielack S. Chemotherapy for osteosarcoma. *Semin Orthop.* 1988;3:48-58..[1]

Osteosarcoma: Review of the Past, Impact on the Future. The American Experience

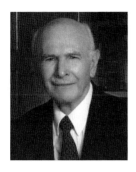

Norman Jaffe

Abstract Major advances have been achieved in the treatment of osteosarcoma with the discovery of several chemotherapeutic agents that were active in the disease. These agents comprise high-dose methotrexate with leucovorin rescue, Adriamycin, cisplatin, ifosfamide and cyclophosphamide. The agents were integrated into various regimens and administered in an effort to destroy silent pulmonary micrometastases which are considered to be present in at least 80% of patients at the time of diagnosis. Their efficacy in achieving this goal was realized and their use was further extended to the application of preoperative (neoadjuvant) chemotherapy to destroy the primary tumor and achieve safe surgical resections. Disease free survival was escalated from <20% prior to the introduction of effective chemotherapy to 55–75% and overall survival to 85%. Further, the opportunity to perform limb salvage was expanded to 80% of patients. Of interest also was an attempt in one series to treat the primary tumor exclusively with chemotherapy, and abrogation of surgery.

Adding to these advances, varieties of subsequently discovered agents are currently undergoing investigations in patients who have relapsed and/or failed conventional therapy. The agents include Gemcitabine, Docetaxel, novel antifolate compounds, and a liposome formulation of adriamycin (Doxil). A biological agent, muramyl tripeptide phosphatidyl ethanolamine (MTPPE) was also recently investigated in a 2×2 factorial design to determine its efficacy in combination with chemotherapy (methotrexate, cisplatin, Adriamycin and ifosfamide).

In circumstances where the tumor was considered inoperable, chemotherapy and radiotherapy were advocated for local control. High dose methotrexate, Adriamycin and cisplatin and Gemcitabine interact with radiation therapy and potentiate its therapeutic effect. This combination is also particularly useful in palliation. Occasionally, the combination of radiation and chemotherapy may render a tumor

N. Jaffe (✉)
Children's Cancer Hospital, University of Texas M.D. Anderson Cancer Center, 1515 Holcombe Boulevard, Unit #87, Houston, TX, 77030-4009, USA
e-mail: njaffe@mdanderson.org

suitable for surgical ablation. Samarium,[153] a radio active agent, is also used as palliative therapy for bone metastases.

However, despite the advances achieved with the multidisciplinary application of chemotherapy, radiotherapy and surgical ablation of the primary tumor over the past 3½ decades, the improved cure rate reported initially has not altered. Particularly vexing is the problem of rescuing patients who develop pulmonary metastases after receiving seemingly effective multidisciplinary treatment. Approximately 15–25% of such patients only are rendered free of disease with the reintroduction of chemotherapy and resection of metastases. Extrapulmonary metastases and multifocal osteosarcoma also constitute a major problem. The arsenal of available agents to treat such patients has not made any substantial impact in improving their survival. New chemotherapeutic agents are urgently required to improve treatment and outcome. Additional strategies to be considered are targeted tumor therapy, anti tumor angiogenesis, biotherapy and therapy based upon molecular profiles.

This communication outlines sequential discoveries in the chemotherapeutic research of osteosarcoma in the United States of America. It also describes the principles regulating the therapeutic application of the regimens and considers the impact of their results on the conduct in the design of future investigations and treatment

Introduction

During the past half century, therapeutic research has identified several chemo- therapeutic agents that are effective in the treatment of osteosarcoma. These agents were incorporated into a number of therapeutic regimens. With their application in innovative multimodal strategies, cure rates were escalated from <20% prior to the 1907s to current levels of 65–75%. Accompanying this escalation has been the ability to offer limb salvage to approximately 80% of patients.

The principal agents currently in use comprise high-dose methotrexate with leucovorin rescue, doxorubicin (Adriamycin), cisplatin, cyclophosphamide, and ifosfamide. Earlier investigations with nitrogen mustard, mitomycin C, and vincristine had yielded minimal response, and these agents were abandoned.[1]

Con*p*adri/Com*p*adri Series

In the early 1960s, Sutow and coworkers[2] demonstrated anti-tumor activity in osteosarcoma with L-phenylalanine mustard. Temporary regression in 10–43% of patients was achieved.[2] This result prompted an investigation of L-phenylalanine mustard as adjuvant chemotherapy for patients with nonmetastatic osteosarcoma after ablation of the primary tumor, and a disease-free survival rate of 14% was achieved.[3] In 1969, the combination of vincristine, dactinomycin (actinomycin D), and cyclophosphamide (VAC) was demonstrated to be effective in treating rhabdomyosarcoma.[4] The success achieved in rhabdomyosarcoma prompted Sutow et al[5] to investigate the efficacy of the regimen as adjuvant treatment for osteosarcoma after ablation of the primary tumor. During this same period, osteosarcoma was shown to be responsive to cyclophosphamide (as discussed below).[6] To potentiate the efficacy of the VAC regimen, Sutow administered cyclophosphamide in an intensive intermittent pulse schedule based on studies reported by Finklestein et al.[7] This regimen designated "pulse VAC," was administered to 12 patients and resulted in a 33% disease-free survival rate in all of them.[8]

With the demonstration that doxorubicin was effective in the treatment of osteosarcoma, [9] Sutow elected to substitute doxorubicin for dactinomycin in the pulse VAC regimen and to augment its efficacy with the addition of L-phenylalanine mustard. This regimen [pulsed cyclophosphamide, vincristine (Oncovin), L-phenylalanine mustard, and doxorubicin (Adriamycin)] was designated "Conpadri" or Conpadri I.[10] It yielded a 55% disease-free survival rate. Sequential changes in the composition and acronym of the Conpadri regimen followed. Methotrexate was incorporated and it was designated "Compadri," commencing with Compadri II. Each successive number indicated an evolution in the regimen.[11] Sutow also observed that pulmonary metastases were appearing later in patients treated with the Compadri regimen.[12] This change in the pattern of development of pulmonary metastases inaugurated new concepts in the treatment of patients with metastatic osteosarcoma. The conceptual development and the evolution of programs designed for this purpose were outlined in two publications.[13,14] Prior to 1970, the survival rate for patients with metastases was considerably less than 2%. After 1970, according to Sutow, it improved to approximately 40%.[13] The best postmetastatic survival rates occurred in patients whose metastatic lesions developed at least 13 months after initial treatment; the worst rates occurred when metastases were present at diagnosis.[11] Sutow's observation was confirmed by Jaffe et al,[15] who noted an alteration in the pattern of relapse in several patients treated with adjuvant chemotherapy: metastases in these patients appeared later than in untreated or inadequately treated patients. They also tended to be single or isolated.[15] This development permitted successful multidisciplinary intervention in an increasing number of patients.

The Compadri II and III regimens yielded disappointing results. It was surmised that their lack of efficacy was due to reduced doses of doxorubicin, and the approach was adjusted in Compadri IV and Compadri V: high-dose methotrexate and doxorubicin were intensified, and aggressive "front loading" was adopted. Unfortunately, Wataru Sutow's untimely death precluded evaluation of the last two Compadri studies. However, before he died, an updated review of the Compadri I, II and III regimens was published: 81 of 200 patients (41%) were alive without evidence of disease, 18 months and longer after diagnosis.[16]

The Compadri regimens represented the first rational attempt to promote the use of combination chemotherapy as adjuvant therapy in osteosarcoma. They comprised different agents with different modes of action and minimal overlapping toxicity. Compadri was later superseded by other chemotherapeutic regimens.

High-Dose Methotrexate with Leucovorin Rescue

The use of methotrexate against osteosarcoma was initiated in the 1970s (see Chap. 11). Methotrexate binds stoichiometrically and irreversibly to dihydrofolate reductase, thereby inhibiting the formation of tetrahydrofolate from dihydrofolate. This inhibition interferes with the de novo biosynthesis of purine and pyrimidine. Ultimately, thymidylate biosynthesis is inhibited; this is the key event leading to cell death. The antidote to methotrexate is leucovorin (5-formyl tetrahydrofolate). Within the cell, leucovorin is converted to 5,10 methylene tetrahydrofolate and 5-methyl tetrahydrofolate, thereby replenishing the product surceased by methotrexate.

The methotrexate-leucovorin "rescue" regimen (MTX-L) took wing following publications by Jaffe et al.[17–20] Methotrexate is usually administered intravenously in doses of 10–12.5 G/m^2 over 4–6 h, with leucovorin "rescue" commencing 24 h after the initiation of the methotrexate infusion. When deployed as single-agent therapy for "intensification" or "consolidation," MTX-L should optimally comprise 4–8 doses administered at 10–14-day intervals. When combined with other agents, the interval between MTX-L and the other agents (generally doxorubicin, which may be administered 8–10 days after MTX-L) is usually extended to 21–28 days before initiating the next MTX-L dose.

MTX-L administered postoperatively as the sole agent to patients with osteosarcoma after ablation of the primary tumor, yielded a 40% disease-free survival.[18] When MTX-L was combined with other agents as pre- and post-operative therapy for osteosarcoma, a disease-free survival rate of 65–75% was achieved.[17–27]

The Children's Cancer Study Group considered high-dose MTX-L and intermediate-dose MTX-L in combination with doxorubicin as adjuvant therapy for nonmetastatic osteosarcoma; no benefit was observed for patients who received MTX-L. The overall outcome in these patients was not superior to that in patients who received doxorubicin alone.[28] Two Osteosarcoma studies, one in Europe and the other in the United Kingdom, found an inferior disease-free survival rate in patients who received a three-drug regimen: doxorubicin, cisplatin and MTX-L as compared with the rate in patients who received the regimen without MTX-L.[29,30] Several factors could possibly account for the inferior results achieved with high- or intermediate-dose MTX-L in these studies. The factors include inadequate tumoricidal concentrations due to substandard doses (vide the Children's Cancer Study Group investigation), and dilution of methotrexate because of the excessive hydration that was designed to eliminate the drug. Other factors, including age and pharmacokinetics, also influence serum methotrexate levels and tumor response.[21,31–33]

It has been suggested that methotrexate levels of 700–1,000 µmol/L at 4–6 h (generally 1,000 µmol/L) after initiation of the infusion are required for optimum results.[31,32] However, for unexplained reasons, inter- and intra-patient variability in methotrexate concentration is often encountered, despite administration of a standard dose, and optimum levels are not constantly obtained. In the author's experience, a methotrexate concentration of 1,500 µmol/L or higher at 4–6 h is desirable. This concentration is more likely to be obtained by limiting pre- and intra-therapeutic intravenous (alkaline) hydration to 3 L/m^2/24 h.

Efforts to increase the therapeutic effect of methotrexate by enhancing the local concentration at the tumor site using the standard dose with intra-arterial, rather than intravenous, administration were unsuccessful.[34] Apparently, response requires a critical dose, and any dose escalation above this level will not enhance therapeutic efficacy. Similarly, in pharmacokinetic and clinical studies of a 24-h infusion of high-dose methotrexate with leucovorin administered after completion of the infusion, the efficacy of the drug did not improve over that of a shorter 4–6-h infusion.[35] These observations indicate that the optimum therapeutic tumoricidal concentration is achieved with the intravenous dosages described above.

With the optimum dosage administered over 4–6 h and the appropriate hydration, the following peak methotrexate levels may be anticipated at specific time intervals after initiation of the infusion (Fig. 1):

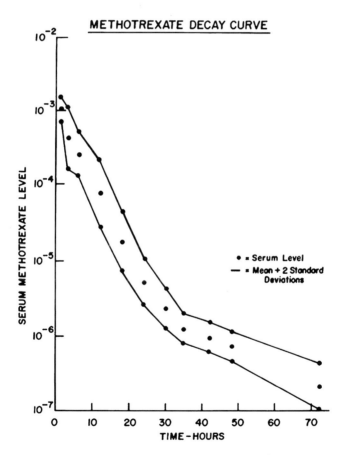

Fig. 1 Methotrexate decay curve following a 6-h infusion at 7.5 G/m² dissolved in 600 cc of 5% dextrose water administered over 6 h. Reproduced with permission from Advances in Chemotherapy. Jaffe N. Antifolate rescue use of high-dose methotrexate and citrovorum factor. In: Rossowsky A, ed. *Advances in Chemotherapy*. New York and Basel: Marcel Decker Inc.; 1979:111-141

- 24 h 30–300 μmol/L
- 48 h 3–30 μmol/L
- 72 h <0.3 μmol/L

Values in excess of these concentrations, particularly at the 48-h level, portend potential toxicity.[35–38]

Leucovorin is administered according to specially designed algorithms that are available in most institutions. The algorithm generally advocates an intravenous dose of 10 mg after completion of the methotrexate infusion and a similar dose every 6 h until the methotrexate level is ≤0.1 μmol/L. This usually occurs at 72 h and requires 12 doses. However, it may be necessary to prolong the leucovorin administration if the ≤0.1 μmol/L methotrexate level is not attained at 72 h. In some institutions, a methotrexate level of ≤0.3 μmol/L may be an acceptable endpoint.

Prerequisites for MTX-L therapy include normal renal and hepatic function, a normal hemogram, and absence of infection. The prerequisites are usually determined by obtaining a corrected creatinine clearance rate, a serum electrolyte study, urinalysis, liver function studies, and a complete blood count prior to each course of therapy. Collections of fluid (pleural, pericardial and peritoneal effusions) may cause a delay in methotrexate excretion by sequestering methotrexate into the fluid collection and are contraindicated in MTX-L treatment.

Toxic reactions are infrequent. They are generally induced by incomplete (delayed) renal clearance and are usually associated with methotrexate precipitation in the renal tubules. This reaction manifests with gastrointestinal mucosal ulceration, myelosuppression, and hepatorenal failure. Measures for aborting or treating toxic reactions may comprise any or all (usually the latter) of the following:

1. Increasing fluid intake to 4 L/m^2/24 h.
2. Increasing leucovorin dose to 50–100 mg (or higher) every 6 h, as stipulated by the institution's algorithm.
3. Administering carboxypeptidase G-2 if the serum 24- or 48-h methotrexate level is extremely high and/or anuria or oliguria appears to be developing.
4. Considering high-flux renal dialysis at any time in the above circumstances.

In addition to its efficacy as a pre- and post-operative agent, methotrexate potentiates the tumoricidal effects of radiation therapy.[39–42] The effects are limited to the portals of radiation and include dermatologic reactions. Radiation effects are more likely to occur if the methotrexate administration coincides with radiation or is juxtaposed with the immediate postradiation period. With longer intervals between radiation and methotrexate, response and skin reactions are less observed. The combination of radiation therapy and methotrexate may be used for treatment of resistant pulmonary metastases and inoperable primary tumors. This combination is also extremely useful in alleviating cord compression and relieving bone pain.

Doxorubicin

Doxorubicin came into use for treatment of osteosarcoma in the early 1970s. The agent intercalates into DNA and induces topoisomearase II-mediated single- and double–strand breaks in the DNA. Initial studies in which doxorubicin was administered intravenously, alone or in combination with dacarbazine [dimethyldiethyl triazeno imidazole carboxamide, (DTIC)] produced responses in 35–40% of patients with pulmonary metastases.[43-45] Responses included complete disappearance of lung lesions and a 40% reduction in tumor volume. The onset of the responses occurred within 1–2 months with doses of 30–35 mg/m^2 administered daily for 3 days, at 3–4-week intervals. When administered as the sole agent after ablation of the primary tumor, doxorubicin also improved survival rates in patients with osteosarcoma.[8,43-47]

Doxorubicin can also potentiate the therapeutic effects of radiation therapy.[48] In one study, doxorubicin was administered intra-arterially over 24 h in combination with radiation (3.5 Gy) to treat the primary tumor. More than 75% tumor destruction was reported in 24 of 36 patients.[49] However, the procedure was complicated by erythema and ulceration of the skin and subcutaneous tissue in several patients. Selective entry of the drug into a small vessel was implicated, and it was suggested that the complication could possibly be prevented by positioning the catheter in a large-caliber vessel proximal to the tumor. Ulceration precludes limb-salvage procedures, and consequently intra-arterial doxorubicin is generally not advocated as local treatment for potential limb-salvage candidates.[50]

Doxorubicin may induce cardiac failure. To prevent this complication, the cumulative dose is generally limited to 300 mg/m^2 in children under 6 years of age and to 450–500 mg/m^2 in adolescents. However, based on experiences with adult patients with breast cancer, the cumulative dose may possibly be extended to 600 mg/m^2 (or more) with liposomal formulations of the drug (e.g., Doxil[51]). Dexrazoxane has also been administered in combination with doxorubicin to prevent cardiac failure.[52] The potential salubrious effect of the agent in preventing cardiac complications in long-term survival remains to be determined.

Doxorubicin has been claimed to be the most effective agent for the treatment of osteosarcoma.[53] It is incorporated in most combination chemotherapy regimens used for this disease. A cardiac assessment comprising an electrocardiogram and echocardiogram should optimally be obtained prior to the administration of each course. Cardiac assessments should also be obtained at regular intervals in long term survivors.

Cisplatin

Cisplatin (*cis*-diamminedichloroplatinum II) was first used for treatment of osteosarcoma in the 1970s. It exerts its cytotoxic action by platination of DNA. It may be administered intravenously or intra-arterially. In a series of studies in which cisplatin was administered intravenously, it produced responses of 30–50%.[54–56] The responses were obtained in patients with unresectable or metastatic disease who received the agent alone or in combination with doxorubicin. In contrast, in studies in which cisplatin was administered intra-arterially as the sole agent for treatment of the primary tumor, response rates were 60–90%.[57,58] The intra-arterial route achieves higher local cytotoxic concentrations which improves penetration across the cell membrane.[57] This strategy was investigated principally at The University of Texas M.D. Anderson Cancer Center.[58–62] The procedure, which involved general anesthesia or conscious sedation of the patient, required placement of an arterial catheter via the Seldinger technique through the brachial or femoral artery (Fig. 2) under fluoroscopic guidance. Concurrently, a systemic intravenous infusion was initiated to provide hydration at 3 $L/m^2/24$ h and Manitol. The tip of the arterial catheter was positioned into a vessel that supplied the neoplasm. A pulsatile infusion pump was used to induce turbulence of the cisplatin with saline[59]; this turbulence prevented laminar flow and reduced the possibility of a "platinum burn" because of selective entry of high platinum concentrations into small vessels. Occasionally, tumor embolization may be performed to improve the direction and concentration of chemotherapy to the tumor, if excessive neovascularity is present.

In the initial studies, the dosage was 150 mg/m^2 administered with Mannitol over 2 h at 3-week intervals.[57,58] Four preoperative courses were administered. In more recent studies, 120 mg/m^2 cisplatin is administered intra-arterially over 4 h, and concurrently 95 mg/m^2 doxorubicin is administered over 24 h. In a schedule similar to the sole treatment with intra-arterial cisplatin, four preoperative courses are administered at 4-week intervals.

Pharmacokinetic studies were conducted as part of the initial study of 150 mg/m^2 cisplatin administered intra-arterially. Evaluation of the local venous effluent and concurrent systemic venous concentrations demonstrated consistently higher cisplatin concentrations in the local vein than in the peripheral vein[57] (Fig. 3, *left* and *right* respectively). The highest single concentrations in the local vein were 10 and 9 µg/mL at 60 and 90 min, respectively, as opposed to the highest concentrations in the peripheral vein, which were 1.7 and 3.9 µg/mL at 30 and 120 min, respectively. From 90 min, the local venous concentrations plotted on a log scale were linear by curve fitting. The concentration in the systemic circulation was sufficiently tumoricidal to destroy pulmonary metastases. Figure 4 demonstrates complete disappearance of pulmonary metastases after two courses of 150 mg/m^2 intra-arterial cisplatin administered for a primary tumor in the distal femur. These pharmacokinetic and clinical studies contradict the claim that the systemic concentration following intra-arterial administration is insufficient to destroy pulmonary metastases.[63] Systemic concentrations in these studies were also sufficient to cause adverse side effects, including auditory and renal dysfunction.[64,65]

The efficacy of intra-arterial therapy may be demonstrated by angiographic study with the disappearance of tumor neovascularity and staining (Fig. 5). It is also capable of inducing a complete response in patients with pathological fractures (Fig. 6).

Osteosarcoma 247

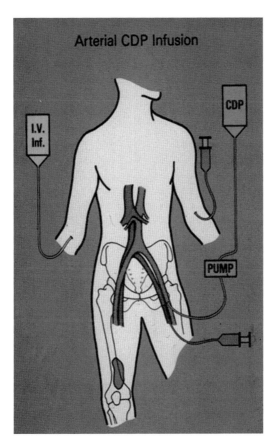

Fig. 2 Arterial catheter containing cisplatin (CDP) attached to pulsatile infusion pump (PUMP) inserted into left femoral artery and directed to the tumor in the contralateral limb via the bifurcation of the aorta. Systemic hydration and Mannitol are provided through a venous catheter (I.V.Inf) in the right antecubital fossa. The diagram also depicts sites of venous catheters inserted to determine cisplatin concentrations in the local tumor draining vein and systemic circulation. I.V. Inf = Intravenous in fusion; CDP = Cisplatin; PUMP = Pusatile Infusion Pump

Tissue determinations of cisplatin levels were obtained in the tumor and the surrounding tissues in some patients (Fig. 7). These revealed that concentrations of 17–40 µg/g were associated with tumor destruction of 60–100%

Figure 8 demonstrates 100% tumor destruction after four courses of intra-arterial cisplatin. This result contrasted sharply with those for concentrations of 12 µg/g or less, which were associated with tumor destruction of less than 60%. The difference in the mean cisplatin tumor concentrations between the groups with greater than 60% tumor destruction and those with less than 60% destruction was 16.7 µg/g. Using the one-tailed t-test, this difference was significant at a level of <0.025

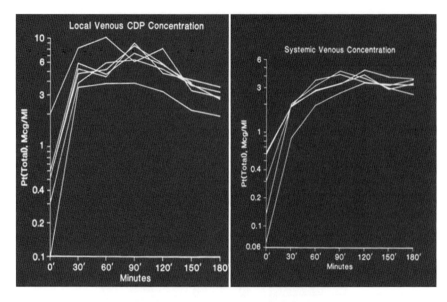

Fig. 3 *Left*: Local venous cisplatin concentrations (tumor draining vein). *Right*: Systemic venous cisplatin concentrations. *CDP* cisplatin; *Pt* total platinum (Mcg/ml)

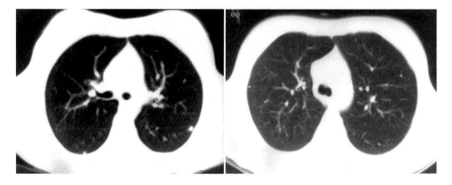

Fig. 4 Computer scan of lungs demonstrating pulmonary metastases (*left*) and disappearance of pulmonary metastases (*right*) following two courses of intra-arterial cisplatin 150 mg/m^2

Cisplatin uptake also varied with tumor subtype in this study. Smaller concentrations were detected in patients with telangiectactic osteosarcoma and malignant fibrocystic histiocytoma, as opposed to chondroblastic osteosarcoma. In patients with malignant fibrocystic histiocytoma, 60% tumor destruction was noted with a cisplatin concentration of 2.4 μg/g.[57] Cisplatin tumor concentration and tumor destruction were also related to the number of infusions: the percentage of tumor destruction was greater with three or more infusions than with two infusions.[58]

TREATMENT OF LOCAL RECURRENCE

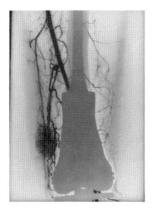 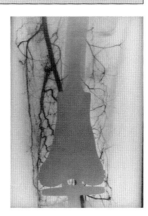

Fig. 5 Arteriogram demonstrating recurrent tumor in the distal end of the femur manifesting with neovascularity and stain (*left*). Complete disappearance of tumor neovascularity was obtained with after four courses of intra-arterial cisplatin, 150 mg/m^2/course (*right*). Pathological examination of resected tissues demonstrated absent tumor or complete tumor necrosis in sites where minimal residual tumor was suspected to be present

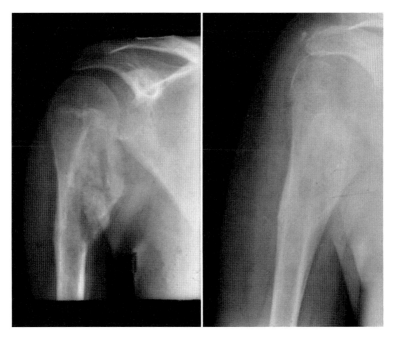

Fig. 6 Pathological fracture of the humerus at diagnosis (*left*) and complete healing after four courses of intra-arterial cisplatin, 150 mg/m^2/course (*right*)

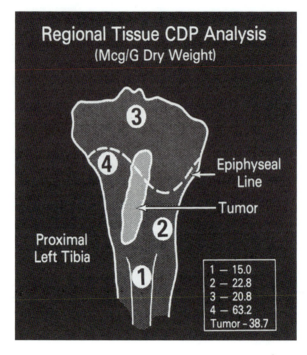

Fig. 7 Tissue cisplatin determinations in the proximal tibia following four course of intra-arterial cisplatin, 150 mg/m^2/course

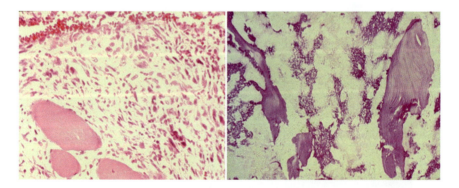

Fig. 8 Photomicrograph of tumor at diagnosis (*left*) and specimen obtained after treatment with four courses of intra-arterial cisplatin, 150 mg/m^2/course (*right*). Complete necrosis was induced. There is a complete absence of tumor cells in the specimen comprising residual bone trabeculae

Patients whose tumors initially respond and later relapse may experience a response again with reinstatement of cisplatin at the same dose (Fig. 5 shows an example). Intra-arterial therapy is extremely useful when an immediate response is desired, particularly in the treatment of pathological fractures[72] (Fig. 6) or with the threat of tumor invasion and potential imminent compromise to the neurovascular bundle.

A review of the results of treatment with intra arterial cisplatin in several publications revealed an average sensitivity of 95% and a specificity of 87%.[66–71]

The tumoricidal effects achieved with the first or second course of intra-arterial cisplatin may also be achieved with conventional intravenous therapy administered over a more prolonged period (several courses). In contrast, intra-arterial cisplatin is capable of producing a rapid definitive attack on the primary tumor. The rapidity and immediacy of response with intravenous cisplatin are not as impressive as that achieved with the first or second course of intra-arterial cisplatin. In addition, the efficacy of intra-arterial treatment may also be assessed reasonably early on the arteriogram by observing the reduction of tumor neovascularity and staining after the first or second course.

Oxazaphosphorines

The oxazaphosphorines, cyclophosphamide and ifosfamide, are alkylating agents that require hepatic microsomes for activation. They possess moderate to high efficacy in the treatment of osteosarcoma.[5,6,73–75] Cyclophosphamide was probably the first agent discovered to have activity in osteosarcoma[5] (Fig. 9). In 1962, Pinkel[6] stated that he knew of no reports concerning responses of "osteogenic sarcoma to other alkylating agents" at that time.

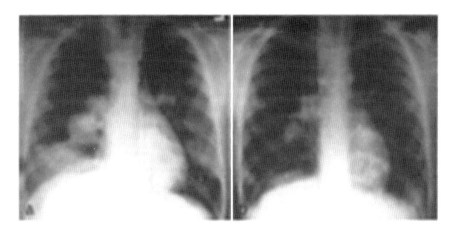

Fig. 9 Chest radiograph demonstrating pulmonary metastases from osteosarcoma (*left*) and partial response to oral cyclophosphamide (*right*). The latter manifested with disappearance and reduction of tumor masses. This material is reproduced with permission of Wiley-Liss, Inc., a subsidiary of John Wiley & Sons, Inc. (Pinkel[6]: Figs. 3a,b)

Cyclophosphamide may be administered in combination with etoposide (VP-16), which is thought to augment the efficacy of the alkylating agent through a synergistic interaction. An early study of this combination yielded a 58% response rate in various malignant diseases, including osteosarcoma.[76] A follow-up of the study concluded that the combination of cyclophosphamide and etoposide was effective therapy for both primary and metastatic osteosarcoma.[77] Eighty-eight percent of the patients experienced complete or partial responses. Because of its putative synergistic effect, etoposide is also frequently combined with ifosfamide.

Cyclophosphamide and ifosfamide produce a metabolite, acroline, that causes hemorrhagic cystitis. This complication can be prevented with the administration of Mesna. The latter absorbs the acroline, providing uroprotection. This strategy permits the administration of high doses of cyclophosphamide and ifosfamide. The intake of liberal amounts of fluid is another means of preventing hemorrhagic cystitis.

The activity of the alkylating agents, particularly ifosfamide, can be augmented by fractionating the dose. The efficacy can also be enhanced by dose escalation. Investigators have reported initial responses of 10–40% with doses of 6–9 g/m^2 [78–80]; escalating the dose to 12 or 14 g/m^2 yielded enhanced responses of 60%.[81–84] These results were noted in patients who had had relapses or in whom conventional therapy had failed. This experience, however, was not observed by Harris et al,[85] who noted a complete and partial response rate of only 30% with a dose of 12 g/m^2. The alkylating agents also are not cross-resistant: in patients who have relapses after treatment with a specific alkylating agent, responses may again be achieved by substituting an alternative alkylating agent (e.g., ifosfamide for cyclophosphamide or vice versa).

Goorin et al[86] treated patients with newly diagnosed osteosarcoma in a "therapeutic window" at 3–4-week intervals and achieved a 59% response rate with a combination of ifosfamide (3.5 g/m^2/day for 5 days, for a total of 17.5 g/m^2) and etoposide (100 mg/m^2/day for 5 days). This experience was duplicated by investigators at M. D. Anderson Cancer Center. However, in contrast to the patients treated by Goorin et al, patients at M.D. Anderson had been heavily pretreated with high-dose methotrexate, doxorubicin, cisplatin, and ifosfamide (9 g/m^2). Etoposide was usually omitted. The response of one such patient with pulmonary metastases who was treated with ifosfamide only is illustrated in Fig. 10. The total dose of ifosfamide, 17.5 g/m^2, was associated with moderate myelosuppression and mild renal dysfunction. In addition, two other patients developed moderate renal failure following the fifth course of 17.5 g/m^2 ifosfamide. Thus, the use of high-dose ifosfamide (17.5 g/m^2) should probably be limited to four courses. If there is evidence of renal dysfunction, cyclophosphamide, which is unlikely to affect the kidneys, may be substituted for ifosfamide at an equivalent dose. This is determined by dividing the ifosfamide dose (17.5 g/m^2) by 3.5. The resulting dose of cyclophosphamide (3–4 g/m^2) may be administered over two consecutive days (i.e., 1.5–2 g/m^2/day) at 3–4-week intervals with Mesna.

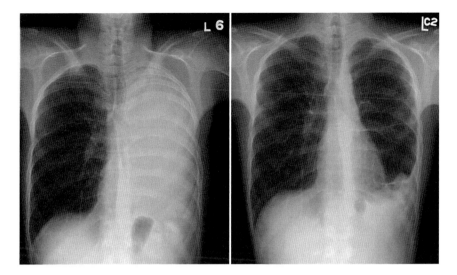

Fig. 10 Chest radiograph of patient who responded to four courses of Ifosafamide 17.5 G/m^2/course administered over 5 days (3.5 G/m^2/dx5). The patient had previously been treated with, and responded to, Ifosfamide 14 G/m^2 and later relapsed

Less Frequently Employed Chemotherapeutic Agents

Carboplatin, has been used in several combination regimens.[87–90] In a study of patients with metastatic lung lesions, a regimen containing 560 mg/m^2/day carboplatin was not as effective as 100 mg/m^2/day cisplatin.[88] Petrilli et al[90] investigated intra-arterial carboplatin (Study III) in a series of patients. They were also treated with epirubicin, ifosfamide and MTX-L. In contrast, in Study IV, intravenous carboplatin in conjunction with cisplatin, doxorubicin and Ifosfamide was employed. The overall survival rate for Study III and Study IV in patients who had nonmetastatic osteosarcoma at the time of their original diagnosis, was 60.5%, and the event-free survival rate, 45.5% at 5 years. Since other agents in addition to carboplatin were employed, the contribution of the latter to the final result cannot be assessed.

Novel antifolate agents, including trimetrexate, have been investigated in patients who have had relapses. Although these agents produced isolated responses, they have not been evaluated in formal clinical trials. In addition, gemcitabine, which has been reported to produce responses in osteosarcoma, awaits further investigation.[91,92]

High-dose radioactive samarium^{153} [^{153}Sm-EDTMP (Quadramet)] has been used to treat bone metastases and has afforded patients appreciable relief with regard to symptoms.[93] However, this treatment is usually complicated by severe myelosuppression and may require peripheral blood or stem-cell support.

A 2×2 factorial design study using two chemotherapy regimens, one standard and one experimental, was employed in conjunction with liposomal muramyl tripeptide phosphatidyl ethanolamine (L-MTPPE).[94] The latter induces infiltration of inflammatory macrophages into lung metastases. The study was designed to evaluate the activity of L-MTPPE in osteosarcoma. As such, each standard and experimental arm included or did not include L-MTPPE. All patients received identical cumulative doses of cisplatin, doxorubicin, and MTX-L. The results published in the initial report found no statistically significant advantage for L-MTPPE in disease-free survival, the primary endpoint, although the trend favored the combination of ifosfamide and L-MTPPE. Overall survival, which was not prespecified in the protocol, showed a 76% six year survival rate for patients who received L-MTPPE with ifosfamide, compared with a rate of 66% for patients who did not receive the combination ($p = 0.183$).

The U.S.Food and Drug Administration[95] concluded that the L-MTPPE single study did not provide substantial evidence of effectiveness: the results for the primary endpoint did not reach statistical significance, and the overall survival analysis was not part of the study plan. The report stated: "Follow-up data have not been rigorously collected and are incomplete with insufficient follow-up for a significant proportion of patients."[95] L-MTPPE was not sanctioned for general clinical distribution.

In a follow-up report of the above study the authors confirmed a trend for improved event free survival ($p = 0.08$) and improved overall survival ($p = 0.03$) for the MTPPE arm.[96] These results were discussed in several letters to the Editor of the Journal of Clinical Oncology.[97–99] It was suggested that additional investigation be performed to substantiate the utility of MTPPE and define its exact role in the treatment of osteosarcoma. The agent is available through a Compassionate Investigational New Drug (CIND) application and in certain investigational trials.

Inhalation therapy with granulocyte-macrophage colony-stimulating factor (GM-CSF) is currently under investigation by the Pediatric Oncology Group for treating pulmonary metastases.

Chemotherapy Regimens

Spawned by the efficacy of chemotherapy, combination regimens were devised for treating patients with osteosarcoma. Currently most regimens, following the principles and example provided by Sutow, comprise agents with different mechanisms of action and minimal or non overlapping toxicity. An important additional principle in the construction of each regimen is the attempt to deliver agents at maximum dose intensity. Chemotherapy is integrated into a multidisciplinary approach to assist surgical extirpation of the primary tumor and resection of pulmonary metastases. Chemotherapy may also potentiate the action of radiation therapy in resistant and recurrent tumors.

The results obtained with most regimens have been similar. Except for an occasional publication, [71] there does not appear to be a regimen which can claim superiority over those published in most communications. With current strategies, utilizing pre- and postoperative chemotherapy, cure rates of 60–75% in newly diagnosed nonmetastatic patients have been reported.[17–20,22,27,30,71] Limb salvage and, occasionally, rotationplasty have been reported in as many as 80% of the patients in these studies and in several communications devoted specifically to this topic.[100–102] In this context, an attempt was made to perform limb salvage exclusively with chemotherapy and abrogating surgery.[103] It was successful in three patients only: Figs. 11 and 12 demonstrate the result in one of these patients.

Inadequacy of Chemotherapy

While chemotherapy has produced remarkable successes in osteosarcoma, it has also been marred by failures. The survival rate for patients with pulmonary metastases following aggressive multimodal treatment is of the order of 25–30%.[104–113]

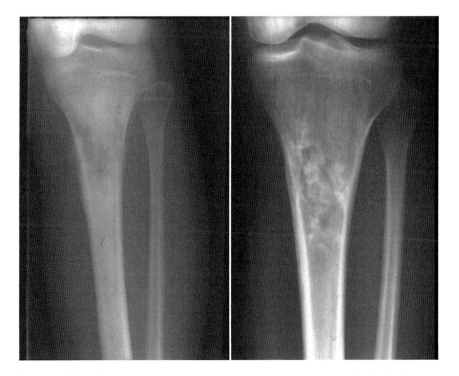

Fig. 11 Initial radiograph of patient with osteosarcoma of the proximal tibia (*left*). There is a mixed osteoblasic and osteolytic lesion. Follow-up after seven courses of high dose methorexate (7.5 G/m^2/course) demonstrates healing by calcification of the medulary lytic lesions and solid periosteal bone formation (*right*). This was accompanied clinically by a complete absence of symptomatology. This material is reproduced with permission of Wiley-Liss, Inc., a subsidiary of John Wiley & Sons, Inc. (Jaffe N et al: *Cancer* 1985;56:461-466)

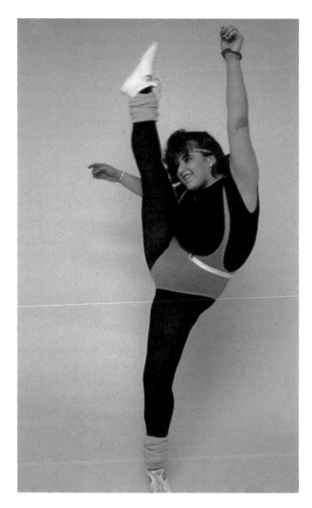

Fig. 12 Photograph of patient with lesion depicted in Fig. 11 10 years after completion of treatment exclusively with chemotherapy. The patient has remained alive and well without recurrent tumor 28 years after diagnosis and therapy

It has not improved over the past quarter century. Bielack et al reported that overall and event-free survival rates, respectively, were 16% and 9% for second, 14% and 0% for third, 13% and 6% for fourth, and 18% and 0% for fifth recurrences: "The exact role of retreatment with chemotherapy, particularly in the adjuvant situation, remains to be defined."[114]

Patients with partially treated tumors in whom survival has been prolonged, have also developed extrapulmonary metastases in uncommon sites, notably the kidneys, brain, heart, mediastinum, and epidural space.[115–117] Such metastases may cause severe complications, and considerable pain and discomfort, and require extensive palliative maneuvers. Attempts to prevent and eradicate such extra pulmonary metastases constitute a major challenge. New therapy for patients with multifocal (sclerosing) osteosarcoma must also be developed.

Conspectus: Impact on the Conduct of Future Investigation and Treatment

Despite major discoveries in the chemotherapeutic pantheon for osteosarcoma over the past 35 years, the survival rate has plateaued. This is due principally to the fact that the arsenal of available effective chemotherapeutic agents over this period has not changed substantially . New agents and alternative strategies for the conquest of this malignancy are urgently required. Employing new paradigm shifts should receive serious consideration, while acquisition of new agents might include biotherapy, gene therapy, anti-angiogenic agents, targeted therapy, and attempts to harness the power of the immune system.

The reviews and reports cited above make no mention of identification markers to detect silent pulmonary micrometastases. Biomarkers or mechanisms with reliable specificity and sensitivity to identify such metastases would constitute a significant saltation in planning new strategies of treatment. Molecular profiles with rigorous characterization, gene expression patterns and phenotypes of osteosarcoma could afford an opportunity for planning risk-adjusted or personalized chemotherapy with reduced toxicity. Identification of patients free of micrometastases would permit treatment with chemotherapy limited to downstaging the primary tumor for surgical extirpation.

Despite the absence of major advances in chemotherapy and of any significant improvement in survival during the past 35 years, the ability to offer limb salvage to approximately 80% of newly diagnosed patients is noteworthy. Further, although the attempt to treat patients exclusively with chemotherapy, avoiding surgical ablation of the primary tumor was not entirely unsuccessful[102], three of the 31 patients were cured with this approach. With new and more effective agents, the ability to cure osteosarcoma without surgical ablation of the primary tumor may yet be realized. The ability to rescue most patients with recurrent pulmonary metastases may also be attained. Considering the phenomenal strides made in the treatment of this disease over the past 35 years, the current lack of new agents notwithstanding, these possibilities may become a reality in the new century.

References

1. Jaffe N, Traggis D, Enriquez C. Evaluation of a combination of mitomycin C (NSC-26980), phenylalanine mustard (NSC-16210) and vincristine (NSC-6757) in the treatment of osteogenic sarcoma. *Cancer Chemother Rep.* 1971;55:181-191.
2. Sullivan MP, Sutow WW, Taylor G. L-phenylalanine mustard as treatment for metastatic osteogenic sarcoma in children. *J Pediatr.* 1963;63:227-237.

3. Sutow WW, Sullivan MP, Fernbach DJ, et al. Adjuvant chemotherapy in primary treatment of osteogenic sarcoma. *Cancer*. 1975;36:1598-1602.
4. Wilbur JR, Sutow WW, Sullivan MP, et al. Successful treatment of rhabdomyosarcoma with combination chemotherapy and radiation therapy. *Proc ASCO*. 1971;7:56.
5. Sutow WW, Sullivan MP, Wilbur JR, et al. The study of adjuvant chemotherapy in osteogenic sarcoma. *J Clin Pharmacol*. 1975;15:530-533.
6. Pinkel D. Cyclophosphamide in children with cancer. *Cancer*. 1962;15:42-49.
7. Finklestein J, Hittle RE, Hammond CD. Evaluation of a high-dose cyclophosphamide regimen in childhood tumors. *Cancer*. 1969;23:1239-1242.
8. Sutow WW. Chemotherapeutic management of childhood rhabdomyosarcoma. In: Taylor G, Sutow WW, eds. *Neoplasia in Childhood*. Chicago: Year Book Medical Publishers; 1969: 201-208.
9. Cortes EP, Holland JF, Wang JJ, et al. Chemotherapy of advanced osteosarcoma. In: Price CHG, Ross FCM, eds. *Colston Paper N.24 Bone-Urban Aspects of Neoplasia*. London: Buttersworth; 1972:265-280.
10. Sutow WW. Combination chemotherapy with Adriamycin (NSC-123127) in primary treatment of osteogenic sarcoma (Part III). *Cancer Chemother Rep*. 1975;6:315-317.
11. Sutow WW, Gehan EA, Dyment PC, et al. Multi-drug adjuvant chemotherapy in osteosarcoma. *Interim report of the Southwest Oncology Group studies. Cancer Treat Rep*. 1978;62: 265-269.
12. Sutow WW. Late metastases in osteosarcoma. *Lancet*. 1976;1:856.
13. Sutow WW, Herson J, Perez C. Survival after metastasis in osteosarcoma. *Natl Cancer Inst Monogram*. 1981;56:227-231.
14. Perez C, Herson J, Kimball JC, et al. Prognosis after metastases in osteosarcoma. *Cancer Clin Trials*. 1978;1:315-320.
15. Jaffe N, Smith E, Abelson HT, Frei E III. Osteogenic sarcoma: Alterations in the pattern of pulmonary metastases with adjuvant chemotherapy. *J Clin Oncol*. 1983;1:251-254.
16. Herson J, Sutow WW, Elder K, et al. Adjuvant chemotherapy in non metastatic osteosarcoma A Southwest Oncology Group Study. *Med Pediatr Oncol*. 1980;8:343-352.
17. Jaffe N, Link M, Traggis D, et al. The role of high-dose methotrexate in osteogenic sarcoma. Sarcomas in soft tissue and bone in childhood. *Natl Cancer Inst Monogr*. 1981;56:201-206.
18. Goorin AM, Delorey M, Gelber RD, et al. The Dana-Farber Cancer Institute/The Children's Hospital adjuvant chemotherapy trials for osteosarcoma: Three sequential studies. *Cancer Treat Symp*. 1986;3:155-159.
19. Rosen G, Marcove RC, Huvos AG, et al. Chemotherapy en bloc resection, and prosthetic bone replacement in the treatment of osteogenic sarcoma. *Cancer*. 1976;37:1-11.
20. Rosen G. Role of chemotherapy in the treatment of primary osteogenic sarcoma. A five-year follow-up of T-10 neoadjuvant chemotherapy. In: Kimura K, Wang Y-M, eds. *Methotrexate in Cancer Therapy*. New York: Raven Press; 1986:227-238.
21. Delepine N, Delepine G, Jasmine C, et al. Importance of age and methotrexate dosage: Prognosis in children and young adults with high-grade osteosarcoma. *Biomed Pharmacother*. 1988;42:257-262.
22. Winkler K, Beron G, Dilling G, et al. Neoadjuvant chemotherapy of osteosarcoma. Results of Randomized Cooperative Trial (COSS-82) with salvage. Chemotherapy based on histologic tumor response. *J Clin Oncol*. 1988;6:329-337.
23. Bacci G, Picci P, Ruggeri P, et al. Primary chemotherapy and delayed surgery (neoadjuvant chemotherapy) for osteosarcoma of the extremities: The Instituto Rizzoli Experience in 127 patients treated preoperatively with intravenous methotrexate (high versus moderate doses) and intra-arterial cisplatin. *Cancer*. 1990;65:2539-2553.
24. Meyers PA, Heller G, Healey JH, et al. Chemotherapy for non-metastatic osteogenic sarcoma: The Memorial Sloan-Kettering experience. *J Clin Oncol*. 1992;10:5-15.
25. Bacci G, Picci P, Avella M, et al. The importance of dose intensity in neoadjuvant chemotherapy of osteosarcoma: A retrospective analysis of high-dose methotrexate, cisplatinum and adriamycin used preoperatively. *J Chemother*. 1990;2:127-135.

Osteosarcoma 259

26. Provisor AJ, Ettinger LJ, Nachman JB, et al. Treatment of non-metastatic osteosarcoma of the extremity with preoperative and postoperative chemotherapy: A report from the Children's Cancer Group. *J Clin Oncol.* 1997;15:76-84.
27. Meyers PA, Gorlick R, Heller G, et al. Intensification of preoperative chemotherapy for osteogenic sarcoma: Results of the Memorial Sloan-Kettering (T-12) protocol. *J Clin Oncol.* 1998;16:2452-2458.
28. Krailo M, Ertel I, Makley J, et al. A randomized study comparing high-dose methotrexate with moderate-dose methotrexate as components of adjuvant chemotherapy in childhood nonmetasatic osteosarcoma: A report from the Children's Cancer Study Group. *Med Pediatr.* 1987;15:69-77.
29. Bramwell VH, Berger SM, Sneath R, et al. A comparison of two short intensive adjuvant chemotherapy regimen in operative osteosarcoma of limbs in children and young adults: The first study of the European Osteosarcoma Intergroup. *J Clin Oncol.* 1992;10:1579-1591.
30. Souhami RL, Craft AW, Vander Eijken JW, et al. Randomised trial of two in operable regimens of chemotherapy inoperable osteosarcoma: A study of the European Osteosarcoma Intergroup. *Lancet.* 1997;350:911-917.
31. Grem J, King S, Whittes R, et al. The role of methotrexate in osteosarcoma. *J Natl Cancer Inst.* 1988;80:626-655.
32. Graf N, Winkler K, Betlemovic M, et al. Methotrexate pharmacokinetics and prognosis in osteosarcoma. *J Clin Oncol.* 1994;12:1443-1451.
33. Wang Y-N, Sutow WW, Romsdahl MM, et al. Age related pharmacokinetics of high-dose methotrexate in patients with osteosarcoma. *Cancer Treat Rep.* 1979;63:405-410.
34. Jaffe N, Prudich J, Knapp J, et al. Treatment of primary osteosarcoma with intra-arterial and intravenous high-dose methotrexate. *J Clin Oncol.* 1983;7:428-431.
35. Cohen H, Jaffe N. Pharmacokinetic studies of 24-hour infusions of high-dose methotrexate. *Cancer Chemother Pharmacol.* 1978;1:61-64.
36. Wang YM, Lantin E, Sutow WW. Blood, urinary and cerebral spinal fluid methotrexate levels in children after high-dose methotrexate infusion. *Clin Chem.* 1976;22:1053-1056.
37. Wang YN, Kim PY, Lantin E, et al. Degradation and clearance of methotrexate in children with osteosarcoma receiving high-dose infusion. *Med Pediatr Oncol.* 1978;4:221-229.
38. Perez C, Wang Y-M, Sutow WW, et al. Significance of 48-hour plasma level in high-dose methotrexate regimens. *Cancer Clin Trials.* 1978;1:107-111.
39. Jaffe N, Farber S, Traggis D, et al. Favorable response of metastatic osteogenic sarcoma to past high-dose methotrexate with citrovorin rescue and radiation therapy. *Cancer.* 1973;31:1367-1373.
40. Rosen G, Tefft M, Martinez A, et al. Combination chemotherapy and radiation therapy in the treatment of metastatic osteogenic sarcoma. *Cancer.* 1975;35:622-630.
41. Machak GN, Tkachev SI, Solovyev YN, et al. Neoadjuvant chemotherapy and local radiotherapy for high grade osteosarcoma of the extremities. *Mayo Clin Proc.* 2003;78:147-155.
42. Ozaki T, Flege S, Kevric M, et al. Osteosarcoma of the pelvis: Experience of the Osteosarcoma Study Group. *J Clin Oncol.* 2003;21:334-341.
43. Bonnadonna G, Monfardi S, De Lena M, et al. Phase I and preliminary phase II evaluation of Adriamycin (NSC/123127). *Cancer Res.* 1970;30:2527-2582.
44. Middleman E, Luce L, Frei E. Clinical trials with Adriamycin. *Cancer.* 1971;28:844-850.
45. O'Bryan RN, Luce JK, Talley R, et al. Phase II evaluation of Adriamycin in human neoplasia. *Cancer.* 1973;32:1-7.
46. Cortes EP, Holland JF, Wang JJ, et al. Amputation and Adriamycin in primary osteosarcoma. *New Engl J Med.* 1974;291:998-1000.
47. Cortes EP, Holland JF, Glidewell O. Osteogenic studies by the Cancer and Leukemia Group B. *Natl Cancer Inst Monogr.* 1975;56:207-209.
48. Cassady JR, Richter NP, Piro AJ, et al. Radiation, Adriamycin interactions – Preliminary clinical observations. *Cancer.* 1975;36:946-949.
49. Eilber FR, Grant T, Morton C. Adjuvant chemotherapy of osteosarcoma: Preoperative treatment. *Cancer Treat Rep.* 1978;62:213-216.

50. Jaffe N, Watts H, Fellows KE, et al. Local en bloc resection for limb preservation. *Cancer Treat Rep.* 1978;62:217-273.
51. Basser RI, Green MD. Strategies for prevention of anthracycline cardiotoxicity. *Cancer Treat Rev.* 1994;19:57-77.
52. Seifert CF, Nesser ME, Thompson DF. Dexrazoxane in the prevention of doxorubicin-induced cardiotoxicity. *Ann Pharmacother.* 1994;28:1063-1072.
53. Smith MA, Ungerleider RS, Horowitz ME, et al. Influence of doxorubicin dose intensity on response and outcome for patients with osteogenic sarcoma and Ewing's sarcoma. *J Natl Cancer Inst.* 1991;83:1460-1470.
54. Baum E, Greenberg L, Gaynon P, et al. Use of *Cis*-diamminedichloroplatinum-II (CPDD) in Osteogenic Sarcoma (OS) in Children (Abstract C-315). *Proc AACR-ASCO.* 1978;19:385.
55. Nitschke R, Starling KA, Vats T, et al. *Cis*-diamminedichloroplatin-II (NSC 119875) In Childhood Malignancies. A Southwest Oncology Group Study. *Med Pedatr Oncol.* 1978;4:127-132.
56. Ochs JJ, Freeman AR, Douglass HO Jr, et al. *Cis*-diamminedichloroplatinum (II) in advanced osteogenic sarcoma. *Cancer Treat Rep.* 1978;62:239-245.
57. Jaffe N, Knapp J, Chuang VP, et al. Osteosarcoma intra-arterial treatment of the primary tumor with Cis-diamminedichloroplatinum-II (CDP). Angiographic, pathologic and pharmacologic studies. *Cancer.* 1983;51:402-407.
58. Jaffe N, Raymond AK, Ayala A, et al. Effect of cumulative courses of intra-arterial *Cis*-diamminedichloroplatinum II on the primary tumor in osteosarcoma. *Cancer.* 1989;63:63-67.
59. Wright KC, Wallace S, Kim EE, et al. Pulse arterial infusions. Chemotherapeutic complications. *Cancer.* 1986;57:1952-1956.
60. Chuang VP, Benjamin RS, Jaffe N, et al. Radiographic and angiographic changes in osteosarcoma after intra-arterial chemotherapy. *Am J Radiol.* 1982;139:1065-1069.
61. Shirkoda A, Jaffe N, Wallace S, et al. Computed tomography of osteosarcoma following intra-arterial chemotherapy. *Am J Radiol.* 1985;144:95-99.
62. Pan G, Raymond AK, Carrasco CH, et al. Osteosarcoma: MR imaging after preoperative chemotherapy. *Radiology.* 1990;174:517-526.
63. Meyers PA. Osteosarcoma In Pediatric Bone and Soft Tissue Sarcomas. In: Pappo A, ed. *Pediatric Bone and Soft Tissue Sarcomas.* Berlin, Heidelberg, New York: Springer; 2005:219-233.
64. Ruiz L, Gilden J, Jaffe N, et al. Auditory function in pediatric osteosarcoma patients treated with multiple doses of *cis*-diamminedichloroplatinum-II (CDP). *Cancer Res.* 1989;49:742-744.
65. Jaffe N, Keifer R III, Robertson R, et al. Renal toxicity with cumulative doses of cis-diamminedichloroplatinum-II in pediatric patients with osteosarcoma. *Cancer.* 1987;59:1577-1581.
66. Kawai A, Sugihara S, Kunisada T, et al. Imaging assessment of the response of bone tumors to preoperative chemotherapy. *Clin Orthop Relat Res.* 1997;Apr(337):216-225.
67. Kunisada T, Ozaki T, Kawai A. Imaging assessment of the responses of osteosarcoma patients to preoperative chemotherapy: Angiography compared with thallium-201 scintigraphy. *Cancer.* 1999;86(6):949-956.
68. Carrasco CH, Charnsangavej C, Raymond AK, et al. Osteosarcoma: Angiographic assessment of response to preoperative chemotherapy. *Radiology.* 1989;170:839-842.
69. Lang P, Vahlensieck M, Matthay KK. Monitoring neovascularity as an indicator to response to chemotherapy in osteogenic and Ewing sarcoma using magnetic resonance angiography. *Med Pediatr Oncol.* 1996;26(5):329-333.
70. Kumpan W, Lechner G, Wittich GR. The angiographic response of osteosarcoma following pre-operative chemotherapy. *Skeletal Radiol.* 1986;15(2):96-102.
71. Wilkins RM, Cullen JW, Odom L, et al. Superior survival in treatment of primary nonmetastatic pediatric osteosarcoma of the extremity. *Ann Surg Oncol.* 2003;10:498-507.
72. Jaffe N, Spears R, Eftekhari F, et al. Pathologic fracture in osteosarcoma: Effect of chemotherapy in primary Tumor and survival. *Cancer.* 1987;59:701-709.

Osteosarcoma

73. Antman KH, Montella D, Rosenbaum C, et al. Phase II Trial of ifosfamide with mesna in previously treated metastatic osteosarcoma. *Cancer Treat Rep.* 1985;69:499-504.
74. Bowman LG, Mayer WN, Douglass EC, et al. Activation of ifosfamide in metastatic and unresectable osteosarcoma (Abstract). *Proc ASCO.* 1987;C-214:844.
75. Meyer WH, Pratt CB, Farham D, et al. The activity of Ifosfamide (IFOS) in previously pretreated patients with osteosarcoma (OS): Preliminary results of SJCRHOS-86 Study. *Proc ASCO.* 1988;7:261.
76. Grana N, Graham-Pole J, Cassano W, et al. Etoposide (VP-16) infusion plus Cyclophosphamide (CY) pulses: An effective combination for refractory cancer. *Proc ASCO.* 1989;8:300.
77. Saleh R, Graham-Pole J, Cassano W, et al. Response of osteogenic sarcoma to the combination of rtoposide and cyclophosphamide as neoadjuvant chemotherapy. *Cancer.* 1990;65:861-865.
78. Pratt CB, Luo X, Fay L, et al. Response of pediatric malignant solid tumors following ifosfamide or ifosfamide/carboplatin/etoposide. *A single hospital experience. Med Pediatr Oncol.* 1996;27:145-148.
79. Harris MB, Cantor AB, Goorin AM. Treatment of osteosarcoma with ifosfamide: Comparison of response in pediatric patients with recurrent disease versus patients previously untreated: A Pediatric Oncology Group study. *Med Pediatr Oncol.* 2002;20:426-433.
80. Pratt CB, Meyer WH, Dauglass EC, et al. A phase I study of ifosfamide with Mesna given daily for 3 consecutive days to children with malignant solid tumors. *Cancer.* 1993;71: 3661-3665.
81. Chawla S, Rosen G, Lowenbraun S, et al. Role of high-dose ifosfamide in recurrent osteosarcoma. *Proc ASCO.* 1990;9:310.
82. Patel S, Vadhan-Raj S, Papadopolous N, et al. High-dose ifosfamide in bone and soft tissue sarcomas: Results of a Phase II and Pilot Studies – dose-response and schedule dependence. *J Clin Oncol.* 1997;15:2378-2384.
83. Berrak S, Pearson P, Berbergoglu S, et al. High-dose ifosfamide in relapsed pediatric osteosarcoma: Therapeutic effects and renal toxicity. *Pediatr Blood Cancer.* 2005;44:215-219.
84. Pratt CB, Meyer WH, Rao BN, et al. Osteosarcoma studies at St Jude Children's Research Hospital from 1968 through 1998. *Cancer Treat Res.* 1993;62:323-326.
85. Harris MB, Gieser P, Goorin AM, et al. Treatment of metastatic osteosarcoma at diagnosis: A Pediatric Oncology Group Study. *J Clin Oncol.* 1998;16:3641-3648.
86. Goorin AM, Harris MB, Bernstein M, et al. Phase II/III trial of etoposide and high-dose ifosfamide in newly diagnosed metastatic osteosarcoma: A Pediatric Oncology Group Trial. *J Clin Oncol.* 2002;20:426-433.
87. Daw NC, Billups CA, Rodroguez-Galindo C, et al. Metastatic osteosarcoma. *Cancer.* 2006;106:403-412.
88. Meyer WH, Pratt CB, Poquette CA, et al. Carboplatin/Ifosfamide window therapy for osteosarcoma: Results of the St Jude Children's Research Hospital OS-91 Trial. *J Clin Oncol.* 2001;19:171-182.
89. Fergusen WS, Harris MB, Goorin AM, et al. Presurgical window of carboplatin and surgery and multi-drug chemotherapy for the treatment of newly diagnosed metastatic or unresectable osteosarcoma: Pediatric Oncology Group trial. *J Pediatr Hematol Oncol.* 2001;23:340-348.
90. Petrilli AS, de Camargo B, Filho VO, et al. Results of the osteosarcoma treatment group studies III and IV: Prognostic factors and impact on survival. *J Clin Oncol.* 2006;24:1161-1168.
91. Merimsky O, Meller I, Flusser G, et al. Gemcitabine in soft tissue or bone sarcoma resistant to standard chemotherapy: A phase II study. *Cancer Chemother Pharmacol.* 2000;45:177-181.
92. Navid F, Willert JR, Mc Carville MB, et al. Combination of gemcitabine and docetaxel in the treatment of children and young adults with refractory bone sarcoma. *Cancer.* 2008;113:419-425.
93. Anderson PM, Wiseman GA, Dispenzieri A, et al. High-dose samarium-153 ethylene diamine tetramethylene phosphonate: Low toxicity of skeletal irradiation in patients with osteosarcoma and bone metastases. *J Clin Oncol.* 2002;20:189-196.

94. Meyers P, Schwartz CL, Krailo M, et al. Osteosarcoma: A randomized prospective trial of the addition of ifosfamide and/or muramyl tripeptide to cisplatin, doxorubicin, and high-dose methotrexate. *J Clin Oncol.* 2005;23:2004-2011.
95. Lu L, Lu L. Junovan fails to win ODAC nod for osteosarcoma treatment. *ONI.* 2007;16:1632.
96. Meyers PA, Schwartz CL, Krailo MD, et al. Osteosarcoma: The addition of muramyl tripeptide to chemotherapy improves overall survival – a report from the Children's Oncology Group. *J Clin Oncol.* 2008;26:633-638.
97. Bielack SS, Marina N, Ferrari S, et al. Osteosarcoma: The same old drugs or more? *Journal Clin Oncol.* 2008;26:3192-3193.
98. Hunsberger S, Freidlin B, Smith MA. Complexities in interpretation of osteosarcoma clinical trial results. *Journal Clin Oncol.* 2008;26:3193-3194.
99. Meyers PA, Schwartz CL, Krailo MD, et al. In Reply Journal. *Clin Oncol.* 2008;26:3194-3195.
100. Gitelis S, Neel MD, Wilkins RM, et al. The use of a closed expandable prosthesis for pediatric sarcomas. *Chir Organi Mov.* 2003;88:327-333.
101. Hudson M, Jaffe MR, Jaffe N, et al. Pediatric osteosarcoma: Therapeutic strategies, results and prognostic factors derived from a 10-year experience. *J Clin Oncol.* 1990;8:1988-1997.
102. Hosalkar HS, Dormans JP. Limb sparing surgery for pediatric musculoskeletal tumors. *Pediatr Blood Cancer.* 2004;42(4):295-310.
103. Jaffe N, Carrasco H, Raymond K, et al. Can cure in patients with osteosarcoma be achieved exclusively with chemotherapy and abrogation of surgery? *Cancer.* 2002;95:2202-2210.
104. Kaste SC, Pratt CB, Cain AM, et al. Metastases detected at the time of diagnosis of primary pediatric extremity osteosarcoma at diagnosis: Imaging features. *Cancer.* 1999;86(8):1602-1608.
105. Meyers PA, Heller G, Healy JH, et al. Osteogenic sarcoma with clinically detectable pulmonary metastases at initial presentation. *J Clin Oncol.* 1993;11:449-453.
106. Su WT, Chewning J, Abramson S, et al. Surgical management and outcome of osteosarcoma patients with unilateral pulmonary metastases. *J Pediatr Surg.* 1994;39(3):1849-1858.
107. Meyer WH, Schell MJ, Kumar AP, et al. Thoracotomy for pulmonary metastatic osteosarcoma. An analysis of prognostic indicators of survival. *Cancer.* 1987;59(2):374-379.
108. Skinner KA, Eilber FR, Holmes E, et al. Surgical treatment and chemotherapy for pulmonary metastases from osteosarcoma. *Arch Surg.* 1992;127(90):1065-1070. discussion 1070-71.
109. Chou AJ, Merola P, Wexler LH, et al. Treatment of osteosarcoma at first recurrence after contemporary therapy: The Memorial Sloan-Kettering Cancer Center experience. *Cancer.* 2005;104(10):2214-2221.
110. Harting MT, Blakely ML, Jaffe N, et al. Long-term survival after aggressive resection of pulmonary metastases among children and adolescents with osteosarcoma. *J Pediatr Surg.* 2006;41(1):194-199.
111. Ward WG, Mikaelian K, Dorey F, et al. Pulmonary metastases of stage IIB extremity osteosarcoma and subsequent pulmonary metastases. *J Clin Oncol.* 1994;12(9):1849-1858.
112. Bacci G, Ferrari S, Bertoni F, et al. Long-term outcome for patients with nonmetastatic osteosarcoma of the extremity treated at the Istituto Ortopedico Rizzoli/osteosarcoma-2 protocol: An updated report. *J Clin Oncol.* 2000;18(24):4016-4027.
113. Nathan SS, Gorlick R, Bukata S, et al. Treatment algorithm for locally recurrent osteosarcoma based on local disease-free interval and the presence of lung metastasis. *Cancer.* 2006;107(7):1607-1616.
114. Bielack SS, Kempf-Bielack B, Branscheid D, et al. Second and subsequent recurrences of osteosarcoma: Presentation and treatment outcomes of 249 Consecutive Cooperative Osteosarcoma Study Group patients. *J Clin Oncol.* 2008;27:557-565.
115. McCarten KM, Jaffe N, Kirkpatrick JA. The changing radiographic appearance of osteosarcoma. *Ann Radiol.* 1980;23:203-208.
116. Lockhart SK, Coan JD, Jaffe N, et al. Osteosarcoma metastatic to the kidney. *Clin Imaging.* 1989;13:154-156.
117. Baram TZ, Van Tassel P, Jaffe N. Brain metastases in osteosarcoma: Incidence, clinical and neurological findings and management options. *J Neuro Oncol.* 1988;6:45-52.

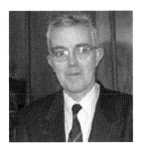

Osteosarcoma: The European Osteosarcoma Intergroup (EOI) Perspective

Alan W. Craft

Abstract In the late 1970s, there was confusion regarding the best management for osteosarcoma. The benefit of chemotherapy had not been established and which chemotherapy could be used was even more uncertain. The European Osteosarcoma Intergroup (EOI) was established in order to conduct randomised studies to determine the best treatment for this tumour. Their first study 80831 established that a two drug combination of CDDP/DOX was safe and improved the survival rate over previous regimes with suboptimal chemotherapy. The CDDP/DOX was superior to a less intense CDDP/DOX/MTX regime. The second study 80861 compared the CDDP/DOX arm with a multi-drug Rosen-T10 regime. In almost 400 patients, there was the difference in outcome between the two arms. However, adherence to the protocol and completion of allocated treatment was substantially less good in the prolonged 42 week multi-drug regime compared to the two drug arm.

The third study 80961 investigated interval compression i.e. if the CDDP/DOX when given every 2 weeks with GCSF superior to the same two drugs given every 3 weeks. There was no difference in survival between the arms, although there was a better histologic response rate in the compressed arm.

Three randomised controlled trials on this rare disease have taken more than 20 years to accrue a sufficient sample of patients. The overall outcome has changed little in this time. Large multinational studies are needed to be able to answer these important questions in a timely fashion

Introduction

In the late 1970s there was confusion surrounding the management of osteosarcoma. Doctors were faced with a series of conflicts. The Mayo Clinic reported that with surgery alone they had been able to improve the survival rate from 20% to almost

---

A.W. Craft (✉)
Northern Institute for Cancer Research, Newcastle University, Newcastle upon Tyne, NE1 7RU, UK
e-mail: a.w.craft@ncl.ac.uk

50%,[1] while at the same time, the early promise of chemotherapy as initially reported by Jaffe[2] had been logically extended by Rosen[3] in a series of ground breaking studies, culminating in the spectacular results of T10 where over 90% of patients were disease free at 2 years.[4] Before the advent of chemotherapy, there was general agreement that amputation alone would result in no more than 20%[5] long term survival. The EORTC in parts of continental Europe, and the Medical Research Council in the United Kingdom, undertook studies using chemotherapy, but the results were very disappointing.[6,7] In retrospect, it is clear that the dose and dose intensity of chemotherapy were inadequate.

It was against this background that a number of European cancer study groups met and formed the European Osteosarcoma Intergroup (EOI). These groups were the Medical Research Council and the United Kingdom Children's Cancer Study Group (UKCCSG), the Bone and Soft Tissue Sarcoma Group of the EORTC and the International Paediatric Oncology Society (SIOP). Later, the group was joined by the Canadian Sarcoma Group (CSG). The Institut Gustave Roussy of Paris was involved in the initial discussions but ultimately decided not to participate in the EOI studies and undertook a Rosen T10 approach.

The MIOS and UCLA studies[8,9] settled the question of the benefit of chemotherapy in two separate randomised controlled trials. The EOI was, therefore, able to concentrate its efforts on the determination of optimum chemotherapy.

First EOI Study (80831)[10]

The initial intention of the EOI was to study two short intensive chemotherapy regimes with a view to adopting one to compare in a randomised trial with a Rosen type T10 regime. This began as a randomised Phase II trial where cisplatin and doxorubicin were compared to the same two drugs with the addition of methotrexate. The study scheme is shown in Fig. 1.

The study was set up as a toxicity and response study but accrued patients very rapidly so that it was expanded into a formal Phase III study with survival and disease free survival as additional end points. Between 1983 and 1986, 207 eligible patients with limb primaries and no metastases were evaluable for the trial. Seventy-nine percent successfully completed the designated chemotherapy, with the remainder stopping early either because of toxicity or early relapse. The outcome, according to treatment arm, is shown in Fig. 2 for overall survival and in Fig. 3 for disease free survival. The DFS was significantly better for the two-drug arm than the three-drug arm ($P < 0.02$). There was an excess of toxicity in the MTX containing arm.

The conclusion of this study was that both treatment arms were tolerable with no serious differences in toxicity. DFS was better for the two-drug arm without methotrexate. It was, however, not a true comparison of the addition of MTX as the total dose and dose intensity in the two arms were substantially different. Those randomised to the three-drug arm received only 66% of the DDP/DOX and the

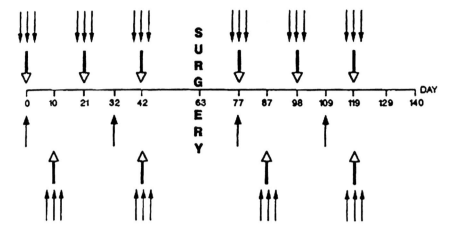

Fig. 1 Chemotherapy regimens. ↑↑↑, DOX 25 mg/m² IV daily times 3; , CDDP 100 mg/m² 24-h infusion; ↑HDMTX 8 g/m² 6-h infusion plus LU rescue at 24 h 12 mg/m² 6 h times 10. Hydration regimens: DOX/CDDP, Pretreatment: 400 mL/m² isotonic saline (0.9 NaCl) during a 2-h period and, 400 mL/m² 5% dextrose (D5W) during a 2-h period. Chemotherapy: total dose CDDP in 2,400 mL/m² 0.9 NaCl during a 24-h period plus 80 mEq/L KCL plus 32 g/m² mannitol. Posttreatment: 600 mL/m² D5W plus 8 g/m² mannitol plus 20 mEq/L KCl during a 6-h period; 600 mL/m² 0.9 NaCl plus 20 mEq/L KCL plus 2 mmol/L magnesium sulphate plus 0.6 mmol/L calcium gluconate during a 6-h period. 600 mL/m² D5W, additives as previously mentioned during a 12-h period; and furosemide 20-40 mg IV if diuresis <400 mL/m² per 6 h. HDMTX, Pretreatment: 750 mL/m² 0.9 NaCl:D5W plus 20 MEq/L KCL during a 6-h period. Chemotherapy: total dose HDMTX in 1,000 mL D5W during a 6-h period. Posttreatment: alternating litres D5W plus 0.9 NaCl 3,000 mL/m² plus 60 mEq/L KCL during a 24-h period; alkalinisation with oral bicarbonate 3 g 6 h (1 mmol/kg/24 h oral sodium citrate 0.3 mol/L liquid for pediatric patients) was commenced 12 h before treatment and continued with IV sodium bicarbonate 167 mmol/L until serum MTX level was below 10^{-8} mol/L

DDP/DOX pulses were 31 rather than 21 days apart. The final conclusion of this study, therefore, was that the total dose and dose intensity are important predictors of outcome. It was decided to take forward the two-drug arm into the next study.

The Second EOI Study (80861)[11]

This was a randomised trial of two chemotherapy regimes in the treatment of operable non metastatic osteosarcoma. The two arms were those containing two drugs from the 80831 study and a multi-drug regime designed to be similar to the Rosen T10 regime. However, there was no switch of chemotherapy after surgery, depending on the histological response, as there had been in the T10 regime. In the 80861 multi-drug arm, there was a "fixed switch" to DDP/DOX after surgery, independent of the postchemotherapy histology. The aim of the study was to determine whether a short intensive chemotherapy lasting 18 weeks differed in terms of survival and disease free survival from a more prolonged regime lasting 42 weeks. The study scheme is shown in Fig. 4.

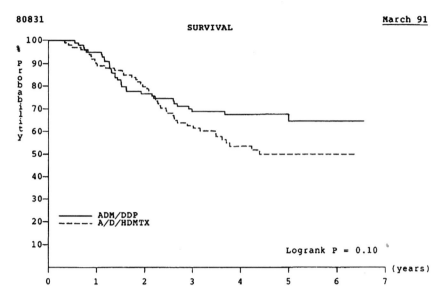

Fig. 2 The survival according to treatment arm. The median follow-up is 40 months

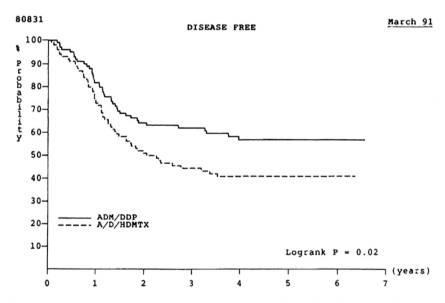

Fig. 3 The disease-free survival according to treatment arm. The median follow-up is 40 months

A total of 391 eligible patients were entered. 199 were randomised to the two drug arm and 167 of these completed all of the protocol treatment. 192 entered the multi-drug arm but only 72 completed all of the pre designated treatment. However, the analysis was done on an 'intention to treat' basis. The main reasons for terminating the protocol chemotherapy are given in Table 1.

Osteosarcoma: The European Osteosarcoma Intergroup (EOI) Perspective

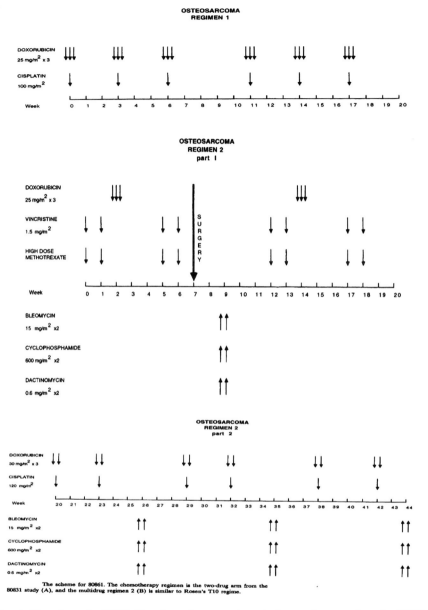

Fig. 4 The scheme for 80861. The chemotherapy regimen is the two-drug arm from the 80831 study (A) and the multidrug regimen 2 (B) is similar to Rosen's T10 regime

The survival and disease free survival by treatment group are shown in the Figs. 5 and 6. The histopathological response rate was determined in 69% of the patients and a good response was similar in both arms i.e. 29%. As was to be expected, there was a significant difference in survival between good and bad responders as shown in Fig. 7.

Table 1 Reasons for termination of protocol chemotherapy (80861)

	Two-drug group ($n=199$)	Multi-drug group ($n=192$)	
		To cycle 6	After cycle 6
Treatment completed	167 (83.4%)		72 (37.5%)[a]
Treatment terminated			
Progression	14	10	22
Toxic effects	10	5	30
Refusal	3	3	24
Postoperative complications	2	0	3
Change from protocol schedule	2	6	14
Lost to follow up	1	1	2
Total	32	25	95

[a]Includes nine patients who missed one or more cycles during treatment period

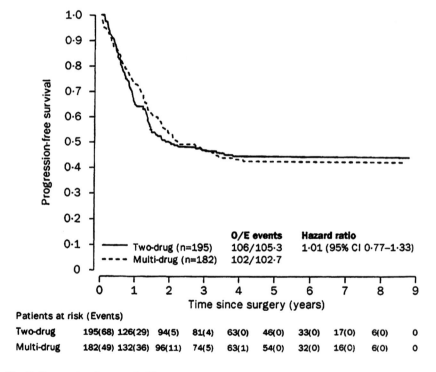

Fig. 5 Progression-free survival by treatment group

This trial was designed to answer a very practical clinical question i.e. whether a short chemotherapy could be equivalent to a longer and more complex regime. No evidence of any difference was found in either event free survival or overall survival, although a difference of 10% could not be excluded, even given the large size of the randomised trial. Not surprisingly, the cost of drugs was substantially greater for the multi-drug regime (about 9,000$) than for the two drug regime (about

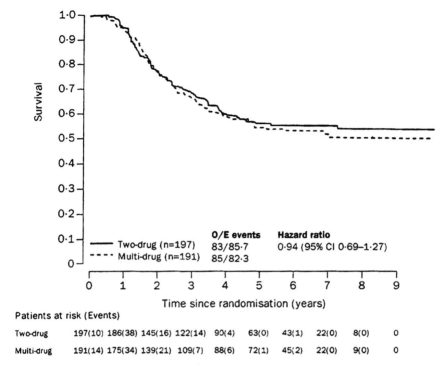

Fig. 6 Survival from randomisation by treatment group

3,000$). Length of time in hospital and bed occupancy was also higher. Given the lack of any difference in survival between the two regimes and the economic and social benefit of the shorter regime, the conclusion was that the shorter treatment regime was preferable. The lack of compliance to chemotherapy in the multi-drug regime came in for much criticism following the publication of the results. In retrospect, we believe that the very large perceived difference (by the patients and physicians) between the two arms was a major factor in encouraging patients to stop treatment early.

Further analysis of the data suggested that the dose intensity in the two-drug arm was higher than that of the multi-drug regime, at least for cisplatin and doxorubicin.

Dose Intensity in 80831 and 80861 Studies[12]

The first decade of EOI studies had suggested that dose intensity of chemotherapy might be an important prognostic factor in the management of osteosarcoma. A separate analysis was undertaken of 287 patients who had been randomised to

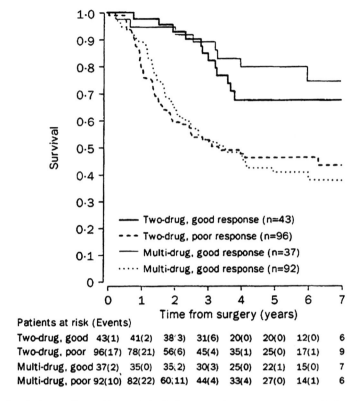

Fig. 7 Survival according to histopathological response by treatment group calculated from date of surgery

DOX/CDDP in the first two studies, and who had received at least one cycle of chemotherapy. 232 (81%) had received all six cycles of chemotherapy. On an average, 79% of the intended dose of DOX and 80% of the intended dose of CDDP was given. However, the mean time to complete chemotherapy was 1.27 times that specified by the protocol. The mean Received Dose Intensity (RDI) for DOX was 0.64 (SD=0.19), and for CDDP it was 0.65 (SD=0.18). The progression free survival was lower in those who completed less than six cycles with a hazard ratio of 1.69: 95% confidence interval, 1.03–2.78. Although survival and progression free survival were lowest for patients with RDI less than 0.6, these differences were not statistically significant. There was no clear evidence of preoperative dose or dose intensity influencing the histological response.

The conclusion was that a clear survival benefit could not be established for increasing the received dose or dose intensity and that the hypothesis that increasing the dose intensity improves the outcome required prospective evaluation.

Pilot Study of Interval Compression[13]

The feasibility of delivering the two drug standard EOI arm in 2 weeks, with GCSF support, instead of 3 weeks was tested in a pilot Phase II study reported in 1994. Twenty-four patients were treated with an accelerated schedule of chemotherapy. The conclusion was that the two weekly chemotherapy was feasible; even so, only 75% of the intended dose intensity of DOX and CDDP could be given. Not surprisingly, the main side effects were thrombocytopenia and neutropenic sepsis.

Third EOI Randomised Study: MRC B006 and EORTC 80931[14]

This study built on the previous EOI experience. It took forward the "standard" two drug CDDP/Dox regime given every 3 weeks, with the same two drugs given every 2 weeks supported by granulocyte colony stimulating factor. The plan of treatment is given in Fig. 8. Between May 1993 and September 2002, 497 eligible patients

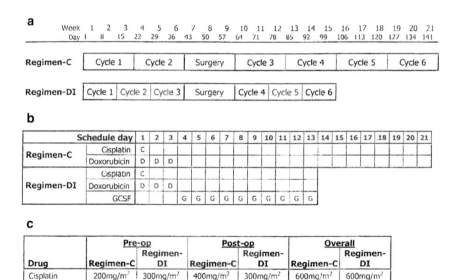

Fig. 8 Schedule of drug treatment and surgery and planned dosage in the trial. (**a**) Schedule of drug treatment cycles and surgery for the conventional regimen (Regimen-C) and the dose-intensive regimen (Regimen-D1) that were compared in the trial. (**b**) Schedule of drug doses within each cycle. In both regimens, C=administration of cisplatin as a 100 mg/m² 24-h infusion, D=administration of doxorubicin as a 25 mg/m² 4-h intravenous infusion, and G=granulocyte colony-stimulating factor (GCSF) given as a 5 µg/kg injection. Cisplatin infusion was preceded by 4 h of predehydration followed by a 24-h posthydration schedule, which included a forced mannitol diuresis. (**c**) Planned total doses of each drug according to regimen in preoperative, postoperative, and full period of treatment

were randomly allocated to one of the two regimes. Six cycles of chemotherapy were completed by 78% of patients in regime C (conventional) and 80% in regime DI (dose intense). The delivered preoperative median dose intensity of cisplatin was 86% in regime C and 111% in regime DI (when compared to that planned for the conventional three weekly regime). The dose intense regime was associated with lower risks of severe leucopenia and neutropenia but higher levels of thrombocytopenia and mucositis. A good histological response (greater than 90% tumour necrosis) was seen in 36% of regime C patients and 50% of regime DI ($P=003$). However, although there was an improvement in the histological response, which normally equates to improvement in survival, there was no evidence of any difference in overall survival (hazard ratio=0.94, 95% CI=0.71–1.24: $P=0.64$). Similarly, there was no difference in disease free survival Fig. 9

The EOI concluded that planned intensification of chemotherapy with cisplatin and doxorubicin increased the received dose intensity and resulted in a statistically

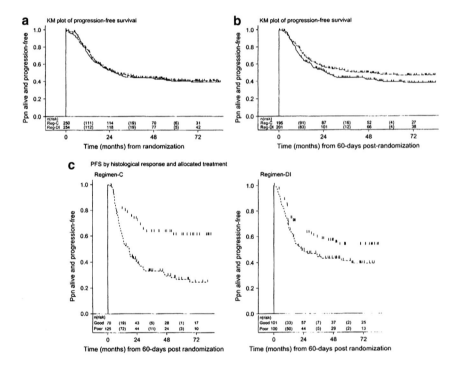

Fig. 9 Progression-free survival according to allocated treatment. Progression-free survival (PFS) for patients treated with conventional regimen (Regimen-C [*solid line*]) and dose-intensive regimen (Regimen-Dl [*dashed line*]) was calculated from the time of randomisation (hazard ratio [HR]=0.98, 95% confidence interval [CI]=0.77-1.24) (**a**) or from 60 days after randomisation (HR=0.82 95% CI=0.63-1.08) (**b**) when histologic response was known. (**c**) Progression-free survival for patients allocated to Regimen-C (*left panel*) or Regimen-DI (*right panel*) according to histologic response (good [*solid line*] or poor [*dashed line*]). Hatch marks denote censoring events. Numbers at risk are shown below each graph

significant increase in favourable histological response rate but not in increased progression free or overall survival. They concluded that the results called into question the use of histological response as a surrogate outcome measure in trials of this disease.

Conspectus

The EOI carried out three successive randomised controlled trials, each of which accrued around 400 patients. In order to do this, there was multinational collaboration. However, several European groups were undertaking single arm studies at this time, and in the US, the POG and COG had an intergroup osteosarcoma study. The three EOI studies took almost 20 years to complete.

The standard EOI treatment of two drugs, CDDP/DOX was equivalent to a multi-drug regime containing methotrexate in a randomised study. However, although the results of the two-drug arm are consistent across all of the EOI studies, when compared to other group studies, most of which contain methotrexate, the results do not compare favourably.

The EOI studies clearly demonstrate the difficulties of undertaking RCTs in a rare disease, and even more multi-national collaboration is needed. They also demonstrate the undue length of time it takes to accrue sufficient patients, and once again, more international collaboration would help.

Finally, these studies demonstrate that there has been little improvement in the management of osteosarcoma over the past 20 years or so, and new ideas are needed.

In view of all of these conclusions, it was decided that the next EOI study should be a combined one with as many groups as possible to collaborate. This resulted in EURAMOS, which, it is hoped, will address many of the issues raised by EOI studies.

Acknowledgements The continuing support of all EOI colleagues is acknowledged along with the generous support of funding bodies to the individual groups.

References

1. Edmondson JH, Green SJ, Ivins JC, et al. A controlled pilot study of high-dose methotrexate: a postsurgical adjuvant treatment for primary osteosarcoma. *J Clin Oncol.*. 1984;2:156.
2. Jaffe N, Frie E III, Watts H, Raggis D. High-dose methotrexate in osteogenic sarcoma: a 5-year experience. *Cancer Treat Rep.*. 1978;6:259-264.
3. Rosen G, Nirenberg A. Chemotherapy for osteogenic sarcoma: an investigative method, not a recipe. *Cancer Treat Rep.*. 1982;66:1687-1697.
4. Rosen G, Caparros B, Huvos AG, et al. Preoperative chemotherapy for osteogenic sarcoma. *Cancer.*. 1982;49:1221-1230.

5. Friedmann MA, Carter S. The therapy of osteogenic sarcoma: current status and thoughts for the future. *J Surg Oncol.*. 1972;4:482-510.
6. Medical Research Council (MRC). A trial of chemotherapy in patients with osteosarcoma (a report to the Medical Research Council by their Working Party on Bone Sarcoma). *Br J Cancer.*. 1986;53:513-518.
7. Burgers JMV, Van Glabbeke M, Busson A, et al. Osteosarcoma of the limbs: report of the EORTC-SIOP 03 trial 20781 investigating the value of adjuvant treatment with chemotherapy and/or prophylactic lung irradiation. *Cancer.*. 1988;5:1024-1031.
8. Link MP, Gorrin AM, Miser AW, et al. The effect of adjuvant chemotherapy on relapse-free survival in patients with osteosarcoma of the extremity. *New Engl J Med.*. 1986;134:1600-1606.
9. Eilber F, Giuilano A, Eckardt J, Patterson K, Moseley S, Goodnight J. Adjuvant chemotherapy for osteosarcoma: a randomised prospective trial. *J Clin Oncol.*. 1987;5:21-26.
10. Bramwell VH, Burgers M, Sneath R, et al. A comparison of two short intensive adjuvant chemotherapy regimens in operable osteosarcoma of limbs in children and young adults: the first study of the European Osteosarcoma Intergroup. *J Clin Oncol.*. 1992;10:1579-1591.
11. Souhami RL, Craft AW, Van der Eijken JW, et al. Randomised trial of two regimens of chemotherapy in operable osteosarcoma: a study of the European Osteosarcoma Intergroup. *Lancet.*. 1997;350:911-917.
12. Lewis IJ, Weeden S, Machin D, Stark D, Craft AW. Received dose and dose-intensity of chemotherapy and outcome in nonmetastatic extremity osteosarcoma. European Osteosarcoma Intergroup. *J Clin Oncol.*. 2000;18:4028-4037.
13. Ornadel D, Souhami RL, Whelan J, et al. Doxorubicin and cisplatin with granulocyte colony-stimulating factor as adjuvant chemotherapy for osteosarcoma: phase II trial of the European Osteosarcoma Intergroup. *J Clin Oncol.*. 1994;12:1842-1848.
14. Lewis IJ, Nooij MA, Whelan J, et al. Improvement in histologic response but not survival in osteosarcoma patients treated with intensified chemotherapy: a randomised Phase III trial of the European Osteosarcoma Intergroup. *JNCI*. 2007;99:112-128.

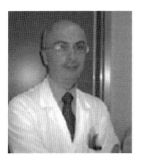

The Treatment of Nonmetastatic High Grade Osteosarcoma of the Extremity: Review of the Italian Rizzoli Experience. Impact on the Future

Stefano Ferrari, Emanuela Palmerini, Eric L. Staals, Mario Mercuri, Bertoni Franco, Piero Picci, and Gaetano Bacci

Abstract The Bone Tumor Center of the "Istituto Ortopedico Rizzoli" was established in 1955 with the aim of studying and treating the musculoskeletal tumors. Between 1959 and 2006, 1245 patients with high grade nonmetastatic osteosarcoma of the extremity were treated at our Institute. Most of them were enrolled in study protocols.

In the "prechemotherapy era", the cure rate was 11%, with an amputation rate of 90%. Our first experience with adjuvant chemotherapy was in 1972. A total of 223 patients received adjuvant chemotherapy, with a disease-free survival (DFS) ranging from 45% to 53%, according to the chemotherapy protocol used. With the introduction of neoadjuvant chemotherapy, the resection rate increased and reached 94%, when high dose fosfamide was added to standard doses of methotrexate, cisplatin, and adriamycin.

In the last few years, the results of treatment of nonmetastatic osteosarcoma of the extremity have reached a plateau (64% five-year DFS), and strategies of dose intensification are not able to improve the prognosis. Not only new active drugs, but also different approaches to the disease, are needed.

In this regard, we are now investigating tumor microenvironment-targeted agents and chemotherapy protocols based on prospective biological stratification of patients.

Collaborative projects with international groups and institutions are crucial for this rare disease.

Introduction

The Bone Tumor Center was established at the "Istituto Ortopedico Rizzoli" in Bologna in 1955 by Professor Italo Federico Goidanich. Since then, our Institute has been particularly devoted to the treatment and study of musculoskeletal tumors.

S. Ferrari (✉)
Sezione di Chemioterapia, dei Tumori dell' Apparato Locomotore, Istituto Ortopedico Rizzoli, via Pupilli 1, Bologna, 40136, Italy
e-mail: stefano.ferrari@ior.it

Osteosarcoma is one of the most common primary bone tumors and between 1959 and 2006, 1.245 patients with nonmetastatic osteosarcoma of the extremity were diagnosed and treated at our Institute.

In the present review, starting from the historical approach to the disease, our clinical experience, the current standard of treatment, and the future perspectives of osteosarcoma care will be reported.

Prechemotherapy Era

Patients Treated Only with Surgery

In the prechemotherapy era, surgery alone was the standard approach to osteosarcoma. Between 1959 and 1970, 127 patients with nonmetastatic osteosarcoma of the extremity were treated only by surgery, at our Institute; the majority were amputated, with a cure rate of 11%.[1] The percentage of cure was 14% in a group of 70 patients who refused chemotherapy and were treated only by surgery, in a more recent period, from 1971 to 1998 (unpublished data). In a series of 160 patients treated at the M.D. Anderson Cancer Center between 1956 and 1968, the cure rate was 13%,[2] and similar results were reported at the Memorial Sloan-Kettering Cancer Center: 14% cure rate in 145 patients treated between 1949 and 1965.[3] More recently, a retrospective analysis conducted at the Mayo Clinic has been published: the percentage of long-term survivors of osteosarcoma treated in the prechemotherapy era was 17.8%.[4]

Amputation According to the Cade Method

Another approach to the local treatment of osteosarcoma was the Cade method.[5] The patients were not immediately operated, but initially underwent radiotherapy at very high doses (10.000 rad). If no metastases developed during the following 6 months, the patients underwent amputation. The rationale of the method was to avoid amputation in patients with a short life expectancy. At the Rizzoli Institute, 16 patients were treated according to the Cade method in the 1970s. Metastases developed after 6 months in 10 out of the 16 patients, but an amputation was necessary anyway in 8 of these 10 metastatic patients for the severe and painful local sequelae of high dose radiotherapy.

Prophylactic Irradiation of Lungs

In 1971, 6 patients were treated with prophylactic irradiation of lungs in addition to amputation.[1] The rationale for this strategy was based on a hypothetical effect of

The Treatment of Nonmetastatic High Grade Osteosarcoma of the Extremity 277

radiation therapy on micrometastases. The method was proposed by Jenkin et al. in the early 1970s.[6] In our Institute, in order to decrease the risk of severe respiratory complications associated with bilateral lung irradiation, only the right lung was treated at a dose of 1,5 Gy. In all the 6 patients treated, metastases appeared in the irradiated lung very early (from 2 to 5 months).[1]

Immunotherapy with Autologous Vaccine

Beginning from 1971, 16 patients who underwent surgery (amputation in 13 cases and limb salvage in 3) for nonmetastatic osteosarcoma of the extremity were also treated with an autologous vaccine. The vaccine was obtained from resected tumor cells, previously irradiated with 12.000 rad.[1] Only 2 of the 16 patients survived, 13 patients died of metastases and one, surgically treated with a limb-salvage resection, had a local recurrence after 8 years. The patient refused an amputation and died of disease 10 months later. The cure rate was 12%, not different from the cure rate achieved by surgery alone. However, it is interesting to notice that the mean time to relapse was 16 months, and the mean survival was 26 months. In the same period, patients managed with surgery alone showed a mean time to recurrence of 8 months and a mean survival of 16 months.[1] A similar experience was reported at the Memorial Sloan-Kettering Cancer Center.[7] No further research in this field was pursued at our Institute, but the results seem to suggest a relation between immunomodulation and metastatic behavior in osteosarcoma.

Chemotherapy Era

Adjuvant Chemotherapy

In the early 1970s, the use of chemotherapy drastically changed the prognosis and the treatment strategy for osteosarcoma. The first reports on the efficacy of chemotherapy were mainly based on the use of methotrexate and doxorubicin.[8,9]

The first osteosarcoma patient to receive chemotherapy at the Rizzoli Institute was admitted in 1972. Chemotherapy was given after surgery as adjuvant treatment. Since then, 223 patients with nonmetastatic osteosarcoma of the extremity have been treated with surgery and adjuvant chemotherapy according to 4 different protocols. 117 patients received treatment based on methotrexate, vincristine and doxorubicin from 1972 to 1978, and the probability of 5-year DFS was 45%.[1] The percentage of limb-salvage was very low, with about 90% of patients undergoing amputation.[1] In the subsequent years (1979–1983), 106 patients with nonmetastatic osteosarcoma of the extremity were enrolled in a randomized study comparing different doses of methotrexate (200 mg/m^2 vs. 2 g/m^2) added to doxorubicin and vincristine.[10] The DFS at 5 years was 53% and no differences were found according to the dose of methotrexate.[10] The resection rate was 22%. The higher rate of limb-salvage reflected an increased expertise and confidence acquired by our orthopedic surgeons. Furthermore, a more accurate staging and surgical treatment planning was possible thanks to the use of modern radiological techniques.

Neoadjuvant Chemotherapy

A further step in the treatment of osteosarcoma was the primary use of chemotherapy. New challenges emerged due to improved prognosis after chemotherapy introduction. The increased percentage of long term survivors called attention to patients' quality of life. In an attempt to reduce the rate of amputation and, at the same time, to start immediately with an effective systemic treatment against the disease, a chemotherapy protocol based on primary chemotherapy was activated at the Rizzoli Institute in 1983.[11] Exciting data on this topic had already been reported by the end of the 1970s by Rosen et al.[12,13] From 1983 to 1986, the first neo-adjuvant study at the Rizzoli Institute recruited 127 patients who were further randomized to receive either a moderate (750 mg/m^2) or high (7.5 g/m^2) dose of methotrexate added to cisplatin, doxorubicin and bleomycin, cyclophosphamide and dactinomycin. In the primary phase, cisplatin was intra-arterially delivered. The updated results of the study were reported in 1997.[14] The 12-year DFS was 46% (high dose methotrexate 52%, moderate dose 38%) (Fig. 1), and the multivariate analysis performed showed a significant advantage for patients treated with high dose methotrexate. These results strongly supported the use of methotrexate in osteosarcoma and also indicated a relation between the dose of methotrexate and its efficacy. In terms of survival, the data were not different from those achieved with adjuvant chemotherapy, but the increase of the resection rate was impressive, reaching 72%. In this study, the predictive significance of the histological response to the primary chemotherapy was clearly shown, supporting evidences previously reported by Rosen.[13]

A subsequent study was carried out at the Rizzoli Institute from 1986 to 1989.[15] The endpoints were to increase the percentage of patients with a good histologic response ($\geq$90% chemotherapy-induced tumor necrosis) to primary chemotherapy and to improve the prognosis of poor responder patients.

In the primary phase, doxorubicin was added to methotrexate and intra-arterially delivered cisplatin. In the adjuvant treatment, poor responder patients (<90% chemotherapy-induced tumor necrosis) were given ifosfamide in addition to methotrexate, cisplatin and doxorubicin. This second neo-adjuvant study (IOR/OS-2) recruited 164 patients. The rate of good histologic response was 71%, and the percentage of patients treated with limb-salvage surgery was 84%. The 5-year DFS was 65% and the 5-year overall survival (OS) was 74% (Fig. 2). According to the histological response, good responder patients had a 5-year DFS of 67%, whereas the poor responder patients obtained a 5-year DFS of 51% ($p=0.08$).[15]

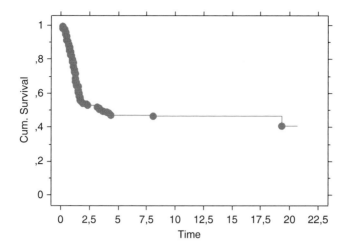

Fig. 1 Result of IOR/OS-1 neoadjuvant chemotherapy protocol: 127 patients treated with methotrexate cisplatin doxorubicin, bleomycin, dactinomycin and cyclophosphamide. 12-year DFS: 46%[14]

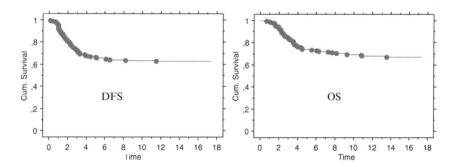

Fig 2 Result of IOR/OS-2 neoadjuvant chemotherapy protocol: 164 patients treated with doxorubicin, methotrexate and intra-arterially delivered cisplatin+ifosfamide in poor responders. 5-year DFS: 65%; 5-year OS: 74%[15]

The same strategy of treatment, three drugs preoperatively and addition of ifosfamide in poor responder patients, was adopted in the third neo-adjuvant study, performed to investigate the role of the infusion route of cisplatin.[16] In 1990 and 1991, 95 patients were randomly assigned to receive intra-arterial or intravenous cisplatin preoperatively. The results obtained showed a significantly ($p=0.05$) higher percentage of good responders (≥90% chemotherapy-induced tumor necrosis) in patients treated with intra-arterial cisplatin (64%), compared with those who received intravenous cisplatin (43%). However, the infusion route did not significantly affect the outcome.[16] It is interesting to note that similar results were reported by the COSS group in the same period.[17]

In the following years, two studies were carried out at the Rizzoli Institute.[18,19] In the last one (1993–1995) 133 patients received ifosfamide, together with methotrexate, cisplatin and doxorubicin, after the primary phase.[19] The resection rate reached 94%, but none of these protocols was able to improve the outcome achieved in the IOR/OS-2 study.

In 1997, the Rizzoli Institute established the Italian Sarcoma Group (ISG), in order to promote a large Italian cooperation for the treatment of sarcoma patients. All the Italian Institutions involved in the treatment of patients with sarcoma joined this cooperative group. The first ISG protocol was carried out in collaboration with the Scandinavian Sarcoma Group (ISG/SSG I). The chemotherapy strategy was essentially based on a treatment intensification with the use of high dose ifosfamide (15 g/m^2) added to methotrexate, cisplatin and doxorubicin in the preoperative phase. Due to the planned intensity of the chemotherapy treatment, the protocol was preceded by a study performed at our Institute to evaluate its feasibility.[20] ISG/SSG I recruited 182 patients from 1997 to 2000 and obtained a 5-year DFS of 64%[21] (Fig. 3). Once again, the DFS achieved was not better than that of the IOR/OS-2 neo-adjuvant study. However, the percentage of patients undergoing limb-salvage surgery was remarkable: 94%, the highest percentage ever reported in a multicentric study for nonmetastatic osteosarcoma of the extremity.

The failure of the dose intensification strategy and the lack of new active agents were the starting points for the subsequent study of the Italian Sarcoma Group. The evaluation of chemotherapy toxicity and quality of life in patients with osteosarcoma were the main objectives of ISG/OS-1.[22] In this randomized study, the drugs and cumulative doses were the same in each arm, but they were delivered according to different schedules. This study was activated in June 2001 and closed in December

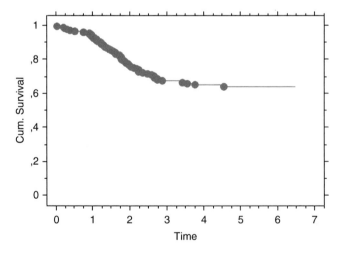

Fig 3 Result of ISG/SSG-1 neoadjuvant chemotherapy protocol: 182 patients treated with doxorubicin, methotrexate and high dose Ifosfamide. 5-year DFS: 64%[21]

Prognostic Factors

The tumor, the patient and the treatment-related factors influencing the prognosis were evaluated in our patients. A first analysis was conducted on 300 patients treated according to the same chemotherapy strategy: methotrexate, cisplatin and doxorubicin preoperatively, with ifosfamide added postoperatively in poor responder patients.[23] After multivariate analysis, tumor volume >150 mL, age <13 years and osteoblastic and chondroblastic histologic subtypes were found to be factors significantly affecting the prognosis. Interestingly, the histological response, which was statistically significant at the univariate analysis, lost its value after the multivariate analysis. This suggests that the use of ifosfamide is effective as "salvage chemotherapy" in patients who are poor responders to methotrexate, cisplatin and doxorubicin.

In a larger and more recent retrospective study including 789 patients (300 of them from the previous analysis), age and tumor volume as well as the serum alkaline phosphatase level, the adequacy of surgical margins and the histological response were factors significantly influencing the prognosis.[24] Data reported in Table 1

The retrospective analysis of prognostic factors in nonmetastatic osteosarcoma is useful for the clinical practice. However, risk-adapted chemotherapy protocols have never been designed so far.

A better understanding of the biological characteristics of osteosarcoma has been reached in more recent years. Our research group focused on the role of P-glycoprotein overexpression in osteosarcoma.[25–27] In our experience, the overexpression of P-glycoprotein can be considered an important prognostic factor.

Table 1 Multivariate analysis on 789 patients with nonmetastatic osteosarcoma patients of the extremity; Cox regression with iterative Wald model[24]

Variable		Relative risk	p
Serum alkaline phosphatase	Normal	1	<0.0005
	High	2.31	
Volume	≤200 ml	1	<0.004
	>200 ml	1.26	
Chemotherapy	Neoadjuvant	1	<0.0005
	Adjuvant	1.66	
Histologic response	Good	1	<0.0005
	Poor	1.87	
Surgical margins	Adequate	1	<0.024
	Inadequate	1.34	

Multivariate analysis on 789 patients with nonmetastatic osteosarcoma patients of the extremity; Cox regression with iterative Wald model[24]

However, there is no general consensus on this topic, since conflicting data have been reported.[28-31] Nonetheless, in a Rizzoli study evaluating the expression of P-glycoprotein, ErbB2, p53 and Bcl-2 in patients who developed lung metastases, the expression of P-glycoprotein in lung metastases was higher than that observed in the corresponding primary tumors.[31] The role of P-glycoprotein overexpression in osteosarcoma, not only as a marker of chemo-resistance to doxorubicin, but also as a prognostic factor is shown in a retrospective analysis of the ISG/SSG I study.[32] In fact, in the population treated according to the protocol ISG/SSG I, mainly characterized by the use of high dose Ifosfamide, the 5-year event free survival (EFS) was 47% in patients showing overexpression of P-glycoprotein and 82.5% in those without P-glycoprotein overexpression.[32] These data, added to similar data obtained in 186 patients previously reported,[25-27] confirm that the P-glycoprotein status influences the prognosis of osteosarcoma patients and could be used for a biologic stratification of patients in future chemotherapy protocols.

Postrelapse Survival

All the patients treated at our Institute are followed up in our outpatient clinic for both orthopedic and oncologic aspects. Over the years, the patients have been followed according to different schedules and modalities. In the last 15 years, for patients with nonmetastatic osteosarcoma of the extremity, follow-up visits were performed every 3 months in the first 3 years, every 4 months in the fourth and fifth year, and every 6 months subsequently. The oncologic follow-up is based on a chest computed tomography and X-rays of the involved limb. The late effects of chemotherapy are assessed by means of routinely performed blood tests, echocardiograms, and audiograms.

Tumor recurrence is an adverse event, but it can be successfully managed, at least in selected patients. In our experience, the 5-year postrelapse survival (PRS) is 28%.[33] In case of complete surgical remission, the PRS is 39%, whereas for those who can not reach a complete surgical remission, the survival at 3 years drops to 0%. Several factors can influence the PRS: the relapse-free interval (RFI) (better survival in case of RFI longer than 24 months), the site of relapse (better survival in case of lung metastases vs. nonpulmonary metastases), and the number of lung metastases (better survival in case of 1 or 2 lung metastases). In our experience, the addition of a second line chemotherapy treatment (mainly high dose ifosfamide) in surgically free patients did not influence the survival. On the contrary, patients with unresectable recurrence benefit from a second-line chemotherapy. The strategy of dose-intensification was also pursued in relapsed patients . A high-dose chemotherapy study in relapsed osteosarcoma patients was carried out by the Italian Sarcoma Group at the end of 1990s.[34] The chemotherapy consisted of high dose carboplatin and etoposide followed by stem-cell rescue. The study recruited 32 relapsed osteosarcoma patients. One patient died of transplantation-related adverse effects, and the 3-year survival rate was 20%. After this experience, the use of high dose chemotherapy with stem cells support in relapsed osteosarcoma was abandoned by our group.

A specific issue is represented by the local recurrence. In our experience, the overall incidence of local recurrence is 5.4%.[35] It is interesting to note that in patients treated with immediate surgery and adjuvant chemotherapy, the incidence of local recurrence was 33% in case of resection, and 4.9% in case of amputation.[1] In resected patients treated from 1983 to 1999 with neoadjuvant chemotherapy, the incidence of local recurrence was 6% [36] and 4% in more recent experience.[21] The median time to local recurrence is 2.3 years, but it is important to stress that local recurrence can develop very late (up to 17 years in our experience). This fact, together with the evidence of very late recurrence in osteosarcoma,[37] recommends a prolonged follow-up of osteosarcoma patients.

Patients with local recurrence have a very poor prognosis: the 5-year post local relapse survival in our series is only 16%. The main factor influencing local control is the adequacy of the surgical margins, but the chemotherapy-induced tumor necrosis also plays an important role.[35]

Late Effects

The late effects of chemotherapy are carefully monitored in our patients by means of a strict and centralized follow-up.

Hearing loss, as evaluated by audiograms, was detected in about 40% of our patients after a cumulative cisplatin dose of 600 mg/m^2. Nevertheless, the hearing loss mainly involves the high frequencies without significant clinical impairment.[21] The incidence of clinically evident cardiomyopathy in our population was 1.7%, and it was related to the cumulative doxorubicin dose.[38] As expected, a higher incidence of renal toxicity was reported in patients who received high dose ifosfamide added to methotrexate and cisplatin, and chronic renal tubular toxicity was reported mainly in pediatric patients.[39]

The fertility in male and female patients was also evaluated. In female patients, the reproductive function and their newborns' health were not affected by the chemotherapy received.[40] On the contrary, the incidence of infertility was high in male patients and was related to the cumulative dose of ifosfamide.[41]

Twenty-six patients developed a second malignant neoplasm from 1 to 25 years (median 8 years) after the start of treatment.[42] Of these patients, only two had a family history of cancer. Two patients had a third tumor. The second malignancies were: leukemia in ten patients (nine cases of AML and one of ALL); breast cancer in 7; lung cancer in 2; renal cancer in 2; CNS tumors in 2; and soft tissue sarcoma, parotidis cancer and colon cancer in one patient each. The risk to develop a second neoplasm was 1.5% at 5 years, 4.2% at 10 years and 4.5% at 15 years. In comparison with the normal population, the cumulative risk at 10 years to develop a second malignancy was 1.8 times higher for solid tumors and 4.5 times higher for leukemia. It is important to underline that only a few patients received etoposide (the poor responder patients of our second neo-adjuvant study), and none of them developed leukemia. The rate of second tumor was significantly higher in females than in males ($p < 0.02$), and the time to second malignancy was significantly shorter in hematologic than in solid tumor (2.5 year vs. 9.4 years, $p < 0.01$). No second malignancies were seen in 176 patients aged 10 or younger at the time of chemotherapy.[42]

Future Directions

The results of the treatment of nonmetastatic osteosarcoma of the extremity have reached a plateau. With the use of the classic four drugs (methotrexate, cisplatin, doxorubicin and ifosfamide), a 5-year DFS of 65% can be expected. Strategy of dose intensification, even based on high dose treatment and stem-cell rescue, are not able to improve the prognosis.

We certainly need new active drugs, but at the same time, different approaches to the disease have to be planned.

In this regard, we are now investigating the possibility to modify the tumor microenvironment in order to increase the chemosensitivity of tumor cells. Researchers from the Istituto Superiore di Sanità (Rome, Italy) reported that proton pump inhibitor pretreatment can decrease the resistance of solid tumor to cytotoxic drugs.[43] A study, sponsored by the Italian agency for drugs (AIFA) (http://oss-sper-clin. agenziafarmaco.it/) and using a proton pump inhibitor pretreatment as chemosentitizer during primary chemotherapy for nonmetastatic osteosarcoma, is ongoing.

The new chemotherapy protocol for nonmetastatic osteosarcoma of the extremity will be characterized by a biologic stratification based on the P-glycoprotein expression. Patients who do not overexpress P-glycoprotein will receive the standard chemotherapy with the classic three drug combination (methotrexate, cisplatin, doxorubicin) in the primary phase and "standard dose" ifosfamide in poor responder patients. At least 75% probability of a 5-year EFS is expected in this group. A more aggressive chemotherapy treatment, mainly characterized by the use of "high dose" ifosfamide, is planned for patients who overexpress P-glycoprotein.

A final remark on a key factor for modern clinical research has to be addressed. National and international cooperation are pivotal for the development of our knowledge, especially in the field of rare diseases such as sarcomas. In recent years, the Rizzoli Institute has intensified collaborative projects with international institutions. Interesting studies on new drugs are ongoing or are being activated with Sarcoma Alliance for Research through Collaboration (SARC) (www.sarctrials. org/public/pag1.aspx) or Innovative Therapy for Children with Cancer (ITCC) consortium (http://www.itcc-consortium.org/index). A nonrandomized prospective intergroup study for patients older than 40 years with high grade osteosarcoma or other spindle cell sarcomas (EURO.B.O.S.S European bone over 40 sarcoma study) is ongoing. This study is being carried out with the cooperation of the Italian Sarcoma Group, the Cooperative Osteosarcoma Study Group (COSS) and the Scandinavian Sarcoma Group (SSG).

Conclusions

The vast majority of patients with nonmetastatic osteosarcoma of the extremity can undergo conservative surgical procedures with a low (<5%) incidence of local recurrence and good functional results, when treated in experienced centers.

With the use of the classic four drugs (methotrexate, cisplatin, doxorubicin and ifosfamide), a 5-year DFS of 65% can be expected. Strategy of dose intensification, even based on high dose treatment and stem-cell rescue, are not able to improve the prognosis. The outcome of patients with nonmetastatic osteosarcoma of the extremity has reached a plateau: new drugs and innovative approaches to the disease are needed.

The centralization of patients in experienced centers and the development of international cooperation projects are key factors in the management and study of these rare diseases.

References

1. Campanacci M, Bacci G, Bertoni F, Picci P, Minutillo A, Franceschi C. The treatment of osteosarcoma of the extremities: twenty years experience at the Istituto Ortopedico Rizzoli. *Cancer.* 1981;48:533-542.
2. Uribe-Botero G, Russel WO, Sutow WW, Martin RG. Primary osteosarcoma of bone: clinicopathological investigation of 243 cases, with necroscopy studies in 54. *Am J Clin Pathol.* 1977;67:427-435.
3. Marcove RC, Mike V, Hajek JV, Levin AG, Hutter RV. Osteogenic sarcoma below the age of twenty-one. A review of one hundred and forty five cases. *J Bone Joint Surg Am.* 1970;52:411-423.
4. Gaffney R, Unni KK, Sim FH, Slezak JM, Esther RJ, Bolander ME. Follow-up study of long-term survivors of osteosarcoma in the prechemotherapy era. *Hum Pathol.* 2006;37:1009-1014.
5. Cade S. Osteogenic sarcoma: a study based on 133 patients. *J R Coll Surg Edinb.* 1955;1:79-111.
6. Jenkin RD, Allt WE, Fitzpatrick PJ. Osteosarcoma. An assessment of management with particular reference to primary irradiation and selective delayed amputation. *Cancer.* 1972;30:393-400.
7. Marcove RC, Miké V, Huvos AG, Southam CM, Levin AG. Vaccine trials for osteogenic sarcoma. A preliminary report. *CA Cancer J Clin.* 1973;23:74-80.
8. Jaffe N. Recent advances in the chemotherapy of metastatic osteogenic sarcoma. *Cancer.* 1972;30:1627-1631.
9. Cortes EP, Holland JF, Wang JJ, et al. Doxorubicin in disseminated osteosarcoma. *JAMA.* 1972;221:1132-1138.
10. Bacci G, Gherlinzoni F, Picci P, et al. Adriamycin-methotrexate high dose versus adriamycin-methotrexate moderate dose as adjuvant chemotherapy for osteosarcoma of the extremities: a randomized study. *Eur J Cancer Clin Oncol.* 1986;22:1337-1345.
11. Bacci G, Picci P, Ruggieri P, et al. Primary chemotherapy and delayed surgery (neoadjuvant chemotherapy) for osteosarcoma of the extremities. The Istituto Rizzoli Experience in 127 patients treated preoperatively with intravenous methotrexate (high versus moderate doses) and intraarterial cisplatin. *Cancer.* 1990;65:2539-2553.

12. Rosen G, Marcove RC, Caparros B, Nirenberg A, Kosloff C, Huvos AG. Primary osteogenic sarcoma: the rationale for preoperative chemotherapy and delayed surgery. *Cancer*. 1979;43:2163-2177.
13. Rosen G, Caparros B, Huvos AG, et al. Preoperative chemotherapy for osteogenic sarcoma: selection of postoperative adjuvant chemotherapy based on the response of the primary tumor to preoperative chemotherapy. *Cancer*. 1982;49:1221-1230.
14. Ferrari S, Bacci G, Picci P, et al. Long-term follow-up and post-relapse survival in patients with non-metastatic osteosarcoma of the extremity treated with neoadjuvant chemotherapy. *Ann Oncol*. 1997;8:765-771.
15. Bacci G, Ferrari S, Bertoni F, et al. Long-term outcome for patients with nonmetastatic osteosarcoma of the extremity treated at the istituto ortopedico rizzoli according to the istituto ortopedico rizzoli/osteosarcoma-2 protocol: an updated report. *J Clin Oncol*. 2000;18:4016-4027.
16. Ferrari S, Mercuri M, Picci P, et al. Nonmetastatic osteosarcoma of the extremity: results of a neoadjuvant chemotherapy protocol (IOR/OS-3) with high-dose methotrexate, intra-arterial or intravenous cisplatin, doxorubicin, and salvage chemotherapy based on histologic tumor response. *Tumori*. 1999;85:458-464.
17. Winkler K, Bielack S, Delling G, et al. Effect of intra-arterial versus intravenous cisplatin in addition to systemic doxorubicin, high-dose methotrexate, and ifosfamide on histologic tumor response in osteosarcoma (study COSS-86). *Cancer*. 1990;66:1703-1710.
18. Bacci G, Ferrari S, Longhi A, et al. Neoadjuvant chemotherapy for high grade osteosarcoma of the extremities: long-term results for patients treated according to the Rizzoli IOR/OS-3b protocol. *J Chemother*. 2001;13:93-99.
19. Bacci G, Briccoli A, Ferrari S, et al. Neoadjuvant chemotherapy for osteosarcoma of the extremity: long-term results of the Rizzoli's 4th protocol. *Eur J Cancer*. 2001;37:2030-2039.
20. Bacci G, Ferrari S, Longhi A, et al. Italian Sarcoma Group/Scandinavian Sarcoma Group. High dose ifosfamide in combination with high dose methotrexate, adriamycin and cisplatin in the neoadjuvant treatment of extremity osteosarcoma: preliminary results of an Italian Sarcoma Group/Scandinavian Sarcoma Group pilot study. *J Chemother*. 2002;14:198-206.
21. Ferrari S, Smeland S, Mercuri M, et al. Italian and Scandinavian Sarcoma Groups. Neoadjuvant chemotherapy with high-dose Ifosfamide, high-dose methotrexate, cisplatin, and doxorubicin for patients with localized osteosarcoma of the extremity: a joint study by the Italian and Scandinavian Sarcoma Groups. *J Clin Oncol*. 2005;23:8845-8852.
22. ISG/OS-1 Protocol at: www.controlled-trials.com/ISRCTN21335128.
23. Ferrari S, Bertoni F, Mercuri M, et al. Predictive factors of disease-free survival for non-metastatic osteosarcoma of the extremity: an analysis of 300 patients treated at the Rizzoli Institute. *Ann Oncol*. 2001;12:1145-1150.
24. Bacci G, Longhi A, Versari M, Mercuri M, Briccoli A, Picci P. Prognostic factors for osteosarcoma of the extremity treated with neoadjuvant chemotherapy: 15-year experience in 789 patients treated at a single institution. *Cancer*. 2006;106:1154-1161.
25. Baldini N, Scotlandi K, Barbanti-Bròdano G, et al. Expression of P-glycoprotein in high-grade osteosarcomas in relation to clinical outcome. *N Engl J Med*. 1995;333:1380-1385.
26. Baldini N, Scotlandi K, Serra M, et al. P-glycoprotein expression in osteosarcoma: a basis for risk-adapted adjuvant chemotherapy. *J Orthop Res*. 1999;17:629-632.
27. Serra M, Scotlandi K, Reverter-Branchat G, et al. Value of P-glycoprotein and clinicopathologic factors as the basis for new treatment strategies in high-grade osteosarcoma of the extremities. *J Clin Oncol*. 2003;21:536-542.
28. Gorlick R, Huvos AG, Heller G, et al. Expression of HER2/erbB-2 correlates with survival in osteosarcoma. *J Clin Oncol*. 1999;17:2781-2788.
29. Schwartz CL, Gorlick R, Teot L, et al. Children's Oncology Group. Multiple drug resistance in osteogenic sarcoma: INT0133 from the Children's Oncology Group. *J Clin Oncol*. 2007;25:2057-2062.
30. Serra M, Picci P, Ferrari S, Bacci G. Prognostic value of P-glycoprotein in high-grade osteosarcoma. Comment on: *J Clin Oncol*. 2007;25:2057-2062.

The Treatment of Nonmetastatic High Grade Osteosarcoma of the Extremity

31. Ferrari S, Bertoni F, Zanella L, et al. Evaluation of P-glycoprotein, HER-2/ErbB-2, p53, and Bcl-2 in primary tumor and metachronous lung metastases in patients with high-grade osteosarcoma. *Cancer*. 2004;100:1936-1942.
32. Serra M, Pasello M, Manara MC, et al. Can P-glycoprotein status be used to stratify high-grade osteosarcoma patients? Results from the Italian/Scandinavian Sarcoma Group 1 treatment protocol. *Int J Oncol*. 2006;29:1459-1468.
33. Ferrari S, Briccoli A, Mercuri M, et al. Postrelapse survival in osteosarcoma of the extremities: prognostic factors for long-term survival. *J Clin Oncol*. 2003;21:710-715.
34. Fagioli F, Aglietta M, Tienghi A, et al. High-dose chemotherapy in the treatment of relapsed osteosarcoma: an Italian sarcoma group study. *J Clin Oncol*. 2002;20:2150-2156.
35. Bacci G, Forni C, Longhi A, et al. Local recurrence and local control of non-metastatic osteosarcoma of the extremities: a 27-year experience in a single institution. *J Surg Oncol*. 2007;96:118-123.
36. Bacci G, Briccoli A, Ferrari S, et al. Neoadjuvant chemotherapy for osteosarcoma of the extremity: long-term results of the Rizzoli's 4th protocol. *Eur J Cancer*. 2001;37:2030–2039.
37. Ferrari S, Briccoli A, Mercuri M, et al. Late relapse in osteosarcoma. *J Pediatr Hematol Oncol*. 2006;28:418-422.
38. Longhi A, Ferrari S, Bacci G, Specchia S. Long-term follow-up of patients with doxorubicin-induced cardiac toxicity after chemotherapy for osteosarcoma. *Anticancer Drugs*. 2007;18:737-744.
39. Ferrari S, Pieretti F, Verri E, et al. Prospective evaluation of renal function in pediatric and adult patients treated with high-dose ifosfamide, cisplatin and high-dose methotrexate. *Anticancer Drugs*. 2005;16:733-738.
40. Longhi A, Porcu E, Petracchi S, Versari M, Conticini L, Bacci G. Reproductive functions in female patients treated with adjuvant and neoadjuvant chemotherapy for localized osteosarcoma of the extremity. *Cancer*. 2000;89:1961-1965.
41. Longhi A, Macchiagodena M, Vitali G, Bacci G. Fertility in male patients treated with neoadjuvant chemotherapy for osteosarcoma. *J Pediatr Hematol Oncol*. 2003;25:292-296.
42. Bacci G, Ferrari C, Longhi A, et al. Second malignant neoplasm in patients with osteosarcoma of the extremities treated with adjuvant and neoadjuvant chemotherapy. *J Pediatr Hematol Oncol*. 2006;28:774-780.
43. Luciani F, Spada M, De Milito A, et al. Effect of proton pump inhibitor pre-treatment for resistance of solid tumor to cytotoxic drugs. *J Natl Cancer Inst*. 2004;96:1702-1713.

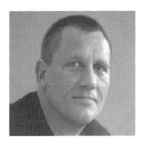

Osteosarcoma: The COSS Experience

Stefan Bielack, Herbert Jürgens, Gernot Jundt,
Matthias Kevric, Thomas Kühne, Peter Reichardt,
Andreas Zoubek, Mathias Werner, Winfried
Winkelmann, and Rainer Kotz

Abstract COSS, the interdisciplinary Cooperative German–Austrian–Swiss Osteosarcoma Study Group, was founded in 1977 and has since registered some 3,500 bone sarcoma patients from over 200 institutions. For the purpose of the Pediatric and Adolescent Osteosarcoma Conference in Houston, March 2008, the outcomes of 2,464 consecutive patients with high-grade central osteosarcoma, who had been diagnosed between 1980 and 2005 and had been treated on neoadjuvant COSS protocols, were reviewed. Intended treatment had included surgery and multidrug chemotherapy, with high-dose methotrexate, doxorubicin, cisplatin, and ifosfamide being used in most protocols. After a median follow-up of 7.31 years for 1,654 survivors, 5- and 10-year survival estimates were 0.748/0.695 for 2,017 patients with localized extremity tumors and 0.369/0.317 for 444 patients with axial tumors or/and primary metastases, respectively. Tumor response to preoperative chemotherapy was of independent prognostic significance. Over the years, there was a major shift from amputation towards limb-salvage. This development was least evident for patients below the age of 10. While survival expectancies improved from the first to the second half of the recruitment period, no further improvement was evident within the latter period. In the manuscript, the results described above are discussed based on the findings of the previous analyses of our group.

Introduction

The Cooperative Osteosarcoma Study Group COSS

COSS, the Cooperative Osteosarcoma Study Group, was founded in 1977 as an interdisciplinary, collaborative, German-language group with members from all specialties involved in the treatment of osteosarcoma and related bone tumors

---

S. Bielack (✉)
Klinikum Stuttgart, Zentrum für Kinder- und Jugendmedizin - Olgahospital, Pädiatrie 5 (Onkologie, Hämatologie,Immunologie), Bismarckstr. 8, D-70176, Stuttgart, Germany
e-mail: coss@olgahospital-stuttgart.de

(founding chairman: Kurt Winkler, Hamburg, Germany).[1] Over the past 30 years, COSS has recruited some 3,500 bone sarcoma patients from over 200 institutions, mainly from Germany, Austria, and Switzerland.[1-13] According to German Pediatric Cancer Registry data, COSS has reliably recruited almost 100% of all German pediatric osteosarcoma patients for many years.[14]

Registration Policy

The COSS-registration policy may be unique among multicentric groups: Registration has never been restricted to patients recruited into prospective, randomized trials (usually young patients with localized extremity osteosarcoma), but the group has always tried to also include all other patients with conventional osteosarcoma, its variants, and biologically related bone tumors, such as malignant fibrous histiocytoma of bone or leiomyosarcoma of bone, into its database. For some of these, treatment guidelines are given in appendices of the COSS-Protocols; for others, the COSS-Center is available for guidance. Follow-up is intended to be indefinite for all patients. This policy has allowed COSS to build one of the largest bone tumor databases worldwide, making it possible to address questions regarding various aspects of presentation and treatment, with reasonably large patient numbers even when evaluating relatively uncommon situations.

Aims

From the very beginning, COSS has pursued two aims: The first was and is to advance the knowledge about the optimal treatment of osteosarcoma by performing clinical trials. The second aim, no less important, is to build and maintain a population based, multicentric, multidisciplinary infrastructure for treatment of osteosarcoma and other biologically related bone sarcomas, guaranteeing that each and every patient can receive treatment according to current interdisciplinary standards. In the latter context, the COSS-Center acts as a referral institution to which participating institutions can address questions related to all aspects of systemic or local treatment, both during first-line therapy and in the relapse setting. The COSS-Center then coordinates the responses by expert panels from imaging, pathology, bone and thoracic surgery, radiotherapy, and pediatric and medical oncology.

Scope of this Paper

For the purpose of the Pediatric and Adolescent Osteosarcoma meeting, we aimed to give an overview of 25 years of multicentric, multidisciplinary collaboration within the COSS group, to describe the outcomes obtained during this period, and to put these results into perspective by reviewing the previously published experience of our group.

25 "Neoadjuvant COSS Years": Patients and Methods

Patients

For the "Pediatric & Adolescent Osteosarcoma" meeting, an analysis of all consecutive non-pretreated (except primary surgery) COSS patients from 1980–2004 in whom a diagnosis of high-grade central osteosarcoma of any region except craniofacial bones was made between the end of 1979 (start of the first neoadjuvant trial, COSS-80) and Dec. 31, 2004, was performed. Primary metastatic tumors were included. Tumors were only counted as primary metastatic if the metastases were proven by surgery or progression.

Treatment Strategy

Ever after a first trial, COSS-77, which was based on postoperative, adjuvant therapy only,[1] all COSS-regimens have included a uniform treatment concept of preoperative, neoadjuvant induction chemotherapy followed by surgery of the primary tumor and adjuvant chemotherapy. Procedures used to define the extension of the primary tumor, included conventional radiography in all studies, while other methods (CT, MRI) varied with time and availability. The minimum requirements for exclusion of primary metastases were a negative chest X-ray and a negative 99Tc-methylene diphosphonate bone scan. After 1991, computed tomography of the chest was also mandatory. During follow-up, radiograms of the chest and the primary tumor were to be repeated at regular intervals specified in the respective treatment protocols.[2–13] Based on the groundbreaking studies of Norman Jaffe,[15,16] all neoadjuvant COSS-protocols have included high-dose methotrexate at 12 g/m² per course with leucovorin rescue. In addition, doxorubicin at 60–90 mg/m² per course, cisplatin at 90–150 mg/m² per course, ifosfamide at 6–10 g/m² per course, carboplatin/etoposide, and/or BCD (bleomycin, cyclophosphamide, dactinomycin) were used in varying combinations. All protocols since 1986 were based on the four-drug concept of study COSS-86,[5,7] with slight variations (Table 1). The scheduled duration of chemotherapy ranged from 24–38 weeks. Definitive surgery was scheduled to take place between weeks 9 and 18, in study COSS-80 and between weeks 9 and 11, in all other protocols.[2–13] The type of surgery was not specified, but complete removal of the tumor with wide or radical surgical margins was always to be attempted. Response to preoperative chemotherapy was assessed histologically

Table 1a Chemotherapy in the neoadjuvant COSS trials 1980–2004

		Preoperative					Surgery	Postoperative				
	Recruitment	DOX mg/m²	MTX g/m²	DDP mg/m	IFO g/m²	Other	Response	DOX mg/m²	MTX g/m²	DDP mg/m	IFOg/m²	Other
(a)												
COSS-80	12/79–08/82	*bolus i.v.*1× (2×45)	*4 h i.v.* 4×12	*5 h i.v.* 1×120	–	–1×BCD	G/PG/P	*bolus i.v.*3× (2×45)	*4 h i.v.* 10×12	*5 h i.v.* 3×120	–	–3×BCD
DDP-Arm		1×(2×45)	4×12					3×(2×45)	10×12			
BCD-Arm												
COSS-82	08/82–11/84	*bolus i.v.*– 2×(2×30)	*4 h i.v.* 4×12	*40′ i.v.* 2×(90–120)	–	2×BCD–	GP	*bolus i.v.*– 6×(2×30)	*4 h i.v.* 4×12	*30′(40′) i.v.*– 6×(90–120)	*120 h i.v.*–	.2×BCD
BCD-Arm			4×12				G	2×(2×30)	4×12	2×(90–120)		–
DDP/DOX-Arm							P	–		3×(5×20)	3×10	3×BCD
COSS-86	02/86–11/88	*30′ i.v.*1× (2×45)	*4 h i.v.* 2×12	*1–5 h i.v.* f.i.a.	*1 h i.v.*– 2×(2×3)	–	GP	*30′ i.v.*3× (2×45)	*4 h i.v.* 10×12	*5 h i.v.* 2×120	*1 h i.v.*– 3×(2×3)	–
Low risk		1×(2×45)	2×12	2×120			G/P	4×(2×45)	12×12	3×120	3×(2×3)	–
High risk				2×(120–150)				4×(2×45)	12×12	3×120		
COSS-86B	12/88–11/90	*48 h i.v.* 1×90	*4 h i.v.* 2×12	*5 h i.v.* 2×120	*1 h i.v.*– 2×(2×3)	–	GP	*48 h i.v.* 3×90	*4 h i.v.* 10×12	*5 h i.v.* 2×120	*1 h i.v.*– (2–)3× (2×3)	–
Low risk		1×90	2×12	2×120			G/P	(3–)4×90	(10–)12×12	(2–)3×120	(2–)3× (2×3)	–
High risk								(3–)4×90	(10–)12×12	(2–)3×120	(2–)3× (2×3)	
COSS-91	12/90–4/92	*1 h i.v.*2× (2×30)	*4 h i.v.* 2×12	*5 h vs. 72 h i.v.* 2×120	*1 h i.v.*2 x(2×3)	–	G/P	*1/2 h i.v.*2× (2×30)	*4 h i.v.* 6×12	*5 h vs. 72 h i.v.* 2×120	*1 h i.v.*2× (2×3)	–
COSS-86C	05/92–6/96	*48 h i.v.*1 ×90	*4 h i.v.* .2×12	*5 h vs. 72 h i.v.* 2×120	*1 h i.v.*2 x(2×3)	–	G/P	*48 h i.v.* 3×90	*4 h i.v.* 8×12	*5 h vs. 72 h i.v.* 2×120	*1 h i.v.*2× (2×3)	–
COSS-96	06/96–12/02	*48 h i.v.*1 ×90	*4 h i.v.* 2×12	*72 h i.v.* 2×120	*1 h i.v.*2 x(2×3)	–	LRSR1	*48 h i.v.* 1×90	*4 h i.v.* 4×12	*72 h i.v.* 1×120	*1 h i.v.*1× (2×3)	–
							SR2	3×90	8×12	2×120	2×(2×3)	–
							HR	2×90	10×12	1×120	1×(2×3)	5×CE
								1×90	2×12	–		
COSS-Interim	01/03–04/05	*48 h i.v.*1 ×90	*4 h i.v.* 2×12	*72 h i.v.* 2×120	*1 h i.v.*2 x(2×3)	–	G/P	*48 h i.v.* 3×90	*4 h i.v.* 8×12	*72 h i.v.* 2×120	*1 h i.v.*2 x(2×3)	–

Table 1b Cumulative drug dosages in the neoadjuvant COSS trials 1980–2004

	Response	DOXmg/m²	MTXg/m²	DDP mg/m	IFO g/m²	CARBO mg/m²	VP16mg/m²	BLEO mg/m²	CYCg/m²	ACTO-Dmg/m
COSS-80	G/P	360	168	480	–	–	–	–	–	–
DDP-Arm BCD-Arm	G/P	360	168	–	–	–	–	96	48	3,6
COSS-82	G	–	96	–	–	–	–	120	48	4,8
BCD-Arm	P	240	48	540–	–	–	–	60	24	2,4
DDP/DOX-Arm	GP	240120	9648	720360–480480–540	–30	–	–	–90	–36	–3,6
COSS-86	G	360	144	480	–	–	–	–	–	–
Low risk	P	450	168	600	18	–	–	–	–	–
High risk	G/P	450	168	600	30	–	–	–	–	–
COSS-86B	GP	360360–450	144144–168	480480–600	–12–18	–	–	–	–	–
Low risk High risk	G/P	360–450	144–168	480–600	24–30	–	–	–	–	–
COSS-91	G/P	240	96	480	24	–	–	–	–	–
COSS-86C/ COSS-Interim	G/P	360	120	480	24	–	–	–	–	–
COSS-96	LR	180	72	360	18	–	–	–	–	–
	SR1	360	120	480	24	–	–	–	–	–
	SR2	270	144	360	18	–	–	–	–	–
	HR	180	48	240	12	3,000	3,000	–	–	–

DOX doxorubicin, *MTX* high-dose methotrexate, *DDP* cisplatin, *IFO* ifosfamide, *BCD* bleomycin/cyclophosphamide/dactinomycin, *BLEO* bleomycin, *CYC* cyclophosphamide, *ACTO-D* actinomycin D, *CE* carboplatin/etoposide. Response: *G* good, *P* poor. *LR/SR/HR* risk-groups of study COSS-96 according to the six-grade scale of Salzer-Kuntschik et al, in which grade 1 denotes no viable tumor, while grade 6 means no effect of chemotherapy, with grades 2–5 lying in between.[17] A good response was defined as less than 10% viable tumor (response grades 1–3). All primary metastases were also to be removed surgically, whenever feasible, in the months following surgery of the primary tumor. All COSS studies were accepted by the local ethics committee and/or the Protocol Review Committee of the German Cancer Society. Informed consent was required from all patients and/or their legal guardians, depending on their age.

Statistical Analyses

For the purpose of this analysis, all patients were evaluated on an intention to treat basis. Overall survival was calculated using the Kaplan–Meier-Method,[18] from the date of the diagnostic biopsy until death from any cause. The log-rank test was used to compare survival curves.[19] Multivariate analyses of overall survival was carried out using Cox's proportional hazards model.[20] An analysis of the types of surgery used (limb-salvage, rotation-plasty, or amputation) in relation to various factors, was performed on patients with extremity primaries who had received induction chemotherapy. SPSS software, version 15.0, was used for statistical calculations.

25 "Neoadjuvant COSS Years": Results

Patient Characteristics

Overall, 2,464 patients fulfilled the inclusion criteria (Tables 2 and 3). Their median age was 15.6 years (range: 2.18–74.56), and 77.6% of all patients (1,913) fell into the "pediatric and adolescent" category (below 20 years of age). There were 1,440 males (58.4%) and 1,024 females (41.6%); 2,287 extremity (92.8% – femur 1,229 [49.9%], tibia 636 [25.8%], fibula 129 [5.2%], humerus 245 [9.9%], radius 24 [1.0%], ulna 9 [0.4%], foot 12 [0.5%], hand 3 [0.1%]), and 225 axial primaries (7.2% – pelvis including sacrum 128 [5.2%], mobile spine 14 [0.6%], rib 21 [0.9%], clavicle 5 [0.2%], scapula 9 [0.4%]); 2,162 osteosarcomas (87.7%) were counted as localized and 299 as primary metastatic (12.1%). Two-thousand-seventeen osteosarcomas (81.9%) fell into the "localized extremity" category. Fifty-three osteosarcomas arose as secondary malignancies (2.2%).

Response to Induction Chemotherapy

Of the 2464 patients, 212 had received primary surgery and 81 no surgery. Response data was available for 1,929 of the remaining 2,171 (88.9%), and the exact grade of regression according to Salzer-Kuntschik et al[17] for 1,883 (86.7%). There were

Table 2 Outcome of 2,464 COSS patients with non-pretreated, high-grade central osteosarcoma according to risk factors

			Age	Follow-up (years median)		Status		Survival probability (standard error)		
	n	Percent	(median)	All	Survivors	Alive	Died	5 year	10 year	p^a
Total	2,264	100%	15.6	4.91	7.32	1,654	810	0.680 (0.010)	0.628 (0.010)	
Age										
≤Median	1,233	50.0%	12.6	5.49	8.21	836	397	0.694 (0.014)	0.645 (0.015)	0.050
>Median	1,231	50.0	19.2	4.36	6.44	818	413	0.665 (0.015)	0.609 (0.016)	
0–9	302	12.3%	8.2	5.23	8.72	204	98	0.687 (0.028)	0.655 (0.029)	<0.001
10–19	1,611	65.4%	15.1	5.36	7.67	1,091	520	0.692 (0.012)	0.638 (0.013)	
20–29	324	13.1%	23.0	4.51	6.50	220	104	0.689 (0.028)	0.615 (0.032)	
30–39	117	4.7%	34.6	3.50	4.68	73	44	0.581 (0.052)	0.541 (0.056)	
40–49	57	2.3%	44.7	3.47	5.07	40	17	0.670 (0.052)	0.541 (0.056)	
50–59	37	1.5%	55.4	2.02	3.50	20	17	0.422 (0.071)	n.a.	
60–69	12	0.5%	63.7	1.15	1.80	4	8	0.318 (0.149)	n.a.	
≥70	4	0.2%	73.2	1.25	1.40	2	2	n.a.	n.a.	
Gender										
m	1,440	58.4%	16.2	4.82	7.32	952	488	0.671 (0.013)	0.616 (0.014)	0.287
f	1,024	41.6%	14.8	5.10	7.31	702	322	0.692 (0.015)	0.645 (0.017)	
Tumor site										
Limb	2,287	92.8%	15.3	5.19	7.38	1,576	711	0.699 (0.010)	0.648 (0.011)	<0.001
Femur	1,229	49.9%	15.3	4.76	7.33	819	410	0.668 (0.014)	0.624 (0.016)	
Tibia	636	25.8%	15.4	6.06	7.67	482	154	0.784 (0.017)	0.727 (0.020)	
Fibula	129	5.2%	16.2	5.52	7.52	97	32	0.750 (0.040)	0.705 (0.046)	
Humerus	245	9.9%	15.1	4.20	6.82	141	104	0.576 (0.534)	0.508 (0.036)	
Radius	24	1.0%	14.0	7.24	9.93	18	6	0.774 (0.115)	0.619 (0.166)	
Ulna	9	0.4%	17.2	7.05	6.98	8	1	1.000	1.000	
Hand/foot	15	0.6%	23.5	6.03	6.15	11	4	0.774 (0.115)	0.619 (0.166)	
Axial	177	7.2%	20.8	2.61	5.75	78	99	0.424 (0.040)	0.362 (0.042)	
Pelvis	128	5.2%	20.9	2.33	4.42	48	80	0.344 (0.046)	0.287 (0.047)	
Mobile spine	14	0.6%	20.0	3.37	4.64	10	4	0.673 (0.136)	0.673 (0.136)	

(continued)

Table 2 (continued)

	n	Percent	Age (median)	Follow-up (years median) All	Follow-up (years median) Survivors	Status Alive	Status Died	Survival probability (standard error) 5 year	Survival probability (standard error) 10 year	p^a
Rib	*21*	*0.9%*	*23.8*	*2.34*	*8.91*	*10*	*11*	*0.501 (0.112)*	*0.430 (0.117)*	
Clavicle	*5*	*0.2%*	*56.3*	*6.17*	*6.27*	*4*	*1*	*1.000*	*0.750 (.217)*	
Scapula	*9*	*0.4%*	*17.9*	*4.06*	*7.57*	*6*	*3*	*0.667 (0.157)*	*0.667 (0.157)*	
Primary metastases										
Absent	2,162	87.7%	15.7	5.48	7.38	1,552	610	0.731 (010)	0.677 (0.011)	<0.001
Present	299	12.1%	15.3	1.95	6.04	99	200	0.310 (0.029)	0.269 (0.029)	
No data	*3*									
Secondary osteosacoma										
No	2,411	97.8%	15.6	4.94	7.34	1,628	783	0.682 (0.010)	0.632 (0.011)	0.011
Yes	53	2.2%	19.4	4.25	6.59	26	27	0.580 (0.070)	0.435 (0.078)	
Response[b]										
Good	1,087	56.4%	14.8	6.09	7.35	860	229	0.805 (0.013)	0.763 (0.015)	<0.001
Grade 1	*254*	*13.5%*	*14.7*	*7.43*	*8.32*	*210*	*44*	*0.862 (0.023)*	*0.817 (0.027)*	*<0.001*
Grade 2	*367*	*19.5%*	*14.7*	*6.16*	*7.17*	*306*	*61*	*0.852 (0.020)*	*0.801 (0.025)*	
Grade 3	*447*	*23.7%*	*15.1*	*5.57*	*7.13*	*334*	*113*	*0.744 (0.022)*	*0.709 (0.024)*	
Poor	842	43.6%	16.1	4.04	7.10	472	370	0.575 (0.018)	0.506 (0.020)	
Grade 4	*426*	*22.6%*	*15.8*	*4.26*	*6.45*	*261*	*165*	*0.620 (0.025)*	*0.539 (0.029)*	
Grade 5	*339*	*18.0%*	*16.6*	*3.47*	*7.42*	*177*	*162*	*0.540 (0.029)*	*0.488 (0.030)*	
Grade 6	*50*	*2.7%*	*16.0*	*2.98*	*8.00*	*24*	*26*	*0.438 (0.076)*	*0.409 (0.076)*	

[a]Log-rank
[b]See text for definitions and evaluability

Table 3 Survival estimates according to year of osteosarcoma diagnosis, p=log-rank test

	n	Percent	Age (median)	Follow-up (years median)		Status		Survival probability (standard error)	
				All	Survivors	Alive	Died	5 year	10 year
All 2,464 patients (p=0.002)									
Before 1985	394	16.0%	14.9	7.20	14.66	213	181	0.594 (0.025)	0.544 (0.026)
1985–1989	413	16.8%	15.8	9.52	11.81	259	154	0.688 (0.023)	0.634 (0.024)
1990–1994	491	19.9%	15.5	7.01	9.48	320	171	0.679 (0.022)	0.644 (0.023)
1995–1999	586	23.8%	16.1	6.04	7.20	404	182	0.708 (0.019)	0.652 (0.022)
2000–2004	580	23.5%	15.6	2.90	3.10	458	122	0.704 (0.026)	n.a.
Localized limb tumors only (p<0.001)									
All	2,017	81.9%	15.4	5.66	7.43	1,480	537	0.748 (0.010)	0.695 (0.012)
Before 1985	*327*	*13.3%*	*14.8*	*9.29*	*14.63*	*196*	*131*	*0.658 (0.027)*	*0.607 (0.028)*
1985–1989	*364*	*14.8%*	*15.8*	*9.80*	*11.77*	*244*	*120*	*0.725 (0.024)*	*0.674 (0.025)*
1990–1994	*411*	*16.7%*	*15.4*	*7.80*	*9.41*	*299*	*112*	*0.761 (0.023)*	*0.721 (0.023)*
1995–1999	*461*	*18.7%*	*15.8*	*6.54*	*7.19*	*357*	*104*	*0.794 (0.020)*	*0.739 (0.024)*
2000–2004	*454*	*18.4%*	*15.3*	*3.01*	*3.15*	*384*	*70*	*0.770 (0.028)*	*n.a.*
Axial or primary metastatic tumors only (p=0.059)									
All	444	18.0%	16.4	2.37	5.98	171	273	0.369 (0.023)	0.317 (0.025)
Before 1985	*67*	*2.7%*	*15.5*	*1.80*	*15.46*	*17*	*50*	*0.282 (0.056)*	*0.235 (0.053)*
1985–1989	*49*	*2.0%*	*16.1*	*1.95*	*12.22*	*15*	*34*	*0.408 (0.070)*	*0.339 (0.069)*
1990–1994	*80*	*3.2%*	*16.1*	*2.44*	*10.17*	*21*	*59*	*0.271 (0.050)*	*0.258 (0.049)*
1995–1999	*125*	*5.1%*	*17.6*	*3.13*	*8.01*	*47*	*78*	*0.396 (0.045)*	*0.341 (0.045)*
2000–2004	*123*	*5.0%*	*17.0*	*2.24*	*3.09*	*71*	*52*	*0.463 (0.056)*	*n.a.*

1,087 good responders (56.4%) and 842 poor responders (43.6%). Complete nonresponse (grade 6) was very rare ($n=50$; 2.0%) (Table 2).

Type of Surgery

After excluding 177 patients with axial primaries, 174 who had primary surgery, 69 patients without surgery (25, radiotherapy, 44, no local treatment) and 44 with insufficient information about local therapy, exactly 2,000 patients were evaluable for an analysis of types of surgery in patients with extremity osteosarcoma pretreated by induction chemotherapy. Of these, 1,156 (57.8%) had received limb-salvage surgery; 359 (18.0%) rotation plasties, and 485 (24.3%), amputations. Over the years, there was a strong tendency to move away from amputations towards limb-salvage, with the major shift happening around 1990 (Fig. 1, Table 4). In the latter years of the period evaluated, considerably less than 10% of all femoral or humeral osteosarcomas resulted in amputations, while such procedures were still used for more than one quarter of patients with tibia or fibula tumors (Table 4).

Overall Outcome and Causes of Death

After a median follow-up of 4.91 years for all 2,462 patients (range: 0.04–26.08) and 7.31 years for survivors, 1,654 patients were alive, for 5, 10, 15, and 20 year survival probabilities of .680 (standard error: 0.010), 0.628 (0.011), 0.601 (0.013), and 0.561 (0.022), respectively. Of the 1,654 survivors, 1,125 had been followed for more than 5 years, 521 for over 10, 190 for over 15, and 41 for over 20 years.

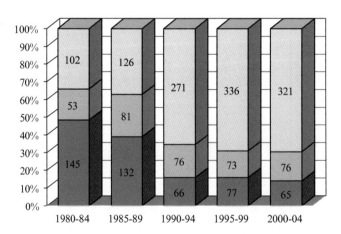

Fig. 1 Distribution of surgical techniques in 2,000 extremity osteosarcomas by period of diagnosis

Osteosarcoma: The COSS Experience

Table 4 Choice of definitive surgical procedures according to primary tumor site, patient age, and year of osteosarcoma diagnosis

	Evaluable	Limb–salvage	Rotation–plasty	Amputation
All patients	2,000	1,156 (57.8%)	359 (18.0%)	485 (24.3%)
1980–1984	*300*	*102 (34.0%)*	*53 (17.7%)*	*145 (48.3%)*
1985–1989	*339*	*126 (37.2%)*	*81 (24.4%)*	*132 (39.8%)*
1990–1994	*413*	*271 (65.6%)*	*76 (18.4%)*	*66 (16.0%)*
1995–1999	*486*	*336 (69.1%)*	*73 (15.0%)*	*77 (15.8%)*
2000–2004	*462*	*321 (69.5%)*	*76 (16.5%)*	*65 (14.1%)*
Femur	1,090	582 (53.4%)	337 (30.9%)	171 (15.7%)
1980–1984	*175*	*48 (27.4%)*	*50 (28.6%)*	*77 (44.0%)*
1985–1989	*178*	*60 (33.7%)*	*76 (42.7%)*	*42 (23.6%)*
1990–1994	*230*	*139 (60.4%)*	*73 (31.7%)*	*18 (7.8%)*
1995–1999	*243*	*163 (67.1%)*	*66 (27.2%)*	*14 (5.8%)*
2000–2004	*264*	*172 (65.2%)*	*72 (27.3%)*	*20 (7.6%)*
Tibia	550	292 (53.1%)	21 (3.8%)	237 (43.1%)
1980–1984	*78*	*21 (26.9%)*	*3 (3.8%)*	*54 (69.2%)*
1985–1989	*98*	*27 (27.6%)*	*4 (4.1%)*	*67 (68.4%)*
1990–1994	*101*	*60 (59.4%)*	*3 (3.0%)*	*38 (37.6%)*
1995–1999	*158*	*106 (67.1%)*	*7 (4.4%)*	*45 (28.5%)*
2000–2004	*115*	*78 (67.8%)*	*4 (3.5%)*	*33 (28.7%)*
Fibula	100	70 (70.0%)	1 (1.0%)	29 (29.0%)
1980–1984	*11*	*6 (54.5%)*	*–*	*5 (45.5%)*
1985–1989	*22*	*11 (50.0%)*	*1 (4.5%)*	*10 (45.5%)*
1990–1994	*27*	*25 (92.6%)*	*–*	*2 (7.4%)*
1995–1999	*17*	*11 (64.7%)*	*–*	*6 (35.7%)*
2000–2004	*23*	*17 (73.9%)*	*–*	*6 (26.1%)*
Humerus	223	190 (85.2%)	–	33 (14.8%)
1980–1984	*32*	*27 (84.4%)*	*–*	*5 (15.6%)*
1985–1989	*36*	*25 (69.4%)*	*–*	*11 (30.6%)*
1990–1994	*48*	*42 (87.5%)*	*–*	*6 (12.5%)*
1995–1999	*57*	*49 (86.0%)*	*–*	*8 (14.0%)*
2000–2004	*50*	*47 (94.0%)*	*–*	*3 (6.0%)*
Age <10 years	259	103 (39.8%)	102 (39.4%)	54 (20.8%)
1980–1984	*42*	*13 (30.2%)*	*11 (26.2%)*	*18 (41.9%)*
1985–1989	*34*	*10 (29.4%)*	*16 (47.1%)*	*8 (23.5%)*
1990–1994	*57*	*28 (49.1%)*	*22 (38.6%)*	*7 (12.3%)*
1995–1999	*59*	*21 (35.6%)*	*25 (42.4%)*	*13 (22.0%)*
2000–2004	*67*	*31 (46.3%)*	*28 (41.8%)*	*8 (11.9%)*
Age 10–19 years	1,371	793 (57.8%)	226 (16.5%)	352 (25.7%)
1980–1984	*233*	*79 (33.9%)*	*40 (17.2%)*	*114 (48.9%)*
1985–1989	*242*	*84 (34.7%)*	*57 (23.6%)*	*101 (41.7%)*
1990–1994	*273*	*184 (67.4%)*	*46 (16.8%)*	*43 (15.8%)*
1995–1999	*322*	*230 (71.4%)*	*41 (12.7%)*	*51 (15.8%)*
2000–2004	*301*	*216 (71.8%)*	*42 (14.0%)*	*43 (14.3%)*
Age >19 years	370	260 (70.3%)	31 (8.4%)	79 (21.4%)
1980–1984	*25*	*10 (40.0%)*	*2 (8.0%)*	*13 (52.0%)*
1985–1989	*63*	*32 (50.8%)*	*8 (12.7%)*	*23 (36.5%)*

(continued)

300 S. Bielack et al.

Table 4 (continued)

	Evaluable	Limb–salvage	Rotation–plasty	Amputation
1990–1994	83	59 (71.1%)	8 (9.6%)	16 (19.3%)
1995–1999	105	85 (81.0%)	7 (6.7%)	13 (12.4%)
2000–2004	94	74 (78.7%)	6 (6.4%)	14 (14.9%)

Among the 810 deceased patients, the median time to death was 2.18 years (range: 0.08–19.85). Overall, 715 patients died in the first 5 years, 75 in years 6–10, 14 in years 11–15, and 6 thereafter. Causes of death were osteosarcoma in 705 (87.0%), others in 83 (10.2%), and unknown in 22 (0.9%, mostly with progressive disease at last follow-up). Death from osteosarcoma occurred after a median of 2.20 years (range: 0.15–16.27), with 629 patients dead within the first 5 years, 63 in years 6–10, 10 in years 11–15, and three thereafter.

Death from causes other than osteosarcoma occurred during primary treatment in 37 patients (1.6% of all patients, 4.6% of all deaths). Causes were myelotoxicity (27: infection 22, hemorrhage 2, multi-organ-failure 3 – last drugs administered: methotrexate 10, ifosfamide/cisplatin 5, doxorubicin 5, doxorubicin/cisplatin 1, BCD 1, cisplatin 1, ifosfamide 1, carboplatin/etoposide 1, not documented 2); cardiac failure (2); perioperative complications including infection, bleeding, and embolic disease (7: primary tumor, biopsy or definitive surgery 6, metastases 1); and suicide because of progressive osteosarcoma (1). Twenty-three patients died in the first remission after the end of therapy. Causes were secondary malignancy (12: hematologic cancer 8, solid tumors 4); cardiomyopathy (7); accidents (2); AIDS (1); and cerebral hemorrhage (1). Another 23 patients died from causes other than osteosarcoma after having experienced a recurrence; for these, causes of death were myelotoxicity (10), perioperative complications after metastasectomy (4), cardiomyopathy (3), secondary hematologic malignancy (2), and hepatitis, anorexia, pulmonary fibrosis, and thrombosis in one each.

All but one (a patient who received additional therapy because of recurrence) of the total of 12 deaths from cardiac failure occurred in patients diagnosed before 11/88. The median time to death from cardiomyopathy in first remission (7 patients) was 4.84 years (range: 1.12–15.69).

In 14 patients, who died from secondary malignancy after treatment for osteosarcoma, the median time to death was 4.78 years (range: 1.05–19.85). It was 3.90 years (1.05–7.24) for 10 patients with hematologic cancers and 10.18 (2.95–19.85) in four patients, who died from secondary solid tumors. Osteosarcoma had already been a secondary malignancy in 4 of the 14.

Prognostic Factors

Upon univariate testing, secondary osteosarcomas did worse than primary osteosarcomas ($p = 0.011$). Primary metastases ($p < 0.001$, log-rank) and axial site

($p<0.001$) predicted inferior survival probabilities, leading to major differences in survival probabilities between patients with localized extremity osteosarcoma and others, the 5- and 10 year survival estimates being 0.748/0.695 and 0.369/0.317, respectively ($p<0.001$, Table 3, Fig. 2). Among extremity primaries, those of the humerus were associated with the lowest survival probability. Increasing age was of negative prognostic significance when evaluated by decade ($p<0.001$) and of borderline significance when dichotomized at the median ($p=0.050$). Good responders to induction chemotherapy had a significantly more favorable prognosis than poor responders ($p<0.001$). A further subdivision of response into the six regression grades of Salzer-Kuntschik et al[17] revealed prognostic differences between the individual grades ($p<0.001$) (Table 2, Fig. 3). When evaluating survival probabilities by 5-year periods from 1980 until 2004, outcomes improved overall ($p=0.002$) and for localized extremity primaries ($p>0.001$), while no improvement was obvious for axial or metastatic primaries ($p=0.059$) (Table 3).

Upon multivariate analysis, tumor site (axial vs. limb), primary metastases (present vs. absent), and treatment period (first vs.second half of the recruitment period), retained independent prognostic significance, while age and the presence of osteosarcoma as a secondary malignancy did not. When response was added to the equation, this was also of independent prognostic significance (Table 5).

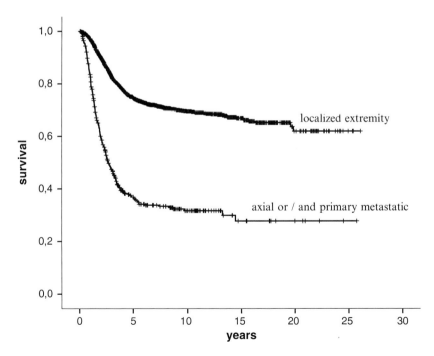

Fig. 2 Survival estimates for 2,017 patients with localized extremity osteosarcoma and 444 patients with axial or/and primary metastatic tumors

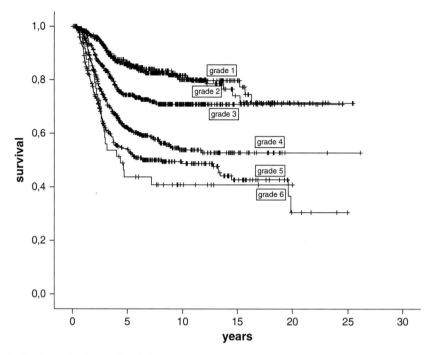

Fig. 3 Survival estimates in relation to response to preoperative chemotherapy (regression grades 1–6 according to Salzer-Kuntschik et al[17])

Discussion

This analysis of 2,464 patients with previously untreated, high-grade central osteosarcoma of the extremities or axial skeleton is, to our knowledge, the largest ever performed by any collaborative treatment group. It confirms and expands results obtained by a previous analysis of 1,702 patients diagnosed until 1998.[10] The COSS group now follows well over a thousand 5-year survivors and over five hundred 10-year survivors. The survival probability at 10 years approached 70% for patients with localized extremity osteosarcomas, but hovered below one-third for others – patients with axial or primary metastatic tumors-despite identical treatment guidelines.

Local Therapy

Surgery remains the mainstay of local therapy in osteosarcoma. In the COSS experience, the paramount importance of complete surgery has been repeatedly confirmed, be it for localized extremity disease,[8,10] for tumors of the axial skeleton[6,11,12] or craniofacial bones,[21] for primary metastatic tumors,[13,22] or for recurrent osteosarcoma.[23] In all of these situations, complete surgery emerged almost as a prerequisite for cure. We could, however, also demonstrate that radiotherapy to lesions which could not be removed with sufficient margins correlated with prolonged survival in osteosarcomas situated at unfavorable sites such as the spine[11] or pelvis[12], and in recurrent osteosarcoma,[23] hence our group's current recommendation is to irradiate lesions which cannot be removed with wide margins.

Picci et al have convincingly demonstrated that the local failure rate in osteosarcoma correlates with both the quality of the surgical margins and the extent of tumor response to induction chemotherapy.[24] We were able to confirm the latter finding, and also observed that local failure rates were particularly high in patients who had been treated by limb-salvage surgery despite a poor response, pointing out that surgeons should be particularly sure about their margins when thinking about whether to perform limb-salvage in tumors which might turn out to be poor responders.[25] This strategy seems to have been implemented within our group: In our analysis of 1,702 patients with osteosarcomas of the limbs or trunk treated between 1980 and 1998,[10] limb-salvage was reported for 61% of operated good responders, but only for 39% of operated poor responders. Using such a strategy, local recurrences were rare, and only developed in 84 of 1,589 patients, who had been rendered free of their primary tumor (5.3%).[10]

As local control is so frequently achieved in patients with extremity osteosarcoma, the debate is whether to use limb-salvage – thereby maintaining body image and integrity – in almost every patient, probably accepting a slightly higher rate of local recurrences and an increased rate of operative complications along the way, or to use other, functionally more or less equivalent; techniques,[26] such as rotation-plasty. There are many aspects which influence the answer to this question, and the choice of surgical techniques has, of course, not remained static over time. Overall, we observed a strong shift away from amputations, and in the past 15 years, most COSS patients with extremity primaries received limb-salvage surgery, with amputations restricted mostly to the distal extremities (Tables 4 and 5). Conventional expandable endoprostheses used to be associated with the necessity for multiple reoperations and a very high complication rate,[27] while rotation-plasties, though cosmetically challenging, frequently led to excellent functional and even psychosocial results.[26,28] Consequently, even rather recently, children below the age of 10 years were treated by limb-salvage much less frequently than older patients (Table 5). It may be assumed that this difference will become less marked with the advent of modern, noninvasive expanding devices and techniques.[27,29,30]

Mortality

Systemic multiagent chemotherapy as administered in the COSS-protocols was effective, resulted in a good response (<10% viable tumor) in 56.4% of 1,883 evaluable tumors and, together with surgery, contributed to the favorable survival rates detailed above. Osteosarcoma was by far the most frequent cause of death in this cohort, and, while almost 90% of all osteosarcoma related deaths occurred within the first 5 years,

Table 5 Multivariate analyses of factors associated with survival

Variable	Relative risk	p	Relative risk	p
Primary metastases (present)	4.166 (3.546–4.902)	<0.001	3.690 (3.012–4.505)	<0.001
Site (axial)	2.563 (2.051–3.202)	<0.001	1.967 (1.409–2.747)	<0.001
Secondary osteosarcoma	1.192 (0.803–1.767)	0.384	1.534 (0.925–2.538)	0.097
Sex (male)	1.135 (0.983–1.309)	0.084	1.088 (0.920–1.287)	0.323
Age (>median)	1.063 (0.921–1.226)	0.404	0.999 (0.845–1.181)	0.991
Response (poor)			2.538 (2.146–3.003)	<0.001
Period (before 07/92)	1.327 (1.152–1.529)	<0.001	1.199 (1.016–1.416)	0.032

tumor related fatalities continued to occur as late as 16 years from the initial diagnosis. Multimodal therapy was, however, toxic, as exemplified by 27 deaths due to myelotoxic complications of the first-line treatment. Interestingly, even though usually relatively devoid of myelotoxicity, methotrexate was the drug most frequently associated with such acute and devastating complications. It must be stressed that high-dose methotrexate therapy should never be administered casually, that supportive care must be meticulous, and that severe toxicity may arise unpredictably despite optimal support.

Secondary malignancy was the most frequent cause of death for patients who died in complete remission after the completion of first-line treatment however; it was responsible for less than 2% of all deaths overall. Based on a detailed review of the literature available at the time,[31] COSS switched from short to continuous, 48 h doxorubicin administration, around 1990 and also limited the cumulative dose to 360 mg/m² (Table 1). All but 1 of 12 cardiac deaths occurred in patients diagnosed before these changes took place, the only exception being a patient who had received further chemotherapy for recurrent disease; so, we may assume that the strategy was rather efficacious against cardiomyopathy, at least in the short and intermediate run.

Prognostic Factors

As in our previous analysis of 1,702 patients diagnosed until 1998,[10] axial tumor site, primary metastases, and poor response to primary chemotherapy were confirmed as important and independent negative prognostic factors. Within the framework of our multi-institutional group's treatment guidelines, there was no clear cut impact of patient age or gender (Table 6). We have previously demonstrated that patients with osteosarcoma arising as a secondary cancer may have survival chances similar to those of otherwise comparable (age, tumor site) patients with primary osteosarcoma,[9] and this was again confirmed here by multivariate testing.

Why do patients with axial and primary metastatic tumors do so poorly? In osteosarcoma of the axial skeleton or the craniofacial bones, achieving and maintaining local control is still a very big challenge. In our group's published experience, 47/67 pelvic,[12] 15/22 vertebral (including sacral),[11] and 25/49 craniofacial osteosarcomas[21] failed to remain in permanent local control, and patients in whom this was the case almost all died. Patients who were permanently rendered free of their primary tumors, on the other hand, had outcomes which were similar to those of patients with extremity lesions.[6,11,12,21] Similarly, patients with primary metastases only very rarely become long-term survivors unless the primary tumor and all metastases are removed by surgery.[13] We were recently able to expand this observation to patients with skip metastases, a cohort long believed to have a particularly poor prognosis; they, in fact, seem to do reasonably well if all lesions are removed within a multidisciplinary treatment framework.[22]

In our group's first neoadjuvant trial, COSS-80, no differences in outcomes between either cisplatin or the BCD combination, when given in combination with doxorubicin and HD-MTX, were observed.[2] As a byproduct of that trial, our group for the first time confirmed the prognostic relevance of tumor response to induction chemotherapy,[2] and has done so repeatedly ever since.[3,7,10] Here, a very large group of 1,883 primaries evaluable for response allowed us to clearly demonstrate once more that the effect of response is not an "all or nothing" between good and poor, but that more subtle variations – like that between regression grades 1 through 6, according to Salzer-Kuntschik et al[17] - allow for a further subdivision of prognostic groups, and that even very minor responses – grade 5 (more than 50% viable tumor remaining) – are associated with a better prognosis than grade 6 (no histologic evidence of a chemotherapy effect[17]). Fortunately, the group of tumors with no histologic chemotherapy effect at all was very small (2.7%). Despite its outcome being worse than that of all the others, the observed 10-year survival expectancy of 0.409 is still higher than reported for patients treated without chemotherapy,[32–34] warning against uncontrolled abandonment of standard treatment even in patients with a very poor chemotherapy response.

Unfortunately, multiple efforts by various groups to alter the prognosis of poor responders by postoperative chemotherapy modifications have so far not led to convincing improvements.[35] In fact, trying to start out with relatively low-intensity induction chemotherapy (MTX plus BCD) and later to salvage poor responders to this preoperative protocol by an intensive, doxorubicin and cisplatin-containing postoperative regimen led to inferior outcomes compared to starting out with these drugs in a randomized trial, COSS-82.[3] From this experience, our group concluded that deficiencies of induction chemotherapy which result in a suboptimal response rate cannot be made up for by postoperative treatment modifications. An attempt to further increase the proportion of good responders by intra-arterial compared to intravenous cisplatin as part of multiagent treatment failed.[5,7]

Here, we were happy to observe that, in addition to the shift away from amputation, treatment in the latter half of the 25-year recruitment period was also associated with a somewhat improved survival expectancy. Unfortunately, however, patients with axial or metastatic primaries seemed to have been more or less excluded from this positive development, and, even for patients with localized extremity osteosarcomas, there was no clear cut evidence of further survival improvements within the later period. This is by no means specific for the COSS trials, but unfortunately very characteristic of the situation in osteosarcoma in general, as perhaps best exemplified by a large cumulative analysis of 59 cancer registries, recently, in which the 5-year survival rates for pediatric and adolescent osteosarcoma throughout Europe showed almost no improvement since 1983, still hovering around 60%.[36]

Treatment of Recurrent Disease

The analyses discussed above focused on the primary treatment of osteosarcoma, and most patients who become long-term survivors indeed do so without ever having to experience disease recurrence. Nevertheless, some 30–50% of all osteosarcoma patients will develop recurrent disease, and most of these will succumb to their cancer. In a COSS analysis of 576 consecutive patients with osteosarcoma recurrences after multimodal treatment, 5- and 10-year post-recurrence survival were only 23% and 18%, respectively. A long recurrence-free interval and the presence of a solitary manifestation of recurrence predicted superior outcomes. Complete surgery was once again as much a prerequisite for cure. Interestingly, the use of chemotherapy was associated with limited survival benefits both in the palliative and the adjuvant situation,[23] so that our group continues to favor the use of second-line chemotherapy. An analysis of outcomes after 409 second and subsequent recurrences again demonstrated surgical clearance to be of paramount importance.[37]

Conclusions

COSS has succeeded in building and maintaining a large and successful, multicentric, multidisciplinary osteosarcoma treatment network. Our registration policy which was never restricted to "young, localized extremity osteosarcoma" patients has allowed us to develop an almost population-based database and to perform analyses on large groups of patients with classical presentation and on still reasonably sized cohorts of patients with special disease features. While major advances have occurred in the surgical field, progress in chemotherapy – at least as far as cure rates are concerned – has been very limited for years, and important questions, such as that of the role of salvage therapy for poor responders to induction treatment, remain unanswered. Future progress is likely to remain slow unless new drugs become available through translational research. Proof of efficacy requires confirmation in large, prospective, randomized trials, and our group has joined others in the European and American Osteosarcoma Study Group EURAMOS so that such studies might be performed within reasonably short recruitment periods.

Acknowledgements We thank all the patients who contributed to the COSS studies, and acknowledge the physicians, nurses, data managers, and support staff of the collaborating centers for their active participation, and the Deutsches Kinderkrebsregister for the exchange of follow-up information and data on secondary malignancies. We particularly appreciate the dedicated work of the staff of the COSS study center and of the members of the COSS reference panels. The COSS studies on which these analyses are based received support from Deutsche Krebshilfe, Bundesministerium für Forschung und Technologie, and Fördergemeinschaft Kinderkrebszentrum Hamburg.

References

1. Winkler K, Beron G, Schellong G, et al. Kooperative Osteosarkomstudie COSS-77: Ergebnisse nach über 4 Jahren. *Klin Pädiatr.* 1982;194:251-256.
2. Winkler K, Beron G, Kotz R, et al. Neoadjuvant chemotherapy for osteogenic sarcoma: results of a cooperative German/Austrian study. *J Clin Oncol.* 1984;2:617-623.
3. Winkler K, Beron G, Delling G, et al. Neoadjuvant chemotherapy of osteosarcoma: results of a randomized cooperative trial (COSS-82) with salvage chemotherapy based on histological tumor response. *J Clin Oncol.* 1988;6:329-337.
4. Bielack S, Beck J, Delling G, et al. Neoadjuvant chemotherapy of osteosarcoma. Results of the cooperative studies COSS-80 and COSS-82 after 7 and 5 years. *Klin Padiatr.* 1989;201:275-284.
5. Winkler K, Bielack S, Delling G, et al. Effect of intraarterial versus intravenous cisplatin in addition to systemic doxorubicin, high dose methotrexate, and ifosfamide on histologic tumor response in osteosarcoma (Study COSS-86). *Cancer.* 1990;66:1703-1710.
6. Bielack S, Wulff B, Delling G, et al. Osteosarcoma of the trunk treated by multimodal therapy: experience of the cooperative osteosarcoma study group COSS. *Med Pediatr Oncol.* 1995;24:6-12.
7. Fuchs N, Bielack S, Epler D, et al. Long-term results of the co-operative German–Austrian–Swiss osteosarcoma study group's protocol COSS-86 of intensive multidrug chemotherapy and surgery for osteosarcoma of the limbs. *Ann Oncol.* 1998;9:893-899.
8. Bielack S, Kempf-Bielack B, Schwenzer D, et al. Neoadjuvante Therapie des lokalisierten Osteosarkoms der Extremitäten. Erfahrungen der Cooperativen Osteosarkomstudiengruppe COSS an 925 Patienten. *Klin Padiatr.* 1999a;211:260-270.
9. Bielack SS, Kempf-Bielack B, Heise U, Schwenzer D, Winkler K. Combined modality treatment for osteosarcoma occurring as a second malignant disease. *J Clin Oncol.* 1999;17:1164-1174.
10. Bielack SS, Kempf-Bielack B, Delling G, et al. Prognostic factors in high-grade osteosarcoma of the extremities or trunk: an analysis of 1,702 patients treated on neoadjuvant Cooperative Osteosarcoma Study Group protocols. *J Clin Oncol.* 2002;20:776-790.
11. Ozaki T, Flege S, Liljenqvist U, et al. Osteosarcoma of the spine: experience of the Cooperative Osteosarcoma Study Group (COSS). *Cancer.* 2002;94:1069-1077.
12. Ozaki T, Flege S, Kevric M, et al. Osteosarcoma of the pelvis: experience of the Cooperative Osteosarcoma Study Group (COSS). *J Clin Oncol.* 2003;21:334-341.
13. Kager L, Zoubek A, Pötschger U, et al. Primary metastatic osteosarcoma: presentation and outcome of 202 patients treated on neoadjuvant Cooperative Osteosarcoma Study Group (COSS) protocols. *J Clin Oncol.* 2003;21:2011-2018.
14. Kaatsch P, Spix C, et al.: Jahresbericht 2005: Deutsches Kinderkrebsregister. Mainz, Germany, Johannes-Gutenberg-Universität, Institut für Medizinische Statistik und Information; 2006
15. Jaffe N, Paed D, Farber S, et al. Favorable response of metastatic osteogenic sarcoma to pulse high-dose methotrexate with citrovorum rescue and radiation therapy. *Cancer.* 1973;31:1367-1373.
16. Jaffe N, Frei E 3rd, Traggis D, Bishop Y. Adjuvant methotrexate and citrovorum-factor treatment of osteogenic sarcoma. *N Engl J Med.* 1974;291:994-997.
17. Salzer-Kuntschik M, Brand G, Delling G. Bestimmung des morphologischen Regressionsgrades nach Chemotherapie bei malignen Knochentumoren. *Pathologie.* 1983;4:135-141.
18. Kaplan EL, Meier P. Nonparametric estimation from incomplete observations. *J Am Stat Assoc.* 1958;53:457-481.

19. Mantel M. Evaluation of survival data and two new rank order statistics arising in its consideration. *Cancer Chemother Rep*. 1966;50:163-170.
20. Cox DR. Regression models and life-tables [with discussion]. *J R Stat Soc [B]*. 1972;34:187-220.
21. Jasnau S, Meyer U, Potratz J, et al. Craniofacial osteosarcoma Experience of the cooperative German–Austrian–Swiss osteosarcoma study group. *Oral Oncol*. 2008;44:286-294.
22. Kager L, Zoubek A, Kastner U, et al. Skip metastases in osteosarcoma: experience of the Cooperative Osteosarcoma Study Group. *J Clin Oncol*. 2006;24:1535-1541.
23. Kempf-Bielack B, Bielack SS, Jürgens H, et al. Osteosarcoma relapse after combined modality therapy: an analysis of unselected patients in the Cooperative Osteosarcoma Study Group (COSS). *J Clin Oncol*. 2005;23:559-568.
24. Picci P, Sangiorgi L, Rougraff BT, et al. The relationship of chemotherapy-induced necrosis and surgical margins to local recurrence in osteosarcoma. *J Clin Oncol*. 1994;12:2699-2705.
25. Bielack S, Kempf-Bielack B, Winkler K. Osteosarcoma: relationship of response to preoperative chemotherapy and type of surgery to local recurrence. *J Clin Oncol*. 1996;15:683-684.
26. Hillmann A, Hoffmann C, Gosheger G, Krakau H, Winkelmann W. Malignant tumor of the distal part of the femur or the proximal part of the tibia: endoprosthetic replacement or rotationplasty. Functional outcome and quality-of-life measurements. *J Bone Joint Surg Am*. 1999;81:462-468.
27. Abudu A, Grimer RJ, Tillman R, et al. The use of prostheses in skeletally immature patients. *Orthop Clin North Am*. 2006;37:75-84.
28. Hardes J, Gebert C, Hillmann A, et al. Die Möglichkeiten und Grenzen der Umkehrplastik im operativen Behandlungsplan der primär malignen Knochentumoren. *Orthopäde*. 2003;32:965-970.
29. Kotz RI, Windhager R, Dominkus M, Robioneck B, Müller-Daniels H. A self-extending paediatric leg implant. *Nature*. 2000;406:143-144.
30. Krepler P, Dominkus M, Toma CD, Kotz R. Endoprosthesis management of the extremities of children after resection of primary malignant bone tumors. *Orthopade*. 2003;32:1013-1019.
31. Bielack S, Erttmann R, Winkler K, Landbeck G. Doxorubicin: effect of different schedules on toxicity and anti-tumor efficacy. *Eur J Cancer Clin Oncol*. 1989;25:873-882.
32. Friedman MA, Carter SK. The therapy of osteogenic sarcoma: current status and thoughts for the future. *J Surg Oncol*. 1972;4:482-510.
33. Jaffe N, Frei E. Osteogenic sarcoma: advances in treatment. *CA Cancer J Clin*. 1976;26:351-359.
34. Link MP, Goorin AM, Miser AW, et al. The effect of adjuvant chemotherapy on relapse-free survival in patients with osteosarcoma of the extremities. *N Engl J Med*. 1986;314:1600-1606.
35. Bielack SS, Machatschek JN, Flege S, Jürgens H. Delaying surgery with chemotherapy for osteosarcoma of the extremities. *Expert Opin Pharmacother*. 2004;5:1243-1256.
36. Stiller CA, Bielack SS, Jundt G, Steliarova-Foucher E. Bone tumours in European children and adolescents, 1978–1997. Report from the Automated Childhood Cancer Information System project. *Eur J Cancer*. 2006;42:2124-2135.
37. Bielack S, Kempf-Bielack B, Branscheid D, et al. Second and subsequent recurrences of osteosarcoma: Presentation, treatment, and outcomes of 249 consecutive Cooperative Osteosarcoma Study Group patients. *J Clin Oncol*. 2009;27:557–65.

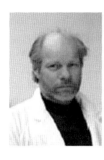

Treatment of Osteosarcoma. The Scandinavian Sarcoma Group Experience

Øyvind S. Bruland, Henrik Bauer, Thor Alvegaard, and Sigbjørn Smeland

Abstract Results from four consecutive trials, conducted from 1982 by members of the Scandinavian Sarcoma Group, are reviewed. A total of 330 classical osteosarcoma patients were enrolled. In all trials chemotherapy was based on the three active drugs, methotrexate, doxorubicin and cisplatinum and for the latter trials also ifosfamide. Post-operative chemotherapy was stratified by histological response to up-front treatment.

Introduction

Despite the fact that osteosarcoma (OS) is the most common primary solid bone tumor, it is a rare disorder that displays considerable heterogeneity and appears in clinical entities showing a considerable span in tumor biology and prognosis.[1-4] Most commonly, OS strikes children and young adults as classical OS; i.e., extremity-localized primary tumor, of high-grade histology, with no overt metastasis detectable at diagnosis and at age below 40 years of age – the cohort studied in most OS clinical trials.

Evidence from the prechemotherapy era has revealed that micrometastases were present in the majority of OS-patients[5] who usually died despite primary amputation.[6] This constitutes the rationale for the adjuvant chemotherapy currently given to all patients with high-grade histology.[7]

The Scandinavian Sarcoma group (SSG) was established in 1979 and comprises multidisciplinary teams with oncologists, both adult and pediatric; surgeons; radiologists; pathologists; nuclear medicine specialists; and tumor biologists from the Nordic countries. These countries have similar social structures, modern medical care paid by the government and an effective registration of all cancer patients. The aims of SSG are

---

Ø.S. Bruland (✉)
The Norwegian Radium Hospital, University of Oslo, Oslo, N-0310, Norway
e-mail: oyvind.bruland@medisin.uio.no

the timely referral of all sarcoma patients to centralized centers with complete facilities and experience for multidisciplinary care to improve the outcome of these patients.

Ongoing protocols have defined the standard treatment of OS in Scandinavia. This paper attempts to briefly review the SSG experience in treating OS-patients, with the focus on the results obtained in the various clinical trials in classical-OS run by this organization. Experiences from the still ongoing trial Euroboss, bone sarcoma in patients above 40 years of age, and the recently closed ISG/SSG-2; only published in abstract[8] for patients with pelvic OS or primary metastatic disease, will not be addressed.

Materials and Methods

Since 1982, members of the SSG have enrolled 330 classical OS patients into four consecutive trials (Tables 1 and 2). Results from three of these trials have been published.[9–12] In all the trials, chemotherapy was based on the three active drugs, methotrexate (MTX), doxorubicin, and cisplatinum (cis-Pt), and for the latter three trials, ifosfamide was also used. Postoperative chemotherapy was stratified by histological response to up-front treatment.

SSG II. This trial was based on Rosen's T-10 protocol[7] of four courses of high-dose MTX given preoperatively. "Good Responders" continued with MTX postoperatively with the addition of BCD (bleomycin, cyclophosphamide and dactinomycin). "Poor Responders" were salvaged by a combination of doxorubicin and cis-Pt.[9] Of the 114 pts. included in the period 1982–1989, 97 were eligible for analyses.

SSG VIII. This was the second OS-trial, running from 1990 to 1997; 113 patients were enrolled and eligible.[10] Here, both doxorubicin and cis-Pt were given in addition to high-dose MTX preoperatively. Good responders continued the three drug combination postoperatively, whereas the poor responders were shifted to courses of standard dose ifosfamide and etoposide.

ISG/SSG I. The low incidence of OS is a strong argument for international collaboration. From 1997 to 2000 a total of 177 eligible pts. were included in ISG/SSG I conducted in collaboration with the Italian Sarcoma group.[11] A total of 57 pts. were recruited from SSG centers. The trial was undertaken to explore the effect of adding high-dose ifosfamide (15 g/m^2) to MTX, cis-Pt and doxorubicin also in the preoperative phase. Patients were scheduled for surgery at week 13, and 58% achieved a good histological response according to the Huvos grading system.

Table 1 SSG osteosarcoma clinical trials

SSG II (classical) 1982–1989
SSG VIII (classical) 1990–1997
ISG/SSG I (classical) 1997–2000
ISG/SSG II (high-risk) – closed/unpublished
SSG XIV (classical) 2001–2005
Euroboss (>40 years) – ongoing

Table 2 Summary of osteosarcoma trials conducted by the Scandinavian Sarcoma Group

Trial	No. of pts.	5 years MFS %	5 years EFS %	5 years OS %	No. LR
SSG II	97	55	54	64	5
SSG VIII	113	63	61	74	8
ISG/SSG 1	57	60	59	72	3
SSG XIV	63	69	65	77	2

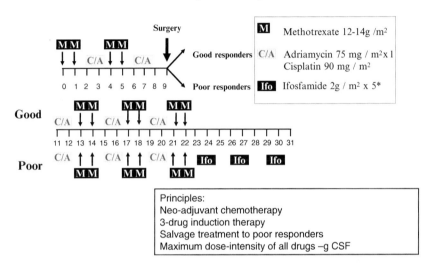

Fig. 1 Osteosarcoma protocol, SSG XIV

SSG XIV. Our last OS-trial was activated in February 2001, as an interim protocol before the start of Euramos 1. Chemotherapy was then considered standard therapy based on SSG's own experience as well as from international experience (Fig. 1). The design was based on a 3-drug combination given up-front – Mtx, Doxo, CDP (as in SSG VIII)– and not a 4-drug regimen with ifosfamide (as in ISG/SSG 1). Salvage therapy for poor responders consisted of the addition of high-dose ifosfamide and not a replacement (as in SSG VIII).

The rationale was to keep a maximum dose-intensity of all three proven active drugs. The use of g-CSF was according to ASCO guidelines, and was given to patients after a previous episode of neutropenic fever or delayed recovery. Based on hematological nadir values, a 20% dose increase of ifosfamide was recommended. However, this was feasible only in four patients.

Out of 63 eligible patients, 34 (55%) were from Sweden (6 centers), 25 (40%) from Norway (3 centers; my own Institution recruited 17 pts), three from Finland, and one from Iceland. The mean age was 16 years (8–39), with three patients above 30 years of age. The male/female ratio was 1.8. The anatomical site of the OS was the femur in 34 cases, the tibia in 15, the humerus in 6, the fibula in 4, and other sites in 3 cases; one case was with missing information.

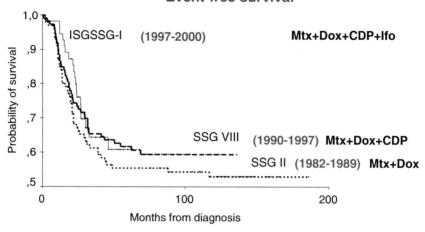

Fig. 2 Clinical trials in osteosarcoma

Results

The results from the three previously published OS-trials are illustrated in Fig. 2. A steady increase in the rate of limb salvage surgery has been documented within SSG, as in other collaborative groups, and with an acceptably low number of local recurrences (Fig. 3).

SSG II. Results from this first OS-trial of SSG showed an event-free survival, EFS, of 54%, at 5 years, a metastasis free survival, MFS of 55% and an overall survival, OS, of 64%. Only 17% of the pts. were classified as good responders, and a 25% difference in MFS between good and poor responders was demonstrated.[9] Hence, in contrast to the original report by Rosen et al., the salvage approach did not improve the outcome for the poor responders. Furthermore, the importance of MTX administration/elimination was emphasized by the correlation between serum levels of MTX and histological response.[9]

SSG VIII. In this second trial an MFS of 63%, at 5 years, an EFS of 61%, and an OS of 74% were obtained.[10] With the three active drugs given up front, 58% of the patients were classified as good responders histologically. Although some improvement in outcome was observed when compared to SSG II, the substantial increase in the percentage of good responders did not translate into a similar improvement in the outcome. Unfortunately, the poor responders were not adequately salvaged, and their inferior survival of 53% may indicate that discontinuation of the three active drugs postoperatively is not justified.

ISG/SSG I. Results from the complete trial have already been published.[11] Results for the 57 SSG-pts showed an MFS of 60%, an EFS of 59% and an OS of

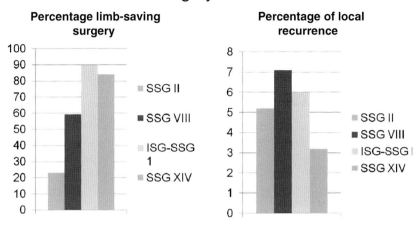

Fig. 3 Surgical development

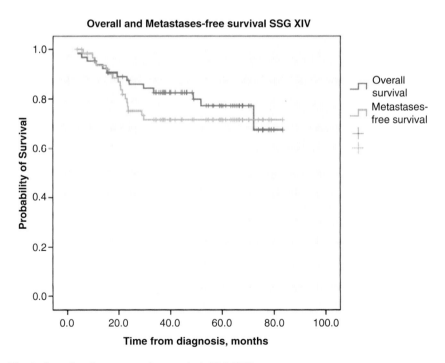

Fig. 4 Overall and metastases-free survival, SSG XIV

By response

		M+	M–	Log rank p
Poor	33pts (54%)	15	18	0.003
Good	27pts (46%)	3	24	

By gender

		M+	M–	p
Male	40	12	28	0.72
Female	23	6	17	

Metastases-free survival by Response — X: 2pts primary amp.+ 1 tox. death

Survival Functions

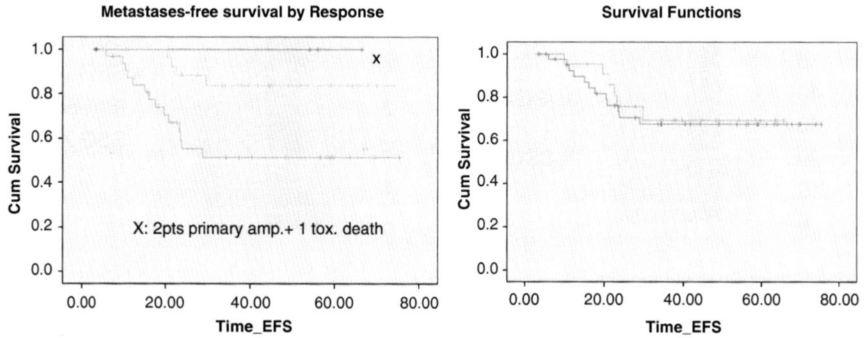

Fig. 5 Metastases-free survival by response to chemotherapy and gender, SSG XIV

72% (Table 2 and Fig. 2). Thus, the addition of high-dose ifosfamide up front seemingly improved neither histological response nor outcome.

SSG XIV. The latest clinical trial conducted by SSG over the period 2001–2005; SSG XIV enrolled 71 pts., 6 of whom had overt metastases at diagnosis and two had a non-osteosarcoma histology upon histopathological revision, leaving 63 eligible pts. As many as 30% of the patients had a longer time-course of completing chemotherapy than what was prespecified in the protocol.

The projected MFS at 5 years was 69%, EFS was 65% and OS, 77% (Fig. 4). This is, seemingly, the best outcome observed in the trials run by SSG (Table 2) with 49 patients alive; of these, 41 are in CR 1. Differences in the outcome based on response to chemotherapy and gender are presented in Fig. 5.

Out of the 63 eligible patients, 41 were alive and with NED at a mean follow up of 64 months. Eleven died of OS, three succumbed to a treatment related event (see below), one died in an accident with NED, and one patient was lost to follow up. Twenty-two events were registered: 17 metastases, 2 local recurrences (one coinciding with metastases) and 3 toxic deaths. In all three cases, it was a neutropenic fever with sepsis, in two of which a severe colitis was the suspected cause. Unfortunately, two of the patients did not receive adequate antibiotic treatment/management: one due to patient delay, and the other due to a doctor's delay. A 15 year old female patient experienced a grade IV cardiotoxicity, but has since recovered.

In SSG XIV, a limb salvage procedure was performed in 90% of the pts, compared to 27%, 58% and 88% in the three former studies. The local recurrence rate was 3% in SSG XIV compared to 5%, 7%, and 5% in the other trials, respectively (Fig. 3).

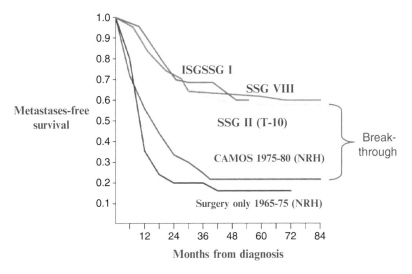

Fig. 6 Historical evolution in osteosarcoma outcome. The Scandinavian Sarcoma Group (SSG) and The Norwegian Radium Hospital (NRH) experience

Discussion

Major achievements have been obtained in the treatment of OS over the past three decades.[1,2] This was made possible through well designed clinical trials and by establishing multidisciplinary teams, by centralization and international collaboration. For SSG, the breakthrough in chemotherapy came in the early 1980s with the introduction of SSG II; but since then, improvement has been modest. Further improved management of OS has been possible through advances in imaging and orthopedic surgery. Compared to historical controls from my own Institution, the gain in survival is unquestionable (Fig. 6), in agreement with international experience.[1,2] This refinement has been made despite the lack of recent randomized controlled clinical trials. The results from the SSG OS-trials compare well with the best published data.[12] Nevertheless, additional endpoints to survival such as long term toxicity and quality of life are lacking in most published reports.

The prognosis for OS-patients with primary metastatic disease and also in cases of primary tumors located in the axial skeleton is still poor.[5,13] The scope beyond the classical OS is not often reported. Seeing adult patients as well, my Institution quite frequently experiences the many faces of this disease. The gruesome outcome of patients with axial OS, often dying from lack of local control without metastases, and the chemo resistant subclinical disease in patients presenting with overt metastases, remain two unsolved clinical challenges. The poor tolerance to toxic chemotherapy in the elderly also remains an obstacle.

The Scope Beyond the Classical OS-Patient

Table 1. Patient categories

Classical osteosarcoma	**69 patients (45%)**
Non-classical osteosarcoma	**84 patients (55%)**
Age >40 only	14
Non-extremity only	18
Metastatic only	20
Several factors	32

Fig. 7 Reprinted from the "Osteosarcoma Odyssey" (153 OS-pts, single Institution 1980-1997) From ref. 14

"Inadequate Treatment - 1"

Table 2. Patients who received inadequate treatment

	Incidence	Reason for inadequacy		
		Surgery	Chemotherapy	Both
Classical osteosarcoma	6/69 (9%)	0	6 (100%)	0
Non-classical osteosarcoma	61/84 (73%)	18 (30%)	9 (15%)	34 (56%)
Age >40 only	11/14 (79%)	0	7 (64%)	4 (36%)
Non-extremity only	12/18 (66%)	8 (67%)	1 (8%)	3 (25%)
Metastatic only	10/20 (45%)	8 (80%)	0	2 (20%)
Several factors	28/32 (88%)	2 (7%)	1 (4%)	25 (89%)

Fig. 8 Inadequate treatment defined as complete surgery with non-contaminated margins + at least 6 cycles of chemotherapy containing at least 2 of 4 active drugs

We have earlier published our single institution experience in such patients in the modern chemotherapy era,[13,14] from the Norwegian Radium Hospital. In this unselected material, it is seen that, in fact, more than 50% of the patients are not presenting with classical-OS (Fig. 7), and that inadequate treatment is very common (Fig. 8). Nonclassical OS-patients, as a group, have a dismal prognosis (Fig. 9a). However, among those few patients that did receive adequate treatment, the overall survival was approximately 50% (Fig. 9b).

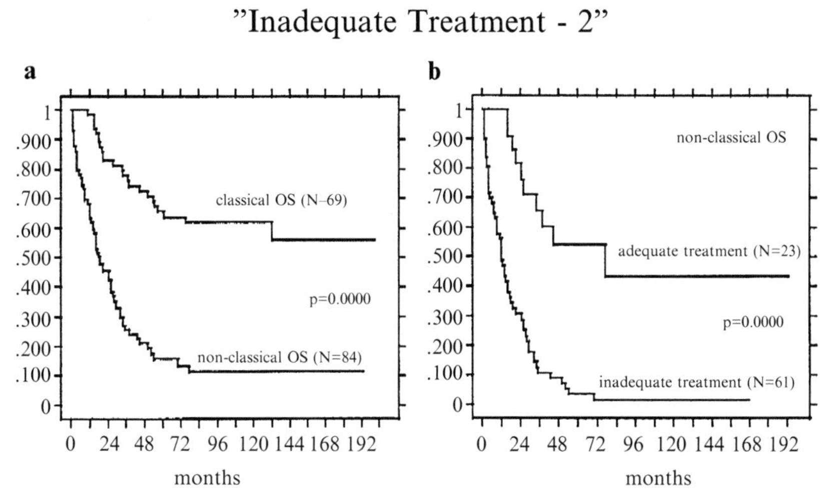

Treatment of Osteosarcoma. The Scandinavian Sarcoma Group Experience

"Inadequate Treatment - 2"

Fig. 9 Outcome in classical and non-classical osteosarcoma patients (**a**). Impact of adequate treatment or not (**b**). From Ref. 14

Conspectus

Further improvements in the outcome are unlikely with the currently available drugs. Novel treatment approaches based on knowledge of the tumor-biology of OS are required; they must be ideally individualized and more effectively tailored to combat chemo-resistant micrometastatic disease.[5,15] The continued efforts require a broad international collaboration.

References

1. Malawer MM, Helman LJ, O'Sullivan B. Sarcomas of bone. In: Devita VT, Hellman S, Rosenberg SA, eds. *Cancer – Principles & Practice of Oncology*. 7th ed. Philadelphia: Lippincott-Raven Publishers; 2005:1638-1686.
2. Souhami R, Cannon SR. Osteosarcoma. In: Peckham M, Pinedo HM, Veronesi U, eds. *Oxford Textbook of Oncology*. Oxford: Oxford University Press; 1995:1969-1976.
3. Huvos AG. Osteogenic sarcoma. In: Huvos AG, ed. *Bone Tumors. Diagnosis, Treatment and Prognosis*. Philadelphia: WB Saunders; 1991:85-155.
4. Dahlin D, Unni K. Osteogenic sarcoma of bone and its important recognizable varieties. *Am J Surg Pathol*. 1977;1:61-72.
5. Bruland OS, Pihl A. On the current management of osteosarcoma. A critical evaluation and a proposal for a modified treatment strategy. *Eur J Cancer*. 1997;33(11):1725-1731.
6. Cade S. Osteogenic sarcoma: a study based on 133 patients. *J R Coll Surg Edinb*. 1955;1:79-111.
7. Rosen G, Marcove RC, Caparros B. Primary osteogenic sarcoma: the rationale for preoperative chemotherapy and delayed surgery. *Cancer*. 1979;43:2163-2177.
8. Del Prever AB, Smeland S, Tienghi A, et al. High-risk osteosarcoma (OS): preliminary results of the ISG-SSG II protocol. *ASCO Meet Abstr*. 2005;23(26):9002.

9. Saeter G, Alvegard TA, Elomaa I, Stenwig AE, et al. Treatment of osteosarcoma of the extremities with the T-10 protocol, with emphasis on the effects of preoperative chemotherapy with single-agent high-dose methotrexate: a Scandinavian Sarcoma Group study. *J Clin Oncol.* 1991;9:1766-1775.

10. Smeland S, Muller C, Alvegard TA, et al. Scandinavian Sarcoma Group Osteosarcoma Study SSG VIII: prognostic factors for outcome and the role of replacement salvage chemotherapy for poor histological responders. *Eur J Cancer.* 2003;39:488-494.

11. Ferrari S, Smeland S, Mercury M, et al. Neoadjuvant chemotherapy with high-dose Ifosfamide, high-dose methotrexate, cisplatin, and doxorubicin for patients with localized osteosarcoma of the extremity: a joint study by the Italian and Scandinavian Sarcoma Groups. *J Clin Oncol.* 2005;23:8845-8852.

12. Alvegård TA, Rydholm A, eds. The Scandinavian Sarcoma Group. 25 years' experience. *Acta Orthop Scand.* 2004;75(Suppl 311):1-114.

13. Saeter G, Bruland OS, Follerås G, et al. Extremity and non-extremity high-grade osteosarcoma – the Norwegian Radium Hospital experience during the modern chemotherapy era. *Acta Oncol.* 1996;35(Suppl 8):129-134.

14. Sæter G and Bruland, ØS. High-grade osteosarcoma: The scope beyond the classical patient. 21-23 In: *Towards the Eradication of Osteosarcoma Metastases – An Odyssey*; 1998. ISBN 82-91929-02-5

15. Bruland ØS, Kleppe H, Sæter G, et al. Hematogenous micrometases in osteosarcoma patients. *Clin Cancer Res.* 2005;11(13):4666-4673.

Childhood Osteosarcoma: Multimodal Therapy in a Single-Institution Turkish Series

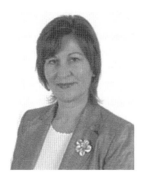

İnci Ayan, Rejin Kebudi, and Harzem Özger

Abstract Between January 1990 and December 2006, 123 patients ≤16 years with the histopathologic diagnosis of osteosarcoma were treated with a chemotherapy regimen comprising epirubicin, cisplatin, and ifosfamide. The mean follow-up time was 36 months (range 2-219 months). Among the 94 patients analyzed, 68 patients (72.3%) were alive at the time of the analysis. A total of 26 patients (13 each with nonmetastatic and metastatic disease) died; 20 of these (9 with nonmetastatic disease and 11 with metastatic disease) died of disease; 5, of chemotherapy toxicity, and 1, of nonmetastatic disease from acute nonlymphoid leukemia 13 months following the cessation of osteosarcoma therapy. The estimated 5- and 10-year Overall Survival (OS) rates for all patients were 64.7% (95% confidence interval [95% CI] 74.8-52.94%) and 62.2% (95% CI 74.6-49.9%), respectively. The Event Free Survival (EFS) rate for all patients was 51.8% (95% CI 40.2-63.4%) at both 5 and 10 years. The estimated 5- and 10-year Overall Survival (OS) rates for patients with nonmetastatic disease were 78.3% (95% CI 66.9-89.7%) and 75.1 (95% CI 62.6-87.6%), respectively; this 5-year rate was significantly superior to that of patients with metastatic disease, 13.5% (95% CI 0-30.8%) ($p<0.001$). The estimated EFS rate for patients with nonmetastatic disease was 62.4% (95% CI 49.9-79.9%) at both 5 and 10 years and was significantly better than the 5-year EFS of 6.9% (95% CI 0-19.9%) in patients with metastatic disease ($p<0.001$). Progression during preoperative chemotherapy was encountered in 18 patients (19.1%), 11 of whom had metastatic disease at diagnosis. Four patients (three with nonmetastatic disease and one with metastatic disease) underwent salvage treatment consisting of early surgical intervention and preoperative radiation. The estimated 5- and 10-year OS rates were 13% (95% CI 0-29.7%) for patients who had progression during treatment; this rate was significantly inferior to both the 5- and 10-year OS rates for patients without progressive disease, which were 78.2% (95% CI 66.1-90.4%) and 75% (95% CI 61.9-83.1%), respectively ($p<0.001$). A total of 33 patients experienced relapse and/or progression at a median time of 9 months (range 0-40 months).

İ. Ayan (✉)
Department of Pediatric Oncology, Institute of Oncology, İstanbul University, İstanbul, Turkey
e-mail: inciayan@gmail.com

Histologic response (<90% necrosis vs. ≥90%) was significantly correlated with the 5-year EFS (31% vs. 67.6%, respectively, $p=0.023$) but not with OS (57.7% vs. 76.5%, respectively, $p=0.13$). The presence of metastases at diagnosis was found to be the most significant single characteristic influencing the outcome. The rate of histologically good response to preoperative chemotherapy was 64.5%, which is comparable with the 28-85% response rates given in the literature. Our results demonstrate that the combination of epirubicin, cisplatin, and ifosfamide is an active and reasonably well-tolerated regimen for childhood osteosarcoma.

Introduction

The history of effective chemotherapy for osteosarcoma extends from the early 1970s, when promising results with doxorubicin, and with high-dose methotrexate with citrovorin factor rescue were first described by Cortes et al. and Jaffe et al., respectively.[1,2] Many investigations were conducted in the United States and Europe to identify the most effective agents, regimen, and setting for achieving the best results in terms of long-term survival. Preoperative chemotherapy using multiple agents was conceived in an effort to improve survival and make limb-salvage surgery possible. Current treatment protocols include the four most effective drugs: cisplatin, anthracyclines, ifosfamide, and high-dose methotrexate – in a pre- and postoperative setting, while en bloc excision of the primary and metastatic tumors remains the cornerstone of treatment.[3–14]

The role of radiotherapy in the management of primary osteosarcoma is limited to patients with unresectable tumors or with positive microscopic margins following surgery. Prophylactic irradiation of the lungs, as an adjuvant to primary tumor surgery, has demonstrated only marginal benefit. In metastatic or progressive disease, radiotherapy may provide palliation when given in addition to second-line chemotherapy and/or surgery.[15–19]

The results of multicentric trials reported recently from the United States and Europe indicate that about 60-75% of patients with nonmetastatic osteosarcoma of the extremity survive with no evidence of disease. Unfortunately, the prognosis of patients with axial tumors and/or metastatic tumors remains dismal.[12–14]

Increased knowledge of cytomorphological characteristics and biologic behavior, recognition of the role of pathology in determining histologic response as a prognostic criterion, and a multidisciplinary approach and multicentric studies have also contributed to improve the prognosis.

According to the Turkish Pediatric Oncology Group Tumor Registry data, the annual incidence of pediatric cancers in Turkey is 115.6 per million, and about 2,500 new cancer cases are estimated to be diagnosed in children (<16 years) each year. In 2002, data from 33 centers in Turkey demonstrated 1,073 pediatric malignant solid tumors, of which 60 (5.6%) were osteosarcoma.[20] İstanbul University Institute of Oncology (İUIO) is one of the leading centers for patients with bone and soft-tissue tumors in Turkey. Between 1990 and 1995, a total of 498 pediatric patients with solid tumors were treated, 40 (8%) of which were osteosarcoma.[21]

Childhood Osteosarcoma: Multimodal Therapy in a Single-Institution Turkish Series 321

Osteosarcoma constituted the fourth most common malignancy treated following brain tumors, lymphomas, and soft-tissue sarcomas.

With the incorporation of the Pediatric Oncology Unit at İUIO in 1989, new institutional protocols were designed for pediatric patients in accordance with the principles of what had been learned from national experiences and international studies. By 1990, a treatment protocol of pre- and postoperative multiagent chemotherapy consisting of a combination of epirubicin, ifosfamide, and cisplatin, and wide en-bloc resection of the primary tumor, was implemented for pediatric osteosarcoma patients. The main reasons for choosing a nonmethotrexate regimen were the lack of feasibility of detecting and monitoring methotrexate levels in the early 1990s and the overall expenses of high-dose methotrexate treatment.

In this chapter, we report the data for osteosarcoma patients treated between 1990 and 2006 at a single institute in Turkey using this multimodality protocol. Our goals were to identify the demographic features of this patient population, to assess the activity of the selected chemotherapy regimen in terms of clinical and histologic response, to assess the impact on outcome of combining surgery with pre- and postoperative chemotherapy, and to determine prognostic factors for patients with extremity osteosarcomas.

Patients and Methods

Patients and Pretreatment Work-Up

Patients younger than 16 years with newly diagnosed, biopsy-proven high-grade, metastatic or nonmetastatic osteosarcomas of the extremity were eligible for the study. They were referred mainly from the Department of Orthopedics, İstanbul School of Medicine, but other clinics from all over Turkey also enrolled patients. Evaluations of techniques and specimens for biopsies that had been undertaken at other clinics were performed in İstanbul School of Medicine's Departments of Orthopedics and Pathology, respectively. Biopsies were repeated when necessary, and a *tru-cut* technique was preferred for diagnostic material.

Following histopathologic diagnosis, each patient underwent a pretreatment evaluation, which included a complete medical history and physical examination with measurement of the largest diameter of the primary tumor. Initial laboratory studies and those prior to each chemotherapy cycle consisted of a complete blood count and biochemical analysis, including renal- and hepatic-function tests, alkaline phosphatase (AP) level, lactic dehydrogenase (LDH) level, electrolyte levels, urinalysis, and creatinine clearance. Patients were required to have a serum creatinine level ≤ 1.5 mg/dL, creatinine clearance ≥ 60 mL/min/1.73 m^2, a bilirubin level ≤ 1.5 mg/dL, an aspartate aminotransferase–to–alanine aminotransferase ratio $\leq 2.5 \times$ normal, a hemoglobin level of ≥ 10 g/dL, a white blood cell count $\geq 2,000$/dL, an absolute neutrophil count (ANC) $\geq 1,000$/dL, a platelet count $\geq 100,000$/dL, normal electrocardiogram findings, and an echocardiogram with an ejection fraction $\geq 60\%$.

Imaging studies at diagnosis included X-ray, computed tomography (CT), and/or magnetic resonance imaging (MRI) of the primary site, CT of the chest, and a Tc-99 whole-body bone scan.

Informed consent was obtained from each patient's legal guardian prior to study entry.

Treatment

Chemotherapy

Patients were given three 4-day cycles of epirubicin (90 mg/m^2/day intravenously on day 1), ifosfamide (1.8 g/m^2/day intravenously on days 1-3) with mesna for uroprotection (2 g/m^2/day intravenously on days 1-3), and cisplatin (100 mg/m^2/day intravenously on day 4) preoperatively. They were given the same three cycles postoperatively. The interval between cycles was designed as 3 weeks (Fig. 1). Special care was given to commence the first cycle of chemotherapy as soon as the histopathologic diagnosis was reported and to commence the subsequent cycles as soon as the blood and biochemistry parameters were eligible. Patients received the first postoperative chemotherapy cycle when the surgical wound had completely healed.

Chemotherapy was administered at full dosage whenever possible. If the neutrophil count was <1,000/dL and the platelet count was <100,000/dL at the beginning of a treatment, chemotherapy was delayed until a repeat count indicated recovery. For transient renal-function impairment, treatment was delayed until recovery of the creatinine level and creatinine clearance.

Supportive treatment included transfusions with red-blood-cell suspensions when the hemoglobin values were ≤7 g/dL and with platelet suspensions when the

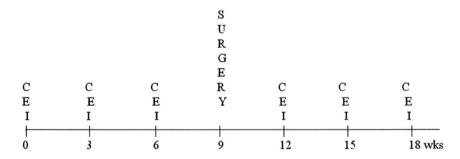

Fig. 1 The treatment schedule for the study

platelet counts were ≤30,000/dL and/or in the event of bleeding. All the blood products were irradiated with a dose of 15-20 Gy. Primary prophylaxis for neutropenia with granulocyte colony-stimulating factor (G-CSF) and prophylaxis for infection with trimethoprim sulfamethoxazole were not given, but some patients with febrile neutropenia received G-CSF (5-10 µg/kg/day) as part of their treatment and continued to receive it as secondary prophylaxis thereafter. Febrile neutropenia was treated according to institutional protocol in an algorithm designed for all pediatric cancer patients in that time period. Central venous catheters were not routinely used in pediatric patients with solid tumors.

Surgery

Surgery was carried out between 9 and 11 weeks after commencement of chemotherapy or earlier when progressive disease was detected. The time to surgery was defined as the interval between the commencement of the first preoperative chemotherapy cycle and the date of surgery. The decision for surgical intervention was made by the multidisciplinary bone-tumor team consisting of orthopedic oncologic surgeons, pediatric oncologists, radiation oncologists, radiologists, and pathologists. The aim of the surgery was to remove the tumor and achieve wide margins. Limb-salvage surgery was the treatment of choice whenever possible. Amputation/ disarticulation was restricted to those for whom limb-salvage surgery could not yield wide margins or adequate function. Reconstructive techniques used included endoprotheses, plates, external fixation, and autograft fixation. Pulmonary and bone metastases were resected, whenever possible, after primary-tumor resection.

Radiotherapy

Radiotherapy was not a part of the protocol, but a few patients who had progression during preoperative chemotherapy, who had positive microscopic margins following surgery, who could not have surgery for any reason, or who had lung metastases were given radiotherapy before, after, or instead of surgery. The dose, fractionation, and technique were decided on a case-by-case basis following the discussion of risks and benefits, at the Bone Tumor Board meeting of the Oncology Institute. A total dose of 30-50 Gy, depending on age, site, and disease status, was given for the primary tumor, and 14 Gy was given for lung metastases.

Characteristics and Variables

The following characteristics and variables were evaluated at the diagnosis and/or during the course of disease: age at diagnosis, sex, primary tumor site, size of the primary tumor with respect to maximum diameter (<10 cm vs. ≥10 cm), presence or absence of pathologic fracture, histopathologic subtype (conventional vs. other [telangiectatic, chondroblastic, or fibroblastic]), presence or absence of metastases at diagnosis, serum AP level at diagnosis (<500 U/L vs. ≥500 U/L), serum LDH level at diagnosis (<500 U/L vs. ≥500 U/L), clinical response to preoperative chemotherapy (response vs. progression), time to surgery (≤11 weeks vs. >11 weeks), type of surgery (limb salvage or amputation), surgical margins (free of tumor or showing microscopic disease), histologic response (<90% tumor necrosis vs. ≥90% necrosis), time to progression or relapse (≤1 year after completion of therapy vs. >1 year after completion), and type of progression or relapse (local, distant, or local and distant).

Assessment of Response

Clinical response to preoperative chemotherapy was defined by the regression or cessation of pain and any reduction of tumor mass determined by clinical and radiologic (CT/MRI) measurements. Progression was defined as >25% enlargement of any tumor mass or the appearance of disease at a new site and/or consistency of pain. Histologic response was categorized as good if there was ≥90% necrosis or poor if there was <90% necrosis. Patients with nonmetastatic disease were considered to be in complete remission on the date of primary tumor resection, and patients with metastases were considered to be in complete remission on the date of resection of all the tumor sites.

Toxicity

Toxic effects were graded according to National Cancer Institute Common Toxicity Criteria. For toxic effects related to cardiac, renal, audiological, or other system functions that necessitated long-term follow-up, we consulted with the relevant departments.

Statistical Analysis

Frequency tables were created and statistical analysis was performed with SPSS 16.0 software (SPSS Inc., Chicago, IL). Patient characteristics were evaluated, and the variables were correlated with survival. Overall survival (OS) was defined as the time between the date of biopsy (histologic diagnosis) and the most recent clinical visit or death from any cause. Event-free survival (EFS) was defined as the time from surgery (limb salvage or amputation) to disease recurrence or death from any cause. If recurrence or death had not occurred, patients' OS and EFS durations were censored at the patient's last contact. The Kaplan–Meier method was used to

Childhood Osteosarcoma: Multimodal Therapy in a Single-Institution Turkish Series   325

estimate the OS and EFS distributions. Differences between survival curves were analyzed using the log-rank (Mantel–Cox) test. Cox regression analysis was performed to determine the prognostic variables. P values of less than 0.05 were considered statistically significant.

Follow-Up

Patients were followed up by clinical, hematologic, biochemical, cardiological, and radiologic assessments for the primary site, metastatic sites, and lungs every 3 months for the first 2 years, every 6 months for the next 3 years, and once a year thereafter.

Results

Demographic and Disease-Related Data

Between January 1990 and December 2006, a total of 123 patients ≤16 years with the histopathologic diagnosis of osteosarcoma were referred to the Pediatric Oncology Unit, Institute of Oncology, Istanbul University. A total of 94 patients constituted the study population; 29 patients were excluded from the clinical and survival analyses. These patients were those who were referred for a second opinion ($n=18$), who had axial tumors ($n=2$), or whose histopathologic review revealed mesenchymal chondrosarcoma ($n=4$) or small-cell osteosarcoma ($n=5$). Among the 94 eligible patients, there were 53 male and 41 female patients (male-to-female ratio 1.29) with an age range of 5-16 years (median 13 years). Patient and disease characteristics are shown in Table 1. The most common primary tumor site was the femur (46 patients, or 48.9%), followed by the tibia (29 patients, or 30.8%). The most common histopathologic osteosarcoma subtype was conventional osteosarcoma (57 patients, or 60.6%). Seventy-seven patients (81.9%) had nonmetastatic disease; among the 17 patients (18.1%) with metastases, the sites of metastasis were the lung, bone, and lymph nodes.

Treatment Results

Preoperative Chemotherapy and Response

Of 77 patients with nonmetastatic disease, 75 had one to five cycles of preoperative chemotherapy. Forty-eight patients (62.3%) received three cycles of preoperative

Table 1 Patient and Disease Characterstics

Characteristic	Number of patients	%
Total	94	100
Sex		
Male	53	56.4
Female	41	43.6
Primary tumor location		
Femur (distal)	46 (43)	48.9 (45.7)
Tibia (proximal)	29 (26)	30.8 (27.6)
Fibula (proximal)	7 (7)	7.4 (7.4)
Humerus (proximal)	6 (5)	6.4 (5.3)
Radius (proximal)	2 (1)	2.1 (1.1)
Ulna (proximal)	2 (1)	2.1 (1.1)
Multifocal	2	2.1
Primary tumor diameter		
≥10cm	49	52.1
<10cm	45	47.9
Pathologic fracture		
yes	12	12.8
NO	82	87.2
Histopathologic subtype		
Conventional	57	60.6
Chondroblastic	17	18.1
Plemorphic	8	8.5
Fibroblastic	7	7.4
Telangiectatic	5	5.3
Disease stage		
Nonmetastatic	77	81.9
Metastatic	17	18.1
Metastatic sites (n=17)		
Lung	7	41.2
Lung = bone	6	35.3
Bone	2	11.8
Lymph node	2	11.8
Serum LDH (n=78)		
≥ 500 U/L	22	28.2
≥ 500 U/L	56	71.8
Missing data	16	
Serum AP (n=78)		
≥ 500 U/L	25	32.1
≥ 500 U/L	53	67.9
Missing data	16	

chemotherapy. Because of delay for surgical needs, 20 (26%) received four cycles, and three (3.9%) received five cycles of preoperative chemotherapy. Four patients had fewer than three cycles of chemotherapy, and two patients had no preoperative chemotherapy because of primary amputation due to a huge tumor mass. Clinical and radiologic response was achieved in 67 (89.3%) of 75 patients who received preoperative chemotherapy. Progressive disease was identified in seven patients (9.3%). There was one toxicity-related death, due to febrile neutropenic septicemia, before surgery.

All 17 patients with metastatic disease received preoperative chemotherapy (four had less than three cycles, four had three cycles, five had four cycles, and four had greater than or equal to five cycles). Five patients (29.4%) responded, 11 (64.7%) had progressive disease, and 1 died because of a septic biopsy wound during the second neutropenic period.

For the whole series, 92 patients (97.9%) received preoperative chemotherapy, and the response rate was 78.3%. Data for the preoperative chemotherapy cycles and clinical response are summarized in Tables 2 and 3, respectively.

Surgery

A total of 86 patients (91.5%) underwent surgery. Surgery could not be performed in eight patients (five with metastatic disease and three with nonmetastatic disease) because of progression of disease or treatment complications. Seventy-eight of the 86 (90.7%) had limb salvage. There were 68 patients with nonmetastatic disease and 10 patients with metastatic disease in this group. Reconstruction was per-

Table 2 Chemotherapy cycles received before surgery

Patient group	Number of cycles					
	0	1-2	3	4	≥ 5	Total
Pts. with nonmetastatic disease	2*	4	48	20	3	77
Pts. with metastatic disease	0	4	4	5	4	17
Whole series (%)	2 (2.1)	8 (8.5)	52 (55.3)	25 (26.6)	7 (7.4)	94 (100)

* Patiets with primary amputation

Table 3 Clinical Response to Preoperative Chemotherapy in 90 Patients*

Patient group	Clinical response	Clinical progression	Total
Pts. with nonmetastatic disease (%)	67 (90.5)	7 (9.5)	74 (100)
Pts. with metastatic disease (%)	5 (31.2)	11 (68.8)	16 (100)
Whole series (%)	72 (80.0)	18 (20.0)	90 (100)

* Four patients excluded from "Clinical response to preoperative chemotherapy" evaluation: These are the 2 patients with nonmetastatic disease who had primary amputation and the other 2 patients (one of each nonmetastatic and metastatic group) who died of therapy related toxicity.

formed by endoprosthetic replacement (using a Kotz, Turkish Musculoskeletal Tumor Society [TMTS], or Finn system, or a Modular Universal Tumor and Revision System [MUTARS]) in 41 patients (52.6%). Biologic reconstruction techniques were used for 37 patients (47%); these included vascularized fibula grafting ($n=24$), fibular transposition or reposition and grafting ($n=2$), osteosynthesis with plate ($n=1$), fresh-frozen allograft implantation ($n=3$), autoclavized graft implantation ($n=2$), destruction epiphysiodesis and external fixator placement ($n=3$), and rotationplasty ($n=2$). Amputation/disarticulation was performed in eight patients (9.3%). Six of these patients had nonmetastatic disease, and two had metastatic disease. Two patients in the nonmetastatic group had primary amputation outside Istanbul University, due to huge tumor masses. Patients underwent surgery between 3 and 38 weeks after the commencement of chemotherapy The mean time until surgery was 10 weeks. A total of 50 patients had surgery before 11 weeks, while 34 patients had surgery after 11 weeks.

Histopathologic evaluation confirmed that 73 patients (84.9%) had wide surgical margins that were free of tumor cells. In seven patients, microscopic disease was detected, and in six patients, no information about margins existed. The surgical characteristics and histopathologic data for the 86 patients who underwent surgery are given in Table 4.

Table 4 Surgical Characteristics and Histopathologic Data for 86 Patients Who Underwent Surgery

Characteristic	Number of patients	%
Surgery	86	100
Limb salvage	78	90.7
Amputation	8	9.3
Disease stage for limb-salvage patients (n=78)		
Nonmetastatic	68	87.2
Metastatic	10	12.8
Type of limb salvage (n=78)		
Endoprosthetics	41	52.6
Biologic reconstruction	37	47.4
Disease stage for patients with amputation (n=8)		
Nonmetastatic (primary amput.)	6 (2)	
Metastatic	2	
Time to surgery 0 wks (primary amput.)	2	2.3
≤ 11 wks	50	58.1
> 11 wks	34	39.5
Surgical margins (n=80)[1]		
Free of tumor	73	91.2
Microscopic disease	7	8.8
Histopathologic response (n=76)[2]		
≥ 90% necrosis	49	64.5
< 90% necrosis	27	35.5

[1]Missing data for surgical margins in 6 patients
[2]Missing data for histopathologic response in 10 patients

Radiotherapy

Although it was not a part of the treatment protocol, ten patients received radiotherapy. Among these, seven patients with disease progression received radiotherapy following preoperative chemotherapy either to improve tumor control so that limb-salvage surgery could be performed or to palliate symptoms. Limb salvage was possible for four of the patients who had preoperative radiotherapy. Postoperative radiotherapy was given to three patients who had microscopically positive surgical margins. Radiotherapy doses ranged between 30 and 50 Gy with standard fractionation.

Postoperative Chemotherapy

Seventy-nine patients (84%) completed a total of six cycles of chemotherapy. Six patients suffered from drug toxicity and progression and could not receive all six cycles.

Granulocyte Colony Stimulating Factor (G-CSF) was given to 53% of patients for secondary prophylaxis and/or treatment of febrile neutropenia.

Histologic Response

Histologic response, which was defined in terms of proportion of tumor necrosis, was reported in 76 of 86 patients who underwent surgery. Forty-nine (64.5%) of these had $\geq$90% necrosis and were considered to have had a good response. Twenty-seven of the 76 had <90% necrosis and were considered to have had a poor response.

Treatment Complications

Chemotherapy Dose Intensity and Acute Toxicity

A pilot study was conducted to assess the dose intensity and acute toxicity of the chemotherapy regimen used during 1990-1996.[22] Thirty-one patients were included, and 147 chemotherapy cycles were analyzed. Results of the dose-intensity analysis yielded a relative dose intensity of 82% for cisplatin, 82% for epirubicin, and 83.6% for ifosfamide. Relative dose intensity was defined as the ratio of received dose to planned dose divided by the ratio of received duration to planned duration, expressed as a percentage of the intended intensity. Planned dose intensity was defined as the total amount of drug planned divided by intended duration, expressed in mg/m^2/day. Received dose intensity was defined as the total amount of drug given divided by received duration, expressed in mg/m^2/day. Received duration was defined as the number of days between day 1 of the first cycle and day 1 of the last cycle plus 21 days. Planned duration was defined as the product of 21 days by cycle number.[23] There was no significant difference between the received dose intensity for patients who received G-CSF (82.4%) and that for patients who did not receive G-CSF (81.6%).

Patients were evaluated for hematologic toxicity on days 1, 10, 14, and 16 of each cycle. Anemia was identified in 72% of cycles; in 39% of these, the anemia was grade 3 or 4 and required red-blood-cell transfusions. Grade 3 or 4 neutropenia occurred in 48% of cycles, and hospitalization for febrile neutropenia was required in 12% of these. Three episodes of documented sepsis developed, two of which resulted in death. Thrombocytopenia occurred in 30% of cycles, and multiple transfusions were given to the patients. Genitourinary toxicity was observed in 26% of cycles; one of the patients had to have continued hemodialysis. In spite of intensive antiemetic treatment, severe nausea and vomiting occurred in 56% of cycles. Ten episodes of hypocalcemic and/or hypomagnesemic tetany and four episodes of seizures associated with hyponatremia occurred. There was no cardiotoxicity during the pilot study; however, one patient had acute myocardial toxicity and died just after completing six cycles of chemotherapy. Hepatic toxicity was minimal. Ototoxicity was not assessed regularly, but two patients demonstrated severe hearing loss. Overall, the acute toxicity was serious, and intensive supportive treatment was required in order to treat the complications and to maintain the dose intensity.[22]

Acute and Late Complications of Surgery

Postsurgical acute- and late-complication data were available in 68 patients. Acute complications were infection in four patients, fibular paralysis in three patients, extension/flexion deficit in three patients, limb-length discrepancy in two patients, and graft fracture in one patient. The most frequent late complication was implant failure (fracture), which was detected in seven patients. Late complications of surgery were extension/flexion deficit in five patients, loosening at the prosthesis in five patients, length discrepancy in three patients, periprosthetic fracture in two patients, periprosthetic infection in two patients, wound infection in two patients, pseudoarthrosis in one patient, and ankle valgus deformity in one patient.

Outcome, Survival, and Prognosis

The mean follow-up time was 36 months (range 2-219 months). Among the 94 patients analyzed, 68 patients (72.3%) were alive at the time of the analysis. A total of 26 patients (13 each with nonmetastatic and metastatic disease) had died; 20 of these (9 with nonmetastatic disease and 11 with metastatic disease) died of disease, 5 (2 with nonmetastatic and 3 with metastatic disease) died of chemotherapy toxicity and 1 with nonmetastatic disease died from acute non lymphoid leukemia 13 months following the cessation of osteosarcoma therapy.

The estimated 5- and 10-year OS rates for all patients were 64.7% (95% confidence interval [95% CI] 74.8-52.94%) and 62.2% (95% CI 74.6-49.9%), respectively. The EFS rate for all patients was 51.8% (95% CI 40.2-63.4%) at both 5 and 10 years. The OS and EFS rates of the whole series are shown in Fig. 2.

The estimated 5- and 10-year OS rates for patients with nonmetastatic disease were 78.3% (95% CI 66.9-89.7%) and 75.1% (95% CI 62.6-87.6%), respectively; this 5-year rate was significantly superior to that of patients with metastatic disease, 13.5% (95% CI 0-30.8%) ($p<0.001$) (Fig. 3). The estimated EFS rate for patients with nonmetastatic disease was 62.4% (95% CI 49.9-79.9%) at both 5 and 10 years, significantly better than both the 5 and 10 year EFS of 6.9% (95% CI 0-19.9%) in patients with metastatic disease ($p<0.001$)

Progression during preoperative chemotherapy was encountered in 18 patients (20%), 11 of whom had metastatic disease at diagnosis. Four patients (three with nonmetastatic disease and one with metastatic disease) underwent salvage treatment consisting of early surgical intervention and preoperative radiation. The estimated 5- and 10-year OS rates were both 13% (95% CI 0-29.7%) for patients who had progression during preoperative treatment; this rate was significantly inferior to both

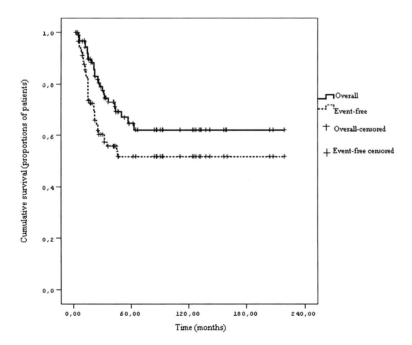

Fig. 2 Overall and event free survival rates of all patients

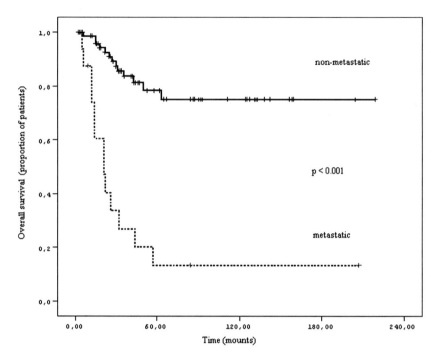

Fig. 3 Overall survival curves of metastatic and non-metastatic patients

the 5- and 10-year OS rates for patients without progressive disease, which were 78.2% (95% CI 66.1-90.4%) and 75% (95% CI 61.9-83.1%), respectively ($p<0.001$).

A total of 33 patients experienced relapse and/or progression at a median time of 9 months (range 0-40 months) from the first day of chemotherapy. These 33 patients include the 18 who had progression before surgery. The sites of relapse were local in 2 patients, pulmonary in 13 patients, both local and pulmonary in 6 patients, multiple (including local, pulmonary, bone, cranial, intraspinal, hepatic, intra-abdominal, adrenal gland, and intracardiac) in 10 patients, isolated bone in 1 patient, and cranial in 1 patient. Fourteen of these patients underwent salvage treatment consisting of metastasectomies, second- and third-line chemotherapy, and radiotherapy. Patients who had complete resection for metastatic foci were given high-dose methotrexate (12 g/m^2/day) with citrovorum rescue every 2-3 weeks for 4-6 cycles. Patients who had incomplete resection for metastasis received high-dose methotrexate (12 g/m^2/day) alternating with high-dose ifosfamide (14 g/m^2/day) every 3-4 weeks for 1 year or until progression. The estimated 5-year OS rate for patients who had progression or relapse was 34.8% (95% CI 14.6-55.0%), whereas the 5- and 10-year OS rate was 97.4% (95% CI 92.5-100%) for patients who had no progression or relapse. Patients who had progression or relapse during the first year had an inferior 5-year OS rate of 17.8% (95% CI 0-39.4%), compared with 61.7% (95% CI 26.4-97.0%) for patients who had relapses later ($p=0.015$).

Childhood Osteosarcoma: Multimodal Therapy in a Single-Institution Turkish Series 333

Table 5 Correlation of Overall and Event-Free Survival with Variables

Variable	OS rate (5 years)	p value	EFS rate (5 years)	p value
All patients	64.7%		51.8%	
Disease stage				
Nonmetastatic	78.3%	< 0.001	62.4%	< 0.001
Metastatic	13.5%		6.9%	
Response to preop chemotherapy				
Clinical response	78.2%	< 0.001		
Progression	13%			
Histologic response				
< 90% necrosis	57.7%	0.13	31.0%	0.023
≥ 90% necrosis	76.5%		67.6%	
Time to relapse or progression				
≤ 1 year	17.8%	0.015		
> 1 year	41.1%			
Age at diagnosis				
< 10 years	100%	0.08	77.8%	0.21
≥ 10 years	61.5%		48.8 5	
Sex				
Male	67.7%	0.5	54.3%	0.81
Female	53.6%		47.8%	
Primary tumor diameter				
<10 cm	64.9%	0.99	40.7%	0.28
≥10 cm	61.8%		59.1%	
Pathologic fracture				
Yes	68.2%	0.54	43.6%	0.39
No	70.1%		57.9%	
Histopathologic subtype				
Conventional	61.6%	0.23	49.9%	0.81
Other	69.0%		51.4%	
Serum AP				
< 500 U/L	65.0%	0.97	50.9%	0.36
≥ 500 U/L	57.0%		43.5%	
Serum LDH				
< 500 U/L	63.3%	0.15	49.8%	0.13
≥ 500 U/L	49.0%		37.7%	
Time to surgery				
≤ 11 weeks	66.4%	0.71	56.2%	0.94
> 11 weeks	69.9%		50.1%	
Type of surgery				
Limb salvage	69.3%	0.57	57.6%	0.7
Amputation	65.6%		45.0%	

Histologic response (<90% necrosis vs. ≥90%) was significantly correlated with 5-year EFS (31% vs. 67.6%, respectively, $p=0.023$) but not with OS (57.7% vs. 76.5%, respectively, $p=0.13$). The statistical workup did not yield any significant correlation between the OS and EFS rate and age ($p=0.08$), sex ($p=0.50$), tumor size ($p=0.99$), pathologic fracture ($p=0.54$), histopathologic subtype ($p=0.23$), serum AP level ($p=0.97$), LDH level ($p=0.15$), or time until surgery ($p=0.71$). The presence of metastases at diagnosis was found to be the most significant single characteristic influencing outcome. Correlation of survival with patient and treatment characteristics is given in Table 5.

Discussion

In this report, we describe the 17-year experience of a single institution in Turkey with 94 pediatric patients treated with a prospectively designed protocol for extremity osteosarcoma. Every effort was given to offer a multidisciplinary diagnostic and treatment approach to each patient. A relatively short (18-week) and easily applicable three-drug chemotherapy regimen, given three cycles before and three cycles after surgery, was used in this study, in order to maximize compliance and to lessen the patients' treatment expenses, length of hospital stay, and number of days away from home. The activity of all the three drugs chosen was well documented in previously published literature.[1,4–7,9–14]

Almost all of the major treatment protocols used for children with osteosarcoma include high-dose methotrexate in addition to the above-mentioned drug combinations. The main reasons for adopting a nonmethotrexate regimen were the lack of feasibility of detecting and monitoring methotrexate levels in the early 1990s and the overall expenses of high-dose methotrexate treatment.

The 5-year OS and EFS rates of the present series were 64.7% and 51.8%, respectively. At presentation, 18.1% of patients had metastatic disease, and OS and EFS rates for these patients were dismal. However, the 5-year OS and EFS rates for patients with nonmetastatic disease were 78.3% and 62.4%, respectively, which were comparable with most of the previously published national and international studies in which high-dose methotrexate was a part of the multidrug regimen.[8,10,12,14,24–28]

The three-drug regimen used in the study described here and the increased experience of orthopedic tumor surgeons on our treatment team enabled the performance of limb-salvage surgery in 90.7% of the patients. Excluding the two patients who underwent primary amputation, only six patients (four with nonmetastatic disease at presentation and two with metastatic disease) underwent amputation. The three studies from Turkey reported amputation rates of 4%, 11%, and 65%.[25–27] In addition to the high rate of limb salvage, surgical margins free of tumor cells were reported in about 85% of patients in our study. Thus, a remarkable improvement in terms of disease control and quality of life was achieved with the application of skillful surgical techniques and multimodality treatment in our patients.

The role of radiotherapy in the multimodality treatment of osteosarcoma has been examined in some studies. Radiotherapy has had a significant benefit in patients with unresectable primary sites and has been helpful in improving the ability to perform limb-salvage surgery.[15–19] In the current study, a total of 10 patients received radiotherapy. In four of seven patients who had progression during preoperative chemotherapy, radiotherapy facilitated limb-salvage surgery, and three of these patients became long-term survivors (survival times 60, 209, and 216 months). Although our experience is very limited due to the small sample size, this observation suggests a benefit of radiotherapy that deserves further investigation in the context of a prospective study.

Several patient and disease characteristics have been studied for determining the prognosis of osteosarcoma. Among these, the presence of metastases at diagnosis has been cited as the most powerful prognostic factor.[10,13,28–30] Our results strongly correlate with this finding as the 5-year OS and EFS rates of patients with metastatic disease at diagnosis were significantly ($p<0.001$) lower than those for patients with nonmetastatic disease. Other characteristics such as age, sex, size of primary tumor, presence of pathologic fracture, histopathologic subtype, and serum AP and LDH levels at diagnosis have also been reported as prognostic factors in some studies.[10,12,13,28–31] None of these variables were found to be an important prognostic factor in our series.

Response to preoperative chemotherapy has been shown to be a strong prognostic indicator, as reported in several studies.[11,13,30,32] Our data demonstrated a significant correlation ($p<0.001$) between clinical response to preoperative chemotherapy and survival. In terms of histologic response, no statistically significant difference was found between necrosis ratio and OS rate ($p=0.13$), but the correlation between necrosis ratio and EFS rate was statistically significant ($p=0.023$). A reasonable explanation for these results might be the cut-off value of 90% for the necrosis ratio. In general, it is accepted that a better prognosis is associated with a Huvos grade of IV (100% necrosis) or a proportion of fewer than 2% residual viable tumor cells in the resected material. However, this finding is not very useful clinically because histologic tumor response is not known before the institution of therapy; furthermore, modification of therapy in poor responders fails to have an impact on outcome. Thus, we believe that new strategies are needed to predict prior to therapy which patients will respond well and which poorly.

A limited number of previous studies exploring the clinical implications as well as prognostic value of biologic markers in our pediatric patients with osteosarcoma yielded no correlation with patient outcome. These markers were immunoreactivity of tumor cells to proliferating cell nuclear antigen (PCNA),[33] serum levels of CD44,[34] and serum levels of intercellular adhesion molecule 1 (ICAM 1).[35] Other treatment-related variables, including type of surgery and time from start of chemotherapy until surgery, did not demonstrate any impact on prognosis.

As an oncologic principle, patients with late relapses do better than patients with early relapses. In our series, the outcome of patients who had late relapses (>1 year after surgery) was significantly better ($p=0.015$) than that of patients who had early relapses (≤1 year). About one-third of our patients who had relapses underwent salvage treatment using multimodality approaches. This result is comparable with those of several studies in which 30-40% of relapsed patients survived more than 5 years after relapse.[36–38] With the improvement of outcome, metastases to less com-

336 İ. Ayan et al.

mon sites, including cranial, [39] intraspinal, hepatic, adrenal gland, intra-abdominal, cardiac, and lymph node were encountered in addition to pulmonary metastases, were encountered in our patients. New treatment strategies are needed to prevent or overcome disease recurrence.

In summary, a 17-year multidisciplinary teamwork approach has improved our understanding and experience in childhood osteosarcoma. Although about two-thirds of children with extremity osteosarcoma were cured of their disease, numerous aspects of care for this patient population need to be addressed. These include the implementation of cooperative multicenter studies in Turkey, with tumor registry, data collection, protocols for each discipline (surgery, pathology, chemotherapy, and radiotherapy), pathology and diagnostic radiology revision, robust statistics, tissue banking, molecular studies, prosthetic device centers, rehabilitation and gain-function centers, long-term follow-up clinics, education and employment of long-term survivors, and hospice centers for end-stage patients. With the expected conditions and with shared information from international studies, we hope to improve the curability of pediatric osteosarcoma patients.

References

1. Cortes EP, Holland JF, Wang JJ, et al. Doxorubicin in disseminated osteosarcoma. *JAMA*. 1972;221:1132-1138.
2. Jaffe N, Farber S, Traggis D, et al. Favorable response of metastatic osteogenic sarcoma to pulse high-dose methotrexate with citrovorum rescue and radiation therapy. *Cancer*. 1973;31:1367-1373.
3. Jaffe N, Frei E III, Traggis D, et al. Weekly high-dose methotrexate-citrovorum factor in osteogenic sarcoma: presurgical treatment of primary tumor and of overt pulmonary metastases. *Cancer*. 1977;39:45-50.
4. Ochs JJ, Freeman AI, Douglass HO Jr, et al. cis-Dichlorodiammineplatinum (II) in advanced osteogenic sarcoma. *Cancer Treat Rep*. 1978;62:239-245.
5. Rosen G, Marcove RC, Caparros B, et al. Primary osteogenic sarcoma: the rationale for preoperative chemotherapy and delayed surgery. *Cancer*. 1979;43:2163-2177.
6. Marti C, Kroner T, Remagen W, et al. High-dose ifosfamide in advanced osteosarcoma. *Cancer Treat Rep*. 1985;69:115-117.
7. Jaffe N, Robertson R, Ayala A, et al. Comparison of intra-arterial cis-diamminedichloroplatinum II with high-dose methotrexate and citrovorum factor rescue in the treatment of primary osteosarcoma. *J Clin Oncol*. 1985;3:1101-1104.
8. Winkler K, Beron G, Delling G, et al. Neoadjuvant chemotherapy of osteosarcoma: results of a randomised cooperative trial (COSS-82) with salvage chemotherapy based on histological tumor response. *J Clin Oncol*. 1988;6:329-337.
9. Winkler K, Bielac S, Delling G, et al. Effect of intra-arterial versus intravenous cisplatin in addition to systemic doxorubicin, high-dose methotrexate, and ifosfamide on histologic tumor response in osteosarcoma (study COSS-86). *Cancer*. 1990;66:1703-1710.
10. Hudson M, Jaffe MR, Jaffe N, et al. Pediatric osteosarcoma: therapeutic strategies, results and prognostic factors derived from a 10-year experience. *J Clin Oncol*. 1990;8:1988-1997.
11. Meyers PA, Gorlick R, Heller G, et al. Intensification of preoperative chemotherapy for osteogenic sarcoma: results of the Memorial Sloan-Kettering (T12) protocol. *J Clin Oncol*. 1998;16:2452-2458.

12. Bacci G, Ferrari S, Bertoni F, et al. Long-term outcome for patients with nonmetastatic osteosarcoma of the extremity treated at the Institute Ortopedico Rizzoli according to the Instituto Ortopedico Rizzoli/Osteosarcoma-2 protocol: an updated report. *J Clin Oncol.* 2000;18:4016-4027.
13. Bielack SS, Kempf-Bielack B, Delling G, et al. Prognostic factors in high-grade osteosarcoma of the extremities or trunk: an analysis of 1,702 patients treated on neoadjuvant Cooperative Osteosarcoma Study Group protocols. *J Clin Oncol.* 2002;20:776-790.
14. Meyers PA, Schwartz C, Krailo M, et al. Osteosarcoma: a randomized, prospective trail of the addition of ifosfamide and/or muramyl tripeptide to cisplatin, doxorubicn, and high-dose methotrexate. *J Clin Oncol.* 2005;23:2004-2011.
15. Pochanugool L, Subhadharaphandou T, Dhanachai M, et al. Prognostic factors among 130 patients with osteosarcoma. *Clin Orthop Relat Res.* 1997;345:206-214.
16. Ozaki T, Flege S, Kevric M, et al. Osteosarcoma of the pelvis: experience of the Cooperative Osteosarcoma Study Group. *J Clin Oncol.* 2003;21:334-341.
17. Claude L, Rousmans S, Carrie C, et al. Standards and options for the use of radiation therapy in the management of patients with osteosarcoma. Update 2004. *Cancer Radiother.* 2005;9:104-121.
18. Dincbas FO, Koca S, Mandel NM, et al. The role of preoperative radiotherapy in nonmetastatic high-grade osteosarcoma of the extremities for limb-sparing surgery. *Int J Radiat Oncol Biol Phys.* 2005;62:820-828.
19. Mahajan A, Woo SY, Kornguth DG, et al. Multimodality treatment of osteosarcoma: radiation in a high-risk cohort. *Pediatr Blood Cancer.* 2008;50:976-982.
20. Kutluk T. First national pediatric cancer registry in Turkey: a Turkish Pediatric Oncology Group (TPOG) study XXXVI. International Pediatric Oncology (SIOP) Meeting, Oslo, Norway, Sept 16–19, 2004. *Med Pediatr Oncol.* 2004;43:146.
21. Topuz E, Ayan I. University of İstanbul, Institute of Oncology: Center Presentation. *Pediatr Hematol Oncol.* 1997;14:315-321.
22. Ayan İ, Kebudi R, Görgün Ö, et al. Assessment of acute toxicity following cisplatin, epirubicin with/without ifosfamide in children with bone sarcomas. *Med Pediatr Oncol.* 1996;27:315.
23. Ornadel D, Souhami RL, Whelan J, et al. Doxorubicin and cisplatin with granulocyte colony-stimulating factor as adjuvant chemotherapy for osteosarcoma: phase II trial of the European Osteosarcoma Intergroup. *J Clin Oncol.* 1994;12:1842-1848.
24. Fuchs N, Bielack SS, Epler D, et al. Long-term results of the co-operative German-Austrian-Swiss osteosarcoma study group's protocol COSS 86 of intensive multidrug chemotherapy and surgery for osteosarcoma of the limbs. *Ann Oncol.* 1998;9:893-899.
25. Kantar M, Çetingül N, Azarsız S, et al. Treatment results of osteosarcoma of the extremity in children and adolescents at Ege University Hospital. *Pediatr Hematol Oncol.* 2002;19:475-482.
26. Özkan A, Celkan T, Apak H, et al. Neoadjuvant chemotherapy for osteogenic sarcoma: results of a single Institute from Turkey. *Australas J Cancer.* 2006;5:325-328.
27. Varan A, Yazıcı N, Aksoy C, et al. Treatment results of pediatric osteosarcoma: twenty-year experience. *J Pediatr Orthop.* 2007;27:241-246.
28. Petrilli AS, de Camargo B, Filho VO, et al. Results of the Brazilian Osteosarcoma Treatment Group Studies III and IV: prognostic factors and impact on survival. *J Clin Oncol.* 2006;24:1161-1168.
29. Provisor AJ, Ettinger LJ, Nachman JB, et al. Treatment of non-metastatic osteosarcoma of the extremity with preoperative and postoperative chemotherapy: a report from the Children's Cancer Group. *J Clin Oncol.* 1997;15:76-84.
30. Davis AM, Bell RS, Goodwin PJ. Prognostic factors in osteosarcoma: a critical review. *J Clin Oncol.* 1994;12:423-431.
31. Özger H, Eralp L, Atalar AC, et al. Survival analysis and the effects of prognostic factors in patients treated for osteosarcoma. *Acta Orthop Traumatol Turc.* 2007;41:211-219.

32. Rosen G, Caparros B, Huvos AG, et al. Preoperative chemotherapy for osteogenic sarcoma: selection of postoperative adjuvant chemotherapy based on the response of the primary tumor to preoperative chemotherapy. *Cancer.* 1982;49:1221-1230.
33. Tokuç G, Doĭan Ö, Ayan İ, et al. Prognostic value of proliferating cell nuclear antigen (PCNA) immunostaining in pediatric osteosarcoma. *Int J Pediatric Hematol Oncol.* 1998;5:373-377.
34. Kebudi R, Ayan İ, Yasasever V, et al. Are serum levels of CD44 relevant in children with pediatric sarcomas? *Pediatr Blood Cancer.* 2006;1:62-65.
35. Kebudi R, Ayan İ, Yasasever V, et al. Serum levels of intercellular adhesion molecule 1 (ICAM 1) in pediatric solid tumors. *J Tumor Marker Oncol.* 2004;19:107-112.
36. Pastorino LI, Gasparini M, Tavecchio L, et al. The contribution of salvage surgery to the management of childhood osteosarcoma. *J Clin Oncol.* 1991;9:1357-1362.
37. Saeter G, Hoie J, Stenwig AE, et al. Systemic relapse of patients with osteogenic sarcoma. Prognostic factors for long term survival. *Cancer.* 1995;75:1084-1093.
38. Ferrari S, Bricolli A, Mercuri M, et al. Postrelapse survival in osteosarcoma of the extremities: prognostic factors for long-term survival. *J Clin Oncol.* 2003;21:710-715.
39. Kebudi R, Ayan İ, Görgün Ö, et al. Brain metastasis in pediatric extracranial malignant tumors. *J Neurooncol.* 2005;71:43-48.

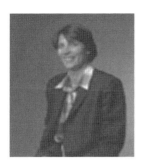

International Collaboration is Feasible in Trials for Rare Conditions: The EURAMOS Experience

N. Marina, S. Bielack, J. Whelan, S. Smeland, M. Krailo, M.R. Sydes, T. Butterfass-Bahloul, G. Calaminus, and M. Bernstein

Abstract The introduction of multi-agent chemotherapy dramatically improved the outcome for patients with osteosarcoma. However, we appear to have reached a plateau in outcome with a long-term event-free survival of 60-70%. Therefore, detection of further improvements will likely require larger numbers of patients. This goal is best achieved via randomized clinical trials (RCTs) requiring large-scale cooperation and collaboration.

With this background, four multinational groups agreed on the merits of collaboration: Children's Oncology Group (COG), Cooperative Osteosarcoma Study Group (COSS), European Osteosarcoma Intergroup (EOI) and Scandinavian Sarcoma Group (SSG); they designed a study to determine whether altering postoperative therapy based on histological response improved the outcome. The study design includes a backbone of 10 weeks of preoperative therapy using MAP (methotrexate, Adriamycin and cisplatin). Following surgery, patients are stratified according to histological response. Patients classified as "good responders" (≥90% necrosis) are randomized to continue MAP or to receive MAP followed by maintenance pegylated interferon, while "poor responders" (<90% necrosis) are randomized to either continue MAP or to receive MAPIE (MAP+ifosfamide, etoposide). The design includes the registration of 1,400 patients over 4 years as well as the evaluation of quality of life using two different instruments. The group has established an efficient infrastructure to ensure successful implementation of the trial. This has included the EURAMOS Intergroup Safety Desk, which has established an international system for SAE, SAR and SUSAR reporting to the relevant competent authorities and ethics committees for each participating country. The group has also developed trial site monitoring and data center audits with funding from the European Science Foundation (ESF). The ESF has also funded three training courses to familiarize institutional staff with the requirements of multinational GCP trials.

N. Marina (✉)
Stanford University Medical Center, 1000 Welch Road, Suite 300, Palo Alto, CA, 94304-1812, USA
e-mail: Neyssa.marina@stanford.edu

We have established a successful collaboration, and as of February 2008, 901 patients have been enrolled (COG 448; COSS 226; EOI 181; SSG 46) from 249 institutions in 16 different countries. As expected, 80% of the patients are <18 years of age, and accrual into the Quality of Life sub-study is proceeding as planned with 90% of the subjects agreeing to participate.

International awareness is increasing and procedures for applicant countries wishing to join the collaboration have been implemented. Details about EURAMOS can be found at www.euramos.org. International trials in rare diseases are practicable with appropriate funding, planning and support. Although the implementation of such trials is difficult and time consuming, it is a worthwhile effort to rapidly complete RCTs and identify interventions that will improve the outcome of all osteosarcoma patients.EURAMOS-1 is the fastest accruing osteosarcoma trial and is already the largest osteosarcoma study conducted.

Introduction

The outcome of patients with osteosarcoma before the use of multi-agent chemotherapy was poor with 2-year survivals of 15-20%.[1-4] Presumptively, most patients have microscopic metastases at the time of diagnosis as 80-90% will develop lung metastases following treatment with surgical resection or radiotherapy alone.[1-4] The most active chemotherapy agents include cisplatin,[5-7] doxorubicin,[8,9] high-dose methotrexate,[10-12] and most recently ifosfamide,[13] alone or combined with etoposide.[14]

Although uncontrolled trials conducted in the 1970s suggested that systemic chemotherapy improved the outcome for osteosarcoma patients when compared with historical controls,[15-19] some investigators were concerned that the improved outcome resulted from patient selection, earlier diagnosis (staging with computerized tomography became a prevalent practice) or improved surgical techniques.[20,21] In the early 1980s, investigators at the Mayo Clinic carried out the first randomized trial of adjuvant chemotherapy for osteosarcoma,[22] and reported a disease-free survival of 40% with no difference among treatment groups, suggesting that the natural history had changed. Two subsequent randomized prospective studies established the importance of adjuvant chemotherapy in the treatment of patients with nonmetastatic osteosarcoma.[23,24] Patients receiving chemotherapy had a significant survival advantage over those treated with surgery and observation (2-year disease-free survival of 66% vs. 17%).[24] The outcome for patients treated with observation in both the studies was no different from that of patients treated in the 1970s, confirming that the natural history of the disease had not changed.

The concept of preoperative chemotherapy introduced by Rosen,[25,26] offered the possibility of developing an endoprosthesis for limb-salvage procedures, as well as early treatment of micrometastases. It has also allowed for the evaluation of histological response to chemotherapy, which has been demonstrated to be a strong predictor of the subsequent outcome.[25,27-29] At the time, a concern with this approach was that delayed tumor removal would lead to chemotherapy resistance. A randomized Pediatric Oncology Group (POG) study, however, revealed an equivalent outcome for patients receiving adjuvant and neo-adjuvant therapy.[30] The use of preoperative therapy, therefore, has become the standard of care, given its advantages of facilitating tumor removal and allowing evaluation of response to chemotherapy. With this approach, most modern series report 3-year event-free survivals (EFS) of 60-70%.[31-34]

Although investigators at Memorial Sloan Kettering Cancer Center initially reported improved outcome when postoperative therapy was adjusted following a poor- histologic response,[35] longer follow-up failed to confirm this improvement,[36] and other studies have been unable to reproduce an improved outcome by altering postoperative therapy based on histological response.[27,28] The intensification of preoperative therapy increases the number of good responders (≥90% necrosis); however, in this setting, the association between histologic response and subsequent outcome is weakened.[37] Although histologic response remains a strong prognostic factor, attempts to improve outcome by increasing the number of good responders or adjusting the postoperative therapy for poor responders have been largely unsuccessful.

Contemporary Results

Although multi-agent chemotherapy has dramatically improved the outcome for patients with localized osteosarcoma, most contemporary series report similar results, [31-34] suggesting that we may have reached a plateau in outcome with 3-year EFS of approximately 70%.

The Cooperative Osteosarcoma Study Group (COSS), including centers in Germany, Austria and Switzerland, has performed a series of studies since 1977, incorporating chemotherapy and surgical resection. These investigators have also recognized the value of histologic response[38] and in COSS-82, attempted to spare patients the toxicity of cisplatin, by administering it only as salvage treatment following a poor histologic response.[27] Unfortunately, this approach was unsuccessful, and patients with a poor histological response had a 4-year metastases-free survival of 41%. The investigators concluded that it was not possible to omit the upfront use of the very active drug pair cisplatin and doxorubicin. COSS's best results, which were reported in a single-arm, nonrandomized study are based on the use of methotrexate, cisplatin, doxorubicin and ifosfamide, with a 10-year survival of 71%.[39] Although the administration of intra-arterial cisplatin offers multiple theoretical advantages,[40,41] a nonrandomized COSS study showed no advantage in the administration of intra-arterial cisplatin in the context of multi-agent chemotherapy.[42]

Meanwhile, many investigators have participated in a series of studies over the last 20 years under the auspices of the European Osteosarcoma Intergroup (EOI): the core of researchers has come from the United Kingdom, Belgium and the

Netherlands, supplemented with researchers from various other countries. Based on a randomized controlled trial, which did not show a survival advantage compared with the three-drug therapy (methotrexate, cisplatin and doxorubicin),[43,44] EOI investigators have used a backbone of six cycles of cisplatin and doxorubicin as their control treatment. Intensification of therapy by administering this combination every 2 weeks did not improve the outcome.[33] Even though the two drug regimen has not been proven inferior to other regimens in a randomized setting, clinicians in EOI were open to adopting a different backbone therapy for future studies. This was because other groups in Europe and the US have reported superior results using regimens including other agents such as methotrexate and ifosfamide.[32,39,45]

The Scandinavian Sarcoma Group (SSG) comprises the Scandinavian countries (Denmark, Finland, Iceland, Norway and Sweden) with a population of about 25 million people. Since 1979, SSG has performed three nonrandomized studies of neo-adjuvant chemotherapy for high-grade osteosarcoma localized to the extremities. The first, SSG II, was based on the Memorial Sloan Kettering's T-10 protocol and included high-dose methotrexate and doxorubicin in the preoperative chemotherapy regimen, and as expected, there was a difference in outcome between good and poor responders.[46] The second osteosarcoma trial (SSG VIII) utilized a three-drug combination of methotrexate, doxorubicin and cisplatin prior to definitive surgery, and the estimated 5-year overall survival was 74%, a 9% improvement compared to the SSG II study.[47] With a relatively low dose of ifosfamide (4.5 g/m^2), the combination of ifosfamide and etoposide failed to improve the outcome for poor histological responders, and the data did not support the strategy used with discontinuation and exchange of all the drugs used preoperatively in the salvage regimen. The following trial, the first joint Italian/Scandinavian study (ISG/SSG I), was undertaken to explore the benefit of adding high-dose ifosfamide (15 g/m^2) to the induction therapy. However, the survival rates in this study were similar to those obtained with the four-drug regimens using standard-dose ifosfamide. [34]

The North American Children's Oncology Group (COG) was formed by the merger of the Children's Cancer Group (CCG), National Wilm's Tumor Study Group (NWTSG), Intergroup Rhabdomyosarcoma Study Group (IRSG), and the POG, in 2000. COG recently reported the results of INT 0133, a 2×2 factorial design study examining whether the addition of ifosfamide and/or muramyl tripeptide (MTP), a biological agent, to a control regimen of methotrexate, doxorubicin, cisplatin (MAP) improved the outcome. The results of INT 0133 have been published, and neither treatment offered an EFS benefit when added to MAP individually. However, there appeared to be a synergistic effect when ifosfamide and MTP were administered together.[32] In an analysis of the trial with a longer period of follow-up, the statistical synergistic interaction between ifosfamide and MTP on risk for EFS-event has diminished.[48] Additionally, the addition of MTP appears to improve overall survival of the combined cohorts. However, longer follow-up continues to show no significant difference in EFS for MTP-treated patients. Although this study suggests that the addition of ifosfamide to standard three drug therapy does not improve the outcome, ifosfamide was administered sub-optimally, the effect of MTP was limited, and it has not been made commercially available. Thus, COG still considers MAP to be the most suitable chemotherapy regimen in this disease.

The standard treatment for patients with nonmetastatic osteosarcoma would definitely include the use of cisplatin and doxorubicin with the addition of high-dose methotrexate by various groups including COG, COSS, SSG and the ISG. Ifosfamide has been included in the treatment of patients by COSS, SSG and the ISG.

Because the survival of patients with osteosarcoma appears to have reached a plateau at approximately 70%, efforts to detect further improvements in outcome may benefit from randomized controlled trials involving a large number of patients. This will provide for the requisite number of *events* that will allow us to detect clinically, relevant differences in survival among treatment arms. This goal can be achieved realistically only through international collaboration. With this goal in mind, investigators from COSS, EOI, SSG and COG agreed on the merits of collaboration. The power of such collaboration lies in the ability to conduct large trials with rapid and effective accrual resulting in the investigation of new treatment strategies. Therefore, European and North American investigators agreed to collaborate in the EURAMOS-1 study (www.EURAMOS.org).

EURAMOS

The EURAMOS investigators recognize the prognostic importance of histological response for patients with osteosarcoma, as well as the controversies surrounding the reports of improved outcome by altering postoperative therapy based on that response.[27,28,35,36] The EURAMOS investigators have, therefore, chosen this large trial to definitively answer this question in the context of neoadjuvant MAP chemotherapy. Their aim is to investigate whether it is feasible to improve outcome for patients whose tumors show either a good or a poor histological response by adding other agents to the postoperative treatment schedule. The investigators agreed on a control arm using cisplatin, doxorubicin and high-dose methotrexate (MAP) and have chosen to address two different questions for patients whose tumors show good or poor histological response to preoperative chemotherapy. Those whose tumors show a poor response are randomized between MAP, and MAP with the addition of ifosfamide and etoposide (MAPIE). Those patients whose tumors show a good response are randomized between MAP, and MAP followed by maintenance therapy with pegylated interferon-α (MAPifn) (see Fig. 1).

Rationale for Ifosfamide and Etoposide

A nonrandomized POG study incorporating ifosfamide with standard multi-agent chemotherapy and surgical resection for patients with clinically detectable metastases

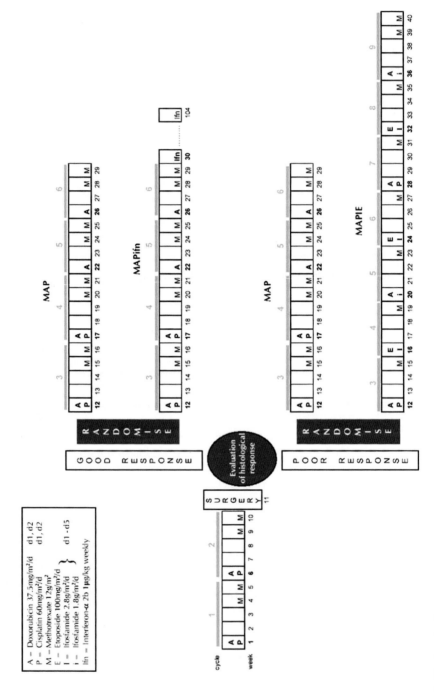

Fig. 1 Treatment schema

at diagnosis resulted in a 5-year (EFS) of 47%.[49] In addition, the EFS for patients treated by COSS investigators using a regimen incorporating ifosfamide, was superior to the standard three-drug regimen with a 10-year survival of 71%.[39,42] Although there was no evidence of a difference in outcome for patients treated in INT-0133 with the addition of ifosfamide, that study prescribed ifosfamide at a lower dose than that given for the treatment of patients with metastatic osteosarcoma.[14,49] Additionally, a number of studies have suggested the presence of a dose-response for ifosfamide, with more favorable responses at dosages >11 g/m^2. Furthermore, a recent trial from POG incorporating high-dose ifosfamide and etoposide into the standard three-drug regimen for patients with initially metastatic osteosarcoma reported a response rate of 62% and a 2-year EFS of 45%.[14] Also, an earlier non-randomized Italian trial reported that the addition of ifosfamide and etoposide to standard chemotherapy for patients with a poor histological response resulted in an outcome similar to that reported for patients with a good histological response.[50] This would suggest that the combination of ifosfamide and etoposide has significant activity and might improve the outcome for patients with a poor histological response.

Thus, although a few studies have evaluated the role of altering postoperative therapy in poor histological responders, the role of high-dose ifosfamide and etoposide in this setting has not been investigated in a large randomized controlled trial. It is important to determine in a randomized controlled trial whether this drug combination improves the outcome for patients with poor histological response since the combination has significant activity in metastatic osteosarcoma, but it also results in added hematological and nonhematological toxicity. This trial proposes a randomization for patients with a poor histological response to chemotherapy, to postoperative therapy with either MAP or MAPIE.

Rationale for Maintenance Therapy with Pegylated Interferon

Evaluation of the patients treated with INT-0133 reveals that 45% had a good histological response (<10% viable tumor) to preoperative therapy, and these patients have a 3-year EFS of 75%. The additional toxicity of ifosfamide and etoposide is difficult to justify in this group. In this subset of patients, EURAMOS investigators have agreed to evaluate the role of interferon-α. Interest in the value of this agent in osteosarcoma has continued since the in vitro effects of interferon-α on osteosarcoma cells were demonstrated more than 20 years ago. Observations since have consistently supported the growth-inhibiting effect in osteosarcoma, both in cell lines and animal models. [51–53] This provides the rationale for the use of this agent in maintaining clinical remission for patients.

As yet, interferon-α has not been widely tested in clinical trials in osteosarcoma although its role as maintenance treatment in other tumors has been extensively studied.[54,55] Most information on the role of this agent in osteosarcoma comes from a Scandinavian series where 64 consecutive patients were treated with interferon-α as a single adjuvant to surgery. Sixty-nine percent (69%) of patients remained in complete remission during the treatment period 1985-1990 (19 patients).[56] A pegylated preparation of interferon-α with an extended half life offers particular advantages, less frequent administration and higher dose delivery.[57] The tolerability of this preparation has now been demonstrated, and there is extensive data on the tolerability of interferon-α in children treated for chronic hepatitis.[58,59] Patients with a good histologic response are randomized to the administration of interferon following the standard three drug therapy (MAP vs. MAPifn).

Rationale for Quality of Life (QL) Evaluation

The medical late effects of therapy have been studied extensively in children[60] and young adults. However, the impact of these late effects on the quality of life (QL) of patients has been less studied, particularly in patients with osteosarcoma.[61–64] Since osteosarcoma survivors are particularly vulnerable to medical late effects because of the intensity of their treatment (surgery and chemotherapy), EURAMOS investigators have agreed to evaluate QL in osteosarcoma patients treated in a single randomized trial. Since no single instrument is approved for use in all countries for all ages, investigators have agreed on the use of one instrument for adults (>16 years; EORTC QLQ-C30) and two different instruments for pediatric patients (Peds QOL in Europe[65] & Peds QL in North America[66]). This is because there is no pediatric QL measure that has been validated in all the participating countries. The assessment of QL within EURAMOS-1 will allow more global concerns to be addressed, for example, whether QL is affected by surgical factors, patient maturity (emotional and physical), and other characteristics such as gender, and site of primary tumor.[67]

Regulatory Concerns

Although the EURAMOS-1 trial offers the opportunity to answer two clinically relevant questions relatively quickly, there were a number of regulatory concerns that the trial investigators and the governing bodies had to overcome for the initiative to be successful. At first, authorities in the United States required that each non-North American participating institution obtain a Federal Wide Assurance number. Recognizing the burdensome nature of this demand, it was subsequently moderated to a request that the overall European sponsor, the Medical Research Council (MRC) in the United Kingdom, renew its Federal Wide Assurance. In addition, the safety desk in Muenster, Germany, had already obtained a Federal Wide Assurance number, to allow COG participation in one stratum of the Euro-E.W.I.N.G.99 study. The Muenster (KKS) safety desk then assumed the responsibility of serving as the EURAMOS-1 Intergroup Safety Desk as well. Data collection for the study as a whole was centralized at the MRC Clinical Trials Unit for analysis, first processed by each participating group's representative Data Centre. This facilitated monthly data transfer, in particular, as the transfer of data from European patients to centers outside of Europe may be problematic under current European guidelines. Common data elements and a common data base were agreed upon by all the investigators and data centers. Therefore, individual participating groups could use their own standard case report forms and collect additional data, if they so chose.

The trial investigators acknowledged the need for an Independent Data Monitoring Committee (IDMC) to provide independent oversight of accumulating trial data.[68,69] The incorporation of so many investigators into EURAMOS-1 posed problems for the establishment of an IDMC, however. Although within the COG, the guidelines allow for investigators not participating in a clinical trial to be members of an IDMC, international guidelines preclude IDMC membership of investigators who are actively participating in the trial. We were able to organize a DMC with members from countries not participating in EURAMOS and from a small number of North American institutions not participating in the study, or investigators no longer actively engaged in clinical oncology practice.

Although the COG had experience with quality control through on-site audits across North America, the COSS, EOI and SSG had not previously been routinely required to conduct such audits. Therefore, we agreed on the establishment of audit procedures to be performed by the various data centers for their own institutional members. In addition, we established procedures for the data centers to audit each other. Moreover, the safety desk has recently undergone audit by the German research infrastructure for clinical trials, the KKS network. We have also successfully developed guidelines for the participation of other European countries that were not part of the original group in which EURAMOS was implemented.

One of the other areas that provided challenges for the study committee was standardization of therapy administration guidelines. As the protocol prescribes doxorubicin to a cumulative dose of 450 mg/m^2, cardioprotection was an important consideration. During the original discussions, we agreed to exclude dexrazoxane from the therapy administration guidelines as this agent was not licensed in Europe at the time. In order to accommodate this while acknowledging the possible long term effects of doxorubicin therapy, North American investigators agreed to administer doxorubicin via continuous infusion as it is the standard of care in Germany. Additionally, as pegylated interferon is not licensed for this indication, we had to cross-file on the investigational new drug (IND) application of Schering Plough with the United States Food and Drug Administration (FDA). Schering Plough agreed to provide the drug free of charge, and we developed procedures for drug delivery across the different countries.

Although the concept and protocol document were developed relatively quickly (within 18 months), it took about 4 years to get the final protocol activated in all the countries. Activation of the trial in Europe was greatly facilitated by the fact that EURAMOS-1 was chosen to receive financial and networking support as part of the European Science Foundation's (ESF) Pan -European Clinical Trial (ECT) EUROCORES. The COSS group was the first group able to activate the study in

April 2005, while COG was the last group to active the study in December 2005. The trial is accruing very well and has now become the largest osteosarcoma trial. There have been three training courses supported by the ESF to help investigators and data managers become comfortable with data collection in the EURAMOS-1 trial. Additionally, that body also supported a sarcoma meeting in Stuttgart, Germany (December 2006) where the political impact of the European Clinical Trials Directive (EC 2001/20) on the care of children with cancer was discussed and publicized.

Accrual: Registration and Randomization

The planned accrual target overall for EURAMOS-1 is to randomize 1,260 patients: 567 good responders and 693 poor responders. We anticipated that we would need to register 1,400 patients in order to randomize 1,260 patients, the attrition primarily because of disease progression and also parent or patient refusal of the postdefinitive surgery randomization. Based on experience in previous trials, the four participating groups expected to ultimately randomize 400 patients per year and accrual was expected to take around 4 years. Accrual in the first 2 years has proceeded as planned. As of February 2008, there are 901 patients enrolled (see Fig. 2). Randomization rates, however, are lower than we had anticipated. The nonrandomization rate had been underestimated at 10% based on prior experience, but the

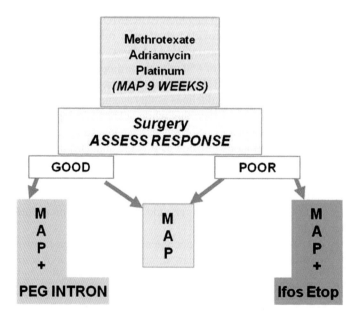

Fig. 2 EURAMOS accrual

delayed randomization after the patient has received approximately 12 weeks of preoperative chemotherapy has likely contributed to the increased nonrandomization rate. We have looked into the reasons for nonrandomization, and we feel that some of these can be addressed in the future. All groups will be implementing measures to try to minimize the number of patients who are not randomized. Enrollment to the trial may need to be extended to obtain the planned 1,260 randomized patients. We will be monitoring this closely.

Conspectus and Conclusion

International collaboration is feasible, particularly for rare diseases where patient numbers limit our ability to answer clinically relevant questions quickly. Although the implementation of such trials is difficult and time consuming, it is worthwhile to complete randomized clinical trials (RCTs) as quickly as possible so that we can provide robust answers that will improve the outcome of such patients. The EURAMOS trial serves as a model for patients with osteosarcoma and is already the largest osteosarcoma trial. The procedures established may facilitate future international trials in osteosarcoma, and perhaps in other rare diseases or subcategories of disease, as well.

In Europe, EURAMOS-1 is supported by the ESF and managed by the European Medical Research Councils Unit (EMRC) under the EUROCORES Programme European Clinical Trials (ECT), through contract No. ERASCT-2003-980409 of the European Commission, DG Research, FP6. Financial support for EURAMOS was generously granted by Fonds National de la Recherche Scientifique (FNRS), Belgium; Fonds voor Wetenschappelijk Onderzoek (FWO), Belgium; Forskningsstyrelsen, Denmark; Suomen Akatemia, Finland; Deutsche Forschungsgemeinschaft (DFG), Germany; Deutsche Krebshilfe, Germany; Semmelweis Foundation, Hungary; Norges forskningsråd (NFR), Norway; ZonMw The Netherlands Organisation for Health Research and Development, The Netherlands; Schweizer Pädiatrisch Onkologische gruppe SPOG, Switzerland;and MRC, United Kingdom.

Bibliography

1. Friedman MA, Carter SK. The therapy of osteogenic sarcoma: current status and thoughts for the future. *J Surg Oncol.* 1972;4:482-510.
2. Marcove RC, Mike V, Hajek JV, et al. Osteogenic sarcoma under the age of twenty-one. A review of one hundred and forty-five operative cases. *J Bone Joint Surg [Am].* 1970;52:411-423.
3. Weinfeld MS, Dudley HR. Osteogenic sarcoma: a follow-up study of the ninety-four cases observed at the Massachusetts General Hospital from 1920 to 1960. *J Bone Joint Surg [Am].* 1962;44A:269-276.

4. Dahlin DC, Coventry MB. Osteogenic sarcoma. A study of six hundred cases. *J Bone Joint Surg [Am]*. 1967;49:101-110.
5. Ochs JJ, Freeman AI, Douglass HO, et al. cis-Dichlorodiammineplatinum (II) in advanced osteogenic sarcoma. *Cancer Treat Rep*. 1978;62:239-245.
6. Gasparini M, Rouesse J, van Oosterom A, et al. Phase II study of cisplatin in advanced osteogenic sarcoma. European Organization for Research on Treatment of Cancer: Soft Tissue and Bone Sarcoma Group. *Cancer Treat Rep*. 1985;69:211-213.
7. Baum ES, Gaynon P, Greenberg L, et al. Phase II trail cisplatin in refractory childhood cancer: Children's Cancer Study Group Report. *Cancer Treat Rep*. 1981;65:815-822.
8. Pratt CB, Shanks EC. Doxorubicin in treatment of malignant solid tumors in children. *Am J Dis Child*. 1974;127:534-536.
9. Cortes EP, Holland JF, Wang JJ, et al. Amputation and adriamycin in primary osteosarcoma. *N Engl J Med*. 1974;291:998-1000.
10. Jaffe N, Frei E, Traggis D, et al. Adjuvant methotrexate and citrovorum-factor treatment of osteogenic sarcoma. *N Engl J Med*. 1974;291:994-997.
11. Pratt CB, Howarth C, Ransom JL, et al. High-dose methotrexate used alone and in combination for measurable primary or metastatic osteosarcoma. *Cancer Treat Rep*. 1980;64:11-20.
12. Pratt CB, Roberts D, Shanks EC, et al. Clinical trials and pharmacokinetics of intermittent high-dose methotrexate-"leucovorin rescue" for children with malignant tumors. *Cancer Res*. 1974;34:3326-3331.
13. Harris MB, Cantor AB, Goorin AM, et al. Treatment of osteosarcoma with ifosfamide: comparison of response in pediatric patients with recurrent disease with patients previously untreated– A Pediatric Oncology Group study. *Med Pediatr Oncol*. 1995;24:87-92.
14. Goorin AM, Harris MB, Bernstein M, et al. Phase II/III trial of etoposide and high-dose ifosfamide in newly diagnosed metastatic osteosarcoma: a pediatric oncology group trial. *J Clin Oncol*. 2002;20:426-433.
15. Pratt C, Shanks E, Hustu O, et al. Adjuvant multiple drug chemotherapy for osteosarcoma of the extremity. *Cancer*. 1977;39:51-57.
16. Pratt CB, Rivera G, Shanks E, et al. Combination chemotherapy for osteosarcoma. *Cancer Treat Rep*. 1978;62:251-257.
17. Sutow WW, Gehan EA, Dyment PG, et al. Multidrug adjuvant chemotherapy for osteosarcoma: interim report of the Southwest Oncology Group Studies. *Cancer Treat Rep*. 1978;62:265-269.
18. Sutow WW, Sullivan MP, Fernbach DJ, et al. Adjuvant chemotherapy in primary treatment of osteogenic sarcoma. A Southwest Oncology Group study. *Cancer*. 1975;36:1598-1602.
19. Goorin AM, Frei E III, Abelson HT. Adjuvant chemotherapy for osteosarcoma: a decade of experience. *Surg Clin North Am*. 1981;61:1379-1389.
20. Taylor WF, Ivins JC, Pritchard DJ, et al. Trends and variability in survival among patients with osteosarcoma: a 7-year update. *Mayo Clin Proc*. 1985;60:91-104.
21. Carter SK. Adjuvant chemotherapy in osteogenic sarcoma: the triumph that isn't? *J Clin Oncol*. 1984;2:147-148.
22. Edmonson JH, Green SJ, Ivins JC, et al. A controlled pilot study of high-dose methotrexate as postsurgical adjuvant treatment for primary osteosarcoma. *J Clin Oncol*. 1984;2:152-156.
23. Eilber F, Giuliano A, Eckardt J, et al. Adjuvant chemotherapy for osteosarcoma: a randomized prospective trial. *J Clin Oncol*. 1987;5:21-26.
24. Link MP, Goorin AM, Miser AW, et al. The effect of adjuvant chemotherapy on relapse-free survival in patients with osteosarcoma of the extremity. *N Engl J Med*. 1986;314:1600-1606.
25. Rosen G, Marcove RC, Caparros B, et al. Primary osteogenic sarcoma: the rationale for preoperative chemotherapy and delayed surgery. *Cancer*. 1979;43:2163-2177.
26. Rosen G, Murphy ML, Huvos AG, et al. Chemotherapy, en bloc resection, and prosthetic bone replacement in the treatment of osteogenic sarcoma. *Cancer*. 1976;37:1-11.
27. Winkler K, Beron G, Delling G, et al. Neoadjuvant chemotherapy of osteosarcoma: results of a randomized cooperative trial (COSS-82) with salvage chemotherapy based on histological tumor response. *J Clin Oncol*. 1988;6:329-337.

International Collaboration is Feasible in Trials for Rare Conditions 351

28. Provisor AJ, Ettinger LJ, Nachman JB, et al. Treatment of nonmetastatic osteosarcoma of the extremity with preoperative and postoperative chemotherapy: a report from the Children's Cancer Group. *J Clin Oncol*. 1997;15:76-84.

29. Bacci G, Picci P, Ruggieri P, et al. Primary chemotherapy and delayed surgery (neoadjuvant chemotherapy) for osteosarcoma of the extremities. The Istituto Rizzoli Experience in 127 patients treated preoperatively with intravenous methotrexate (high versus moderate doses) and intra-arterial cisplatin. *Cancer*. 1990;65:2539-2553.

30. Goorin AM, Schwartzentruber DJ, Devidas M, et al. Presurgical chemotherapy compared with immediate surgery and adjuvant chemotherapy for nonmetastatic osteosarcoma: Pediatric Oncology Group Study POG-8651. *J Clin Oncol*. 2003;21:1574-1580.

31. Bielack SS, Kempf-Bielack B, Delling G, et al. Prognostic factors in high-grade osteosarcoma of the extremities or trunk: an analysis of 1,702 patients treated on neoadjuvant cooperative osteosarcoma study group protocols. *J Clin Oncol*. 2002;20:776-790.

32. Meyers PA, Schwartz CL, Krailo M, et al. Osteosarcoma: a randomized, prospective trial of the addition of ifosfamide and/or muramyl tripeptide to cisplatin, doxorubicin, and high-dose methotrexate. *J Clin Oncol*. 2005;23:2004-2011.

33. Lewis IJ, Nooij MA, Whelan J, et al. Improvement in histologic response but not survival in osteosarcoma patients treated with intensified chemotherapy: a randomized phase III trial of the European Osteosarcoma Intergroup. *J Natl Cancer Inst*. 2007;99:112-128.

34. Ferrari S, Smeland S, Mercuri M, et al. Neoadjuvant chemotherapy with high-dose Ifosfamide, high-dose methotrexate, cisplatin, and doxorubicin for patients with localized osteosarcoma of the extremity: a joint study by the Italian and Scandinavian Sarcoma Groups. *J Clin Oncol*. 2005;23:8845-8852.

35. Rosen G, Caparros B, Huvos AG, et al. Preoperative chemotherapy for osteogenic sarcoma: selection of postoperative adjuvant chemotherapy based on the response of the primary tumor to preoperative chemotherapy. *Cancer*. 1982;49:1221-1230.

36. Meyers PA, Heller G, Healey J, et al. Chemotherapy for nonmetastatic osteogenic sarcoma: the Memorial Sloan-Kettering experience. *J Clin Oncol*. 1992;10:5-15. [see comments].

37. Meyers PA, Gorlick R, Heller G, et al. Intensification of preoperative chemotherapy for osteogenic sarcoma: results of the Memorial Sloan-Kettering (T12) protocol. *J Clin Oncol*. 1998;16:2452-2458.

38. Winkler K, Beron G, Kotz R, et al. Neoadjuvant chemotherapy for osteogenic sarcoma: results of a Cooperative German/Austrian study. *J Clin Oncol*. 1984;2:617-624.

39. Fuchs N, Bielack SS, Epler D, et al. Long-term results of the co-operative German-Austrian-Swiss osteosarcoma study group's protocol COSS-86 of intensive multidrug chemotherapy and surgery for osteosarcoma of the limbs. *Ann Oncol*. 1998;9:893-899.

40. Jaffe N, Knapp J, Chuang VP, et al. Osteosarcoma: intra-arterial treatment of the primary tumor with cis-diammine-dichloroplatinum II (CDP). Angiographic, pathologic, and pharmacologic studies. *Cancer*. 1983;51:402-407.

41. Jaffe N, Robertson R, Ayala A, et al. Comparison of intra-arterial cis-diamminedichloroplatinum II with high-dose methotrexate and citrovorum factor rescue in the treatment of primary osteosarcoma. *J Clin Oncol*. 1985;3:1101-1104.

42. Winkler K, Bielack S, Delling G, et al. Effect of intra-arterial versus intravenous cisplatin in addition to systemic doxorubicin, high-dose methotrexate, and ifosfamide on histologic tumor response in osteosarcoma (study COSS-86). *Cancer*. 1990;66:1703-1710.

43. Souhami RL, Craft AW, Van der Eijken JW, et al. Randomised trial of two regimens of chemotherapy in operable osteosarcoma: a study of the European Osteosarcoma Intergroup. *Lancet*. 1997;350:911-917.

44. Bramwell VH, Burgers M, Sneath R, et al. A comparison of two short intensive adjuvant chemotherapy regimens in operable osteosarcoma of limbs in children and young adults: the first study of the European Osteosarcoma Intergroup. *J Clin Oncol*. 1992;10:1579-1591.

45. Bacci G, Ferrari S, Delepine N, et al. Predictive factors of histologic response to primary chemotherapy in osteosarcoma of the extremity: study of 272 patients preoperatively treated with high-dose methotrexate, doxorubicin, and cisplatin. *J Clin Oncol*. 1998;16:658-663.

46. Saeter G, Alvegard TA, Elomaa I, et al. Treatment of osteosarcoma of the extremities with the T-10 protocol, with emphasis on the effects of preoperative chemotherapy with single-agent high-dose methotrexate: a Scandinavian Sarcoma Group study. *J Clin Oncol*. 1991;9:1766-1775.
47. Smeland S, Muller C, Alvegard TA, et al. Scandinavian Sarcoma Group Osteosarcoma Study SSG VIII: prognostic factors for outcome and the role of replacement salvage chemotherapy for poor histological responders. *Eur J Cancer*. 2003;39:488-494.
48. Meyers PA, Schwartz CL, Krailo MD, et al. Osteosarcoma: the addition of muramyl tripeptide to chemotherapy improves overall survival – a report from the Children's Oncology Group. *J Clin Oncol*. 2008;26:633-638.
49. Harris MB, Gieser P, Goorin AM, et al. Treatment of metastatic osteosarcoma at diagnosis: a Pediatric Oncology Group Study. *J Clin Oncol*. 1998;16:3641-3648.
50. Bacci G, Picci P, Ferrari S, et al. Primary chemotherapy and delayed surgery for nonmetastatic osteosarcoma of the extremities: results of 164 patients preoperatively treated with high doses of methotrexate followed by cisplatin and doxorubicin. *Cancer*. 1993;72:3227-3238.
51. Strander H, Einhorn S. Effect of human leukocyte interferon on the growth of human osteosarcoma cells in tissue culture. *Int J Cancer*. 1977;19:468-473.
52. Brosjo O, Bauer HC, Brostrom LA, et al. Influence of human alpha-interferon on four human osteosarcoma xenografts in nude mice. *Cancer Res*. 1985;45:5598-5602.
53. Bauer HC, Brosjo O, Strander H. Comparison of the growth inhibiting effect of natural and recombinant interferon-alpha on human osteosarcomas in nude mice. *J Interferon Res*. 1987;7:365-369.
54. Allen IE, Ross SD, Borden SP, et al. Meta-analysis to assess the efficacy of interferon-alpha in patients with follicular non-Hodgkin's lymphoma. *J Immunother*. 2001;24:58-65.
55. Bjorkstrand B, Svensson H, Goldschmidt H, et al. Alpha-interferon maintenance treatment is associated with improved survival after high-dose treatment and autologous stem cell transplantation in patients with multiple myeloma: a retrospective registry study from the European Group for Blood and Marrow Transplantation (EBMT). *Bone Marrow Transplant*. 2001;27:511-515.
56. Strander H, Bauer HC, Brosjo O, et al. Long-term adjuvant interferon treatment of human osteosarcoma. A pilot study. *Acta Oncol*. 1995;34:877-880.
57. Bukowski R, Ernstoff MS, Gore ME, et al. Pegylated interferon alfa-2b treatment for patients with solid tumors: a phase I/II study. *J Clin Oncol*. 2002;20:3841-3849.
58. Bunn S, Kelly D, Murray KF. Safety, efficacy and pharmacokinetics of interferon alfa-2b and ribavirin in children with chronic hepatitis C. *J Hepatol*. 2000;32:763.
59. Wozniakowska-Gesicka T, Wisniewska-Ligier M, Kups J, et al. Influence of interferon-alpha therapy on the count and function of T lymphocytes in children with chronic hepatitis C. *Pol Merkur Lekarski*. 2001;11:344-347.
60. Bhatia S, Landier W, Robison L. Late effects of childhood cancer therapy. In: DeVita V, Hellman S, Rosenberg S, eds. *Progress in Oncology 2002*. Sudbury: Jone and Barlett Publications; 2003:171-201.
61. Hudson MM, Tyc VL, Cremer LK, et al. Patient satisfaction after limb-sparing surgery and amputation for pediatric malignant bone tumors. *J Pediatr Oncol Nurs*. 1998;15:60-69. discussion 70-71.
62. Nicholson HS, Mulvihill JJ, Byrne J. Late effects of therapy in adult survivors of osteosarcoma and Ewing's sarcoma. *Med Pediatr Oncol*. 1992;20:6-12.
63. Postma A, Kingma A, De Ruiter JH, et al. Quality of life in bone tumor patients comparing limb salvage and amputation of the lower extremity. *J Surg Oncol*. 1992;51:47-51.
64. Weddington WW. Psychological outcomes in survivors of extremity sarcomas following amputation or limb-sparing surgery. *Cancer Treat Res*. 1991;56:53-60.
65. Calaminus G, Weinspach S, Teske C, et al. Quality of life in children and adolescents with cancer. First results of an evaluation of 49 patients with the PEDQOL questionnaire. *Klin Padiatr*. 2000;212:211-215.

66. Varni JW, Burwinkle TM, Katz ER, et al. The PedsQL in pediatric cancer: reliability and validity of the Pediatric Quality of Life Inventory Generic Core Scales, Multidimensional Fatigue Scale, and Cancer Module. *Cancer*. 2002;94:2090-2106.
67. Nagarajan R, Neglia JP, Clohisy DR, et al. Limb salvage and amputation in survivors of pediatric lower-extremity bone tumors: what are the long-term implications? *J Clin Oncol*. 2002;20:4493-4501.
68. Wilhelmsen L. Role of the Data and Safety Monitoring Committee (DSMC). *Stat Med*. 2002;21:2823-2829.
69. DeMets DL, Yusuf S. The Data and Safety Monitoring Committee: some final thoughts. *Am Heart J*. 2001;141:548-549.

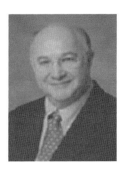

Pediatric and Adult Osteosarcoma: Comparisons and Contrasts in Presentation and Therapy

Robert S. Benjamin and Shreyaskumar R. Patel

Abstract Most data on osteosarcoma is derived from pediatric studies. Although the majority of adult patients with osteosarcoma are young adults, who might be treated in a similar fashion, experience derived from a slightly older population is helpful in directing therapy. We treated a series of 123 patients with osteosarcoma of the extremities with adriamycin and cisplatin as induction therapy. Adriamycin was infused intravenously at 90 mg/m^2 over 96 h. Cisplatin was infused intra-arterially at 120–160 mg/m^2 over 2–24 h. Sequential addition of methotrexate and methotrexate plus ifosfamide in subsequent cohorts improved the continuous relapse-free survival of poor responders such that overall survival improvement was noted in the group where therapy was modified by adding both agents to those with <90% tumor necrosis. Patients with chondroblastic osteosarcoma with poor necrosis had a trend towards improved continuous relapse-free survival compared with other patients with conventional osteosarcoma. Histologic variants of osteosarcoma except telangiectatic osteosarcoma had a worse prognosis than those with conventional osteosarcoma. The variants, especially dedifferentiated parosteal osteosarcoma and dedifferentiated well-differentiated intraosseous osteosarcoma are more common in adults than children, accounting for some of the inferior prognosis in adults. Older patients obviously cannot tolerate the doses of therapy given to children and young adults, again decreasing the chances of successful treatment. Patients with secondary osteosarcoma are often much older as are many with osteosarcomas of the pelvis and jaw. These tumors tend to be less responsive. An attempt to intensify therapy in poor-prognosis patients with a three-drug regimen of adriamycin, cisplatin, and ifosfamide with peripheral stem cell support was unsuccessful at prolonging relapse-free survival, and we no longer use that approach.

R.S. Benjamin (✉)
Dept. of Sarcoma Medical Oncology, The University of Texas M.D. Anderson Cancer Center, 1515 Holcombe Blvd, Unit 450/FC 11.3022, Houston, TX, 77030-4009, USA
e-mail: rbenjami@mdanderson.org

Introduction

Most data on osteosarcoma is derived from pediatric studies. Although the majority of adult patients with osteosarcoma are young adults, who might be treated in a similar fashion, experience derived from a slightly older population is helpful in directing therapy. We describe a consecutive series of patients with primary, high-grade osteosarcoma of the extremities treated at the Department of Melanoma/Sarcoma Medical Oncology (now the Department of Sarcoma Medical Oncology) at the University of Texas M.D. Anderson Cancer Center between May, 1980 and October, 1991, using systemic adriamycin and intra-arterial cisplatin as primary chemotherapy. The series is divided into three groups of patients based on the postoperative chemotherapy given. Preliminary reports of the first two groups of patients have been published[1-5]; but the third group has been reported only at meetings.[6-9] Taken together, the three groups illustrate the advantages of the neoadjuvant strategy.

Except for four, all patients older than 16 with primary, high-grade osteosarcoma of the extremities and no demonstrable metastatic disease treated with preoperative chemotherapy at the University of Texas, M.D. Anderson Cancer Center between May, 1980 and October, 1991 are the subjects of this report. Four patients who declined initial surgery but underwent delayed surgery (including two long-term, disease free survivors) were excluded from the analysis. Otherwise, this represents a consecutive series of 123 patients. They are further divided into three groups depending on the time period in which they were treated and the approach to postoperative chemotherapy.

Age, sex, and skeletal distribution were typical for osteosarcoma, except that patients under age 16, who were treated on our Pediatric service with a different regimen, are excluded. Males outnumbered females by about 3:2; 77% of the patients were below the age of 30; the most commonly involved bone was the femur; and three quarters of the tumors were located around the knee. No significant differences in the demographics of the three groups were detected. Most patients had conventional osteosarcoma (79%) and osteoblastic osteosarcoma was the most frequent subtype. There was an increased proportion of fibroblastic osteosarcoma in the third group.

After informed consent was obtained, all the patients were treated with adriamycin, 90 mg/m^2 by continuous 96-h ambulatory intravenous infusion through a percutaneous silicone elastomer central venous catheter, starting on day 1. At the end of the infusion (day 5), they were admitted to the hospital, and on day 6, underwent an arteriogram with subtraction images and catheter placement. After verification of correct catheter position to infuse the tumor by nuclear flow study, patients received intra-arterial cisplatin.

Group 1 was treated at a dose of 120 mg/m^2, infused over 2 h. Groups 2 and 3 were treated at a dose of 160 mg/m^2 infused over 24 h. All the patients received intensive intravenous hydration ($\geq$250 ml/h) and mannitol diuresis. Intake and output was balanced as needed by infusion of furosemides. After hypomagnesemia was noted in the initial patients, magnesium sulfate ($MgSO_4$) was routinely added to the intravenous fluids. The cisplatin was initially infused in normal saline, but later, it was infused in 3% saline. Chemotherapy cycles were repeated at 4-week intervals.

Patients in group 1 received a median of three courses of preoperative chemotherapy, the time required to obtain a custom prosthesis for most patients. Preoperative chemotherapy was stopped early in the case of disease progression and was extended if the prosthesis could not be obtained by the end of the third course. Postoperatively, patients with $\geq 60\%$ tumor necrosis continued the same chemotherapy intravenously until the development of grade 1–2 peripheral neuropathy. Thereafter, adriamycin was continued and cisplatin was replaced with dacarbazine 750 mg/m^2 as a 96-h infusion (ADIC). Twelve cycles of chemotherapy were administered. Drug doses were decreased for febrile neutropenia with morbidity or documented infection. The doses of cisplatin and dacarbazine were selectively decreased for thrombocytopenia or delayed granulocyte recovery (4 weeks). Hematopoietic growth factors were not used. Grade 2 mucositis was an indication to decrease the duration of the adriamycin infusion to 48 h (and in the first group to 24 h). Only if mucositis $\geq$ grade 2 persisted after the shorter infusion was the dose decreased to 75 and 60 mg/m^2, but never to <60 mg/m^2. Patients in the first group also participated in our studies assessing the cardiac toxicity of continuous-infusion adriamycin and were monitored with endomyocardial biopsies every four courses after a cumulative adriamycin dose of 450 mg/m^2. The five patients with <60% tumor necrosis were felt to have suboptimal response to primary chemotherapy and were allowed to receive alternative treatment at the discretion of their primary physicians. Two received adriamycin and dacarbazine (ADIC), two received high-dose methotrexate, and one received no further chemotherapy.

After the analysis of the patients in group 1 indicated the prognostic importance of obtaining a good response defined as $\geq 90\%$ necrosis in the resected specimen, processed and analyzed by the method of Raymond et al,[2] three modifications were made in the treatment program for group 2. The dose of cisplatin was increased to 160 mg/m^2, the duration of preoperative therapy was increased to four courses, and the postoperative therapy was modified for poor responders (<90% necrosis). Such patients received alternating chemotherapy with four courses of high-dose methotrexate, 8 gm/m^2 with leucovorin rescue repeated every 2 weeks, followed by two courses of ADIC, and then, by two courses of the combination of bleomycin, cyclophosphamide, and actinomycin-D (BCD)[10] at 3-week intervals. The entire cycle of methotrexate, ADIC, and BCD was repeated twice. Good responders continued on adriamycin-cisplatin/ADIC for only three courses. Group 3 received identical primary chemotherapy to that given to group 2. Postoperatively, good responders received three cycles of adriamycin with cisplatin or dacarbazine. Thereafter, they were treated with three cycles of high-dose methotrexate. Poor responders were also treated in the same way as those in group 2; however, ifosfamide 2 g/m^2 given as a 2-h infusion daily for 5 days with continuous infusion mesna 1,200 mg/m^2 qd$\times$5 after a loading dose of 400 mg/m^2 on day 1, replaced BCD.

The median follow-up time for censored patients in groups 1, 2, and 3 respectively as shown in the figures are 134, 91, and 55 months. With the exception of three patients lost to follow-up, the minimum follow-up is 65, 37, and 35 months, respectively. Extending the median and minimum follow-up times to 140, 141, and 120 months and 68, 41, and 51 months (data not shown) did not alter any of the outcomes.

Response to chemotherapy is shown in Table 1. One patient died of pulmonary embolism prior to resection. She is included in the overall relapse-free survival statistics but not in the response rate calculations or the relapse-free survival analyses when stratified by response group. Sixty percent of patients achieved a good response. Of the poor responders, 29% had 60–89% tumor necrosis, and 11% had <60% tumor necrosis. There was no significant difference in the rate of ≥90% necrosis or <60% necrosis between the three groups or between patients who received 120 mg/m² and 160 mg/m² of cisplatin.

Table 1 Response to therapy

Necrosis	Osteoblastic N=53	Chondroblastic N=17	Fibroblastic N=26	Telangiectatic N=11	Other N=15	Total N=122[a]
≥95%	47.2%	35.3%	42.3%	81.8%	33.3%	45.9%
90–94.9%	18.9%	5.9%	7.7%	9.1%	20.0%	13.9%
Good	66%	41.2%	50.0%	90.9%	53.3%	59.8%
80–89.9%	7.5%	23.5%	3.8%	0.0%	6.7%	8.2%
60–79.9%	18.9%	23.5%	23.1%	9.1%	26.7%	20.5%
<60%	7.5%	11.8%	23.1%	0.0%	13.3%	11.5%
Poor	34%	58.8%	50.0%	9.1%	46.7%	40.2%

[a] 1 patient died during induction therapy and did not have surgery

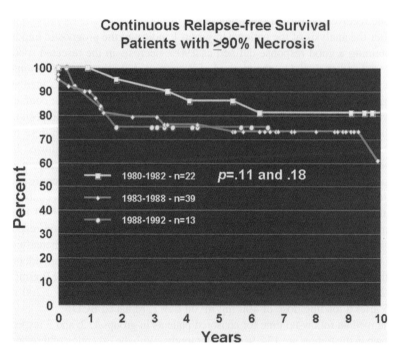

Fig. 1 Continuous relapse-free survival of good responders (>90% necrosis) by treatment group. There are no significant differences between the groups, but there is a suggestion of improvement in the first group

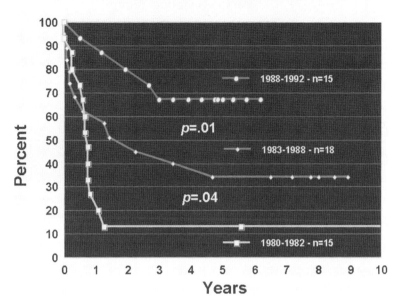

Fig. 2 Continuous relapse-free survival of poor responders (<90% necrosis) by treatment group. Each successive group shows significant improvement

Continuous relapse-free survival for the good responders (>90% necrosis) is shown in Fig. 1. There was no significant difference between any of the three groups. If anything, there was a suggestion that the first group, who got the longest postoperative adriamycin therapy, had the best relapse-free survival. There was no evidence that the addition of methotrexate to group 3 improved the relapse-free survival over that of group 2.

Continuous relapse-free survival for poor responders (<90% necrosis) is shown in Fig. 2. In group 1, only 13% of poor responders have not relapsed, and their continuous relapse-free survival is no different from our historical control series treated with surgery alone (Fig. 3, "historical control"). The addition of methotrexate and BCD in group 2 led to a small but statistically significant improvement in continuous relapse-free survival of 34% (p=0.04). The substitution of ifosfamide for BCD in group 3 led to a further statistically significant improvement in continuous relapse-free survival of 67% (p=0.01).

Continuous relapse-free survival for all patients in groups 1, 2, and 3 is shown in Fig. 4. As a result of the improved continuous relapse-free survival for poor responders in group 3, all the patients in group 3 have a superior continuous relapse-free survival when compared to patients in group 1 (p=0.04). The five-year relapse-free survival for patients in groups 1, 2, and 3 is 54%, 61%, and 70%, respectively.

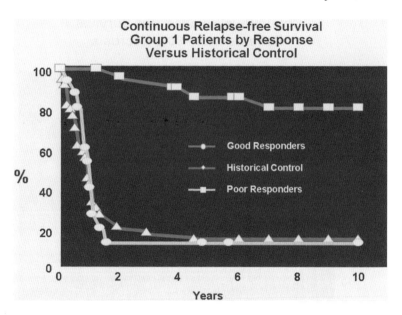

Fig. 3 Continuous relapse-free survival of good and poor responders compared with a historical control (surgery only). The only benefit is in good responders

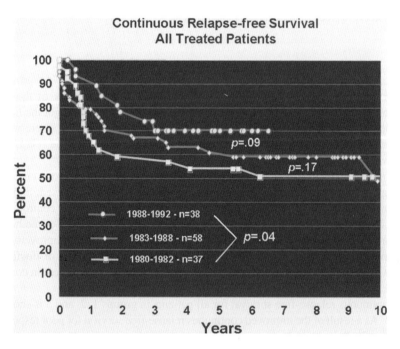

Fig. 4 Continuous relapse-free survival of all treated patients by treatment group. Each successive group shows significant improvement

This series contrasts with other published and unpublished series using alternating chemotherapy with more drugs in the preoperative chemotherapy regimen. With two drugs for induction therapy, we can demonstrate that changing therapy for poor response, a keystone of the neoadjuvant strategy, was indeed effective confirming the original observation by Rosen[11] and the findings of Bacci[12] using an induction chemotherapy similar to ours but with the addition of high-dose methotrexate.

Although the majority of patients in this series were young enough to qualify for pediatric studies, there are some differences seen in the adult population. Patients with secondary osteosarcomas, most commonly post-radiation sarcomas, but also those arising in pre-existing bone disease such as fibrous dysplasia, bone infarcts, or Paget's disease, have a worse prognosis and were excluded from the previous series. Similarly, osteosarcoma of the jaw which is more common in adults and which tends to be locally recurrent rather than metastatic and to have a better prognosis, was also excluded.

Not excluded were more unusual variants of osteosarcoma, which are more common in adults than in children. With the exception of telangiectatic osteosarcoma, which responded in a similar fashion to the conventional subtypes,[13] other high-grade variants fared significantly worse.[14,15] These included dedifferentiated parosteal osteosarcoma, dedifferentiated well-differentiated-intraosseous osteosarcoma, small cell osteosarcoma, and high-grade surface osteosarcoma (Fig. 5).

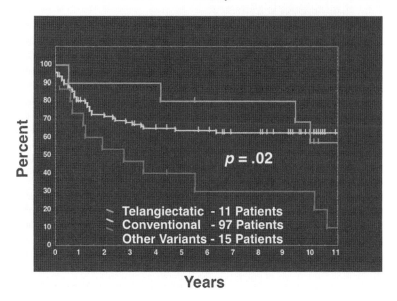

Fig. 5 Continuous relapse-free survival of all treated patients by histologic group. Telangiectatic osteosarcoma has similar relapse-free survival to the conventional subtypes. Other subtypes have significantly inferior prognosis

In an attempt to improve the prognosis of high-risk patients, we imitated a study using full doses of adriamycin, ifosfamide, and cisplatin. This could not be accomplished without stem cell support. Full details of this group of patients are beyond the scope of this manuscript but are published elsewhere.[16] Suffice it to say, while initial results were promising based on initial response to chemotherapy, patients were left with seriously impaired bone marrow reserve after induction therapy, despite stem cell support, and thus could not tolerate sufficient postoperative therapy; so, median relapse-free survival was only 19 months.

This communication also recognizes a recent report in which a worse prognosis was described in patients over 65 years when compared to that in younger patients.[17] The older age group was characterized by a longer time lapse from the onset of symptoms to diagnosis, a larger number of metastatic cases, less use of limb salvage and a reduced number of patients treated with chemotherapy (compare this experience with the above report of impaired bone marrow reserve), and more patients excluded from clinical trials as opposed to the younger age group. Only one of out patients was older than 65, one was 65, and 4 were 57-63. All received chemotherapy.

Conspectus

New drugs are needed to salvage the small proportion of patients who do poorly with our current regimens, and studying these new approaches in patients with poor prognostic characteristics is warranted.

References

1. Benjamin RS, Murray JA, Wallace S, et al. Intra-arterial preoperative chemotherapy for osteosarcoma – a judicious approach to limb salvage. *Cancer Bull*. 1984;36:32-36.
2. Raymond AK, Chawla SP, Carrasco CH, et al. Osteosarcoma chemotherapy effect: a prognostic factor. *Sem Diag Path*. 1987;4:212-236.
3. Benjamin RS. Regional chemotherapy for osteosarcoma. *Semin Onocol*. 1989;16:323-327.
4. Benjamin RS, Chawla SP, Carrasco CH, et al. Primary chemotherapy for osteosarcoma with systemic adriamycin and intra-arterial cisplatin. *Cancer Bull*. 1990;42:314-317.
5. Benjamin RS, Chawla SP, Carrasco CH, et al. Preoperative chemotherapy for osteosarcoma with intravenous adriamycin and intra-arterial cis-platinum. *Ann Oncol*. 1992;3(Suppl 2):S3-S6.
6. Benjamin RS, Patel SR, Armen T, et al. Primary chemotherapy of osteosarcoma of the extremities – long-term follow-up. *Am Soc Clin Oncol*. 1993;12:470.
7. Benjamin RS, Patel SR, Armen T, et al. The value of ifosfamide in postoperative neoadjuvant chemotherapy of osteosarcoma. *Am Soc Clin Oncol*. 1995;14:516.
8. Benjamin RS. Thirty years of progress in the chemotherapy of soft-tissue sarcomas and osteosarcoma in adults and prospects for the future. *J Jpn Ortho Assoc*. 1997;71:S1127.
9. Patel SR, Benjamin RS. Current status of chemotherapy for bone sarcomas. *Indian J Med Ped Onc*. 1997;18:5-8.

10. Mosende C, Gutierrez M, Caparros B, Rosen G. Combination chemotherapy with bleomycin, cyclophosphamide and dactinomycin for the treatment of osteogenic sarcoma. *Cancer.* 1977;40:2779-2786.
11. Rosen G, Caparros B, Huvos AG, et al. Preoperative chemotherapy for osteogenic sarcoma: selection of postoperative adjuvant chemotherapy based on the response of the primary tumor to preoperative chemotherapy. *Cancer.* 1982;49:1221-1230.
12. Bacci G, Picci P, Ferrari S, et al. Primary chemotherapy and delayed surgery for nonmetastatic osteosarcoma of the extremities. Results in 164 patients preoperatively treated with high doses of methotrexate followed by cisplatin and doxorubicin. *Cancer.* 1993;72:3227-3238.
13. Chawla SP, Benjamin RS. Effectiveness of chemotherapy in the management of metastatic telangiectatic osteosarcoma. *Am J Clin Oncol.* 1988;11:177-180.
14. Ayala AG, Ro JY, Raymond AK, et al. Small cell osteosarcoma: a clinicopathologic study of 27 cases. *Cancer.* 1989;64:2162-2173.
15. Sheth DS, Yak AW, Raymond AK, et al. Conventional and dedifferentiated parosteal osteosarcoma: diagnosis, treatment and outcome. *Cancer.* 1996;78:2136-2145.
16. Patel SR, Papadopolous N, Raymond AK, et al. A phase II study of cisplatin, doxorubicin, and ifosfamide with peripheral blood stem cell support in patients with skeletal osteosarcoma and variant bone tumors with a poor prognosis. *Cancer.* 2004;101:156-163.
17. Longhi A, Errani C, Gonzales-Arabio D et al: Osteosarcoma in patients older than 65 years. *J Clin Oncol.* 2008; 28: 5368-73.

Supportive Care and Quality of Life

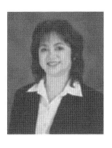 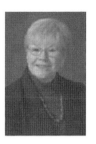

The Role of Physical Therapy and Occupational Therapy in the Rehabilitation of Pediatric and Adolescent Patients with Osteosarcoma

Marissa Punzalan and Gayle Hyden

Abstract The approach to rehabilitation of patients with osteosarcoma has evolved with the many advances in the medical treatment and surgical management of this pediatric and adolescent cancer. In the past, amputation (often radical amputation) was the standard method for treating patients with extremity sarcomas, and rehabilitation was geared toward providing either functional training for patients who had not had limb replacement or prosthetic training for those who had received prostheses. Currently, limb-sparing procedures combined with adjuvant chemotherapy (and occasionally radiotherapy) are used to treat most patients with this disease.
In addition, physical-therapy and occupational-therapy interventions are now tailored to address the multiple physical and psychosocial difficulties these patients will face for the remainder of their lives. Integral parts of the interdisciplinary team, practitioners of these disciplines, provide services that enable patients to achieve their highest functional status to permit them to return to their role in society and hence enjoy dignity and improved quality of life.

Introduction

Osteosarcoma is one of the most common primary malignant bone tumors in the pediatric and adolescent population, with an incidence of 5.6 per 1 million children younger than 15 years.[1] There is a slight predominance in boys, with peak incidence occurring during the adolescent growth spurt[1,2] early, in the second decade of life. The metaphyseal regions of long bones are the most common site affected by this aggres-

---

M. Punzalan (✉)
Senior Physical Therapist, Rehabilitation Services Department, MD Anderson Cancer Center, Houston, TX 77030-4009, USA
e-mail: mpunzala@mdanderson.org

G. Hyden
Senior Occupational Therapist, Rehabilitation Services Department,
MD Anderson Cancer Center, Houston, TX 77030-4009, USA

sive tumor. The cure and survival rates of this patient population have significantly improved as a result of the current standard of treatment: a combination of chemotherapy and surgery, typically, a limb-salvage procedure, and less frequently amputation and rotationplasty.[3–6] However, these surgical interventions result in significant physical, psychosocial, and socioeconomic challenges, which provide rehabilitation specialists a tremendous opportunity to impact upon, in both the acute and the chronic phases, the ability to function, and the quality of life of these young patients. The primary elements of the rehabilitative efforts are physical and occupational therapy. This chapter describes current approaches to each of these disciplines.

The Interdisciplinary Rehabilitation Team

Each pediatric oncology patient ideally has an interdisciplinary team consisting of pediatricians, surgeons, physicians and/or physiatrists, residents, physician assistants, advanced practice nurses, and nursing staff. Members of the therapy team include physical therapists and occupational therapists, speech-language pathologists, and/ or audiologists, as appropriate. In addition, neurophysiologists, psychologists, case managers, social workers, child-life professionals, and chaplains are often included in the team. Cooperation, teamwork, and communication among members of the team are necessary to the success of postsurgical rehabilitation of pediatric/adolescent and young-adult patients.

The Physical Therapist

Physical therapy is a health-care profession concerned with function and movement and with maximizing functional potential. Physical therapists diagnose and treat individuals of all ages, from newborns to the elderly, who have medical problems or other health-related conditions that limit their ability to move or to perform functional activities in their daily lives. In an oncology setting, physical therapists and physical therapy assistants manage patients' musculoskeletal, neuromuscular, integumentary, and cardiopulmonary rehabilitative needs that have resulted from cancer and its treatment. The rehabilitation needs of patients with cancer encompass: (1) acute secondary sequelae of cancer treatment (i.e., surgery, radiotherapy, and chemotherapy), (2) long-term secondary sequelae of treatment, and (3) palliative care.[7]

The Occupational Therapist

Occupational therapy is a health profession that helps individuals maximize their abilities to perform functional activities that are important to them. Functional activities include the self-care, school or work, and leisure activities that people spend their time doing throughout the day, from the time they get up until the time

The Role of Physical Therapy and Occupational Therapy

they go to bed. Occupational therapists aim to enhance patients' development and prevent disability.

The occupational therapist and the certified occupational therapy assistant are trained to help individuals who face physical and mental challenges. Occupational therapists use purposeful activities with patients to maximize their functional performance and independence by reducing the effects of impairments caused by physical or psychological dysfunction.

The Purpose of Rehabilitation in Cancer Care

Patients with cancer often develop functional deficits that adversely affect their ability to participate in desired activities and hence their quality of life. Yadav[8] has listed goals of cancer rehabilitation as:

- Restoring function.
- Minimizing the disability and handicaps caused by cancer and its associated treatments.
- Decreasing the burden of care required by cancer patients to maintain their personal dignity and improve their quality of life.

Historical Overview of Rehabilitation Therapy

Prior to the advent of preoperative and postoperative adjuvant chemotherapy, the survival rate for patients with osteosarcoma was only 10–20% at 5 years.[9] In general, the treatment of choice was radical amputation for lower extremity tumors, hemipelvectomy for pelvic tumors, and amputation or forequarter amputation for high upper extremity tumors. During that time, local resection was not considered curative. Nonsurgical measures such as radiation were considered ineffective and seldom used.[9] Rehabilitation of this population was geared toward providing functional training for all patients and prosthetic training for patients who received prostheses.[10] Physical-therapy interventions consisted of early postsurgical mobility training, restoration of strength and endurance, stump management and pain control, education and training of family members in helping patients with limited mobility and assistance with prostheses.

In 1965, Lambert found that the average prosthetic user among 42 children with osteosarcoma was 3.5 years of age [9] indicating that prosthetic rehabilitation was an important aspect of treatment for this patient population. As patients developed metastatic disease (most commonly in the lungs), physical therapists provided interventions to help them adapt to new restrictions in function and trained them and their families in the use of appropriate assistive devices, for example, if surgical restrictions after thoracotomy necessitated a transition from axillary crutches to forearm crutches or a walker.

Current Rehabilitation Concepts

Rehabilitation intervention is always patient focused, but families are intimately involved in goal setting, treatment planning, and managing patient care. Patient and family participation strongly influences the attainment of optimal functional outcomes for the osteosarcoma patient. In regard to rehabilitation of patients with advanced cancer, Cheville[11] states: "While cancer patients are remarkably adaptive, each impairment may leave them functionally compromised and less resilient for the next challenge. It becomes vital that rehabilitation therapists approach cancer rehabilitation from an anticipatory and preventative stance."

Goals of Physical Therapy

Physical therapists strive to help patients remain as functional as possible by: (1) improving correctable physical impairments, (2) training to enhance strength and endurance, (3) training in using residual function or developing compensatory techniques, (4) correcting balance and coordination impairments, (5) teaching the use of assistive devices, (6) managing pain and fatigue, (7) making recommendations for home modifications that enhance patients' independence, and (8) educating and training family members to assist and enable patients to function independently.

Goals of Occupational Therapy

Survivors of osteosarcoma with salvaged or amputated limbs may live with chronic impairments or disabilities. Occupational therapists focus on restoring skills, teaching adaptive techniques, and recommending adaptive and assistive equipment necessary for self-care, mobility, leisure, and school- or work-related activities. Occupational therapists can also recommend adaptive techniques, energy conservation measures, and specialized equipment to help patients address difficulties such as fatigue, decreased endurance, and physical limitation

Triggers for Referral

Referrals from the medical team begin the physical/occupational therapy process. Triggers for referral encompass functional impairments and the deficits caused by the impairments. Examples are:

- Risk or history of falls.
- Impairment of self-care activities and mobility.

The Role of Physical Therapy and Occupational Therapy 371

- Deficits in function of an extremity.
- Need for assistive equipment.
- Brace/prosthesis training.
- Need for splinting.
- Community re-entry: needs related to work, school, or leisure activities.
- Inability to participate in age-appropriate activities.
- Discharge planning.

Complications that Can Affect Rehabilitation

Rehabilitation of pediatric and adolescent patients with osteosarcoma is complicated by many factors, both intrinsic and extrinsic. Owing to the extensive nature of the surgical intervention and the side effects of chemotherapeutic agents, patients tend to experience pronounced cosmetic changes and functional disabilities after treatment.[12, 13] Common postsurgical impairments are movement and gait dysfunction, compromised strength, limited joint range of motion, and balance and/coordination deficits. The associated psychologic and physiologic challenges that this age group normally experiences are compounded by the complexity of the disease and its treatment. Thus, early physical- and occupational-therapy education of patients and families in regard to the rigorous and potentially lengthy rehabilitation process is of utmost importance.

Referral of patients with osteosarcoma to physical and occupational therapists during the presurgical phase of treatment is sometimes overlooked. This lapse is a significant oversight because in order for physical and occupational therapists to help patients adapt to the challenges of living with cancer, both early intervention and setting of realistic goals need to be discussed presurgically. The assessment of patients' premorbid levels of function should include their levels of age-appropriate physical activities in play and in sports. Compared with more mature patients with osteosarcoma, children and adolescent/young-adult patients tend to participate in more sports-related activities. Hence, physical and occupational therapists need to tailor patients' and their families' expectations to current and functional outcomes. The outcomes include degree of (1) returning to a normal or near-normal gait pattern and mobility,[13] (2) achieving independence in self-care, (3) returning to sports and challenging physical or leisure activities, and (4) returning to school or work activities. A study by Brown et al.[12] suggested that osteosarcoma patients with physically demanding jobs and those living in rural settings have the greatest risk of altered work status.

Most studies comparing the quality of life of patients with osteosarcoma who have undergone limb salvage with that of patients who have had limb amputation demonstrated similar long-term outcomes.[4, 14, 15] Table 1 compares the functional abilities of patients who underwent a limb-sparing procedure with those who had an amputation.[14] When patients and their families are presented with the choice

Table 1 Functional outcomes after limb-sparing procedures and amputation

Functional characteristics	Limb salvage (%)	Amputation (%)
Use of prosthesis or brace	82	91
Use of assistive device for ambulation	53	83
Presence of limp in ambulation	89	78
Difficulty in stair climbing	33	31
Participation in sports	38	39
Ability to drive a car (ages: 21–75 years)	92	90
Employment (ages: 20–60 years)	77	74

between limb salvage and amputation, providing information about the similar long-term outcomes may help in their decision making and long-term goal expectations.

The culture, expectations, and attitudes of patients and their family members can play a significant role in the patients' compliance with the rehabilitation process. Factors that can negatively influence patient participation and compliance with the rigors of physical- and occupational-therapy interventions include emotional factors such as depression, anxiety, fear, peer pressure, altered body image, a sense of lack of control, and overprotective family members.

The consequences of young patients' poor perceptions of self and of their physical impairments can negatively affect their long-term coping mechanisms and successful re-entry into society. In addition, patients' age and reliance on family and caregivers can sometimes result in overly dependent behavior that is easily accepted but should not be condoned or encouraged in the long term. To maximize patients' functional independence, physical and occupational therapists educate and involve patients and family members in a treatment partnership, the importance of which cannot be underestimated.

Current Physical-Therapy Practice

In physical therapy, the first step toward rehabilitation is an initial evaluation in which the therapist gathers information about patients' pertinent medical and physical-activity history. Assessment parameters include both subjective and objective measures of the musculoskeletal, neuromuscular, integumentary, and cardiopulmonary systems. Of particular interest is the kinesiologic assessment of patients' movement and locomotion. The physical therapist observes the patients' quality of movement and records results of objective measures such as goniometric joint range-of-motion testing, isometric and isokinetic manual muscle testing, and functional mobility scoring.[16, 17] In addition, the therapist identifies patients' and families' architectural living situation, the amount of caregiver assistance needed, and the amount of caregiver support available, which assist in goal setting and the development of a plan of care.

The most common physical-therapy interventions used to treat young patients with osteosarcoma are: (1) recommendations for assistive devices such as crutches, walkers, and canes, (2) prescriptions for appropriate orthotic equipment (for example, a long leg brace with hip and knee restriction components for patients who have had proximal femur resection and reconstruction), (3) therapeutic exercises and other interventions designed to improve range of motion, strength and endurance, and balance and coordination, (4) gait-training strategies, and, most important, (5) patient and family education and training in home functional activities and exercise programs. The physical therapist continually reassesses patients' functional abilities and modifies treatment strategies as patients' needs and abilities change.

Presurgical Phase

As mentioned earlier, it is advantageous for physical therapists to be involved in the presurgical phase of treatment for young patients with osteosarcoma. During this phase of treatment, the physical therapist assesses patients' current functional ability, identifying pre-existing impairments, if any,

- Makes recommendations and provides specific physical-therapy interventions to correct limitations or improve current function,
- Identifies needs that may require intervention from other members of the rehabilitation team (i.e., occupational therapy, speech pathology, case management) and makes appropriate referrals to these services,
- Helps patients and families to identify realistic postsurgical and/treatment goals. Patient and family education helps participants understand that successful achievement of their long-term goals is dependent on their participation and compliance with the rehabilitation process.

Postsurgical Phase

The postsurgical phase of the physical-therapy intervention process can be subdivided into three components. The first, or acute, postsurgical phase extends from the day of or day after surgery through 1–2 weeks after surgery. The second phase – the subacute, or intermediate phase extends from the end of the acute phase through 6 weeks after surgery. The third and final postsurgical phase – the chronic, or late, phase of rehabilitation – extends from the end of the subacute phase through, typically, 6 months after surgery, although extended therapy is sometimes necessary. Patients who experience complications such as infections that require surgical intervention, hardware malfunctions, nonunion, and limb-lengthening interventions resulting from growth may need to engage in the rehabilitation process on and off for several years.

The Acute Postsurgical Phase (Postoperative Day 0–2 weeks)

The goals of physical therapy during the acute phase include enabling the patient to be discharged and to return home safely with:

Minimal assistance to modified independence in functional transfers and locomotion

- Appropriate assistive and/or orthotic equipment with patient/family education to enable patients to apply and use this equipment independently (for example, amputees receive a "stump shrinker" and are instructed how to apply and use it properly).
- A referral to appropriate rehabilitation services (a home health service or an outpatient rehabilitation facility) for continuation of care.
- A home program with an understanding of activity precautions and patient demonstration of compliance.
- A return-to-school or return-to-work strategy.

During this postsurgical rehabilitation phase, the affected joint and/or limb must receive maximum protection. Weight-bearing precautions for the patient are determined by the orthopedic surgeon and taught by the physical therapist. Orthotic devices used to protect the limb are prescribed by the surgeon in consultation with the physical therapist and orthotist. Strict adherence to activity precautions is taught. Patients and their families practice these precautions under the supervision of and with the assistance of the physical therapist.[16, 17]

Depending on the site and type of surgical intervention, a continuous passive-motion machine may be used by the physical therapist for early but protected joint mobilization. The therapist also teaches patients how to use available hospital equipment, such as the overhead trapeze, electrical hospital bed, and bed rails, to facilitate their early postsurgical mobilization. Moreover, the therapist teaches patients and families correct body mechanics and pain-relieving strategies for transitional movements.[16, 17] Transfer-training activities and gait training with the appropriate assistive device such as a rolling walker are also started during this phase of recovery. Prior to hospital discharge (usually 5–10 days after surgery, depending on surgical procedure and recovery), bed mobility and transfer techniques are modified to simulate functional movements that are consistent with the patients' home environment (i.e., the use of the overhead trapeze, electrical bed functions, and bed rails is discontinued). Patients receive a home activity-and-exercise program with specific instructions. The therapist obtains, fits, and adjusts the prescribed orthotic device and trains patients and families to put on, take off, use, and care for this equipment. Return demonstrations by the patients and family members ensure that the program is performed appropriately.

The importance of compliance with all components of the acute rehabilitation process is emphasized. Referral to an appropriate rehabilitation service such as home health or outpatient rehabilitation for continuation of care is recommended by the therapist and obtained from the medical team. Patients are expected to make sufficient functional gains during this period so that they can return to school or

The Role of Physical Therapy and Occupational Therapy 375

work, albeit in a limited capacity, in order to comply with postsurgical protected weight-bearing and range-of-motion limitations.

The Subacute or Intermediate Postsurgical Phase (2–6 Weeks after Surgery)

By 2 weeks postoperatively, patients are expected to be managing better from a physical and functional standpoint; pain with activity should be minimal. Patients need to continue their physical-therapy rehabilitation in the outpatient setting. Those who need to be readmitted to a hospital for inpatient chemotherapy should continue with their home exercise program or work with the inpatient physical therapist to continue to make appropriate progress. The goals of physical therapy during this phase may include (1) returning to modified-independent or independent function and mobility at home and at school or work, (2) diminishing the effects of continued chemotherapy after surgery, such as fatigue and general deconditioning, (3) continuing progressive improvement in the functional gains made during the acute phase of treatment, (4) increasing weight bearing and exercises to patients' increased tolerance level, and (5) increasing endurance training.

Depending on the site and extent of surgery, patients may begin to be weaned off their assistive and orthotic devices during this phase. Common physical-therapy treatment strategies and interventions during this period are manual therapy techniques to reduce scar adhesions and restore full joint range of motion, progressive resistance training for strength restoration, endurance training, and progressive gait training that addresses restoration of balance and proprioception on uneven surfaces.

The Chronic or Late Postsurgical Phase (6 Weeks and Beyond as Needed)

Patients' progression in function, strength, and mobility continues during this third postsurgical phase. Those without complications from surgery need to continue physical therapy in the out-patient setting. This is the period of rehabilitation in which patients' life goals can be projected and incorporated into treatment. For young patients who enjoyed and pursued intense sports activities before their diagnosis, alternative choices can be made. Some of the goals of physical therapy at this point are (1) increasing the girth of the affected limb, which indicates increased strength, (2) discontinuing the use of orthotic and assistive devices if this goal has not yet been achieved, (3) advancing strength and endurance training, and (4) incorporating sports-related functional training patterns suitable to patients' status and desire.

Infections, hardware malfunctions, nonunions, tumor recurrences, and metastases can occur postsurgically and require further rehabilitation intervention. Physical-therapy goals and strategies under these conditions are geared toward restoration of joint stability and function as dictated by medical and surgical intervention. Range-of-motion and resistance training gradually progress. Patients are required to adhere strictly to activity restrictions and to continue the use of assistive and orthotic devices prescribed by the therapist.

Another postsurgical challenge associated with limb-salvage procedures in skeletally immature patients is meeting their ongoing growth requirements.[18] Repeated surgical interventions are often required. Achieving limb lengthening by open surgical procedures requires a longer period of rehabilitation than does closed surgical intervention to adjust than endoprosthetic devices. Regardless of the extent of surgery, the three phases of postsurgical physical-therapy intervention – acute, subacute, and chronic, – are again observed. However, this time patients and families are well versed in physical-therapy interventions and strategies and in many cases become advocates of the rehabilitation process.

Physical Therapy After Lower-Extremity Surgery

The treatment and plan of care for osteosarcoma patients can vary according to tumor site and limb-salvage procedure. Table 2 shows expected outcomes, precautions, orthotic recommendations, and special interventions that physical therapists should consider when a lower extremity is involved.

Current Occupational-Therapy Practice

The Occupational-Therapy Assessment

The initial occupational therapy assessment establishes the foundation on which rehabilitation goals are established and treatment interventions are based. The assessment includes a review of the patient's medical history and premorbid status in the areas of fine, gross, and sensorimotor skills, cognitive processing, psycho social adjustment, communication abilities, and social engagement. Emphasis is placed on how these factors interrelate in the patient's participation in daily-living skills at home, at school or work, and in the community. The initial assessment is also the time at which integration of the family members into the rehabilitative process begins. As mentioned earlier, incorporation of family members throughout the process is essential for successful patient outcome.

In forming the intervention plan, the occupational therapist considers the physician's recommendations, the patient's and family's goals and expected outcomes realistic to the procedure, and the amount of caregiver assistance available. Also considered are continuing chemotherapy or radiation treatments, resources available for long-term rehabilitation, and client factors such as degree of fatigue, pain, and anatomic changes.

Table 2 Physical-therapy considerations after lower-extremity surgery

Tumor or operative site	Expected outcomes	Precautions	Orthotic recommendations
Proximal femur	Normal gait	Total hip arthroplasty (for life)	Hip abduction brace. If hip abductors are resected with tumor or if an allograft is used, then hip, knee, ankle, and foot orthosis may be prescribed
Distal femur	Good functional gait, some return to limited sports activities. Use knee support as needed[19, 20]	Limited total knee arthroplasty (long term)	Continuous-passive-motion therapy from after surgery to intermediate phase. Long leg ROM brace with knee component. Range-of-motion limits as dictated by patient status
Total femur reconstruction	Functional gait	Total hip arthroplasty (for life) and limited total knee arthroplasty (long term)	Hip, knee, ankle, and foot orthosis, with hip abduction presets similar to those used after proximal-femur tumor resection
Proximal tibia	Good functional gait; some return to limited sports activities, preferably with use of knee support[19, 20]	Knee immobilization for 6–12 weeks after surgery. Nonweight bearing to touch-down weight bearing during immobilization Limited total knee arthroplasty (long term)	Long leg brace with knee locked in extension during immobilization Lengthy physical therapy intervention after immobilization to regain range of motion and function

Interventions in occupational therapy may include

- Training in activities of daily living.[26]
- Exercises to improve upper-extremity functioning for both fine and gross motor activities.
- Education of patient and family and/or caregiver.
- Training in the use of adaptive equipment.
- Fabrication of splints.
- Training in the use of braces and/or slings.
- Recommendations for home modifications, safety, and driving.
- Coordination with other professionals and agencies.
- Psychological support.

Occupational Therapy and Upper-Extremity

Presurgical Phase

A referral to an occupational therapist is recommended when the planned surgery is scheduled. Interventions at this time include (1) educating and training the patient and the family about rehabilitation services, safety, and adaptive equipment, (2) determining the functional ability of the patient, (3) establishing patient and family goals, and (4) evaluating the preoperative needs for orthotic and assistive devices.

Postsurgical Phase

After the surgery, occupational-therapy interventions may address the following areas related to the patient's physical and functional status:

- Strength of the extremity.
- Range of motion of the affected portion of the extremity.
- Cardiopulmonary function.
- Skin integrity.
- Edema and sensation.
- Bed mobility and transfers.
- Self-care and activities of daily living.
- Current and preoperative functional levels.
- Adaptive equipment needs.
- Previous and anticipated living situations.
- Support system.

The goals of occupational therapy during the postsurgical phase include the following:

- Ensuring safety when the patient is performing.
- Maximizing functional skills.

The Role of Physical Therapy and Occupational Therapy   379

– Educating the family.
– Allowing the healing of soft tissue.
– Reducing pain and inflammation.
– Fostering independence in activities of daily living with modifications and/or adaptations.

The intervention plan should consider the results of the postoperative assessment and the occupational-therapy goals of the patient and family. Table 3 summarizes the overall occupational-therapy treatment programs and expected outcomes for the most common upper-extremity limb-salvage procedures (proximal humerus resection, total humerus replacement, and elbow replacement).

Shared Occupational-Therapy and Physical-Therapy Interventions

Orthotics

Orthotics involving bracing of the affected upper or lower extremity is provided both before and after surgery for joint stabilization or immobilization. The purposes of the orthosis are to prevent deformities and to control pain. A physician's order is necessary for most orthoses. Therapists can construct splints and apply them on the patient. Alternatively, a therapist and an orthotist collaborate to ensure a functional fit.

Amputations and Prosthetics

Pre- and postamputation treatment includes

- Education for the patient and family on stump care to control pain and swelling and to desensitize the stump.
- Exercise to improve the strength and range of motion of the immobile extremity.
- Teaching of techniques to desensitize nerve and phantom limb sensations.
- Residual limb wrapping to promote wound healing and residual limb maturation.
- Skin assessment.
- Strengthening of the remaining extremity
- Preprosthetic training in using the remaining extremity to achieve functional independence in activities of daily living (including, if the dominant hand was amputated, training the uninvolved hand in fine motor skills such as writing).

Table 3 Occupational-therapy considerations after upper-extremity limb-salvage procedures

	Proximal humerus	Total humerus	Elbow
Precautions	Immobilize the shoulder for up to 3 months	Prevent skin breakdown	If a muscle flap is involved, begin passive range-of-motion therapy only after healing
	Prevent skin breakdown in the axilla		
	Avoid sports involving the affected arm or with the potential for falls on the arm	Avoid sports involving the affected arm or with the potential for falls on the arm	If the proximal radius is involved, allow biceps attachment time to heal prior to beginning active elbow flexion
Expected outcomes	Normal distal extremity function	Normal distal extremity function	Fully functional extremity
	Shoulder flexion up to 90°, abduction to 45°	Less active range of motion at the shoulder than seen in proximal humerus resection	
	No active external rotation	No active external rotation	
	Independence or moderate independence in activities of daily living, instrumental activities of daily living and productivity	Moderate independence in activities of daily living and instrumental activities of daily living	
Focus of early rehabilitation	Placement of shoulder immobilizer on the day of surgery	Placement of shoulder immobilizer on the day of surgery	Teaching elevation, positioning, and use of sling
	Instruction in edema management and skin care	Instruction in edema management and" skin care	On postop day 1, passive range-of-motion and/or active assistive range-of-motion therapy
	Use of adaptive equipment for self-care	Use of adaptive equipment for self-care	Progression to active range-of-motion therapy (including the shoulder)
	Active range-of-motion therapy to hand, wrist, and forearm	Active range-of-motion therapy to hand, wrist, and forearm	Activities of daily living training
	Active assistive range-of-motion therapy to affected elbow	Active assistive range-of-motion therapy to affected elbow	Intermediate- Resistive exercises for the hand and/forearm
Focus of late rehabilitation	Passive range-of-motion therapy to shoulder	Passive range-of-motion therapy to shoulder	Progressive resistive exercise for elbow

The Role of Physical Therapy and Occupational Therapy

- Postural-issues training to correct weight bearing imbalance (e.g., the patient leans toward the affected side, causing neck and back problems). Training includes range-of-motion exercises for the neck and trunk and postural exercises using a mirror.

Equipment

Adaptive equipment includes devices that assist a patient in performing activities as safely and independently as possible. Catalogs filled with information about various adaptive equipment for addressing patients' needs are available.

Assistive technology involves using devices to help patients interact with their environment. Assistive-technology devices include environmental controls, computer-access devices, specialized mobility devices, and augmentative and alternative communication devices.

Discharge Recommendations

As members of the discharge-planning team, physical and occupational therapists offer recommendations and inform the team about additional needs patients may have after their hospital discharge.[18]

One recommendation involves continued rehabilitative services. Home health care is recommended when patients have impairments that keep them homebound. The benefits of home health services include the opportunity to obtain a safety evaluation of the home environment with possible home-modification recommendations, and the patients' comfort and security of being in a familiar environment. Recommendations for home modifications can range from installing ramps for access to the home to totally remodeling to provide a safe environment and possibly increased independence for the patient. Outpatient therapy is recommended when patients are able to leave their homes and have transportation to the clinic. The clinic site can be the hospital outpatient department or an outpatient clinic close to home. Physical and occupational therapists can assist with resources, designs, and inspection. They also work with case managers and social workers to identify outside assistance from other sources and the community.

School is the work of children, and resuming their former normal routine is important for their adjustment back into their communities and for their self-esteem, self-worth, and resocialization. The goal is for children to participate in school for as long as possible; those transferring back into school may require accommodations and modifications. As a result of the surgery, students may also have to change how they participate in school activities such as sports programs, which can be especially challenging.[23]

Home instruction may be recommended. This may include therapy services and may involve working with the teacher from the school system. Hospital based schools can provide education to patients during their hospitalization, to outpatients who are away from home, and to patients unable to attend school because of their medical needs.

Future Considerations

Physical- and occupational-therapy interventions are now, more than ever, closely tailored to advances in surgical and medical treatment of various conditions and disease processes, including osteosarcoma. Advances in technology, improvements in surgical and medical management, and improved rehabilitation strategies should address and correct common functional deficits associated with osteosarcoma. Physical therapists need to increase their participation in research projects on the management of osteosarcoma in pediatric and adolescent patients to strongly promote evidence-based practice patterns.

The interdisciplinary team also needs to increase the involvement of occupational-therapy services in addressing age-appropriate life skills as patient mature. Continual awareness is required of advances in orthotics, mobility aids, and assistive technology for inclusion in occupational-therapy practice. The need for advanced training to increase research and expand the use of evidence-based practice patterns will also allow oncology services the benefit of an occupational and physical therapist on their team.

Conclusions

Physical and occupational therapists provide vital services in the treatment and management of pediatric and adolescent patients with osteosarcoma. Successful rehabilitation is a lengthy, complex process in which success is closely linked to the amount of patient and family participation in and commitment to the rehabilitation program. Physical-therapy intervention may need to continue long after the surgical procedure and adjuvant chemotherapy and/or radiotherapy have been completed to meet patients' life goals and to maximize their return to their roles in society.

For the rehabilitation of pediatric and adolescent and young adult patients impaired by their cancer treatment, regaining of their previous functional skills is very important. This patient population is complicated in all aspects (medical, psychological, and social). Functional gains at times may be limited, but reasonable functional outcomes can be expected.

References

1. Lane JM, Christ GH, Khan SN, et al. Rehabilitation for limb salvage patients: kinesiologic parameters and psychological assessment. *Cancer*. 2001;92(4 Suppl):1013–1019.
2. Campanacci MC. Classic osteosarcoma. In: Campanacci MC, ed. *Bone and Soft Tissue Tumors*. Vienna: Springer-Verlag; 1990:455–505.
3. Tunn P-U, Schmidt-Peter P, Pomraenke D, et al. Osteosarcoma in children: long-term functional analysis. *Clin Orthop*. 2004;421:212–217.
4. Ginsberg J, Rai S, Carlson C, Meadows A 2007. A comparative analysis of functional outcomes in adolescents and young adults with lower-extremity bone sarcoma. *Pediatr Blood Cancer*. 2007;49:964–969.
5. Longhi A, Errani C, De Paolis M, et al. Tumor review: primary bone osteosarcoma in the pediatric age: state of the art. *Cancer Treat Rev*. 2006; 32(6):423–426.
6. Hopyan S, Tan J, Graham K, et al. Function and upright time following limb salvage, amputation, and rotationplasty for pediatric sarcoma of bone. *J Pediatr Orthop*. 2006;26:405–408.
7. American Physical Therapy Association. Information for consumers. <http://www.apta.org>; 2007 Retrieved 15.05.2007
8. Yadav R. Rehabilitation of surgical cancer patients at University of Texas M.D. Anderson Cancer Center. *J Surg Oncol*. 2007;95:361–369.
9. Leavitt LA. Rehabilitation problems of the cancer patient. Rehabilitation of the Cancer Patient: A Collection of Papers presented at the 15th Annual Clinical Conference on Cancer; 1970, at the University of Texas M.D. Anderson Hospital and Tumor Institute, at Houston, Texas. Chicago, IL: Year Book Medical Publishers, Inc; 1972:49–55.
10. Cheville A. Rehabilitation of patients with advanced cancer. *Cancer*. 2001;92(suppl 4): 1039–1048.
11. Brown A, Parsons J, Martino C. Work status after distal femoral Kotz reconstruction for malignant tumors of bone. *Arch Phys Med Rehabil*. 2003;84:62–68.
12. Gudas S. Rehabilitation of pediatric and adult sarcomas. *Rehabil Oncol*. 2000;18(3):10–13.
13. Refaat, Y., Gunnoe, J., Hornicek, F et al. Comparison of quality of life after amputation or limb salvage. *Clin Orthop Relat Res*. 2002;397:298–305.
14. Ness, K., Mersten, A., Hudson, M., Wall, M et al. Limitations on physical performance and daily activities among long-term survivors of childhood cancer. *Ann Intern Med*. 2005;143:639–647.
15. Marchese, V., Spearing, E., Callaway, L et al. Relationships among range of motion, functional mobility, and quality of life in children and adolescents after limb-sparing surgery for lower-extremity sarcoma. *Pediatr Phys Ther*. 2006;18(4):238–244.
16. Pakulis, PJ., Young, N., Davis, A. Review: evaluating physical function in an adolescent bone tumor population. *Pediatr Blood Cancer*. 2005;45:635–643.
17. Lewis V. (2005). Limb salvage in the skeletally immature patient. *Curr Oncol Rep Curr Sci*. 1523–3790, 287–292.
18. Tsauo JY, Li WC, Yang RS. Functional outcomes after endoprosthetic knee reconstruction following resection of osteosarcoma near the knee. *Disabil Rehabil*. 2006;28(1):61–66.
19. Benedetti, MG, Catani, F, Donati, D, et al. Muscle performance about the knee joint in patients who had distal femoral replacement after resection of a bone tumor: an objective study with gait analysis. *J Bone Joint Surg*. 2000;82-A(11):1619–1625.
20. Porr SM, Rainville EB. *Pediatric Therapy: A Systems Approach*. Philadelphia, PA: FA Davis Company; 1999.
21. Penfold S. The role of occupational therapist in oncology. *Cancer Treat Rev*. 1996;22:75–81.
22. Cooper J, ed. *Occupational Therapy in Oncology and Palliative Care*. London: Whurt Publishers Ltd; 2003.

23. Shin KY, Gillis TA, Fine SM. *Cancer Rehabilitation: General Principles in Physical Medicine and Rehabilitation Secrets*. Philadelphia, PA: Hanley & Belfus, Inc.; 2002; VII:55.
24. Griffith E. (1981) Rehabilitation of children with bone and soft tissue sarcomas: a physiatrist's viewpoint. *Natl Cancer Inst Monogr*. 36, 137–143.
25. Lenhard RE Jr, Osten RT, Gansler T. *Clinical Oncology*. Atlanta, GA: American Cancer Society; 2001.
26. Yasko A, Reece G, Gillis T, Pollock R. Limb-salvage strategies to optimize quality of life: the M.D. Anderson Cancer Center Experience. *CA Cancer J Clin*. 1997;47:226–238.
27. Varricchio CG, ed. Ades TB, Hinds PS, Pierce M, assoc eds. *A Cancer Source Book for Nurses*, 8th ed. Sudbury, MA: Jones & Bartlett Publishers; 2004.

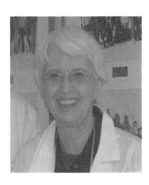

Caring for Children and Adolescents with Osteosarcoma: A Nursing Perspective

Margaret Pearson

Abstract The nurse plays a vital role in caring for patients with osteosarcoma. From the very outset when the disease is explained to the patient and his/her family, the nurse provides comfort and support, as well as enhances and explains the information provided by the physician. All aspects of medical care are addressed, and he/she is frequently the first line of communication when the patient telephones and requests information or wishes to report a problem to the physician. He/She arranges and coordinates appointments to suit the patient's medical, and often social needs to provide comprehensive care with attention to detail. This communication will provide a perspective of the role assumed by the nurse in his/her effort to ensure total care of the patient and the family.

While interviewing a young teen recently, I asked if he had been well prior to his diagnosis. He looked a little startled at the question and quickly replied: "I am still well." It would be a wonderful world if all our patients could have this perception throughout treatment. How can we promote *quality of life* in the face of life-threatening disease and prolonged and difficult treatment? Hinds et al. suggest six domains that have a direct bearing on quality of life for the pediatric patient with cancer. These include symptoms, usual activities, social/family interactions, health status, mood, and the meaning of being ill.[1] As nurses, we are generalists; our scope of practice is broad and frequently overlaps with that of colleagues who are more specialized. In addition, our role affords us the opportunity to spend a good deal of time with our patients and their families, during which we become aware of needs, voiced and observed. For these reasons, frequently in partnership with other disciplines, we are in a wonderful position to influence quality of life for our patients.

M. Pearson (✉)
Advanced Nurse Practitioner for the Solid Tumor Service, Children's Cancer Hospital, The University of Texas M. D., Anderson Cancer Center, 1515 Holcombe Blvd, Houston, TX, 77030-4009, USA

Family-Centered Care

The relationship between the health care team and the patient and his/her family is of utmost importance; we have embraced family-centered care to define that relationship in our institution. "Family-centered care is an approach to health care that shapes health care policies, programs, facility design, and day-to-day interactions among patients, families, physicians, and other health care professionals."[2] The foundation of family-centered care is the understanding that the family is the true expert in the care of their child and the primary source of strength and support. The key concepts include: dignity and respect, collaboration, participation and information sharing.[2,3] It is in the day-to-day interactions that we have the best opportunity to implement the strategies that operationalize these concepts. We need to help prepare and support our patients and their families to be experts in their cancer care.

Developing Patient Tools

When our young patients and their families receive the diagnosis of Osteosarcoma, they enter upon a journey in a world that is foreign and potentially threatening. Our role as patient and family advocates and educators cannot be over emphasized. Identifying ways to help patients understand their disease and its treatment and to organize and build upon initial information requires sensitivity, visual information, and creativity.[4]

One Page Summary

A one page summary, developed by one of our physicians, (Pete Anderson, MD), is an example of an editable Microsoft word document that provides a concise medical history as well as social and contact information. The section for recording the chronologic history of disease status, the treatment, current medications, the patient's problems and future plans, is updated appropriately at each visit. In addition to providing a tool for the patient and his/her family; it is an excellent resource for all providers involved in the care of the patient, i.e., local physicians and specialist consultants. This tool is most useful when it is kept updated. Sending the one page summary with the patient when he has to have an unexpected hospital admission will give the providers receiving the patient an immediate and succinct history, allowing them to attend to the patient in a prepared manner.[4]

Calendars

One of our clinic nurses (Nicole Luckett, RN), was instrumental in developing an editable PDF document in a calendar format. We have found this tool extremely useful in helping patients understand the treatment schedule. Roadmaps are frequently used for this purpose, but the roadmap itself is foreign. The calendar also helps the family integrate the treatment plan with the other events and time demands of the family For each patient on active therapy, a new calendar is prepared each month, printed and a copy given to the family. Because it is editable, if there is a delay in starting a subsequent treatment or if the treatment plan changes, the calendar can be quickly and easily updated.[4] We often share patient calendars with other providers within and outside our institution as a means of making everyone involved and aware of the plan. We discovered recently that the calendar was a sign of hope for a fragile, relapsed patient, and I suspect she is not alone in her thinking. On one of her visits to the clinic, we found that she was not in a suitable condition to receive therapy; she went home without a plan for active treatment until her blood counts recovered. She told us that it made her feel very discouraged not to have a "calendar" plan. Other calendar formats, to help families plan activities and obtain help from other families with regard to care and volunteer coordination, are available on websites (mylifeline.org; lotsahelpinghands.com)

Medication Schedules

Our Pharmacist, (Susannah Koontz, Pharm D) developed a form for the daily dosage of medicines to be given to patients, when they are discharged from the hospital with multiple medications. This tool provides very clear instructions about the time and dose of each medication; the reason for the medication, and a schedule that fits the patient's life schedule. It also helps to avoid administering drugs that are incompatible. In addition to the form being given to the patient, it is faxed from the inpatient unit to the clinic, when the patient is discharged. When we see the patient in the clinic, we can review his/her home medications. We encourage patients to obtain medication boxes; the form helps us in getting the "med boxes" loaded correctly.

Medication Bags ("Tackle Boxes")

A simple tool for ensuring that medications are taken as prescribed is the medication bag (it looks like a lunchbox). Patients bring their home medications to the clinic as part of the review process. This helps us to be sure that the medication was picked up from the pharmacy; also, if the patient is at the clinic at the time a medication is due, there are no missed doses. This process has been especially helpful for non English speaking patients. The insulated medication bags were funded by the Children's Art Project in response to a proposal submitted by the clinic nurses, so we were able to provide these to the patients free of cost. When patients need to travel, the medication bag keeps the medications available in one place so that they can be taken on schedule.

Flash Drive

During the last year, we developed a "Flash Drive" program.[5] At the end of their initial visit, patients are given a flash drive that costs very little : 1 GB is about $7.00. The contents include a one page summary, power point images of the most significant findings of their imaging studies, relevant articles regarding treatment options, the recommended treatment plan in calendar format, patient education documents, and other individualized information. Radiology, pathology, or consult reports can also be added ("cut and paste" into Word")

The objectives of the program were discussed in a recent poster presentation (for availability, contact the author):[5]:

- To increase empowerment and advocacy by providing patients and families an updated copy of the medical record.
- To establish open and transparent communication between patients, families and health care providers.
- To assist patients and families communicate complex medical information to other health care providers.

The flash drive is updated during subsequent visits, and when the clinical status and/or the treatment plan changes. Our plan is to formally evaluate the benefit of the Flash Drive program by asking patients and families to complete a questionnaire. The informal feedback has been extremely favorable.

The tools cited above empower patients and their families to be active participants in their care by providing detailed information in an easily understandable and accessible form.

Outpatient/Home Chemotherapy

Frequent, multiple day hospitalizations have been the usual experience for young people receiving treatment for osteosarcoma. During the last decade, pediatric oncology centers have begun to give some chemotherapy agents, as outpatients and in the home.[6-8] Although a few institutions were motivated by limited inpatient bed capacity, by far the most powerful impetus to embark on a program of out of hospital chemotherapy is quality of life. Feedback from our families and the few studies described in the literature consistently report that outpatient and home treatment are much more supportive of family life and certainly more humane for the patient.[4]

For the last two years, we have been treating the majority of patients receiving high-dose ifosfamide and mesna, either on brief daily visits to the outpatient clinic for chemotherapy bag change or at home with the support of home health care.[9] Initially, our physician, nurse, nurse practitioner and pharmacologist collaborated to develop standardized outpatient continuous infusion ifosfamide and mesna orders; we utilized the experience of Keith Skubitz, MD[10] and made modifications to suit our requirements. Since copious intravenous hydration is not needed; a small daily volume may be used (e.g., 240 or 360 ml; ref.[7]). We use an ifosfamide dose of 2.8 g/m2 mixed 1:1 with mesna, given as a continuous infusion by ambulatory pump over 24 h, daily for 5 days. On the sixth day, a 24 h continuous infusion of Mesna, 2.8 g/m2 is given. The patients come to the outpatient treatment area daily for a chemotherapy bag change; the chemotherapy bag and ambulatory pump fit nicely in a back pack. Most patients receive a daily dose of palonosetron at the same visit. We give pegfilgrastim approximately 24 h after completion of the Ifosfamide.

With the help of our pharmacy staff, we selected a simple and reliable ambulatory pump. We developed a patient /family education brochure that discusses the drugs and their side effects, and tells the patients, their families and the health providers what to watch for; when to call the nurse/physician; how to use the chemotherapy spill kit; and ambulatory pump information, including phone resources for trouble shooting. We developed a calendar (as mentioned earlier) with the days of treatment, schedule of lab checks and the projected next chemotherapy cycle or the next reevaluation scans.

When patients are considered for their first out of the hospital treatment, we discuss the option with their families. The majority of patients are excited about the chance to be able to stay out of the hospital; in fact, after learning about outpatient chemotherapy from other patients, many initiate the request. For a few parents who are uncomfortable, as they are used to their children being hospitalized for treatment, the concept of a "dress rehearsal" may be helpful. Treatment is given as inpatient in the first cycle, or sometimes for just the first 2 or 3 days of the first cycle, and then transitioned to outpatient.

Together with the hematologic and biochemical parameters for chemotherapy, patients should be evaluated for performance status and family/social functioning prior to embarking on outpatient chemotherapy. We have found patients who have poor performance status, i.e., their nutrition level is poor; they have pain and require opioids, may not be good candidates for outpatient therapy. For a few patients, inpatient treatment was preferred because of lack of appropriate family resources to meet the needs of the patient outside the hospital.

We have been able to give high dose methotrexate 12 g/m2. and cisplatin 60 mg/m2/day for two days with the support of ambulatory IV fluids and antiemetics. One of the most important factors for successful outpatient/home chemotherapy is an effective antiemetic regime. Patients are able to carry on their usual activities, including attending school and spending time with family and friends.

Symptom Prevention and Management

To achieve quality of life during treatment, it is imperative to prevent and/or control the symptoms of disease and the side effects of treatment. Pain is the most frequent and potentially, the most troublesome symptom. There are many points along the continuum of care where pain is a symptom requiring intervention.

Nausea and vomiting, fatigue, constipation, and a poor appetite are frequent side effects of treatment.

Disease-related Pain

Pain is frequently the most common symptom for patients with osteosarcoma, and until controlled, it is a major threat to quality of life. For pain due to growth of the localized tumor, at times augmented by pathologic fracture, over the counter analgesics such acetaminophen and ibuprofen become inadequate; medications that combine an analgesic and oral opioid are frequently the next step. The most effective intervention for relief of tumor pain is to begin treatment as quickly as possible.

Initial pain assessment should include a self report (location, character, time of worst and least pain, factors that improve and aggravate pain, and intensity – using a rating scale), parent input, observation of behavior, physical examination and physiologic measures/diagnostic results.[11] Future assessments will often be compared with the baseline initial evaluation. Accurate ongoing pain assessment information is invaluable. If pain resolves quickly after the beginning of treatment, it is thought to be indicative of positive response to therapy. Persistent or worsening pain while receiving chemotherapy is worrisome, for it indicates lack of response to treatment; frequently, imaging and later, pathology confirm it. Onset of acute pain may indicate a new development, i.e., a pathologic fracture, which may occur without accompanying trauma, as in the case of a boy who has just rolled over in bed.

Post Operative Pain

Post surgical pain is fairly predictable; the pain management plan usually incorporates IV or epidural pain medication. The need to continually evaluate the efficacy of treatment cannot be overemphasized, as pain is an individual experience. Patients will recover much more quickly when they are not limited by pain. Post thoracotomy deep breathing and coughing will be done more effectively with good pain management. For patients undergoing local control procedures, including limb salvage and amputation, participation in the rehabilitation program depends on good pain control. Nurses are in a prime position to fine tune the timing of pain medications for the best benefit in the patient's interest.

Progressive Disease Pain

Pain due to progessive disease is a complex problem and requires partnership with the experts. Patients and their families have the right to expect that we will provide the resources to keep pain under control. We are practicing at a time when many new modalities may be brought to bear on the patient with widespread disease. Radiation therapy with radiosensitizing chemotherapy, radiofrequency ablation, cryoablation, nerve blocks as well as pain medications are given in a variety of ways to promote quality of life.

Oral Mucocitis

Pain due to mucocitis significantly affects quality of life; if severe, it may prevent adequate oral intake of food and fluids, and may require hospitalization of the patient for pain control and hydration.[12] This symptom, common to our patient population, has been studied with regard to prevention strategies and treatment regimens. In the prevention realm, oral glutamine supplementation, careful oral hygiene and positive nutrition. have been approaches showing benefit. For a patient with a previous history of HSV, prophylaxis with oral valacyclovir is frequently effective. Once patients have developed mucocitis, we utilize topicals and treatment doses of valacyclovir to prevent progression and promote healing. In the adult world, there has been significant nursing research; in pediatrics, we are making progress, but still have a lot of work to do. Assessment tools to measure the outcomes of proposed interventions specific to our population, are in the development stage.[13]

Nausea and Vomiting

For most patients, the first chemotherapeutic agent they will receive, whether on a protocol or as the "in house" treatment plan, is cisplatin. Dr Jaffe used to say that it is too difficult a drug to receive, but it is also too good a drug to neglect. We have new choices of effective antiemetics, such as palonosetron and aprepitaant, to offer to our patients for acute and delayed nausea.[14-16] Our strategy should be to prevent nausea from the first cycle of chemotherapy. If patients have a good experience in the beginning, it is likely that they will continue to respond well to the antiemetics. If the initial experience is severe nausea and vomiting, the patient will be dealing with anticipatory nausea, as well as the actual effect of the chemotherapy. Saving the "big guns" for when a patient fails is not beneficial.

Nutrition

We can recall well nourished (in some cases over nourished) patients sailing through cycles of chemotherapy without nausea, vomiting, and mucocitis, and never requiring hospitalization for neutropenia and fever. In contrast, we remember poorly nourished kids who experienced a lot of nausea and vomiting, often requiring hospitalization between chemotherapy admissions. They never regain the weight they lose, before the next round of chemotherapy. In short, they begin on a downward spiral. We have also met the teenager who views the loss in weight as a positive aspect of cancer treatment. The role of positive nutrition has been studied in a multitude of patient populations, suggesting decreased infection rates, faster healing, fewer ICU admissions and shorter hospital stays. Recent studies suggest that enteral nutrition is more efficacious and poses less risk than parenteral nutrition.[17] A >5% weight loss is cause for concern for our team; often g-tubes are recommended for a >10% weight loss. TPN is rarely recommended and is considered a poor substitute for enteral nutrition. From the time of diagnosis, we need to assess the nutritional status of the patients and introduce the dietitian. Objective data including the height, weight and BMI, especially in graph form, are helpful as a reality check and can be part of the clinic visit on a regular basis (we can even put it on the calendar as we do lab checks). Promoting positive nutrition may well be one of the most important interventions in preventing or minimizing the side effects of treatment.

Developing Local Experts

One of the most skilled nursing practitioners in our institution (Annette Bisanz RN, CNS), has provided instruction on bowel management. She is unable to attend to every patient in need of her services. She has asked for a volunteer from each inpatient unit and outpatient clinic, and trained the volunteers to be local experts; she conducts bowel management rounds where challenging case studies are presented. She remains available for consultation when needed. This is a model we should consider in our specialty to identify the experts who can in turn develop local experts. This model could be applied within our institutions, and on a larger scale, through our professional organizations.

Maintaining Hope

Two of our multiply relapsed patients have got married within the last two months and another has just got engaged; one patient has trained in skydiving; several have graduated from high school and college, skied, camped in the mountains, travelled to Hawaii all during what we might call the "end of life" period. These young people have made it their business to pack quality into every minute they are given, "the gift of time" that Anderson refers to in his editorial, Osteosarcoma Relapse: Expect the Worst, but Hope for the Best.[18] Dealing with relapsed disease can be daunting for the patient, the family and the care team. Three practices seem particularly important for patients like those cited above: maintaining transparent information sharing throughout the continuum of treatment, keeping patients out of the hospital, and offering strategies to deal with relapsed disease sites causing symptoms or impinging on critical organs (i.e., radiation therapy, radiofrequency ablation, cryoablation) even when cure does not appear possible.

Summary and Conclusions

Family centered care is designed to empower patients and their families to take on the challenges of this disease boldly and become stronger. Our aim is to teach patients and their families about the disease and its treatment; while learning from them how to adapt the plan to their needs and goals. Distilling a lot of information into manageable units gives the art of nursing an opportunity to blossom: our clinic nurse, (Maritza Salazar-Abshire RN) practices the art of patient education at its best! Maintaining as much of the "normal" as possible by providing outpatient and home chemotherapy supports normal development and maintains family life. Symptom management is critical for quality of life and frequently requires a multidisciplinary approach. More new medications, combinations of medications and therapeutic modalities are available to our patients now than ever before.

To quote Norman Jaffe, MD: "I have seen osteosarcoma progress from a terrifying disease…to one that we can now approach undaunted and with cautious optimism."[19]

We are indebted to Dr Jaffe and other "giants", whose passion to save children diagnosed with osteosarcoma, transformed this disease from an almost universally fatal one to one with a cure rate of 65–75%. From the nursing perspective, we may approach the care of our patients with much optimism. There are many opportunities for conducting nursing research and applying this research to our practice. We have unlimited opportunities to be creative in teaching and developing tools to make life easier during treatment. As we use new drugs and care for patients treated with new modalities, we can often learn from our adult counterparts, who have already had some experience. We can become local experts in specific areas of practice and be a resource for others.

References

1. Hinds PS, Gattuso JS, Fletcher A, et al. Quality of life as conveyed by pediatric patients with cancer. *Qual Life Res*. 2004;13:761-772.
2. Eichner J, Johnson B. Family-centered care and the pediatrician's role. *Pediatrics*. 2003;112:691-697.
3. Donnelly JP, Huff SM, Lindsey ML, et al. The needs of children with life-limiting conditions: a healthcare-provider-based model. *Am J Hosp Palliat Care*. 2005;22:259-267.
4. Anderson P, Salazar-Abshire M. Improving outcomes in difficult bone cancers using multimodality therapy, including radiation: physician and nursing perspectives. *Curr Oncol Rep*. 2006;8:415-422.

5. Bell DHM, Triche L, Pearson P, Wells P. Flash drive poster: empowerment of families. *Third Annual Oncology Nursing Symposium: Excellence Through Innovation*. MDACC; 2008
6. Aguilera D, Hayes-Jordan A, Anderson P, et al. Outpatient and home chemotherapy with novel local control strategies in desmoplastic small round cell tumor. *Sarcoma*. 2008;2008:261589.
7. Anderson P, Aguilera D, Pearson M, Woo S. Outpatient chemotherapy plus radiotherapy in sarcomas: improving cancer control with radiosensitizing agents. *Cancer Control*. 2008;15:38-46.
8. Lashlee M, O'Hanlon Curry J. Pediatric home chemotherapy: infusing "quality of life". *J Pediatr Oncol Nurs*. 2007;24:294-298.
9. Pearson M, Salazar-Abshire M, Koontzs S. Continuous infusion ifosfamide/mesna: an opportunity for outpatient therapy. *31st Association of Pediatric Hematology/Oncology Nurses*; 2007:74
10. Skubitz KM, Hamdan H, Thompson RC Jr. Ambulatory continuous infusion ifosfamide with oral etoposide in advanced sarcomas. *Cancer*. 1993;72:2963-2969.
11. Hockenberry-Eaton M. *Pain Management in Children with Cancer*. Texas Cancer Council; 1999:71
12. Tomlinson D, Judd P, Hendershot E, et al. Establishing literature-based items for an oral mucositis assessment tool in children. *J Pediatr Oncol Nurs*. 2008;25:139-147.
13. Tomlinson D, Isitt JJ, Barron RL, et al. Determining the understandability and acceptability of an oral mucositis daily questionnaire. *J Pediatr Oncol Nurs*. 2008;25:107-111.
14. Hunt TL, Gallagher SC, Cullen MT Jr, Shah AK. Evaluation of safety and pharmacokinetics of consecutive multiple-day dosing of palonosetron in healthy subjects. *J Clin Pharmacol*. 2005;45:589-596.
15. Shah AK, Hunt TL, Gallagher SC, Cullen MT Jr. Pharmacokinetics of palonosetron in combination with aprepitant in healthy volunteers. *Curr Med Res Opin*. 2005;21:595-601.
16. Smith AR, Repka TL, Weigel BJ. Aprepitant for the control of chemotherapy induced nausea and vomiting in adolescents. *Pediatr Blood Cancer*. 2005;45:857-860.
17. Grimble RF. Immunonutrition. *Curr Opin Gastroenterol*. 2005;21:216-222.
18. Anderson P. Osteosarcoma relapse: expect the worst, but hope for the best. *Pediatr Blood Cancer*. 2005;47:231-238.
19. Pearson M. Historical perspective of the treatment of osteosarcoma: an interview with Dr Norman Jaffe. *J Pediatr Oncol Nurs*. 1998;15:90-94.

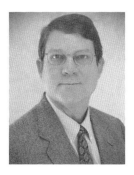

Prosthetics for Pediatric and Adolescent Amputees

Ted B. Muilenburg

Abstract This communication will provide an outline of the variety of prosthetics available to suit the functional (and cosmetic) needs of patients with upper and lower extremity amputations. It will also demonstrate that the prosthetist constitutes a vital role in the rehabilitation of the patient and will respond to his different needs as his requirements for external prosthetic devices change with age and circumstances.

Introduction

Pediatric and adolescent amputees require special custom made external prostheses to combat their infirmity and ensure optimum rehabilitation. During the past quarter century, many changes and modifications in children's prostheses have occurred in response to the challenges they faced with limb loss. The changes were introduced in an effort to contribute to the highest possible standard of life. Many are still being conceived and developed with the discovery of new materials, innovations and inventions. They incorporate expert understanding of the components and socket design, and the accommodations that can be made to the prostheses to improve their life span. Fewer follow-up appointments and adjustment periods are also of importance for well functioning appliances. This is governed by the fact that children, because of their growth and development, will require many prostheses in their lifetime (Figs. 1–3).

This communication will describe prostheses that are available for pediatric and adolescent patients and the factors related to their application. It will cover upper and lower extremity prostheses, the construction methods, the lengthening methods, feet and knee components, socket accommodations for growth, suspension methods and the Van Nes rotationplasty for limb salvage.

T.B. Muilenburg (✉)
Muilenburg Prosthetics Inc., 3900 La Branch Houston, TX, 77004-4094, USA
e-mail: ted@mpihouston.com

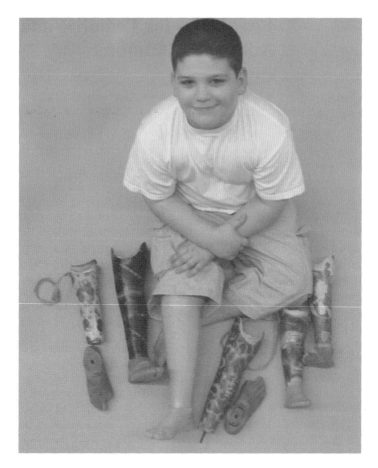

Fig. 1 Seven-year-old boy with several prostheses that he has used over 4 years

General Principles

As part of the rehabilitation team, prosthetists should work closely with the patient, physician, physical and /or occupational therapist, family members and other specialists to establish and achieve treatment goals. Continual focus on emerging technology, advanced equipment and materials of superior performance is essential and will inspire patient confidence and compliance. Innovations, such as precision myoelectric arms and hands, computerized knees, highly functional energy-storing feet and advanced orthotic systems are a specialty, and should preferably be selected for each individual patient's functional needs and unique lifestyle.

On an average, a pediatric or adolescent patient should expect approximately 1–1/2 years of use from a personal prosthesis. A young active adult should expect about 3 years of use from the prosthesis. Older adults, who are not quite as active,

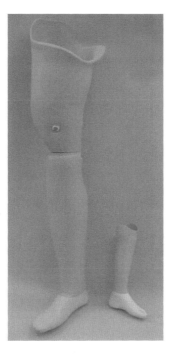

Fig. 2 Two lower extremity prostheses, one for a transfemoral amputation (*Left*) and one for a transtibial amputation (*Right*). Variation in size and design for the different ages and anatomic deficits is noteworthy. These will have to be replaced with growth and development

should expect 5 years of use depending on weight gain or loss. As far as feasible, children with prostheses should be able to participate in the activities and sports they desire. It should also be acknowledged that children will break prostheses, so durability is important. In planning the prosthesis, consideration should be given to adjusting a small size to an adult size with the least number of complications. This process commences before the patient is casted for the prosthesis (Fig. 4). The components should be selected to withstand the expected weight and activity level that can be achieved, and the socket design must be selected appropriately to accommodate for growth. In addition, every effort should be made to adhere to the criteria for construction, fit and comfort. Expert knowledge of the materials used in the construction of the prosthesis is critical, and the advantages and disadvantages should be outlined and discussed with the patient and his/her parents.

Construction of the prosthesis commences with casting to obtain an accurate mold for fit and comfort. The materials are then selected and assembled and construction is initiated. A negative mold of the patient is taken and filled to make a "positive", and it is then modified according to the measurements. A variety of procedures are used to ensure the fit, and the definitive socket is fabricated to attach the selected components. The patient then completes a fitting procedure to ensure the proper alignment and length while ambulating.

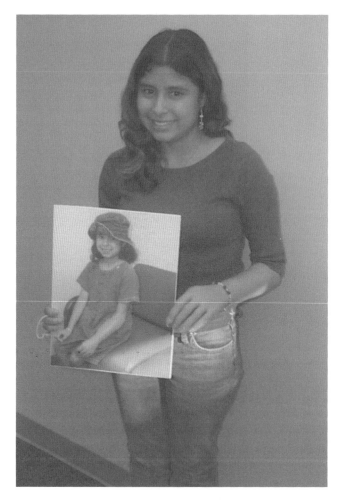

Fig. 3 Eighteen-year-old patient with a myoelectric left upper extremity prosthesis holding a photograph of herself as a child with the prosthesis she utilized at that age

Upper Extremity

Upper extremity prostheses may be of several varieties. Some patients require different types. This is illustrated in Fig. 5. Three upper extremity prostheses were designed for the same active young man and each serves a purpose:

1. The lower prosthesis is a conventional control prosthesis that has a stainless steel work hook and is a voluntary opening terminal device. It has a single control cable that attaches to the forearm, then to the cuff and is activated by the control strap on the figure of 8 harness which is secured to the patient by the axilla loop around the sound side. Also secured on the ring is an anterior support strap that

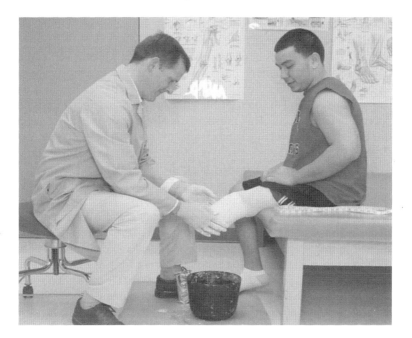

Fig. 4 Cast being applied to commence construction of a lower extremity prosthesis

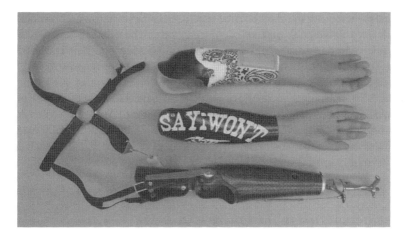

Fig. 5 Three upper extremity prostheses designed for the same active patient. Lower prosthesis: Conventional controlled prosthesis. Center prosthesis: Munster socket which is a self-suspending socket. No harness required. Upper prosthesis: Self-suspending socket with a myoelectrically controlled electric terminal device

extends over the shoulder on the affected side and is attached to the cuff, thus suspending the prosthesis. This is a very durable prosthesis. It is made mostly of waterproof materials; the harness is highly adjustable and the cables and other components can be interchanged or replaced by the patient without the need for immediate socket adjustments and repairs.

2. The center or passive prosthesis has a Munster socket which is self-suspending and does not require a harness. It has a passive hand that is cosmetically acceptable. Many patients wear these appliances for the aesthetics, but they are also functional: they extend the limb enabling the patient to manipulate, position and support different objects. This prosthesis is also appropriate for some contact sports and activities involving submersion in water.

3. The upper prosthesis has the same type of self-suspending socket as the passive prosthesis, but has a myoelectrically controlled electric terminal device. Within the socket are two electrodes: one is over the remnant muscles that flex the wrist and the other over the muscles that extend the wrist. These electrodes pick up electrical impulses produced from the movement of muscles, instructing the hand to open or close. The hand has additional function over the conventional mechanical hand in that it opens further and has a considerable amount of additional pinch force (up to 30 pounds). Ion batteries that last for 1 or 2 days are available. The principal benefit provided by this prosthesis is that the patient is not restricted by a harness to make the terminal device operate. Consequently, the patient can open and close the terminal vice in any position without harness restriction.

Twenty-five years ago, when children were expected to start wearing a prosthesis and continue using a functional aid, there were no small electric or mechanical hands. Consequently, the transradial passive prosthesis, was commonly fitted with a hook terminal device. After the child became used to wearing the prosthesis, a cable would be connected to the hook thus making it functional. These prostheses worked well. The same style prosthesis could be maintained into adult life. This is illustrated in Fig. 6. The young lady continued to wear the same style of prostheses she was originally fitted with. However, today parents and pediatric amputees prefer the more cosmetically appealing myoelectric or mechanical hand. These function well and can be fitted for children as young as 1 year. Figure. 7 is a transradial myoelectric prosthesis made for a 1-year-old. The hand is myoelectrically controlled by electrodes within the socket of the prosthesis. The components of choice that have enabled construction of this small compact prosthesis were batteries of a smaller design.

Construction Design for Lower Extremity

Exoskeletal and endoskeletal designs are illustrated in Fig. 8. The exoskeletal construction design is generally made of wood. The wood is hollowed out and laminated to present a plastic finish, which provides a very strong exterior construction. The endoskeletal design has an internal pylon system, which attaches the foot, knee and socket together, giving it the endoskeletal design. It is covered several times with a soft custom shaped foam and color matched protective skin covering which can be cosmetically appealing. These components have advanced

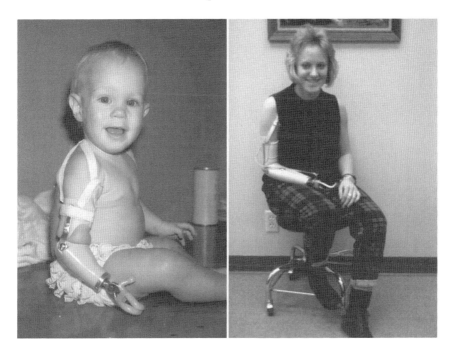

Fig. 6 Young lady with an upper extremity prosthesis (*Right*) of the same style she used as a child (*Left*)

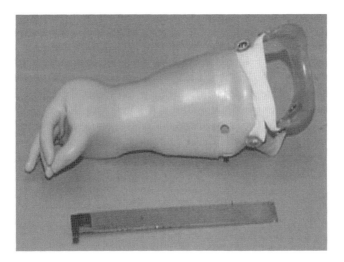

Fig. 7 Transradial myoelectric prosthesis for a 1-year-old. The hand is myoelectrically controlled by electrodes within the socket of the prosthesis

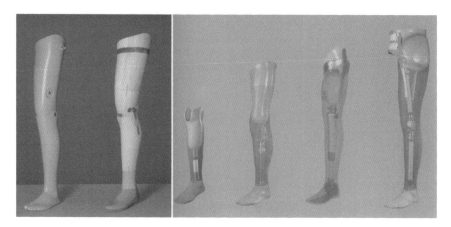

Fig. 8 Exoskeletal (*Left panel*) and Endoskeletal (*Right panel*) types of prostheses. Reprinted with permission from Otto Bock Modular Lower Limb Prosthesis

greatly over the last 15 years while the exoskeletal prostheses have not changed much. In essence, many components of these prostheses have been discontinued because of lack of use. The endoskeletal prostheses are generally used for young active adults whereas in the past the exoskeletal design was the construction method of choice because of their durability. The endoskeletal prostheses are now made with stainless steel, titanium and carbon graphite materials, making them very strong and durable.

Figure 9 demonstrates the components that are available for endoskeletal design from just one of the many manufacturers: 19 different knees and 6 different feet! This permits an opportunity to custom fabricate prostheses to meet specific needs.

In constructing a prosthesis for a child, the ability to lengthen the prosthesis must be taken into consideration. This is not a problem as, in the lower extremity, for example, the exoskeletal design is easily lengthened by removing the foot and placing the appropriate length of wood in between the foot and ankle, and the foot bolts back on (Fig. 10). The wood lengthens the prosthesis. The process is very similar in the endoskeletal design in which a pylon spacer is added within the tube clamp for minimal lengthening. Additional length can be provided by using a longer pylon (Fig. 11). The drawback to this construction is that, with lengthening, a custom shaped "skin" cover must be cut to access the components, and, at times, a considerable amount of time is required to replace or restore the cover to a cosmetically acceptable appearance.

Foot

The first and simplest prosthetic foot is a solid ankle cushion heel foot referred to as the SACH foot seen in the illustrations in Figs. 10–12. SACH is an acronym for **S**olid **A**nkle **C**ushion **H**eel. The foot works at heel strike with the heel compressing

Prosthetics for Pediatric and Adolescent Amputees

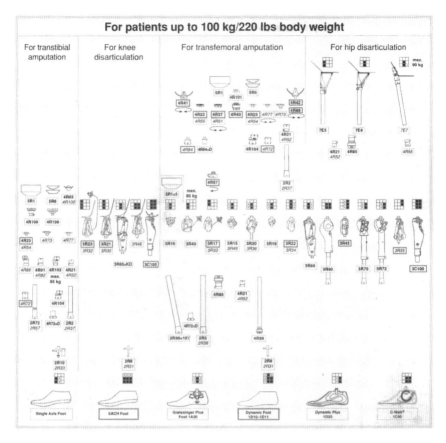

Fig. 9 Components for lower extremity endoskeletal prosthesis. Reprinted with permission from Otto Bock Modular Lower Limb Prosthesis

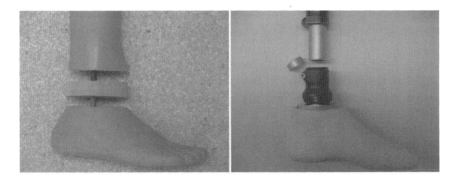

Fig. 10 *Left panel*: Lengthening of exoskeletal prosthesis achieved by removing the foot and placing the appropriate length of wood in between the foot and ankle. The wood lengthens the prosthesis. Foot bolts back on. *Right panel*: Lengthening of endoskeletal prosthesis by bolting metal insertion into tube clamp

and simulating ankle motion. It has a solid ankle keel that gives the patient support at mid-stance. The foot attaches with a single bolt which makes this particular device very adaptable to a number of children; if it breaks, it can be easily replaced. The leg can be lengthened by insertion of wood or metal parts (Fig. 10, panels *left* and *right* respectively). A replacement foot with an ankle bolt wrench can be provided in the event of breakage and the patient can attach the foot without a visit to the prosthetist (Fig. 11). This foot is also manufactured in the smallest design for very young patients and is appropriate for children under 3 years of age. Figure 12 depicts the smallest foot manufactured (10 cm), and beside it is a foot that is a little smaller, demonstrating that a foot can be made.for a child of any size.

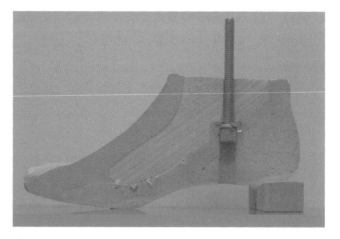

Fig. 11 Cross-section of SACH foot to demonstrate construction and single attachment ankle bolt

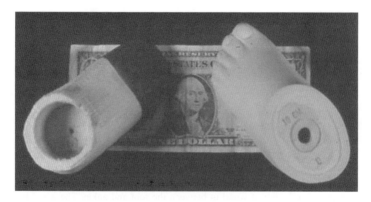

Fig. 12 Smallest manufactured foot, 10 cm (*R*). Adjacent to it is a foot made a little smaller (*L*). Dollar bill utilized to emphasize size

Prosthetics for Pediatric and Adolescent Amputees

The energy storing foot is the dynamic response foot. The Seattle foot was the first foot manufactured with energy storing capabilities (Fig. 13). The white center section is a Delrin plastic material that stores energy. It is shaped like a spring and extends fully forward so that when a patient puts weight on the toe, it flexes upward and the energy that the toe stores springs back immediately, providing a push-off that allows a more efficient step and the ability to run. If the foot is broken, it also has the single bolt attachment and can be easily replaced. This concept has been improved greatly over the years by the use of carbon fibers. Some feet have incorporated shock absorbers (Fig. 14). The tall center prosthesis in Fig. 14 has a hydraulic knee mechanism, making a compact unit for the transfemoral patients.

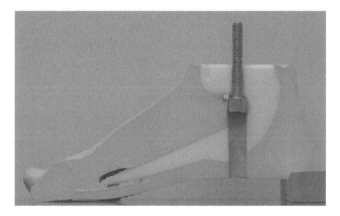

Fig. 13 Seattle foot was the first foot with energy storing capabilities. The white center section is in a spring shape and extends fully forward. When a patient puts weight on the toe, it flexes upward and the energy that the toe stores springs back immediately

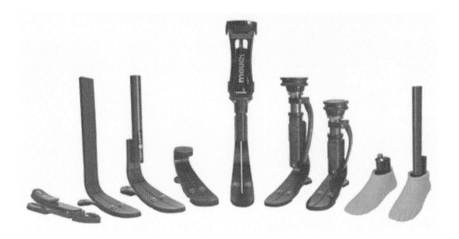

Fig. 14 Energy storing feet. Feet with incorporated shock absorbers. The tall center prosthesis has a hydraulic knee mechanism making a compact unit for transfemoral patients

The Trouper foot (Fig. 15) is a multi-axle and dynamic response foot made specifically for pediatric patients. It can be fit to children as young as 3-years. The main motion of this foot is plantar flexion, which keeps the foot flat, helping to stabilize the prosthetic knee; this is very beneficial for transfemoral amputees. On weight bearing of the toe it flexes upwards, storing energy and providing the patient again with more efficient push-off. This particular foot also incorporates a foot shell with a split toe; so, children can wear different shoes and sandals of their choice.

A transfemoral prosthesis for a 1-year-old (Fig. 16), has a constant friction knee and a SACH foot. Very young children can be fitted when they are learning to pull to a stand, and then they can learn to walk with the prosthesis. The knee is often not appreciated as children do not bend their knees much when walking. However, research has demonstrated that the knee has an important function in certain activities. The prosthesis depicted in Fig. 17 also has a lower section with a geometric locking mechanism. This locks the knee at heel strike. When the patient steps forward, it places weight on the toe, causing an extension movement of the knee, unlocking it and allowing a complete step. Children, in particular, benefit from this knee because there is an inherent stability factor in the design

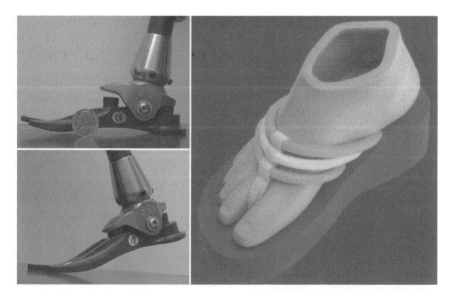

Fig. 15 Trouper foot is a multi-axle and dynamic response foot made specifically for pediatric patients. May be fitted to children as young as 3 years. The main motion is plantar flexion. May be worn with different shoes and sandals of their choice (*R*)

Fig. 16 Transfemoral prosthesis for a 1-year-old, with a constant friction knee and a SACH foot. Length of prosthesis compared to pencil on side

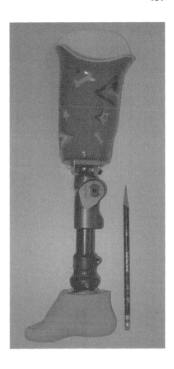

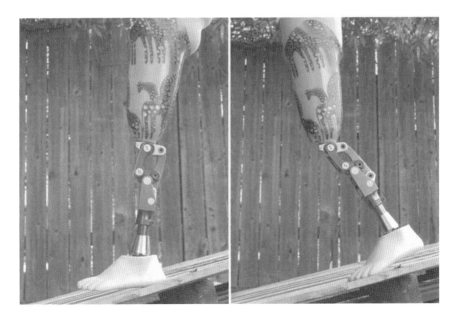

Fig. 17 Transfemoral prosthesis with polycentric knee. Lower section with geometric locking mechanism allows for safe ambulation. There is an inherent stability factor in the design

Knee

Polycentric knees are appropriate for knee disarticulation patients as they allow placement of the knee-center closest to the true anatomical position of the patient (Fig. 18). The microprocessor knee regulates swing and stance resistance, allowing the patient to negotiate steps and walk around objects securely on a wide variety of surfaces, without fear of the knee buckling and /or the patient falling.

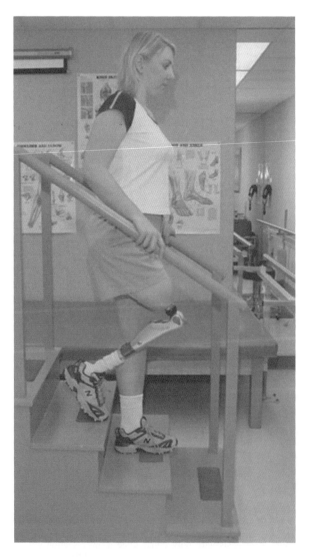

Fig. 18 Microprocessor knee. Regulates swing and stance resistance facilitating ability to descend steps

This particular knee can be fitted to children if their shin is of the appropriate length. The knee is expensive and in ordering the device for children, the possibility of breakage must be considered. Compliance is important.

Socket Accommodations for Growth

The socket of the transtibial prosthesis is often referred to as the "Patella Tendon Bearing Socket" (PTB socket). The major part of the patient's weight can be taken on the mid patella tendon. This is the tendon between the patella and the tibia tubercle that can easily be located on the patient as well as on the prosthesis as observed in a bisected socket. Vertical measurement from the patellar bar provides information on the depth of the socket which is an important component of the prosthesis (Fig. 19). The depth determines how much longitudinal growth of the patient is allowed for in the prosthesis, its utility and its fit. Many patients cannot tolerate any weight bearing on the distal end of their residual limb particularly when bone spurs are present. For these individuals extra depth is also required for high impact sports such as basketball when one bears down hard on the prosthesis.

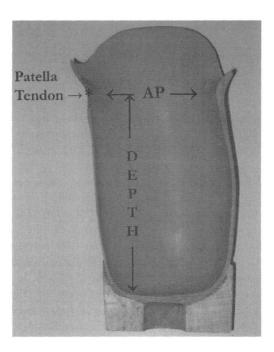

Fig. 19 Cross-section demonstrating Patella Tendon Bearing Socket (PTB socket), a socket of the transtibial prosthesis. The major part of the patient's weight can be taken on the mid patella tendon

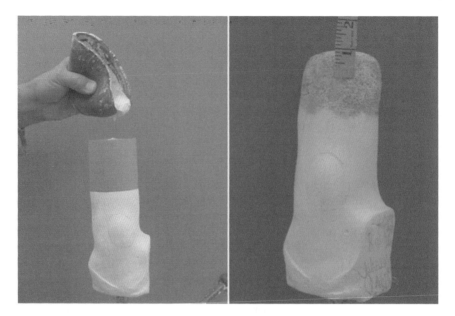

Fig. 20 Method to adjust the depth of the socket. A trouble free approach is simply to add plaster to the end of the cast that is used as the mold to produce the socket (*Left panel*). The end of the cast can be built up at least 1 in. or 25 mm (*Right panel*)

There are many methods to adjust the depth of the socket but most require a visit to the prosthetist. A trouble free approach for the patient is simply to add plaster to the end of the cast that is used as the mold to produce the socket for the patient. The end of the cast is built up at least 1 in. or 25 mm (Fig. 20). When the socket is made, this will produce a void at the distal end that can easily be filled by a removable end pad. As the patient grows into the socket, he may simply remove the distal end pad and replace it with another soft material such as lamb's wool. Patients may also accommodate their growth by using sock management (Fig. 21). The prosthesis can be fit with a 3 or 5 ply sock and as the patient gains weight or grows, a thinner sock may be used to enable the patient to insert the residual limb into the socket. If there is any loss in weight, thicker socks can be worn or doubled up until appropriate support is obtained.

Another component that can be made is a removable soft insert (Fig. 22). It is generally fitted to adult prostheses if scars or boney prominences have developed. This makes the prosthesis more comfortable and adjustable. In pediatric patients, this can also serve another purpose. The removable soft insert is made over a cast that is already elongated. The insert renders the socket extra thick; if a patient gains weight, as may occur after discontinuation of chemotherapy, the insert may be removed. With this strategy, many patients, can continue wearing the same prosthesis with few complications by simply substituting the insert with appropriately thick socks.

Prosthetics for Pediatric and Adolescent Amputees 411

Fig. 21 Patients may accommodate growth by using sock management. A distal end pad is inserted at the end of the socket

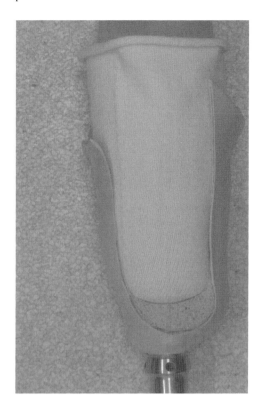

Fig. 22 Removable soft insert. It is fabricated to be placed over a cast that is already elongated

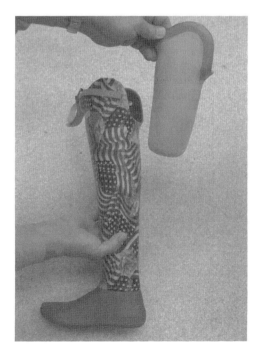

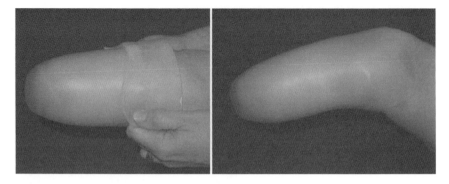

Fig. 23 Cushion liner added to the prosthesis for comfort

Liners

A cushion liner may be added to the prosthesis (Fig. 23). Many adult prostheses are fitted with these cushion liners to add comfort. They are also being used on a more regular basis in children's prostheses. The liner rolls on and is a protective liner for the skin and is particularly helpful to combat severe scarring. If a particular liner is used for a child, selection may be made from a range of thicknesses.

Locking Liner with Pin

This is applied and arranged in the same way as a cushion liner, but it has a nut on the end for a locking pin to be inserted (Fig. 24). It is worn with a sock that has a hole to manage the fit for the pin. Patients simply put the liner and sock on and insert the limb into the prosthesis. The pin attaches to a locking mechanism at the bottom of the socket. The only problem with this prosthesis in children is that it leaves little room for longitudinal growth of the limb. The solution is to fit liners with the removable liner end pad, which is inserted inside the liner **before** the patient is casted. The end pad can simply be removed by the patient when needed.

Suspensions

Cuff suspension strap for transtibial prostheses. This is a common suspension method. It attaches to the proximal sides of the prosthesis. The strap simply leads over the patella and is secured by a second strap that extends around the thigh (Fig. 25). It is easily repaired or replaced and works very well to hold the prosthesis on patients who have a prominent patella.

Prosthetics for Pediatric and Adolescent Amputees 413

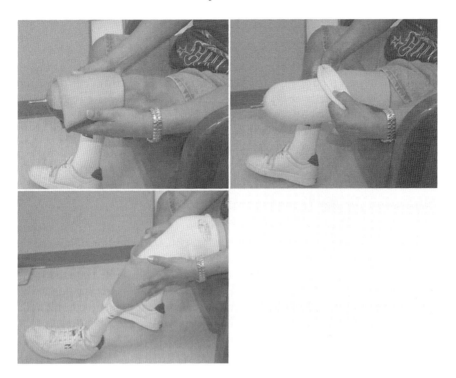

Fig. 24 Locking liner with pin. It is worn with a sock(s) that has a hole for the pin. Patients may wear more than one sock. Panels demonstrate patient putting on liner and inserting limb into prosthesis

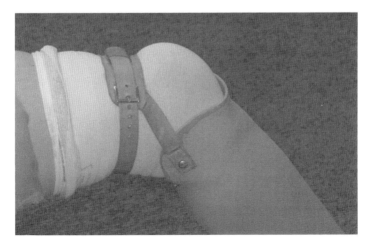

Fig. 25 Cuff suspension strap for transtibial prostheses. Attaches to the proximal sides of the prosthesis. The strap simply leads over the patella and is secured by a second strap that extends around the thigh

Suspension Sleeves

These cover the top of the socket and are pulled up onto the thigh to suspend the prosthesis. They are routinely used on pediatric prostheses instead of cuff suspension straps because the patella has not fully developed, is surrounded by baby fat and slips off. The only side effect is that they are hot and wear out quickly especially when the children crawl. This is easily solved by supplying the patient with two or three liners that they can replace themselves.

Suspension for the Transfemoral Prosthesis

The suspension method of choice is the suction socket. Application of this prosthesis requires the use of a tubular cotton stockinet pulled sock over the residual limb; it is removed through the valve hole as the residual limb is pulled into the socket. The patient is able to wear the prosthesis very well using this true suction method (Fig. 26). The only complication children encounter is related to growth and weight gain and loss which affect the fit and the suspension. Routine adjustments to the socket will be required.

Silesian Belt

This simply attaches around the patient's waist and is secured at the anterior and lateral aspect of the prosthesis to hold it [Fig. 27, (L)]. It works well as demonstrated by the patient swinging on the parallel bars [Fig. 27, (R)]. This type of suspension belt also allows the patient to wear socks. Transfemoral suspension methods that are routinely used comprise the suction socket, the Silesian belt and a locking liner with the pin.

Van Ness Rotationplasty

The Van Nes rotationplasty limb salvage surgery involves rotating the foot 180° (Figs. 28 and 29). This allows the ankle to function well as a knee joint. It also has excellent weight bearing capabilities. Patients have better gait and hip strength than transfemoral amputees, and active proprioseptive feedback is achieved by using the ankle as the knee. The advantages on a functional level far outweigh the cosmesis concerns. Also, because the nerves have not been severed they do not experience phantom sensation or pain. Patients with a Van Ness rotationplasty as opposed to a transfemoral amputation, can function very well as transtibial amputees.

Prosthetics for Pediatric and Adolescent Amputees 415

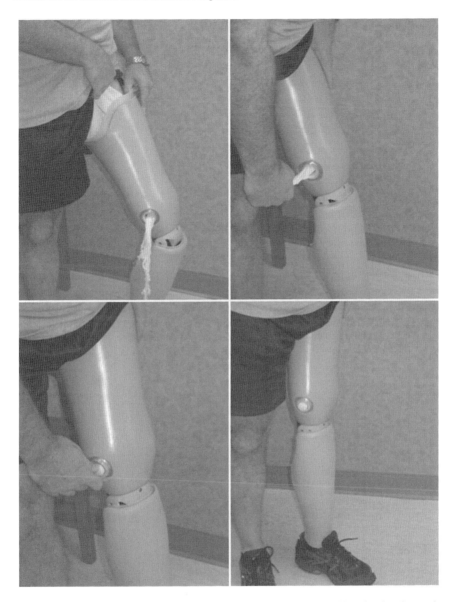

Fig. 26 Suspension suction socket for the transfemoral prosthesis. Stockinet is placed over the residual limb and pulled through the valve hole with the limb concurrently being pulled into the socket (*upper panels*). In the *lower panels* the stockinet has been removed. This is a true suction method and facilitates excellent suspension and use

They can outperform patients who wear a transfemoral prosthesis, even with the best or most expensive knee, when they obtain successful surgery and a well-fitted prosthesis.

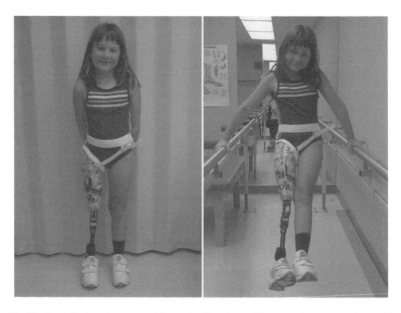

Fig. 27 Silesian belt. Attaches around the patient's waist and is secured at the anterior and lateral side of the prosthesis to hold it (*Left panel*). It works well as demonstrated by the patient swinging on parallel bars (*Right panel*)

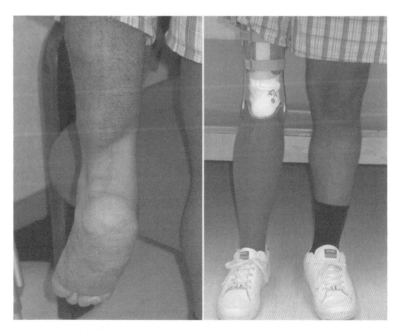

Fig. 28 Van Ness rotationplasty (anterior view). *Left panel*: Right foot rotated 180°. Heel faces anteriorly. *Right panel*: patient fitted with prosthesis

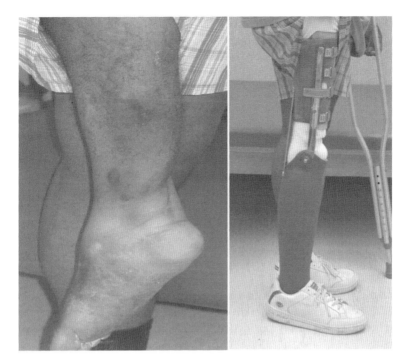

Fig. 29 Van Ness rotationplasty (lateral view). *Left panel*: Right foot rotated 180°. Heel faces anteriorly. *Right panel*: patient fitted with prosthesis

Care of the Prosthesis

Regular cleaning and careful maintenance are important to prolong the useful life of a prosthesis.

Socket

The socket should be wiped daily with a damp cloth, using soap and water. It should not be submerged since water could damage the mechanical components. It should be dried thoroughly and left to air overnight.

Upper Extremity Harness

Cotton and synthetic harness straps should be scrubbed with household cleaner containing ammonia and cleaned whenever soiled as perspiration stains permanently mark harness straps. The prosthesis should be placed on a counter or drainboard protecting it from water and the harness washed in a sink without removing it from the prosthesis. It should then be rinsed and air-dried thoroughly. It should not be placed in a clothes drier or dried with a hair drier to hasten drying.

Control Cable

The control cable to the TD and/or elbow should be examined often for cut or worn areas. Worn cables can be repaired, and spare cables can be manufactured.

A worn-out tension band on a hook terminal device can be cut with scissors and replaced with a new one.

Cosmetic glove

A cosmetic glove should be washed immediately when it becomes soiled. It should be washed daily with a mixture of mild soap and lukewarm water. After rinsing the glove should be allowed to air-dry, resting flat. Wetting the mechanism should be avoided.

Personal Care and Hygiene

Proper care and cleaning are essential to maintaining healthy skin, especially that in contact with the prosthesis. The residual limb should be washed and rinsed daily. Potentially irritating soap film should be completely removed. The skin should be completely dry before putting on the prosthesis. Skin disorders on the residual limb should be reported to the prosthetist or physician.

Conclusion

Children with properly fitting prostheses, therapy and follow-up, can continue to lead normal lives as children. They may participate in many activities of their choice and may ascend to their highest potential (Figs. 30–33)

Fig. 30 Patient with prosthesis rappelling on wall

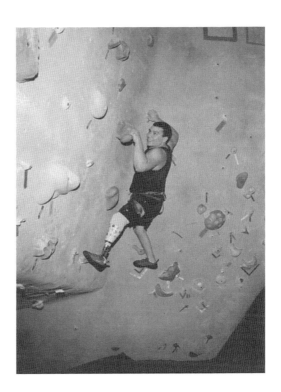

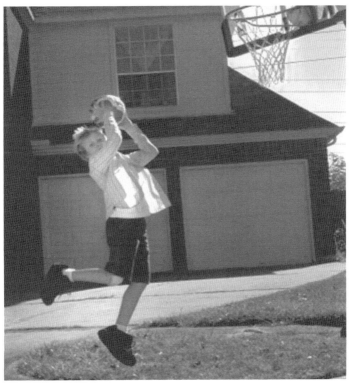

Fig. 31 Patient with prosthesis "shooting basket"

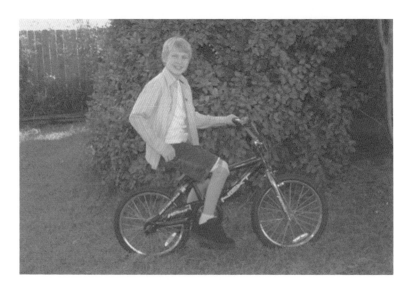

Fig. 32 Patient with prosthesis riding bicycle

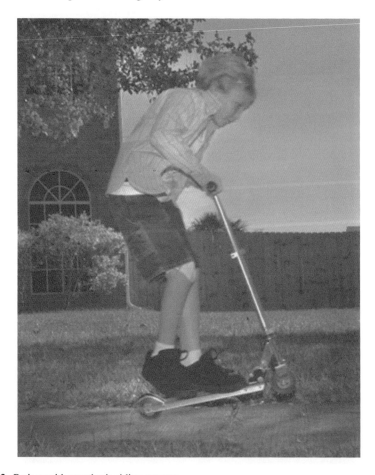

Fig. 33 Patient with prosthesis riding scooter

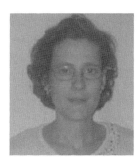

Functional, Psychosocial and Professional Outcomes in Long-Term Survivors of Lower-Extremity Osteosarcomas: Amputation Versus Limb Salvage

Giulia Ottaviani, Rhonda S. Robert, Winston W. Huh, and Norman Jaffe

Abstract As the number of osteosarcoma survivors increases, the impact of quality of life and function needs to be addressed. Limb salvage is the preferred treatment when patients have treatment options; yet, the questionable long-term durability and complications of prostheses, combined with ambiguous function, leave some doubt regarding the best clinical and surgical options. Comparisons between limb salvage patients, amputees and controls also require further investigation. Amputation would leave the patients with a lifelong requirement for an external prosthetic leg associated with an overall limited walking distance. While artificial limbs are much more sophisticated than those used in the past, phantom limb sensations remain a substantial and unpredictable problem in the amputee. Complications such as stump overgrowth, bleeding, and infection, also require further elucidation. Limb salvage surgery using endoprosthesis, allografts or reconstruction is performed in approximately 85% of patients affected by osteosarcoma located in the middle and/or distal femur. One drawback in limb-salvage surgery in the long-term survivor is that endoprostheses have a limited life span with long-term prosthetic failure. The inherent high rate of reoperation remains a serious problem. Replacing a damaged, infected or severely worn-out arthroplastic joint or its intramedullary stem is difficult, especially in the long-stem cemented endoprostheses used in the 1980s. Limb lengthening procedures in patients who have not reached maturity must also be addressed. Periprosthetic infections, compared to other indications for joint reconstruction, were found to be more frequent in patients treated for neoplastic conditions and their outcome can be devastating, resulting in total loss of joint function, amputation, and systemic complications. Quality of life in terms of function, psychological outcome and endpoint achievements such as marriage and employment apparently do not differ significantly between amputee and nonamputee osteosarcoma survivors.

G. Ottaviani (✉)
Children's Cancer Hospital, The University of Texas M.D. Anderson Cancer Center, 77030-4009 Houston, TX, USA
e-mail: giulia.ottaviani@unimi.it

Amputee patients nonetheless appear to have made satisfactory adjustments to their deficits with or without a functional external prosthesis. It also appeared that amputee patients had a similar psychological and quality of life outcome as limb salvage patients. There was no evidence of excessive anxiety or depression or deficits in self-esteem compared with the normal population or matched controls. A number of long-term survivors also achieved high ranking in the professional and commercial work place. These positive aspects should be recognized and emphasized to patients and their parents when discussing the outcome.

Introduction

The prognosis for patients with osteosarcoma has changed radically in recent decades. Historically, the prognosis was poor, with rapid development of metastases and subsequent death common even after amputation. Prior to 1970, amputation was the only surgical treatment prescribed and at least 80% of patients died of metastatic disease, most commonly in the lungs.[1] Treatment strategies adopted over the past three decades, specifically neoadjuvant and postoperative adjuvant chemotherapy, have improved the ability to perform safe limb-sparing resection and to ablate metastases, leading to a significant increase in overall survival rates.[2,3] In the current era, about 70% of patients with osteosarcoma survive.[2,3]

This increased survival success, however, has been marred by the fact that chemotherapy and surgical procedures have long-term consequences that can compromise the quality of life of survivors, i.e., heart problems, hearing loss, osteopenia, osteoporosis, kidney and liver impairments, decreased fertility, functional disability resulting from surgical procedure, hepatitis C, HIV, metachronous skeletal osteosarcoma, second malignant neoplasm.[4-13] Being cognizant of these factors and ensuring optimum quality-of-life in patients are thus important in the treatment of osteosarcoma. These factors may play a dominant role in reaching a decision between amputation and limb-salvage surgery.

In 1986, the Musculoskeletal Tumor Society (MSTS), in a randomized study of nonmetastatic high-grade osteosarcoma of the distal femur, reported that amputation did not result in a survival benefit compared with limb-salvage surgery.[14] Since then, limb-salvage surgery has become the preferred surgical option generally requested by patients when a wide local excision of the bone tumor can be achieved.

The traditional opinion has been that, compared with amputation, limb-salvage surgery would provide a psychological benefit because of the obvious cosmetic difference and the maintenance of reasonably normal function of the preserved limb. However, late complications related to limb salvage are frequent. Many limb-salvage complications, such as nonunion of bone, fracture, poor joint movement, and leg-length discrepancy, are pathologic in nature. Others, such as endoprosthesis failure or aseptic loosening of fixation parts, are mechanically related.[15-20] These late complications can be problematic, and the perceived advantage of limb salvage can be negated by the need for additional operations or, ultimately, an amputation.

On the other hand, if primary or secondary amputation is performed, the patient will have a lifelong requirement for a prosthetic leg. The possibility of stump problems, such as bleeding and infections, and phantom limb sensations should always be considered.[18,21,22]

Unfortunately, there is a paucity of information regarding the inherent risks and benefits of amputation versus limb salvage with regard to the overall function and quality of life of long-term osteosarcoma survivors. Such information would not only facilitate decision making with regard to tnitial treatment, but also, in the event of endoprosthesis failure, help with the difficult and multifaceted decision of whether to undergo additional limb-salvage procedures or ultimately an amputation.

This chapter summarizes the data available on functional outcomes and quality of life after treatment for osteosarcoma of the lower extremity with the two main surgical options, amputation or limb salvage. We review functional outcomes; economic considerations; psychological, social, and professional outcomes; and other late effects of therapy.

Functional Outcomes

Functional or physical outcome comparisons between limb salvage and amputation have been performed using several assessment tools, and the results of the studies have been varied. Studies using the MSTS scoring system have demonstrated improved lower-limb function in limb-salvage patients when compared with amputees.[16–20] However, using the TESS measure, Nagarajan et al[23] did not find any differences in functional outcome based on surgical procedure in 528 adults from the Childhood Cancer Survivor Study cohort. Comparing studies is difficult because many of these studies examine small numbers of patients with different follow-up intervals and use different assessment tools.

Using the MSTS scoring system, Futani et al[24] reported changes in physical function before and after limb-lengthening procedures among survivors of lower-extremity osteosarcoma. A score of 100% indicates optimal function. Prior to lengthening, the mean value was 65%, and after lengthening, the it was 81%. Utilizing TESS, Tunn et al[25] reported the outcome in 78 adults who had been treated for osteosarcoma as children and who survived at least 4 years. Twenty-five of these patients had had endoprosthetic replacements, and 13 had required replacements because of fracture, infection, or aseptic loosening. Patients who had had replacement of distal-femur prostheses reported TESS scores of 51–93% and MSTS scores of 51–83%. Patients who had had replacement of proximal-tibia prostheses reported TESS scores of 42–93% and MSTS scores of 31–83%. Refaat et al[26] reported functional outcomes in 408 patients treated for lower-extremity bone and soft-tissue sarcoma. Among amputees, 91% reported using their prostheses, 83% reported using a walking aid, and 92% reported being able to drive a car.

Van der Windt et al[27] found no difference in energy expenditure in treadmill walking in children who had had rotationplasty, children who had had above-the-knee amputation, and children who had had hip disarticulation. Hann et al[28] noted excellent function in 18 of 22 children who had been treated with rotationplasty.

Lindner et al[17] reported that the functional outcomes of the Van Nes rotationplasty was superior to that of amputation or limb salvage in osteosarcoma survivors. Recently, in a group of sarcoma survivors at a mean time of 10 years after rotationplasty, Sawamura et al[29] have reported vascular compromise as a complication, which resulted in conventional amputation in 12% of cases; late complications included tibial fracture, wound complications, nonunion, and slipped capital femoral epiphysis.

Aksnes et al[30] in a study of 118 sarcoma survivors, concluded that limb-sparing surgery preserved more function than did amputation, as measured by the MSTS score at a mean follow-up of 13 years. Tumors located above the knee resulted in significantly lower MSTS and TESS scores compared with tumors located below the knee.[30]

In essence, as the number of survivors of childhood cancer increases, the impact of functionality and quality-of-life issues needs to be addressed further. Limb salvage is the preferred treatment when patients have treatment options, yet the questionable long-term durability and complications associated with this approach, combined with equivocal functional and quality-of-life outcomes, leave some doubt as to the best clinical and surgical practice advice. A brief review of the impact of these surgical options, on quality of life, the potential complications of these operations, factors related to the decision-making process and quality of life considerations follows.

Amputation

Indications for primary amputation are based on the location and local extent of the tumor and the expected functionality of the extremity after tumor resection.[30-34] Patients who require primary amputation have a higher risk of developing metastases than do patients who undergo limb-salvage procedures, but this risk is associated with the predominantly large size of such tumors.[34] Although amputation is often considered the simplest surgical solution for bone cancer, especially if the cancer is associated with extensive soft-tissue involvement, this treatment option is not always acceptable to patients and their relatives.[15,18,35,36]

Moderate to severe disability accompanies lower-extremity amputation above the ankle regardless of the level of amputation.[37] Amputation leaves patients with a lifelong requirement for a prosthetic leg, which is associated with a claimed overall limited walking distance of 500 m or more.[38] Although artificial limbs today are much more sophisticated than those used in the past, phantom limb sensations remain a substantial and unpredictable problem. The possibility of stump problems, such as bleeding, infections, and bone stump overgrowth, must also be considered[18,21,22,39]

AMPUTATION: complications & drawbacks

- Lifelong requirement for a prosthesis
- Infection of the stump
- Wound breakdown
- Swelling of the stump
- Hip joint flexion contracture
- Pain
- Phantom limb sensation
- Pressure sores from the prosthesis
- Stump bony overgrowths
- Dysfunctionally short stump

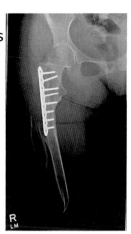

Fig. 1 On the *left*, causes of functional disability as a result of amputation in long-term osteosarcoma survivors are listed. On the *right*, an anteroposterior-view radiogram of the right femoral stump of a Hispanic, female, 16-year-old amputee survivor. Visible are a side plate with multiple screws, as well as disuse osteoporosis and heterotopic bone formation. The patient was 7 years old when a diagnosis of osteosarcoma of the right femur was established. At that time, she was treated with pre- and postoperative chemotherapy and a limb-salvage surgery consisting of a custom expandable total-knee prosthesis. Subsequently, the patient developed problems with wound dehiscence requiring multiple wound debridements. She underwent more than 15 surgeries that that culminated in an above-the-knee amputation at the age of ten. The amputation of the lower leg was completed by the turn-up procedure and internal fixation in an attempt to provide a longer femoral stump

(Fig. 1). The incidence of these complications in long-term survivors awaits further study.

Limb Salvage

Limb-salvage surgery using an endoprosthesis, autograft, allograft, or other reconstruction techniques is performed in about 85% of patients affected by osteosarcoma of the middle and/or distal femur.[32,33]

In patients who undergo primary limb-sparing procedures, there is an increased risk of local recurrence but no increase in overall mortality.[40,41]

The decision to undertake a limb-salvage procedure is usually more acceptable to patients because of their perception that a salvaged limb conforms to "normality" and presumably will result in satisfactory function. All the limb-sparing options after massive bone excision are technically demanding and time consuming for both the patients and the surgeons, needing careful and constant appraisal, especially when the osteosarcoma involves the knee.[15,17,32]

The avoidance of short-term complications and the success of limb salvage depend on the patient following the instructions of the physiotherapist regarding the performing of the prescribed exercises. Special care must be taken with a knee prosthesis, which has a limited range of motion compared with a natural healthy knee. Over time, long-term osteosarcoma survivors with knee prostheses usually undergo repeated revision or replacement operations, which are accompanied by a progressive inexorable deterioration of the extensor apparatus and quadriceps muscle. It is possible to achieve amazing short-term results by reconstructing a resected knee joint using a custom total knee prosthesis. But in time, the device will probably fail because of infection and/or breakage, accompanied by muscle deterioration, and the long-term results are often unfavorable.[15,40–42]

Endoprostheses have a limited life span as many complications may occur (Fig. 2).[15,40–46] Replacing a damaged, infected, or severely worn-out arthroplastic joint is difficult, especially if it has long cemented stems, as did the endoprostheses used in the 1980s[15,45,47] (Fig. 3). Infection represents a major complication of prosthetic joint surgery, despite advances in operating-room design, surgical technique, and antibiotic prophylaxis.[43,44]

Periprosthetic infections may be more frequent in patients treated for a neoplastic condition,[43] and their outcome can be devastating, resulting in total loss of joint

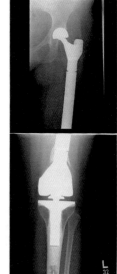

Fig. 2 On the *left*, causes of functional disability as a result of limb salvage in long-term osteosarcoma survivors are listed. On the *right*, an anteroposterior-view radiogram of a left total-femur endoprosthesis in a Hispanic, female, 26-year-old osteosarcoma survivor. Failure of a previous hemiarthroplasty of the left hip was corrected by a total femur replacement.

function, amputation, and systemic complications.[39,43,44] Severe periprosthetic metallosis has also been described.[15,45] Numerous treatments have been proposed; these include irrigation, debridement, prosthesis retention, revision or excision arthroplasty.[15,46] Over time, the endoprosthesis may eventually require replacement or joint arthrodesis to fuse the tibia and femur bones.[15,40]

The application of the Ilizarov method has been gathering increased interest as an important method to save severely damaged limbs.[48,49] In particular, its application in long-term sarcoma survivors, can address not only bone infections and severe bone loss following an endoprosthesis failure, but also correct length discrepancy.[15,48,50]

In favor of limb salvage, is the interesting report by Jeys et al[51] of an increased survival rate in osteosarcoma patients treated for postoperative infections related to endoprostheses. In a study of 547 osteosarcoma patients, the 10-year survival rate for patients who had postoperative endoprosthesis infection was 84.5%, compared with 62.3% for the noninfected group. Infection was identified as a new independent favorable prognostic factor for osteosarcoma; the mechanism of its anti-tumor activity needs further research.[51]

In addition to the problems inherent to limb salvage procedure, little documentation is available on the following complications and their incidence, which may affect the quality of life in limb-salvage patients: delay in scheduled chemotherapy during the initial treatment, a fracture, delayed bone union, bone nonunion or pseudarthrosis, soft-tissue necrosis; inadequate wound coverage and healing, artery, vein, or nerve damage, poor joint movement, malalignment, venous thrombosis; pain, leg-length discrepancy, and deterioration of balance control.[43,52,53]

Reoperation After Limb Salvage

The surgical options and inherent problems in long-term survivors who undergo limb-salvage procedures and then develop a local recurrence or complications are complex. Oncologists and orthopedic surgeons should have detailed discussions with patients and their families regarding the choice of surgical approach, i.e., retention of the salvaged extremity vs. amputation. The choice will depend on the location and local extent of the previously resected tumor, the complications or the extent of the local recurrence, and the expected functional ability of the limb after the proposed operation.[34] As for newly diagnosed bone cancer, and in recurrent bone cancer, survival is not considered to be affected by the type of surgical procedure chosen; amputation and limb-salvage procedures both aim to adequately remove the bone cancer.[14] The training and experience of the attending surgeons may influence the decision to amputate vs. reconstruct a severely affected leg in a patient who has previously undergone a limb-salvage procedure.[15,39,49]

Amputation and limb-sparing techniques have benefits and drawbacks in survivors of osteosarcoma of the lower extremity. One drawback of primary and secondary limb-salvage surgery is that endoprostheses have a limited life span, and long-term

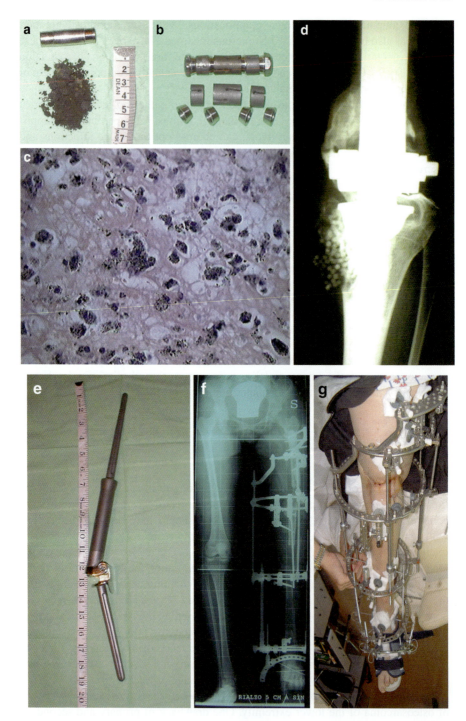

Fig. 3 Long-term osteosarcoma survivor. The patient was 11 years old when a diagnosis of telangiectatic osteosarcoma was established. After a local recurrence and extensive chemotherapy,

prosthetic failure and the inherent high rate of reoperation remain a prolonged and serious problem.[15,32,40,45] Jeys et al[54] reported that the overall risk of subsequent amputation after a limb-salvage surgery with endoprosthesis replacement was 8.9%. Among the 112 patients, amputation was performed because of local recurrence in 63% of cases, infection in 34%, mechanical failure of the prosthesis in 2%, and persistent pain in 1%.[54]

Currently, the most common indication for an arthrodesis of the knee is a failed infected total-knee prosthesis. Other indications for arthrodesis include aseptic loosening, a deficient extensor mechanism, poor soft tissues conditions, instability, pain, and severe metallosis.[15,46] Knee arthrodesis after failed total-knee arthroplasty is a useful salvage procedure, although bone fusion is more difficult to achieve than when arthrodesis is performed as a primary procedure.[46] The problem of severe bone loss due to a failed total-knee replacement can be addressed using an external fixator of the Ilizarov type (Fig. 2). When this method is used, high fusion rates even in cases of extensive bone loss have been reported.[15,46,48]

Most orthopedic surgeons realize that an arthrodesed knee is a stable, painless condition that allows for almost unlimited activity. However, the inability to bend the knee, which interferes with sitting, may be undesirable for the patient. Some patients who have undergone extensive procedures designed to salvage a lower limb believe that they might have been better off with the extremity amputated from the onset of the bone cancer.[42]

Long-term osteosarcoma survivors with an infected or worn-out endoprosthesis may have been subjected to several surgical procedures with little benefit and, together with their families, may be exhausted.

Economic Considerations

The cost difference between amputation and reconstruction in patients with a severely affected leg has been calculated, with a finding of wide variations in surgical

---

Fig. 3 (continued) she underwent en bloc resection of the middle and distal femur and of the proximal tibia with insertion of a modified Guepar-type endoprosthesis. (**a**) Fifteen years later, after metallosis had occurred, the endoprosthesis axle was removed and replaced by a new, custom-made one. Shown is the gross appearance of the metallosis, which was of a powdery consistency, and the original prosthesis axle. (**b**) Custom-made prosthesis expansive axle/pin, especially designed to lock the prosthesis hinge. (**c**) Histologic view of the granuloma with metallosis, showing histiocytes containing abundant metallic debris, abundant fibrosis, and necrosis. Hematoxylin-eosin staining; magnification, 200×. (**d**) Anteroposterior X-rays showing a hydroxyapatite substitute bone graft performed in the proximal tibia where it had been eroded by the granuloma. (**e**) Lateral view of the custom-made prosthesis, modified Guepar-type, removed 17 years after its implantation due to periprosthesic granuloma and infection. After prosthesis removal, femuro-tibial fusion and bone transport, using an Ilizarov frame, were performed. (**f**) Anteroposterior-view radiogram, showing the Ilizarov frame during two-level bone transport, after a femuro-tibial fusion. (**g**) Clinical photograph showing the patient during treatment with the Ilizarov frame to achieve tibial lengthening and internal bone transport and to enhance the femuro-tibial fusion

and medical expenses across hospitals and rehabilitation centers. Bondurant et al[35] suggested that the initial hospitalization costs were considerably less for amputation than limb salvage. Kim et al.,[55] in describing a patient with a large tibial defect treated with ipsilateral fibular transfer using a ring fixator, calculated that the total cost of the multiple procedures was five times more than that of amputation. Conversely, despite studies that showed that the initial hospitalization costs were considerably less for amputation than for limb salvage, Williams[56] noted that the long-term cost of amputation was considerably more than that of a successful reconstruction. These findings have been supported recently by Catagni et al.[39,49]

Psychosocial and Professional Outcomes

Quality-of-life assessments are more difficult to standardize since there are many variables that can be considered, including satisfaction with surgical outcome, body image; self-esteem; psychological, social, spiritual well-being; education level, employment, and marital status. In addition, several assessment tools exist to measure each of these variables, making comparisons across studies difficult, if not impossible. Overall, survivors of osteosarcoma appear to have psychological distress similar to that of the general population. Greenberg et al[57] reported on the psychological outcome of 89 survivors. The sample included persons with amputation and limb salvage. Psychological distress was noted in about 15% of the sample, which is comparable to that in the normal population. Depression, pain, alcohol abuse, and symptoms of traumatic stress were reported.

Sugarbaker et al[58] published one of the first studies examining quality of life with the hypothesis that limb-salvage patients would have better quality of life in terms of psychosocial adjustment than did amputation patients. However, no significant differences were found. Rougraff and colleagues sampled 29 survivors (8 with limb-salvage; 5 with disarticulation at the hip; and 16 with an above-the-knee amputation) and administered standardized psychological measures. No distinctions could be made between the three operative group on the basis of the quality-of-life data.[41]

Postma et al[59] noted that amputees had increased difficulty in finding partners in relationships and were more embarrassed in social settings, but this difference was not corroborated in other studies.[23,26,60]

Quality of life in terms of social and psychological outcomes or achievement endpoints such as marriage and employment does not differ significantly between amputee and nonamputee osteosarcoma survivors.[52,60] Independent of the type of surgical procedure, reduced function and lower quality-of-life scores were associated with poor educational attainment and increased self-reported disability.[26]

A preliminary investigation of pediatric and adult osteosarcoma survivors who had been treated during childhood and adolescence at the Children's Cancer Hospital at The University of Texas M. D. Anderson Cancer Center revealed that they have borne their motor disability reasonably well. It appeared that the limb-salvage patients had a psychological and quality-of-life outcome similar to that of the amputees.

Assessments gleaned from observations at M. D. Anderson Cancer Center's annual ski-rehabilitation program for amputees over the past three decades[61] also have permitted an evaluation of survivors' psychological outlook and participation in recreational and sport activities (Fig. 4). Most of the adult survivors appeared to have economic independence. Family, volunteers in the patients' communities who assisted the patients, and associative environment, such as survivor groups, were of great support. Among the long-term amputee and limb-salvage survivors, seven of 250 had graduated as physicians. Among the other long-term survivors, there were architects, accountants, lawyers, teachers, nurses, and successful business executives.[62] More than 50% of the patients were married and had children.

A recent report by Yonemoto et al[63] noted that among long-term survivors of high-grade osteosarcoma, the percentage who went to college or university was higher in the group who had undergone limb-sparing procedures than in those who had undergone amputation. No difference was noted in the status of employment between the two groups. The overall percentage of survivors who went to college or university and their mean annual income were similar to the national averages.[63]

A study by Aksnes et al[30] noted that, except in physical function, there were no significant differences in quality of life between amputees and those who had had

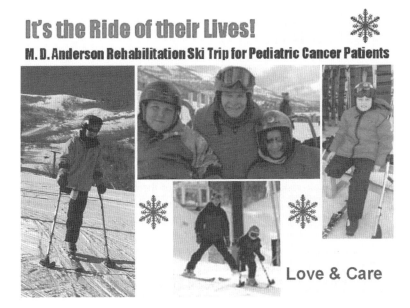

Fig. 4 M.D. Anderson Cancer Center's annual ski-rehabilitation program for amputees was founded by Norman Jaffe, MD, in 1971 and has been held over the past three decades for osteosarcoma patients and survivors from the Department of Pediatrics at M. D. Anderson's Children's Cancer Hospital. This ski program was inspired by Dr. Jaffe's young patient, Ted Kennedy, Jr., who wanted to keep skiing after his amputation. Conquering this physical challenge gives amputees a remarkable boost in self-confidence. Today the trip includes also children and survivors with any type of cancer or physical disability. This program also enables evaluation of the survivors' psychological outlook, as well as their participation in recreational and sport activities

432   G. Ottaviani et al.

limb-sparing surgery. Among the patients, 11% did not work or study. In multivariate analysis, amputation, a tumor location above the knee, and muscular pain were associated with low physical function. The investigators concluded that most of the bone-tumor survivors managed well after adjustment to their physical limitations. A total of 105 of the 108 evaluated survivors were able to work and have an overall good quality of life.[30]

These experiences were not entirely supported by de Boer et al[64] They compared the risk of unemployment of adult survivors of childhood cancer with that of healthy controls. In an extensive literature search of 34 original empirical studies published in the last 40 years that provided data on employment among survivors of childhood cancer, the investigators found that overall, survivors of childhood cancer were nearly twice as likely to be unemployed than were healthy controls. The risk of becoming unemployed was dependent on the cancer diagnosis; the risk was significantly higher among survivors of central nervous system and brain tumors. The risk of unemployment among survivors of blood or bone cancers was elevated but not statistically significant. Eiser et al[65] did not find an excess in deficits in measures of anxiety, depression, or self-esteem in long-term survivors when compared with the normal population or matched controls.

Late Effects of Therapy

There is a paucity of information on the incidence of fractures, aseptic loosening, limb-length discrepancy, implant breakage, poor joint movement, stump problems, skin breakdown, bone overgrowth, sciatic nerve palsy, peroneal nerve palsy, bone nonunion and pseudarthrosis, malalignment, and pain among osteosarcoma survivors. As indicated earlier, the incidence of complications related to amputation also requires further study.

Osteosarcoma survivors, not only have to deal with limb function related problems, but also have an excess risk of mortality because of therapy-related late effects.

Doxorubicin-induced cardiac toxicity is an important side effect of chemotherapy for osteosarcoma.[4,5] It has been reported that several patients have had hearing impairment induced by cisplatin and have required hearing aids.[6] Published investigations have revealed osteopenia, an elevated body-fat index, hyperlipidemia, chronic psychological distress, infertility in men, and premature menopause in women.[7,8,10] Second primary neoplasms and metachronous skeletal osteosarcoma have been described in osteosarcoma survivors.[11–13]

Conclusions

Quality of life in long-term osteosarcoma survivors has been assessed in a number of ways. There are insufficient data to determine overall function and quality of life in survivors, including inherent risks and benefits of amputation and limb-sparing

Functional, Psychosocial and Professional Outcomes in Long-Term Survivors 433

procedures. However, based upon a literature review and a preliminary study of patients treated at the Children's Cancer Hospital at M. D. Anderson Cancer Center, most patients treated by amputation or limb salvage appear to have accepted and adjusted satisfactorily to the resultant deficits. Additional investigation is required to establish the incidence of complications in patients who have undergone amputation and limb-salvage procedures, and to identify the salient factors related to patients' decisions in resolving these complications.

Acknowledgements Dr. Giulia Ottaviani, is the scientific coordinator of the project "Quality of life in long-term osteosarcoma survivors", Joint Mobility Projects for the Exchange of Researchers, joint declaration after the ninth biennial review meeting on scientific and technological cooperation between the Republic of Italy and the United States of America, Washington, DC, Ministry for Foreign Affairs (MAE), 2008–2010.

References

1. Marcove RC, Miké V, Hajek JV, et al. Osteogenic sarcoma under the age of twenty-one. A review of one hundred and forty-five operative cases. *J Bone Joint Surg Am.* 1970;52:411-423.
2. Hudson M, Jaffe MR, Jaffe N, et al. Pediatric osteosarcoma: therapeutic strategies, results and prognostic factors derived from a 10-year experience. *J Clin Oncol.* 1990;8:1988-1997.
3. Mascarenhas L, Siegel S, Spector L, et al. Malignant bone tumors. In: Bleyer A, O'Leary M, Barr R, et al, eds. *Cancer epidemiology in older adolescents and young adults 15 to 29 years of age, including SEER incidence and survival: 1975–2000* (NIH Pub. No. 06-5767). Bethesda, MD: National Cancer Institute; 2006:97-110. Available at: http://seer.cancer.gov/publications/aya/8_bone.pdf. Accessed January 2009
4. Longhi A, Ferrari S, Bacci G, et al. Long-term follow-up of patients with doxorubicin-induced cardiac toxicity after chemotherapy for osteosarcoma. *Anticancer Drugs.* 2007;18:737-744.
5. Berrak SG, Ewer MS, Jaffe N, et al. Doxorubicin cardiotoxicity in children: reduced incidence of cardiac dysfunction associated with continuous infusion schedules. *Oncol Rep.* 2001;8:611-614.
6. Ruiz L, Gilden J, Jaffe N, et al. Auditory function in pediatric osteosarcoma patients treated with multiple doses of cis-diamminedichloroplatinum(II). *Cancer Res.* 1989;49:742-744.
7. Ried H, Zietz H, Jaffe N. Late effects of cancer treatment in children. *Pediatr Dent.* 1995;17:273-284.
8. Mansky P, Arai A, Stratton P, et al. Treatment late effects in long-term survivors of pediatric sarcoma. *Pediatr Blood Cancer.* 2007;48:192-199.
9. Paulides M, Kremers A, Stohr W, et al. Prospective longitudinal evaluation of doxorubicin-induced cardiomyopathy in sarcoma patients: a report of the late effects study surveillance system (LESS). *Pediatr Blood Cancer.* 2006;46:489-495.
10. Vassilopoulou-Sellin R, Brosnan P, Delpassand A, et al. Osteopenia in young adult survivors of childhood cancer. *Med Pediatr Oncol.* 1999;32:272-278.
11. Jaffe N. Metachronous skeletal osteosarcoma after therapy. *J Clin Oncol.* 2004;22:1524.
12. Jaffe N, Pearson P, Yasko AW, et al. Single and multiple metachronous osteosarcoma tumors after therapy. *Cancer.* 2003;98:2457-2466.
13. Inskip PD, Ries LAG, Cohen RJ, et al. New malignancies following childhood cancer. In: Curtis RE, Freedman DM, Ron E, et al, eds. *New malignancies among cancer survivors: SEER cancer registries, 1973-2000* (NIH Publ. No. 05-5302). Bethesda, MD: National Cancer Institute; 2006. Available at: http://seer.cancer.gov/publications/mpmono/Ch18_Childhood.pdf. Accessed January 2009

14. Simon MA, Aschliman MA, Thomas N, et al. Limb salvage treatment versus amputation for osteosarcoma of the distal end of the femur. *J Bone Joint Surg Am.* 1986;68:1331-1337.
15. Ottaviani G, Randelli P, Catagni MA. Segmental cement extraction system (SEG-CES) and the Ilizarov method in limb salvage procedure after total knee cemented prosthesis removal in a former osteosarcoma patient. *Knee Surg Sports Traumatol Arthrosc.* 2005;13:557-563.
16. Ruggieri P, De Cristofaro R, Picci P, et al. Complications and surgical indications in 144 cases of nonmetastatic osteosarcoma of the extremities treated with neoadjuvant chemotherapy. *Clin Orthop Relat Res.* 1993;295:226-238.
17. Lindner NJ, Ramm O, Hillmann A, et al. Limb salvage and outcome of osteosarcoma: the University of Muenster experience. *Clin Orthop Relat Res.* 1999;358:83-89.
18. Davis AM, Devlin M, Griffin AM, et al. Functional outcome in amputation versus limb sparing of patients with lower extremity sarcoma: a matched case-control study. *Arch Phys Med Rehabil.* 1999;80:615-618.
19. Renard AJ, Veth RP, Schreuder HW, et al. Function and complications after ablative and limb-salvage therapy in lower extremity sarcoma of bone. *J Surg Oncol.* 2000;73:198-205.
20. Marulanda GA, Henderson ER, Johnson DA, et al. Orthopedic surgery options for the treatment of primary osteosarcoma. *Cancer Control.* 2008;15:13-20.
21. Krajbich JI. Lower-limb deficiencies and amputations in children. *J Am Acad Orthop Surg.* 1998;6:358-367.
22. Wilkins KL, McGrath PJ, Finley GA, et al. Phantom pain sensations and phantom limb pain in child and adolescent amputees. *Pain.* 1998;7:46-53.
23. Nagarajan R, Clohisy DR, Neglia JP, et al. Function and quality-of-life of survivors of pelvic and lower extremity osteosarcoma and Ewing's sarcoma: the Childhood Cancer Survivor Study. *Br J Cancer.* 2004;91:1858-1865.
24. Futani H, Minamizaki T, Nishimoto Y, et al. Long-term follow-up after limb salvage in skeletally immature children with a primary malignant tumor of the distal end of the femur. *J Bone Joint Surg Am.* 2006;88:595-603.
25. Tunn PU, Schmidt-Peter P, Pomraenke D, Hohenberger P. Osteosarcoma in children: long-term functional analysis. *Clin Orthop Relat Res.* 2004;421:212-217.
26. Refaat Y, Gunnoe J, Hornicek FJ, Mankin HJ. Comparison of quality of life after amputation or limb salvage. *Clin Orthop Relat Res.* 2002;397:298-305.
27. Van der Windt DA, Pieterson I, van der Eijken JW, et al. Energy expenditure during walking in subjects with tibial rotationplasty, above-knee amputation, or hip disarticulation. *Arch Phys Med Rehabil.* 1992;73:1174-1180.
28. Hann SB, Park HJ, Kim HS, et al. Surgical treatment of malignant and aggressive bone tumors around the knee by segmental resection and rotationplasty. *Yonsei Med J.* 2003;44:485-492.
29. Sawamura C, Hornicek FJ, Gebhardt MC. Complications and risk factors for failure of rotationplasty: review of 25 patients. *Clin Orthop Relat Res.* 2008;466:1302-1308.
30. Aksnes LH, Bauer HC, Jebsen NL, et al. Limb-sparing surgery preserves more function than amputation: A Scandinavian sarcoma group study of 118 patients. *J Bone Joint Surg Br.* 2008;90:786-794.
31. Kumta SM, Cheng JC, Li CK, et al. Scope and limitations of limb-sparing surgery in childhood sarcomas. *J Pediatr Orthop.* 2002;22:244-248.
32. Grimer RJ. Surgical options for children with osteosarcoma. *Lancet Oncol.* 2005;6:85-92.
33. Link MP, Gebhardt MC, Meyers PA. Osteosarcoma. In: Pizzo PA, Poplack DG, eds. *Principles and practices of pediatric oncology.* 5th ed. Philadelphia: Lippincott Williams and Wilkins; 2006:1074-1115.
34. Ghert MA, Abudu A, Driver N, et al. The indications for and the prognostic significance of amputation as the primary surgical procedure for localized soft tissue sarcoma of the extremity. *Ann Surg Oncol.* 2005;12:10-17.
35. Bondurant FJ, Cotler HB, Buckle R, et al. The medical and economic impact of severely injured lower extremities. *J Trauma.* 1988;28:1270-1273.
36. Hansen ST Jr. Overview of the severely traumatized lower limb. Reconstruction versus amputation. *Clin Orthop Relat Res.* 1989;243:17-19.

Functional, Psychosocial and Professional Outcomes in Long-Term Survivors

37. MacKenzie EJ, Bosse MJ, Castillo RC, et al. Functional outcomes following trauma-related lower-extremity amputation. *J Bone Joint Surg Am.* 2004;86:1636-1645.
38. Geertzen JH, Bosmans JC, van der Schans CP, et al. Claimed walking distance of lower limb amputees. *Disabil Rehabil.* 2005;27:101-104.
39. Catagni MA, Camagni M, Combi A, et al. Treatment of massive tibial bone loss by fibula transport with the Ilizarov frame. *Clin Orthop Relat Res.* 2006;448:208-216.
40. Grimer RJ, Taminiau AM, Cannon SR, et al. Surgical outcomes in osteosarcoma. *J Bone Joint Surg Br.* 2002;84:395-400.
41. Rougraff BT, Simon MA, Kneils JS, et al. Limb salvage procedure compared with amputation for osteosarcoma of the distal end of the femur. A long-term oncological, functional, and quality-of-life study. *J Bone Joint Surg Am.* 1994;76:649-656.
42. Pritchard DJ. Surgical management of osteosarcoma. In: Unni KK, ed. *Bone tumors.* New York: Churchill Livingstone; 1988:135-148.
43. Jeys LM, Grimer RJ, Carter SR, et al. Periprosthetic infection in patients treated for an orthopaedic oncological condition. *J Bone Joint Surg Am.* 2005;87:842-849.
44. Zeegen EN, Aponte-Tinao LA, Hornicek FJ, et al. Survivorship analysis of 141 modular metallic endoprostheses at early followup. *Clin Orthop Relat Res.* 2004;420:239-250.
45. Ottaviani G, Catagni MA, Matturri L. Massive metallosis due to metal-on-metal impingement in substitutive long stemmed knee prosthesis. *Histopathology.* 2005;46:237-238.
46. Wiedel JD. Salvage of infected total knee fusion: the last option. *Clin Orthop Relat Res.* 2002;404:139-142.
47. Marcove RC. *The surgery of Tumors and Bone Cartilage.* New York: Grune and Stratton; 1981.
48. Catagni MA. Treatment of tibial nonunions. In: Bianchi Maiocchi A, ed. *Treatment of fractures, nonunions and bone loss of the tibia with the Ilizarov method.* Milan, Italy: Il Quadratino; 1998:97-158.
49. Catagni MA, Ottaviani G, Camagni M. Treatment of massive tibial bone loss due to chronic draining osteomyelitis: fibula transport using the Ilizarov frame. *Orthopedics.* 2007;30:608-611.
50. Catagni MA, Ottaviani G. Ilizarov method to correct limb length discrepancy after limb-sparing hemipelvectomy. *J Pediatr Orthop B.* 2008;17:293-298.
51. Jeys LM, Grimer RJ, Carter SR, et al. Post operative infection and increased survival in osteosarcoma patients: are they associated? *Ann Surg Oncol.* 2007;14:2887-2895.
52. Nagarajan R, Neglia JP, Clohisy DR, et al. Limb salvage and amputation in survivors of pediatric lower-extremity bone tumors: what are the long-term implications? *J Clin Oncol.* 2002;20:4493-4501.
53. de Visser E, Deckers JA, Veth RP, et al. Deterioration of balance control after limb-saving surgery. *Am J Phys Med Rehabil.* 2001;80:358-365.
54. Jeys LM, Grimer RJ, Carter SR, et al. Risk of amputation following limb salvage surgery with endoprosthetic replacement, in a consecutive series of 1261 patients. *Int Orthop.* 2003;27:160-163.
55. Kim HS, Jahng JS, Han DY, et al. Immediate ipsilateral fibular transfer in a large tibial defect using a ring fixator. A case report. *Int Orthop.* 1998;22:321-324.
56. Williams MO. Long-term cost comparison of major limb salvage using Ilizarov method versus amputation. *Clin Orthop Relat Res.* 1994;301:156-161.
57. Greenberg DB, Goorin A, Gebhardt MC, et al. Quality of life in osteosarcoma survivors. *Oncology (Williston Park).* 1994;8:19-25.
58. Sugarbaker PH, Barofsky I, Rosenberg SA, et al. Quality of life assessment of patients in extremity sarcoma clinical trials. *Surgery.* 1982;91:17-23.
59. Postma A, Kingma A, De Ruiter J, et al. Quality of life in bone tumor patients comparing limb salvage and amputation of the lower extremity. *J Surg Oncol.* 1992;51:47-51.
60. Nagarajan R, Neglia JP, Clohisy DR, et al. Education, employment, insurance, and marital status among 694 survivors of pediatric lower extremity bone tumors: a report from the childhood cancer survivor study. *Cancer.* 2003;97:2554-2564.
61. Jaffe N, Zietz H. Amputee skiers: lofty ambassadors in the rehabilitation of cancer. *Pediatr Hematol Oncol.* 2004;21:557-562.

62. Huh WW, Jaffe N, Ottaviani G. Adult survivors of childhood cancer and unemployment: a metaanalysis. *Cancer*. 2006;107:2958-2959.
63. Yonemoto T, Ishii T, Takeuchi Y, et al. Education and employment in long-term survivors of high-grade osteosarcoma: a Japanese single-center experience. *Oncology*. 2008;72:274-278.
64. de Boer AG, Verbeek JH, van Dijk FJ. Adult survivors of childhood cancer and unemployment: a metaanalysis. *Cancer*. 2006;107:1-11.
65. Eiser C, Hill JJ, Vance YH. Examining the psychological consequences of surviving childhood cancer: systematic review as a research method in pediatric psychology. *J Pediatr Psychol*. 2000;25:449-460.

Research and Investigation:
New and Innovative Strategies

Bridging the Gap Between Experimental Animals and Humans in Osteosarcoma

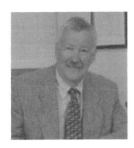
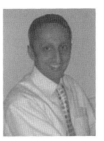

Stephen J. Withrow and Chand Khanna

Osteosarcoma has been reported in virtually all species of mammals (mouse, rat, rabbit, wolf, monkey, cat, dog, horse, ferret, cow, grizzly bear, camel, polar bear, and more), reptiles, fish, birds, and dinosaurs. The pet dog with osteosarcoma shares many similarities with the human condition, including histology, local and metastatic progression, and response to conventional treatment modalities.[1] These similarities, coupled with the high prevalence of osteosarcoma in pet dogs, provide important opportunities to improve our understanding of osteosarcoma biology and therapy through the study of this naturally occurring model (Table 1)[2].

Osteosarcoma is by far the most common primary malignancy affecting the bones of pet dogs.[3] It accounts for over 90% of all primary bone cancers, with estimates of over 10,000 new cases annually in the United States. The median age of onset of osteosarcoma is 7 years with an equal sex distribution and predominantly affects larger and giant breed dogs. Tall shoulder height may also be a risk factor.[4] Most tumors occur in the bones of the leg (appendicular) versus the axial skeleton.[5] The disease is locally aggressive and highly metastatic.

The specific etiology of canine osteosarcoma is unknown, but physical risk factors include heavy weight bearing to "sensitive" metaphyseal sites,[6] malignant transformation around metallic implants, (1 per 10,000 fracture repairs)[7] and ionizing radiation (experimental radionuclides or secondary to therapeutic radiation).[8–10] Much as in the case with human osteosarcoma, no consistent molecular events have been linked to osteosarcomagenesis in the dog. On the contrary, and again consistent with the experience in human osteosarcoma, canine osteosarcoma is characterized by bizarre and irregular karyotypes and marked aneuploidy.[11,12] This finding has led some to suggest that early oncogenic events in this cancer are the result of failures

---

S.J. Withrow (✉)
College of Veterinary Medicine and Biomedical Sciences, Colorado State University, Ft Collins, CO, 80523, USA
e-mail: stephen.withrow@colostate.edu

C. Khanna
Comparative Oncology Program, Center for Cancer Research, National Cancer Institute, Bethesda, MD 20892, USA
e-mail: khannac@mail.nih.gov

Table 1 Comparison of canine and human osteosarcoma (Source: from Dernell et al[1])

Variable	Dog	Human
Mean age	7 years	14 years
Race/breed	Large or giant purebreds	None
Body weight	90% > 20 kg	Heavy
Site	77% long bones	90% long bones
	Metaphyseal	Metaphyseal
	Distal radius > proximal humerus >	Distal femur > proximal tibia > Proximal humerus
	Distal femur > tibia	
Etiology	Generally unknown	Generally unknown
% clinically confined to the limb at presentation	80–90%	80–90%
% histologically high grade	95%	85–90%
DNA index	75% aneuploid	75% aneuploid
Molecular and genetic alterations	See Table 2	See table 2
Prognostic indicators	Young age, alkaline phosphatase	Alkaline phosphatase, MDR1
Metastatic rate without chemotherapy	90% before 1 year	80% before 2 years
Metastatic sites	Lung > bone > soft tissue	Lung > bone > soft tissue
Improved survival with chemotherapy	Yes	Yes
Regional Lymph node metastasis	poor prognosis, < 5%	Poor prognosis

in DNA repair or sensing mechanisms. Telomerase and alternative telomere maintenance strategies appear to be active in canine osteosarcoma.[13] Studies of germline genetic risk factors for osteosarcoma in dogs are underway. The fact that specific breeds and families of dogs are at disproportionate risk for osteosarcoma has allowed for rapid progress in the field. It is likely that ongoing studies in high risk-breeds, such as the Rotteweiler or Scottish Deerhounds, may provide new insight into these heritable and genetic risk factors.[14] For the most part, the genes and pathways found to be dysregulated in human osteosarcoma have been found in the canine disease. Mutations and overexpression of p53 have been documented and are believed to occur in 30–50% of canine tumors.[15,16] Furthermore, dysregulation of either RB or p53 tumor suppressor pathways have been found in most canine osteosarcoma cell lines. Distinctive from the human condition, loss of PTEN function has been observed in a small number of canine osteosarcoma cell lines.[17] The association between canine osteosarcoma and bone growth is supported by the increased prevalence of the disease in large breed dogs and by studies demonstrating the expression of the IGF-I receptor and ligand in canine osteosarcoma cells.[18] The dependence of canine osteosarcoma on IGF-I signaling has been supported by in vitro studies and may represent an important therapeutic target for osteosarcoma patients. Molecular and genetic factors implicated in canine osteosarcoma are summarized in Table 2. It is unclear if there is any association between canine osteosarcoma development and exposure to SV40 antigen or viruses.[19]

Bridging the Gap Between Experimental Animals and Humans in Osteosarcoma 441

Table 2 Molecular and genetic factors associated with OS in dogs (source: from Dernell et al[1])

Factor	Comments
p53	Mutated and/or overexpressed in several investigations
IGF-1/IGF-1R	May contribute to the malignant phenotype
HGF/c-Met	May contribute to the malignant phenotype
*erb*B-2/HER-2	Overexpressed in several canine OS cell lines
PTEN	Mutated or down-regulated in high percentage of canine OS cell lines
sis/PDGF	Overexpressed in some canine cell lines
Matrix metalloproteinases	Overexpressed in canine OS cell lines
Ezrin	A membrane-cytoskeleton linker associated with the metastatic phenotype in canine OS
COX-2	Expression upregulated in some canine OS; prognostic in some investigations, not in others
Angiogenic factors	VEGF measurable in plasma of dogs with OS; angiostatin present in urine of dogs with OS
Telomere maintance system	Upregulated in some canine OS

The vast majority of canine osteosarcoma are high-grade, osteoblastic osteoid-producing malignancies, but they may be histologically subclassified into chondroblastic, fibroblastic, or telangectatic. Support for a primitive mesenchymal origin for canine osteosarcoma is increasing. Recent studies have identified cancer cells with stem-like features from canine osteosarcoma using embryonic stem cell-associated genes.[20] Recent expression microarray studies in canine osteosarcoma have confirmed a strong bone and osteoblastic phenotype (C. Khanna personal communication). The complexity of tumor and normal cell interactions includes cross-talk between osteoblast and osteoclast compartments. This cross-talk in canine osteosarcoma is supported by the clinical presence of the classic mixed bone proliferative and lytic lesions in canine osteosarcoma and the presence and activity of RANK, RANK-ligand, and osteoprotegrin axis in primary tumors and metastatic lesions.[21] Active bone lysis and turnover is evident by elevations in circulating and urine telopeptides.[22] Low grade surface osteosarcoma is rare in dogs. Ewing's sarcoma has not been described in the dog. Soft tissue extension is often moderate to severe (Stage IIb) (Fig. 1) and pathologic fractures may occur. Less than 15% of all osteosarcoma cases can be proven to be metastatic, primarily to lung or bone, at presentation (Stage III). For dogs with osteosarcoma.

Routine staging studies for days with osteosarcoma include regional radiographs, thoracic radiographs (less than 10% positive at presentation), Tc^{99} nuclear scan (less than 10% positive at presentation),[23] regional lymph node metastasis (less than 5% positive),[24] routine CBC and biochemical profile (bone alkaline phosphatase is a negative prognostic indicator),[25] and possibly, a bone biopsy via needle core. Lung CT scan and primary site CT or MRI are occasionally performed.

Local tumor control is generally achieved with amputation (which is very well tolerated in large breed dogs) or limb sparing. Curative intent external beam radiation

Fig. 1 (**a**) Gross, longitudinally split specimen of a proximal femoral osteosarcoma lesion in a dog showing cortical destruction, soft tissue, and osteoid neoplastic components. (**b**) Lateral radiograph of a proximal femoral osteosarcoma lesion from the case in part (**a**). Radiographic features include (*a*) Codman's triangle, (*b*) cortical lysis, (*c*) loss of trabecular pattern in the metaphases, and (*d*) tumor bone extension into the soft tissues in a sunburst pattern (source: courtesy of Dernell et al[1])

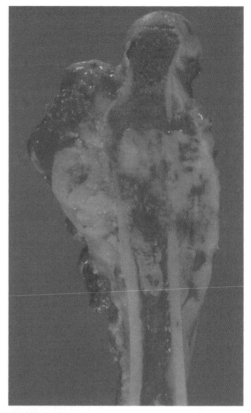

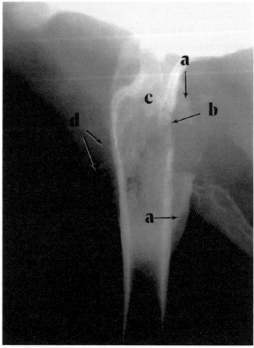

therapy alone rarely achieves durable local control.[26] Palliative measures such as nonsteroidal anti-inflammatories, narcotic analgesics, bisphosphonates, cytotoxic chemotherapy, metronomic chemotherapy radionucleotides such as Samarium, or radiation (8 Gy×3) are alternate choices to the more aggressive surgical options. Newer radiation schemes with stereotactic radiosurgery or image modulated radiation therapy are emerging and may offer local control equivalent to surgery in carefully selected cases without extensive soft tissue extension or impending pathologic fracture.[27]

Limb sparing surgery for dogs with osteosarcoma is restricted to specially trained surgical oncologists and is generally performed with cortical allografts and plate arthodesis of the adjacent joint.[28] Alternate limb spare technologies include metal prosthesis, intra-operative radiation, local bone (ulna) transposition for radius primaries, bone transport, and pasteurized autografts. Limb sparing is clinically successful in 75% of cases. Complications resulting in salvage amputation or poor leg usage include infection, fracture of host bone or allograft, and local tumor recurrence. Preoperative cisplatin chemotherapy (IV or IA) with or without modest radiation doses can result in excellent consolidation and percent necrosis with improved local control.[29,30] Local biodegradable platinum based chemotherapy polymers have reduced local disease recurrence after limb sparing.[31]

Despite effective control of the primary bone tumor, over 90% of dogs are expected to have microscopic metastasis at the time of presentation. These micro-metastasis emerge as gross metastasis, most commonly to the lung, in a median of 3–4 months, after primary tumor control (<10% alive at 1 year with amputation alone). This lung "specific" pattern of progression is characteristic of metastasis in canine osteosarcoma. Adjuvant chemotherapy (after adequate local tumor control) in dogs results in improved disease free intervals and survival. Chemotherapy agents with known activity in the adjuvant setting are doxorubicin, cisplatin, and carboplatin as single agents or in combination. They are often not administered at the equivalent MTDs, cumulative dose or dose intensity for human patients, and this may limit long term survivals. Pooled data assessment of various adjuvant chemotherapy protocols for canine osteosarcoma results in a 10–12 month median survival with a 50% 1 year survival and a 25% 2 year survival.[32-35] Dogs with infected limb spares and adjuvant chemotherapy live longer than dogs without infection, making immunotherapy an intriguing possibility.[36,37]

The process of metastastatic progression in canine osteosarcoma is believed to involve similar steps/processes of metastatic progression in human osteosarcoma. The expression of genes and proteins involved in cellular migration and invasion (e.g., c-met-hepatocyte growth factor axis, matrix metalloproteinases),[38,39] angiogenic factors (e.g., VEGF, b-FGF, COX2),[40,41] and metastatic survival factors (i.e., ezrin)[42] have been identified in canine osteosarcoma. In many of these cases, their expression has been linked to clinical outcome in dogs. Interestingly, the expression of the oncogene, Her2/neu (ERBB2), has been found in canine osteosarcoma.[43] The pattern of expression of Her2/neu in canine and human osteosarcoma is atypical and is characterized by diffuse granular staining of the cytoplasm. There is no evidence for amplification of Her2/neu in either canine or human osteosarcoma; however, its expression intensity (by immunohistochemistry) has been linked to disease free interval in dogs.

The treatment options for gross metastases in dogs are limited in efficacy. Metastectomy may have limited value in selected dogs with slowly progressing disease and minimal tumor burden.[44] Perhaps due to limitations in achievable dose intensity, the use of chemotherapy is associated with a very low response rate in dogs with macroscopic metastatic disease.

Many features of cancers in pet dogs offer an opportunity that may uniquely contribute to our understanding of cancer pathogenesis, progression and therapy.[2] Pet dogs are large and are relatively outbred in comparison to laboratory animals. In addition, the inclusion of dogs from different breeds in clinical trials provides a background genetic diversity similar to that seen in human populations. The recent public release of the canine genome provides evidence of strong similarities with humans; in fact, for cancer-associated gene families, the similarities are significantly closer than the relationship between a mouse and human. Cancers developing in these pet dogs, (i.e., osteosarcoma) are naturally occurring and develop in the context of an intact immune system where tumor, and host and tumor microenvironment are syngeneic. Their intact immune system and the increasing availability of biological reagents for the dog have allowed progress in evaluating novel treatments based on harnessing the immune response against osteosarcoma. Tumor initiation and progression are influenced by similar factors in both human and canine cancers, including age, nutrition, sex, reproductive status, and environmental exposures. The biological complexity of cancers in pet animals captures the essence of cancer in human patients. This is based in large part on the intratumoral (cell-to-cell) heterogeneity seen in these cancers. A natural consequence of this heterogeneity are the same deadly features of human cancers, including acquired resistance to therapy, recurrence, and metastasis.

It is reasonable that the studies that include pet dogs with osteosarcoma will uniquely indicate the development path of new drugs destined for the treatment of human osteosarcoma patients. To support the integration of the dog with cancer into the drug discovery and development path, several national veterinary based clinical trials and tissue archiving cooperatives have been established under the auspices of the National Cancer Institute in the last several years. The Comparative Oncology Trials Consortium engages 18 schools of veterinary medicine and one private not-for-profit institution. Trials may be initiated by the intramural NCI, industry, or collaborative organizations. Individual investigators may initiate trials and conduct translational studies through this trials infrastructure. The Pfizer Canine Comparative Oncology and Genomics Consortia Biospecimen Repository, a complementary tissue archiving initiative, plans to populate a bank of 3,000 tumor and corresponding normal tissues at the NCI in Bethesda, Maryland. Tissue procurement will initially emphasize osteosarcoma, lymphoma, and melanoma and will provide well annotated tissues to maximally utilize the dog model.

Beyond the biological rationale, the evaluation of novel therapeutics with potential activity in osteosarcoma may be rapidly evaluated in dogs. The repeat sampling and surgery opportunities allow biological endpoints to be connected to these studies relatively easily. Pet owners are willing and eager to participate in trials and provide high rates of compliance for studies. The NIH and FDA recognition of the value of the dog cancer models has now caught up with the established interest of the pharmaceutical industry. The increased prevalence of many sarcomas coupled with more

Bridging the Gap Between Experimental Animals and Humans in Osteosarcoma

rapid rates of progression allows longitudinal endpoints of disease free local control and survival to be assessed rapidly. This may be especially important in the evaluation of treatment agents that target metastatic progression. It is likely that further integration of the dog with osteosarcoma into studies of cancer biology and therapy will be informative and will lead to new treatment options for patients.

References

1. Dernell WS, Ehrhart NP, Straw RC, et al. Tumors of the Skeletal System. In: Withrow SJ, Vail DM, eds. *Withrow and MacEwen's Small Animal Clinical Oncology*. 4th ed. St Louis: Saunders Elsevier; 2007:540-582.
2. Paoloni M, Khanna C. Translation of new cancer treatments from pet dogs to humans. *Nat Rev Cancer*. 2008;8:147-156.
3. Withrow SJ, Powers BE, Straw RC, et al. Comparative aspects of osteosarcoma: dog vs. man. *Clin Orthop*. 1991;270:159-167.
4. Ru G, Terracini B, Glickman LT. Host related risk factors for canine osteosarcoma. *Vet J*. 1998;156:31-39.
5. Misdorp W, Hart AA. Some prognostic and epidemiological factors in canine osteosarcoma. *J Natl Cancer Inst*. 1979;62:537-545.
6. Gellasch KL, Kalscheur VL, Clayton MK, et al. Fatigue microdamage in the radial predilection site for osteosarcoma in dogs. *Am J Vet Res*. 2002;63(6):896-899.
7. Stevenson S, Holm RB, Pohler OEM, et al. Fracture-associated sarcoma in the dog. *J Am Vet Med Assoc*. 1982;180:1189.
8. Miller SC, Lloyd RD, Bruenger FW, et al. Comparisons of the skeletal locations of putative plutonium-induced osteosarcomas in humans with those in beagle dogs and with naturally occurring tumors in both species. *Radiat Res*. 2003;160(5):517-523.
9. White RG, Raabe OG, Culbertson MR, et al. Bone sarcoma characteristics and distribution in beagles injected with radium-226. *Radiat Res*. 1994;137(3):361-370.
10. McChesney-Gillette S, Gillette EL, Powers BE, et al. Radiation-induced osteosarcoma in dogs after external beam or intraoperative radiation therapy. *Cancer Res*. 1990;50:54-57.
11. Mayr B, Eschborn U, Loupal G, et al. Characterisation of complex karyotype changes in two canine bone tumours. *Res Vet Sci*. 1991;51(3):341-343.
12. Thomas R, Scott A, Langford CF, et al. Construction of a 2-Mb resolution BAC microarray for CGH analysis of canine tumors. *Genome Res*. 2005;15(12):1831-1837.
13. Campbell SE, Nasir L, Argyle DJ, et al. Cloning of canine IL-1ra, TNFR and TIMP-2. *Vet Immunol Immunopathol*. 2001;78(2):207-214.
14. Phillips JC, Stephenson B, Hauck M, et al. Heritability and segregation analysis of osteosarcoma in the Scottish deerhound. *Genomics*. 2007;90(3):354-363. Epub 2007 Jul 12.
15. Sagartz JE, Bodley WL, Gamblin RM, et al. p53 tumor suppressor protein overexpression in osteogenic tumors of dogs. *Vet Pathol*. 1996;33(2):213-221.
16. van Leeuwen IS, Cornelisse CJ, Misdorp W, et al. P53 gene mutations in osteosarcomas in the dog. *Cancer Lett*. 1997;111(1–2):173-178.
17. Levine RA. Overexpression of the sis oncogene in a canine osteosarcoma cell line. *Vet Pathol*. 2002;39(3):411-412.
18. MacEwen EG, Pastor J, Kutzke J, Tsan R, et al. IGF-1 receptor contributes to the malignant phenotype in human and canine osteosarcoma. *J Cell Biochem*. 2004;92(1):77-91.
19. Owen LN. Transplantation of canine osteosarcoma. *Eur J Cancer*. 1969;5:615-620.
20. Wilson H, Huelsmeyer M, Chun R, et al. Isolation and characterisation of cancer stem cells from canine osteosarcoma. *Vet J*. 2008;175:69-75.
21. Barger AM, Fan TM, de Lorimier LP, et al. Expression of receptor activator of nuclear factor kappa-B ligand (RANKL) in neoplasms of dogs and cats. *J Vet Intern Med*. 2007;21(2):8.

22. Fan TM, de Lorimier LP, Charney SC. Urine N-telopeptide excretion in dogs with appendicular osteosarcoma. *J Vet Intern Med*. 2006;20(2):335-341.
23. Jankowski MK, Steyn PF, Lana SE, et al. Nuclear scanning with 99 m-Tc-HDP for the initial evaluation of osseous metastasis in canine osteosarcoma. *Vet Comp Oncol*. 2003;1:152-158.
24. Hillers KR, Dernell WS, Lafferty MHI, et al. Incidence and prognostic importance of lymph node metastases in dogs with appendicular osteosarcoma: 228 cases (1986–2003). *J Am Vet Med Assoc*. 2005;226(8):1364-1367.
25. Ehrhart N, Dernell WS, Hoffmann WE, et al. Prognostic importance of alkaline phosphatase activity in serum from dogs with appendicular osteosarcoma: 75 cases (1990–1996). *J Am Vet Med Assoc*. 1998;213:1002-1006.
26. Thrall DE, Withrow SJ, Powers BE, et al. Radiotherapy prior to cortical allograft limb sparing in dogs with osteosarcoma: a dose response assay. *Int J Rad Onc Biol Phys*. 1990;18:1354-1357.
27. Farese JP, Milner R, Thompson MS, et al. Stereotactic radiosurgery for treatment of osteosarcomas involving the distal portions of the limbs in dogs. *J Am Vet Med Assoc*. 2004;225(10):1548, 1567-1572.
28. Straw RC, Withrow SJ. Limb-sparing surgery versus amputation for dogs with bone tumors. *Vet Clin North Am*. 1996;26:135-143.
29. Withrow SJ, Thrall DE, Straw RC, et al. Intra-arterial cisplatin with or without radiation in limbsparing for canine osteosarcoma. *Cancer*. 1993;71:2484-2490.
30. Powers BE, Withrow SJ, Thrall DE, et al. Percent tumor necrosis as a predictor of treatment response in canine osteosarcoma. *Cancer*. 1991;67:126-134.
31. Withrow SJ, Liptak J, Straw RC, et al. Biodegradable cisplatin polymer in limb-sparing surgery for canine osteosarcoma. *Ann Surg Oncol*. 2004;11(7):705-713.
32. Berg J, Weinstein MJ, Springfield DS, et al. Response of osteosarcoma in the dog to surgery and chemotherapy with doxorubicin. *J Am Vet Med Assoc*. 1995;206(10):1555-1560.
33. Mauldin GN, Matus RE, Withrow SJ. Canine osteosarcoma treatment by amputation versus amputation and adjuvant chemotherapy using doxorubicin and cisplatin. *J Vet Int Med*. 1988;2:177-180.
34. Kent MS, Strom A, Strom A, London CA, et al. Alternating carboplatin and doxorubicin as adjunctive chemotherapy to amputation or limb-sparing surgery in the treatment of appendicular osteosarcoma in dogs. *J Vet Intern Med*. 2004;18(4):540-544.
35. Withrow SJ, Straw RC, Brekke JH, et al. Slow release adjuvant cisplatin for the treatment of metastatic canine osteosarcoma. *Eur J Musculoskel Res*. 1995;4:105-110.
36. MacEwen EG, Kurzmann ID, Rosenthal RC. Therapy for osteosarcoma in dogs with intravenous injection of liposome-encapsulated muramyl tripeptide. *J Natl Cancer Inst*. 1989;81:935-938.
37. Lascelles BDX, Dernell WS, Correa MT, et al. Improved survival associated with postoperative wound infection in dogs treated with limb-salvage surgery for osteosarcoma. *Annals of Surg Oncol*. 2005;12(12):1073-1083.
38. MacEwen EG, Kutzke J, Carew J, et al. c-Met tyrosine kinase receptor expression and function in human and canine osteosarcoma cells. *Clin Exp Metastasis*. 2003;20(5):421-430.
39. Lana SE, Ogilvie GK, Hansen RA, et al. Identification of matrix metalloproteinases in canine neoplastic tissue. *Am J Vet Res*. 2000;61(2):111-114.
40. Wergin MC, Kaser-Hotz B, Kaser-Hotz B. Plasma vascular endothelial growth factor (VEGF) measured in seventy dogs with spontaneously occurring tumours. *In Vivo*. 2004;18(1):15-19.
41. Mullins MN, Lana SE, Dernell WS, et al. Cyclooxygenase-2 expression in canine appendicular osteosarcomas. *J Vet Intern Med*. 2004;18(6):859-865.
42. Khanna C, Wan X, Bose S, et al. Ezrin, a Membrane - Cytoskeleton Linker, is Necessary for Osteosarcoma Metastasis. *Nat Medicine*. 2004;10(2):182-186.
43. Flint AF, U'Ren L, Legare ME, et al. Overexpression of the erbB-2 proto-oncogene in canine osteosarcoma cell lines and tumors. *Vet Pathol*. 2004;41(3):291-296.
44. O'Brien MG, Straw RC, Withrow SJ, et al. Resection of pulmonary metastases in canine osteosarcoma: 36 cases (1983–1992). *Vet Surg*. 1993;22:105-109.

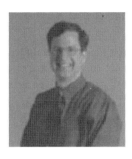

Is There a Role for Immunotherapy in Osteosarcoma?

David M. Loeb

Abstract With the introduction of effective systemic chemotherapy, the prognosis for patients with osteosarcoma has improved dramatically. Estimates of overall survival for osteosarcoma patients prior to 1975 ranged from 5 to 20%, even for patients with localized disease of the extremity treated with amputation. The majority of these patients eventually developed pulmonary metastases and succumbed to their disease. The introduction of effective chemotherapy has dramatically improved the outcome of patients with localized disease, but has not altered the survival of patients with metastatic disease. Moreover, there has been little, if any, improvement in the outcomes of patients with localized disease since the mid-1980s. This has led to the investigation of other treatment approaches, including immunotherapy. Coincident with the initial development of chemotherapy, there were early attempts at immunotherapy. These met with little success. Subsequent approaches to harnessing the immune system have yielded more encouraging results. This chapter will review these various approaches, highlighting the role that immunotherapy might play in the multi-modality treatment of localized and metastatic osteosarcoma.

What Is Immunotherapy?

The term "immunotherapy" broadly refers to any attempt to modulate the immune response for therapeutic gain. This can refer to "active immunotherapy," such as vaccination, or "adoptive immunotherapy," such as the infusion of cytotoxic lymphocytes or pre-formed antibodies. In the context of cancer treatment, immunotherapy can also refer to the use of cytokines or other immunomodulatory agents to affect the treatment of malignant disease. Each of these approaches

---

D.M. Loeb (✉)
Oncology and Pediatrics, Musculoskeletal Tumor Program, Johns Hopkins University, Bunting-Blaustein Cancer Research Building, Room 2M51, 1650 Orleans St, Baltimore, MD, 21231, USA
e-mail: LOEBDA@jhmi.edu

has been evaluated in the treatment of osteosarcoma. The earliest attempts at immunotherapy included tumor vaccines and the use of the transfer factor. More recently, treatment with cytokines and the immune stimulating agent muramyl tripeptide-phosphatidylethanolamine (MTP-PE) have been actively pursued, and monoclonal antibodies have also been investigated. Thus, both active and adoptive immunotherapy are being brought to bear in the fight against osteosarcoma.

To guide the development of osteosarcoma immunotherapy, it was necessary to determine whether patients mount their own immune response to this tumor and to understand the nature of this response. In 1970, Eilber and Morton identified in patients complement-fixing antibodies against sarcoma-specific antigens.[1,2] Wood and Morton demonstrated that some of these antibodies were cytotoxic, at least in vitro.[3] More recently, Théoleyre et al. reported that tumor-infiltrating lymphocytes (TILs) isolated from primary osteosarcoma samples, although CD4-positive, were cytotoxic.[4] Further evidence for an immune response to osteosarcoma comes from a mouse model, wherein SCID (severe combined immune deficiency) mice have a higher rate of metastasis than do immune competent animals.[5] Thus, several lines of evidence point to a role of the immune system in controlling osteosarcoma, and provide the basis for conducting trials of immunotherapy to augment the treatment of this disease.

Historical Overview

The history of immunotherapy dates to the eighteenth century, when it was reported by several physicians that patients with inoperable cancers who develop severe infections can experience tumor regression. In 1742, LeDran reported a patient with inoperable breast cancer whose tumor ulcerated and became infected. The tumor sloughed off, the wound healed, and the patient remained in remission for 8 months. In 1752, Amoureaux treated a patient with an ulcerated breast tumor using a septic dressing. The patient developed fever and inflammation, and the tumor regressed in 4 weeks. In 1783, Trnka reported spontaneous regression of a breast tumor coincident with the development of malaria. This patient had a durable remission. These clinical observations suggested the ability of immune modulating agents (in this case, active infections) to alter the natural history of cancer. It was not until the twentieth century, however, that active attempts to manipulate the immune system were undertaken.

The earliest organized attempts at active immune modulation were undertaken by Coley in the early twentieth century.[6] Coley developed a vaccine using extracts from several bacteria after treating a patient whose tumor regressed coincident with a streptococcal skin infection. He tried numerous formulations, and found that the effective ones all induced both local and systemic inflammation. Because of the inability to explain these observations, "Coley's Toxins" fell into disuse. The approach is being revived, however, in a Phase I trial of Clostridium novyi-NT spores for the treatment of refractory solid tumors being conducted at Johns Hopkins Hospital.

Active Immunotherapy

Active immunotherapy refers to attempts to induce the patient's immune system to respond to a growing tumor. Typically, this involves the use of a vaccine. Various immunogens have been investigated, including whole tumor cells, tumor cell extracts, and tumor-specific peptides.

One of the earliest attempts at active immunotherapy for osteosarcoma utilized allogeneic tumor cells as the immunogen.[7] In this study, osteosarcoma patients were given a tumor implant from another, unrelated, osteosarcoma patient. Leukocytes were isolated from the recipients and infused into the implant donor (Fig. 1). Twenty-eight patients with localized disease treated in this way were compared with 28 "control" patients from other centers, who were treated with surgery alone. The 4-year disease-free survival (DFS) for the immunotherapy patients was 44%, compared with 10% for patients treated with surgery alone, and the mean time to metastasis was 15 ± 2 months compared with 6 ± 2 months.[7] Unfortunately, this promising beginning was not replicated in other trials.

A study conducted at UCLA in the early 1970s enrolled 14 patients with localized disease and 15 patients with metastases. Seventeen were rendered disease-free with surgery (9 localized and 8 metastatic) and were then treated with a live cell vaccine composed of 10^7 SA-2 osteosarcoma cells injected into 4 sites every week for 3 months and then every 2 weeks for 2 years. Extract of Bacillus Calmette-Guerin (BCG) was administered as an adjuvant. Twelve patients served as "controls": 5 had localized disease treated with surgery alone, and 7 had metastatic disease and received adjuvant chemotherapy. No benefit was seen from this immunotherapy.[8] The cause of the discrepancy between these two studies is unclear, although there are several possibilities, including the use of a cell line, rather than a primary tumor, as the immunogen in the UCLA trial, a paradoxical inhibiting effect of BCG (which

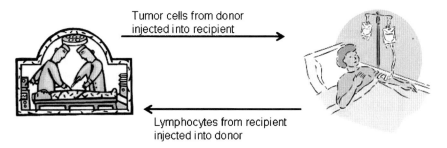

Fig. 1 Schematic of Immunotherapy Protocol. Tumor cells from Patient 1 are injected into Patient 2, and tumor cells from Patient 2 are injected into Patient 1. After a brief period for generation of a cellular immune response, lymphocytes from Patient 2, which should be reactive to Patient 1's tumor, are injected into Patient 1, and lymphocytes from Patient 1 are injected into Patient 2

was used in the latter trial), or simply the fact that both studies used very small patient samples, and thus had correspondingly wide confidence intervals such that the discrepancy could be the result of chance.

Regardless of the explanation, the lack of efficacy in the second study raises a key question: Is osteosarcoma immunogenic? When these two studies were designed and conducted, knowledge of the immune response was rudimentary. Recently, the concept of the immunologic synapse has been proffered to model the complexity of effector/target interactions (Fig. 2). The evidence suggests that target recognition requires more than just the expression of an antigen that can be bound by a T cell receptor on the effector cell. The antigen must be presented appropriately, meaning by MHC antigens, and specific adhesion molecules, such as integrins and intercellular adhesion molecule (ICAM), are also required to generate an effective interaction between effector cell and target cell.[9] A recent study demonstrated that only 12 of 25 osteosarcomas expressed HLA Class I antigens.[10] Interestingly, these patients had superior overall (OS) and event-free survival (EFS) compared with patients whose tumors did not express MHC Class I. The findings that some osteosarcomas express HLA Class I, that TILs can be isolated and are cytotoxic, and that patients generate autologous anti-osteosarcoma antibodies, all suggest that osteosarcoma is sufficiently immunogenic. Thus, early failures to generate an effective tumor vaccine probably reflect inadequate vaccine technology rather than a tumor that cannot be targeted.

Since the reports discussed above, there have been no reports of further attempts at osteosarcoma tumor vaccines in the literature for over 30 years. In 2005, Yu et al. reported laboratory experiments that will underlie the next generation of osteosar-

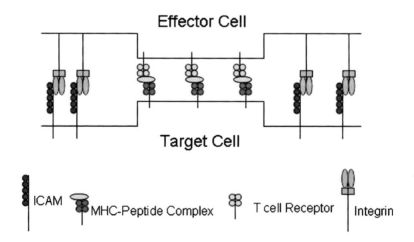

Fig. 2 The Immune Synapse. Proper target cell recognition by cytotoxic T cells requires the formation of a complex interaction region known as the immune synapse. Immunogenic peptides are presented by MHC Class I, and the MHC-peptide complex is recognized by T cell receptors. The cell/cell interaction is strengthened by binding of integrins on the T cell to intercellular adhesion molecule (ICAM) expressed by tumor cells

coma vaccines. Designed to improve the antigenicity of osteosarcoma, this group generated cell fusions between osteosarcoma cells and autologous dendritic cells.[11] Dendritic cells are the body's primary antigen presenting cells, and it is expected that these cell fusions should be more highly immunogenic than unmanipulated tumor cells. Indeed, these cells were very effective activators of cytotoxic T lymphocytes in vitro. More sophisticated approaches such as this will likely result in more effective tumor vaccines and should revive this area of research.

Immune Stimulatory Agents

If active immunotherapy involves directing the immune system to specifically recognize tumor antigens, a related approach involves stimulating the immune system nonspecifically, with the expectation that this will result in a response that spontaneously targets a growing tumor. Unlike active immunotherapy, which seeks to manipulate the adaptive immune system (B and T lymphocytes), immune stimulatory agents frequently work by activating the innate immune system (especially monocytes, macrophages, and natural killer cells).

One of the earliest reported attempts at the therapeutic use of immune stimulatory agents was a clinical trial conducted at the Mayo Clinic in the early 1970s, randomizing patients to treatment with either chemotherapy or Transfer Factor.[12] Transfer factor is a leukocyte dialysate obtained from patients with a delayed-type hypersensitivity (DTH) reaction that transfers this specific sensitivity into a recipient.[13] Thirty-six patients were randomly assigned to receive either chemotherapy or transfer factor, and those who were treated with transfer factor but did not elicit a DTH response, were crossed over to the chemotherapy arm. Neither arm showed a benefit compared with contemporary controls, and neither group did as well as a contemporary group of patients treated with high dose methotrexate.[14]

Concurrently with that study, patients with localized osteosarcoma treated at the Karolinska Institute in Sweden were being offered interferon-α as adjuvant therapy. An early report of this uncontrolled study discussed 11 patients who received adjuvant treatment 3 times per week for 18 months, with an overall survival of 64%, which compared favorably with the 20% survival seen in patients treated with surgery alone.[15] Long-term follow-up of 89 patients with localized disease treated with adjuvant interferon-α between 1971 and 1990 has demonstrated a 10-year metastasis-free survival of 39% and a sarcoma-specific survival of 43%.[16] What is unclear is whether interferon-α was acting as hypothesized (as an immunomodulatory agent), or whether some other activity, such as an effect on tumor angiogenesis,[17] might explain the improved survival these patients experienced compared with contemporary patients treated with surgery alone.

An immunomodulatory agent that shows significant promise in the treatment of osteosarcoma is Muramyl Tripeptide-Phosphatidyl Ethanolamine (MTP-PE). The liposomal formulation of this agent, L-MTP-PE, shows increased uptake by monocytes and macrophages and results in the activation of these cells, as demonstrated by the release of tumor necrosis factor, interleukin-6, and other markers.[18] Preclinical trials of this agent showed substantial promise. In a dog model of osteosarcoma, animals treated with surgery alone had a median remission-free survival (RFS) of 77days, with no dogs surviving beyond 8 months. In contrast, dogs treated with L-MTP-PE had a median RFS of 222 days and 4 out of 14 (29%) of the animals never experienced a relapse.[19] These results led to the design of clinical trials in humans with osteosarcoma.

Based on these preclinical findings, a Phase II study of L-MTP-PE was conducted in patients with relapsed osteosarcoma. The first cohort of patients was treated twice weekly for 12 weeks and had outcomes no better than historical controls. Interestingly, histological evaluation of pulmonary nodules resected from these patients showed a monocytic cellular infiltrate, suggesting some biological activity of the drug, and this led to the decision to extend treatment to a total of 24 weeks. This second cohort of patients experienced extended progression-free survival compared with historical controls (30% long-term progression-free survival, compared with 5%), and this benefit remains even with follow up of 9 to 11 years.[20] These results formed the basis for a Phase III study of L-MTP-PE combined with standard chemotherapy conducted by the Children's Oncology Group.

The Phase III study was designed to test 2 hypotheses: the first was that the addition of ifosfamide would improve the outcome of osteosarcoma patients, and the second was that the addition of L-MTP-PE to adjuvant chemotherapy would improve the outcome. Patients were randomized to receive ifosfamide or not and were independently randomized to receive L-MTP-PE or not. When event-free survival was analyzed, the test of interaction between the two randomizations did not quite rise to the level of statistical significance. In other words, it was not possible to conclusively prove that L-MTP-PE and ifosfamide did NOT interact with each other. However, there was a trend (which did not reach statistical significance) toward improved event-free survival for the patients who received L-MTP-PE compared with patients who did not receive the study drug, regardless of which chemotherapy regimen they received.[21] Recently, the data were re-analyzed for an effect on overall, rather than event-free, survival. In this analysis, the addition of L-MTP-PE improved survival regardless of which chemotherapy was administered, and the benefit did reach statistical significance, with no statistical evidence of interaction between the two randomizations.[22] When compared to SEER data, the survival of patients in this study who received chemotherapy alone did not differ from contemporary patients. In contrast, patients who received L-MTP-PE showed a clinically meaningful and statistically significant improvement in overall survival. Thus, the addition of L-MTP-PE to standard chemotherapy results in improved overall survival and a trend toward improved event-free survival; survival was better than SEER results for the past 20 years.

Another immune stimulatory agent that has been evaluated for the treatment of osteosarcoma is granulocyte-monocyte colony-stimulating factor (GM-CSF). This cytokine not only increases granulocyte and monocyte production in the bone marrow, but also activates monocytes both in vitro and in vivo. A study from the Mayo Clinic examined the possibility that aerosolized GM-CSF would activate pulmonary resident macrophages to treat pulmonary metastases from a variety of solid tumors. A total of 45 patients were treated in this study. Of the 7 patients with osteosarcoma, 4 had stable disease during treatment.[23] This finding prompted a larger, Phase II trial of aerosolized GM-CSF for patients with a first pulmonary relapse of osteosarcoma, currently underway in the Children's Oncology Group.

Another cytokine that has been investigated as a possible therapy for osteosarcoma is interleukin-12 (IL-12). The latter upregulates the expression of both Fas and Fas ligand in osteosarcoma cell lines in vitro, and enhances their sensitivity to 4-HC, the active metabolite of cyclophosphamide.[24] In order to avoid the systemic toxicities associated with IL-12 infusions, localized delivery to the lungs has been investigated, predominantly by way of gene therapy. Intrapulmonary delivery of the IL-12 gene eradicated pulmonary metastases in a mouse model.[25,26] IL-12 delivered in this way also augments the efficacy of ifosfamide.[27] Thus, cytokines may play a role in augmenting the efficacy of standard chemotherapy in addition to having independent activity via modulation of the activity of pulmonary resident macrophages.

Another potential role for IL-12 is as an adjuvant for immunotherapy trials. In addition to upregulating both Fas and Fas ligand,[24] important effectors of cytotoxic T lymphocytes, IL-12 also upregulates ICAM expression in an osteosarcoma cell line.[28] ICAM is a critical component of the immunologic synapse (Fig. 2), and upregulation of ICAM would be expected to make osteosarcoma cells better targets of cytotoxic T cells. IL-12, therefore, has the potential to play a significant role in the treatment of osteosarcoma in the future, as a single agent, as an adjunct to chemotherapy, or as an adjuvant to immunotherapy.

Adoptive Immunotherapy

Adoptive immunotherapy refers to the transfer into the patient of preformed components of an immune response, either antibodies or cells, rather than stimulating the production of these components in the patient de novo (as with a vaccine). An early example of this approach to the treatment of osteosarcoma was reported by Sutherland et al. in 1976.[29] Their report concerned a 14 year old girl diagnosed with osteosarcoma metastatic to the lungs. Coincidentally, she and her mother were HLA identical. Lymphocytes were obtained from the mother by leukopheresis and administered to the patient. This procedure transferred to the patient a DTH response to mumps antigen, and lymphocytes subsequently harvested from the patient efficiently killed osteosarcoma cells in vitro. Unfortunately, there was only a slight and transient improvement in the patient's clinical condition, and loss of in vitro lymphocytotoxicity coincided with rapid deterioration of the patient leading to her death.

A more recent attempt at adoptive immunotherapy involves the use of trastuzumab, a monoclonal antibody that recognizes HER2/erbB-2, a member of the EGF receptor family. In 1999, Gorlick et al. reported overexpression of HER2/erbB-2 in 20 of 47 osteosarcoma samples.[30] They further noted that HER2/erbB-2 expression was inversely correlated with response to chemotherapy and with event-free survival. Subsequent work from other laboratories has been somewhat contradictory. Although this group expanded a retrospective analysis of the prognostic significance of HER2/erbB-2 expression in osteosarcoma, confirming the correlation between high HER2/erbB-2 expression and inferior event-free survival,[31] Thomas et al. were unable to confirm HER2/erbB-2 membrane expression on the surface of osteosarcoma cells by immunohistochemistry, nor were they able to demonstrate HER2 mRNA in these tumors.[32] More recently, Scotlandi et al. appear to have confirmed Gorlick's findings, having reported that a significant fraction of osteosarcomas express HER2/erbB-2 by immunohistochemistry, and that this population has inferior event-free survival.[33] In contrast, a contemporaneous report of tissue microarray-based analysis of HER2/erbB-2 expression in osteosarcoma did not reveal evidence of membrane expression or of gene amplification.[34]

How can these seemingly contradictory reports be reconciled? One discrepancy arises from the ways expression is measured. In breast cancer, where HER2/erbB-2 is most intensely studied, expression is graded based on the strength of membrane-associated immunohistochemical staining.[35] In osteosarcoma, immunohistochemical staining reveals cytoplasmic localization of HER2/erbB-2.[33] Thus, application of the breast cancer grading system to osteosarcoma will yield negative results, but this does not mean the protein is not being expressed. Similarly, in breast cancer, overexpression of HER2/erbB-2 is associated with gene amplification.[35] In osteosarcoma, amplification of this gene has not been reported. There are mechanisms other than gene amplification that can cause overexpression, and one of these may be responsible for high level HER2/erbB-2 expression in osteosarcoma.

To address some of these issues, as well as the potential therapeutic benefit of adoptive immunotherapy targeting HER2/erbB-2 in osteosarcoma, the Children's Oncology Group recently completed a Phase II study of Herceptin (trastuzumab) in combination with standard chemotherapy for the treatment of metastatic osteosarcoma. Although there are no data available regarding the effect of trastuzumab on the survival of osteosarcoma patients with high HER2/erbB-2 expression, the study did demonstrate the safety of combining this agent with standard chemotherapy, including the potentially cardiotoxic doses of anthracycline given to these patients. Data pertaining to HER2/erbB-2 expression in a large cohort of osteosarcoma patients will also become available from this study.

Conclusions and Hope for the Future

The history of immunotherapy for osteosarcoma demonstrates that these approaches hold promise. The early tumor vaccine study reported by Marsh and colleagues did achieve improvements in disease-free survival and median time to metastasis.[7]

Although other studies did not replicate these findings, the approaches were different, and these differences may explain the discrepant results. Moreover, with an improved understanding of the immune system, including what makes a cell a poor target, future tumor vaccine studies may be substantially more successful.

The application of immune modulatory agents has been the most beneficial immunotherapeutic approach to osteosarcoma thus far. Recently published work demonstrates that the addition of L-MTP-PE to chemotherapy improves the survival of patients with localized osteosarcoma,[22] and preclinical work with IL-12 is equally promising. Future trials will undoubtedly seek to apply these agents to patients with metastatic disease, the population for whom chemotherapy alone offers the least benefit.

Finally, adoptive immunotherapy approaches have been investigated. One remaining controversial point here is the appropriate targets for antibody treatment – specifically, whether or not HER2/erbB-2 is a reasonable antigen for targeted treatment. Future work will certainly be aimed at identifying osteosarcoma-specific antigens that can be targeted by monoclonal antibodies, which can then be given either concurrently with or following more standard cytotoxic therapy.

In summary, immunotherapy, either active, adoptive, or via immune modulatory agents, shows substantial promise to improve the outcomes of patients with osteosarcoma. Many challenges remain, including identifying appropriate targets and optimizing the timing of these treatments, but these approaches offer hope that the plateau in survival rates that we have seen since the early 1980s will be temporary, and that improvements in survival simply await the optimization of immunotherapy and its combination with cytotoxic chemotherapy.

References

1. Eilber FR, Morton DL. Demonstration in sarcoma patients of anti-tumor antibodies which fix only human complement. *Nature*. 1970;225(5238):1137-1138.
2. Eilber FR, Morton DL. Sarcoma-specific antigens: detection by complement fixation with serum from sarcoma patients. *J Natl Cancer Inst*. 1970;44(3):651-656.
3. Wood WC, Morton DL. Microcytotoxicity test: detection in sarcoma patients of antibody cytotoxic to human sarcoma cells. *Science*. 1970;170(964):1318-1320.
4. Theoleyre S, Mori K, Cherrier B, et al. Phenotypic and functional analysis of lymphocytes infiltrating osteolytic tumors: use as a possible therapeutic approach of osteosarcoma. *BMC Cancer*. 2005;5:123.
5. Merchant MS, Melchionda F, Sinha M, Khanna C, Helman L, Mackall CL. Immune reconstitution prevents metastatic recurrence of murine osteosarcoma. *Cancer Immunol Immunother*. 2007;56(7):1037-1046.
6. Wiemann B, Starnes CO. Coley's toxins, tumor necrosis factor and cancer research: a historical perspective. *Pharmacol Ther*. 1994;64(3):529-564.
7. Marsh B, Flynn L, Enneking W. Immunologic aspects of osteosarcoma and their application to therapy. A preliminary report. *J Bone Joint Surg Am*. 1972;54(7):1367-1397.
8. Eilber FR, Grant T, Morton DL. Adjuvant therapy for osteosarcoma: preoperative and postoperative treatment. *Cancer Treat Rep*. 1978;62(2):213-216.
9. Friedl P, Storim J. Diversity in immune-cell interactions: states and functions of the immunological synapse. *Trends Cell Biol*. 2004;14(10):557-567.

10. Tsukahara T, Kawaguchi S, Torigoe T, et al. Prognostic significance of HLA class I expression in osteosarcoma defined by anti-pan HLA class I monoclonal antibody, EMR8-5. *Cancer Sci.* 2006;97(12):1374-1380.

11. Yu Z, Ma B, Zhou Y, Zhang M, Qiu X, Fan Q. Activation of antitumor cytotoxic T lymphocytes by fusion of patient-derived dendritic cells with autologous osteosarcoma. *Exp Oncol.* 2005;27(4):273-278.

12. Gilchrist GS, Ivins JC, Ritts RE Jr, Pritchard DJ, Taylor WF, Edmonson JM. Adjuvant therapy for nonmetastatic osteogenic sarcoma: an evaluation of transfer factor versus combination chemotherapy. *Cancer Treat Rep.* 1978;62(2):289-294.

13. Spitler LE, Miller L. Clinical trials of transfer factor in malignancy. *J Exp Pathol.* 1987;3(4):549-564.

14. Jaffe N, Frei E 3rd, Traggis D, Bishop Y. Adjuvant methotrexate and citrovorum-factor treatment of osteogenic sarcoma. *N Engl J Med.* 1974;291(19):994-997.

15. Strander H, Bauer HC, Brosjo O, et al. Long-term adjuvant interferon treatment of human osteosarcoma. A pilot study. *Acta Oncol.* 1995;34(6):877-880.

16. Muller CR, Smeland S, Bauer HC, Saeter G, Strander H. Interferon-alpha as the only adjuvant treatment in high-grade osteosarcoma: long term results of the Karolinska Hospital series. *Acta Oncol.* 2005;44(5):475-480.

17. Lindner DJ. Interferons as antiangiogenic agents. *Curr Oncol Rep.* 2002;4(6):510-514.

18. Kleinerman ES, Jia SF, Griffin J, Seibel NL, Benjamin RS, Jaffe N. Phase II study of liposomal muramyl tripeptide in osteosarcoma: the cytokine cascade and monocyte activation following administration. *J Clin Oncol.* 1992;10(8):1310-1316.

19. MacEwen EG, Kurzman ID, Rosenthal RC, et al. Therapy for osteosarcoma in dogs with intravenous injection of liposome-encapsulated muramyl tripeptide. *J Natl Cancer Inst.* 1989;81(12):935-938.

20. Kleinerman ES, Gano JB, Johnston DA, Benjamin RS, Jaffe N. Efficacy of liposomal muramyl tripeptide (CGP 19835A) in the treatment of relapsed osteosarcoma. *Am J Clin Oncol.* 1995;18(2):93-99.

21. Meyers PA, Schwartz CL, Krailo M, et al. Osteosarcoma: a randomized, prospective trial of the addition of ifosfamide and/or muramyl tripeptide to cisplatin, doxorubicin, and high-dose methotrexate. *J Clin Oncol.* 2005;23(9):2004-2011.

22. Meyers PA, Schwartz CL, Krailo MD, et al. Osteosarcoma: the addition of muramyl tripeptide to chemotherapy improves overall survival – a report from the Children's Oncology Group. *J Clin Oncol.* 2008;26(4):633-638.

23. Rao RD, Anderson PM, Arndt CA, Wettstein PJ, Markovic SN. Aerosolized granulocyte macrophage colony-stimulating factor (GM-CSF) therapy in metastatic cancer. *Am J Clin Oncol.* 2003;26(5):493-498.

24. Duan X, Zhou Z, Jia SF, Colvin M, Lafleur EA, Kleinerman ES. Interleukin-12 enhances the sensitivity of human osteosarcoma cells to 4-hydroperoxycyclophosphamide by a mechanism involving the Fas/Fas-ligand pathway. *Clin Cancer Res.* 2004;10(2):777-783.

25. Jia SF, Worth LL, Densmore CL, Xu B, Duan X, Kleinerman ES. Aerosol gene therapy with PEI: IL-12 eradicates osteosarcoma lung metastases. *Clin Cancer Res.* 2003;9(9):3462-3468.

26. Jia SF, Worth LL, Densmore CL, Xu B, Zhou Z, Kleinerman ES. Eradication of osteosarcoma lung metastases following intranasal interleukin-12 gene therapy using a nonviral polyethylenimine vector. *Cancer Gene Ther.* 2002;9(3):260-266.

27. Duan X, Jia SF, Koshkina N, Kleinerman ES. Intranasal interleukin-12 gene therapy enhanced the activity of ifosfamide against osteosarcoma lung metastases. *Cancer.* 2006;106(6):1382-1388.

28. Liebau C, Merk H, Schmidt S, et al. Interleukin-12 and interleukin-18 change ICAM-I expression, and enhance natural killer cell mediated cytolysis of human osteosarcoma cells. *Cytokines Cell Mol Ther.* 2002;7(4):135-142.

29. Sutherland CM, Krementz ET, Hornung MO, Carter RD, Holmes J. Transfer of in vitro cytotoxicity against osteogenic sarcoma cells. *Surgery.* 1976;79(6):682-685.

30. Gorlick R, Huvos AG, Heller G, et al. Expression of HER2/erbB-2 correlates with survival in osteosarcoma. *J Clin Oncol.* 1999;17(9):2781-2788.

31. Morris CD, Gorlick R, Huvos G, Heller G, Meyers PA, Healey JH. Human epidermal growth factor receptor 2 as a prognostic indicator in osteogenic sarcoma. *Clin Orthop Relat Res.* 2001;382:59-65.

32. Thomas DG, Giordano TJ, Sanders D, Biermann JS, Baker L. Absence of HER2/neu gene expression in osteosarcoma and skeletal Ewing's sarcoma. *Clin Cancer Res.* 2002;8(3):788-793.

33. Scotlandi K, Manara MC, Hattinger CM, et al. Prognostic and therapeutic relevance of HER2 expression in osteosarcoma and Ewing's sarcoma. *Eur J Cancer.* 2005;41(9):1349-1361.

34. Somers GR, Ho M, Zielenska M, Squire JA, Thorner PS. HER2 amplification and overexpression is not present in pediatric osteosarcoma: a tissue microarray study. *Pediatr Dev Pathol.* 2005;8(5):525-532.

35. Torrisi R, Rotmensz N, Bagnardi V, et al. HER2 status in early breast cancer: relevance of cell staining patterns, gene amplification and polysomy 17. *Eur J Cancer.* 2007;43(16):2339-2344.

Molecular Classification of Osteosarcoma

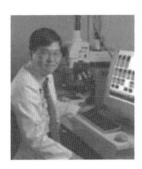

Ching C. Lau

Abstract Genomic technologies are now being used to identify new molecular markers or signatures for both diagnostic and prognostic purposes. Recently, we reported the molecular classification of pediatric osteosarcoma by expression profiling in an attempt to identify a signature that could predict the chemoresistance of a tumor before treatment is initiated. We identified a 45-gene signature that discriminates between good and poor responders to chemotherapy in osteosarcoma. Using this classifier, we can predict with 100% accuracy the chemoresponse of osteosarcoma patients prior to the initiation of treatment. These encouraging results suggest that the genomic approach will revolutionize the diagnosis and prognostication of osteosarcoma patients and improve their outcome through predictive, personalized care.

Introduction

One of the major challenges in the treatment of osteosarcoma is that we have not made much progress in improving the outcome in the past 20 years despite multiple clinical trials by various cooperative groups. This is because of the lack of novel effective chemotherapeutic agents other than the handful that have been used for the past two decades. In addition, there is also a lack of validated prognostic markers that could be used to stratify patients to risk-based therapies. Despite much experience in customizing therapy for leukemia patients based on risk assessment using a combination of clinical and molecular markers, such therapeutic strategies have not been as well developed in the treatment of solid tumors until very recently because of the lack of validated prognostic makers. In the past few years, we and others have tested the feasibility of using comprehensive molecular profiling technologies to

---

C.C. Lau (✉)
Director, Cancer Genomics Program, Texas Children's Cancer Center, 6621 Fannin Street, MC 3-3320, Houston, TX, 77030, USA
e-mail: cclau@txccc.org

identify biomarkers for both diagnostic and prognostic purposes.[1-3] In this chapter, we will illustrate how these biomarkers have been identified and validated. One such application is the use of a multigene signature to predict the response to chemotherapy at the time of diagnosis prior to the initiation of therapy.

Prognostic Markers of Osteosarcoma

Osteosarcoma is the most common malignant bone tumor in children and accounts for approximately 60% of the malignant bone tumors diagnosed in the first two decades of life.[4] After the diagnosis is made by an initial biopsy (IB), standard treatment involves the use of multiagent chemotherapy, followed by definitive surgery (DS) to resect the primary tumor, and postoperative chemotherapy. (Fig. 1) At the time of DS, the resected tumor specimen is evaluated histologically for the degree of necrosis which is subsequently used to guide the choice of postoperative chemotherapy. Degree of necrosis determined at the time of DS as a response to preoperative therapy is a reliable and the only significant prognostic factor in patients with nonmetastatic disease. Patients whose tumors display more than 90% necrosis (good or favorable response) have an excellent prognosis and continue to receive chemotherapy similar to the preoperative regimen. Patients whose tumors display less than 90% necrosis (poor or unfavorable response) have a much higher risk of relapse and poor outcome even after complete resection of the primary tumor.[5] To improve the outcome of the poor responders, attempts are usually made to use postoperative chemotherapy regimens that are different from the preoperative regimen by the addition or replacement of a chemotherapeutic agent. Such attempts in the past have been largely unsuccessful,[4,6] partly because the degree of necrosis is known only after 8–10 weeks of preoperative therapy. It is likely that resistant tumor cells have additional time to either metastasize to the lungs or to evolve further during the period when ineffective preoperative chemotherapy is given. Therefore, there is a need to identify, at the time of initial diagnosis, the patients who are likely to have a poor response to standard preoperative therapy and therefore a poor outcome, eventually. Therapies tailored to improve the outcome for those patients identified at the time of diagnosis to have a poor outcome can then be initiated at the outset when the chance for success is potentially higher. Although a number of other prognostic factors have been proposed for predicting the long-term outcome of osteosarcoma patients, most are still controversial or have not been tested in large prospective studies.[7-14]

Expression Profiling of Osteosarcoma

Recently, we reported the analysis of 34 pediatric osteosarcoma samples by expression profiling.[3] With the goal of identifying molecular signatures that can predict the chemoresistance of osteosarcoma, we first attempted to determine the expression profiles of resistant versus sensitive osteosarcoma cells. We hypothesized that the DS samples from the poor responders should be enriched for resistant tumor cells. Using expression profiles from DS samples would therefore enhance the sensitivity and power to detect the difference between chemosensitive and resistant cell populations as compared to using IB samples in which resistant cells may only be present as a small fraction. Therefore, we predicted that using DS samples would increase the chance of identifying a molecular signature of chemoresistance and if this signature is valid, it could be used to identify the good and poor responders in the IB samples. To test this hypothesis, we designed a genomic profiling study anchored prospectively in a risk-based therapeutic protocol in which all the patients received the same preoperative therapy and either the same postoperative chemotherapy for the good responders or dose-intensified therapy with autologous stem cell rescue for the poor responders. The schema of this protocol is shown in Fig. 1. Tissues were collected for genomic profiling at multiple time points including IB, DS and when lung metastases were surgically resected. Initially, we examined if we could classify good and poor responders using only DS specimens as the training set. We divided the DS samples from 20 patients into two groups, good responders (GR, n=7) and poor responders (PR, n=13). We first identified a set of 45 predictor genes that could discriminate the two classes (GR and PR) in the DS samples using a two-sample t-test with a significance cutoff of $p = 0.005$. Figure 2 shows the relative expressions of these 45 predictor genes in good and poor responders. Most of these genes (91%) were overexpressed in PR specimens.

Various supervised classification algorithms including Compound Covariate Predictor (CCP), K-Nearest Neighbor (K-NN), Nearest Centroid (NC), Support Vector Machine (SVM), and Linear Discriminant Analysis (LDA), were then applied to the training set to test if they could classify GR and PR using p value of 0.005. Leave-One-Out Cross Validation (LOOCV) method was used to test the robustness of each classifier in the training set (Table 1). The correct classification rates of LOOCV using these algorithms were 65–70%. Among the six algorithms,

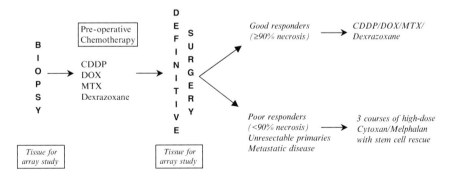

Fig. 1 Treatment schema for osteosarcoma. All patients with localized disease and good response to preoperative chemotherapy will receive the same chemotherapeutic agents in postoperative chemotherapy. Poor risk patients including the poor responders and those that have unresectable primary tumors or metastatic disease will receive more intensive chemotherapy as postoperative therapy

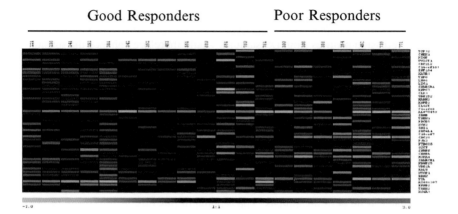

Fig. 2 The 45 predictor genes in the chemoresistance signature were selected based on two-sample t-test to distinguish between good and poor responders in 20 definitive surgery samples at p value of 0.005. Forty-one genes were overexpressed in poor responders, while only four genes were overexpressed in good responders. The color scale at the bottom represents log 2 expression ratios of the genes

SVM had one of the best performances (70% correct classification). Three GR and three PR were misclassified using SVM. Two of the GR (#300 and 394) that were misclassified as PR by the SVM classifier developed recurrent disease, 11 and 9 months respectively, after completion of therapy. This suggested that there may be some residual resistant cells in the DS specimens of these two cases that were recognized by the algorithm based on the predictor gene set. One of the PR (#680) that was misclassified as a GR by the SVM classifier remains free of disease after 30 months of follow-up. The other misclassified PR (#761) had 86% necrosis, which is very close to the cutoff for good response (90%).

Use of Multigene Classifier to Predict Response to Preoperative Chemotherapy in IB

To test the SVM classifier, we divided our validation set of 14 IB samples into two groups. The first group consisted of six samples, which had corresponding DS samples included in the training set (paired samples). Using these six cases, we attempted to verify that our classifier built from DS samples could predict the chemoresistance of the corresponding IB samples, based on the hypothesis that the molecular signature of chemoresistance as recognized in the DS samples was already present in the IB at the time of diagnosis. The second group consisted of eight IB samples that did not have matched DS samples included in the training set, thus representing a totally independent set of samples that had not been used in building the classifier.

Molecular Classification of Osteosarcoma

Table 1 Leave one out cross validation (LOOCV) of 20 definitive surgery osteosarcoma samples

Tumor ID	Histologic response	Concordance of classification with histological response					
		CCP	LDA	1-NN	3-NN	NC	SVM
300	GR	No	No	No	No	No	No
308	GR	Yes	Yes	Yes	Yes	Yes	Yes
386	GR	No	No	No	No	No	No
394	GR	No	No	No	No	No	No
452	GR	Yes	Yes	Yes	Yes	Yes	Yes
759	GR	Yes	Yes	Yes	Yes	Yes	Yes
771	GR	Yes	Yes	Yes	Yes	Yes	Yes
221	PR	Yes	Yes	Yes	Yes	Yes	Yes
236	PR	Yes	Yes	Yes	Yes	Yes	Yes
241	PR	Yes	Yes	Yes	Yes	Yes	Yes
252	PR	Yes	Yes	Yes	Yes	Yes	Yes
311	PR	Yes	Yes	Yes	Yes	Yes	Yes
342	PR	Yes	Yes	Yes	Yes	Yes	Yes
392	PR	Yes	Yes	Yes	Yes	Yes	Yes
483	PR	Yes	Yes	Yes	Yes	Yes	Yes
591	PR	Yes	Yes	Yes	Yes	Yes	Yes
680	PR	No	No	No	No	No	No
691	PR	No	No	No	No	No	No
760	PR	No	Yes	Yes	Yes	No	Yes
761	PR	No	No	No	No	No	No
% Correctly Classified:		65	70	70	70	65	70

LOOCV was carried out with feature selection at each validation to minimize the overoptimistic estimation of error rate. The six classification algorithms used are Compound Covariate Predictor (CCP), Linear Discriminant Analysis (LDA), 1-Nearest Neighbor (1-NN), 3-Nearest Neighbor (3-NN), Nearest Centroid (NC), and Support Vector Machine (SVM). "Yes" denotes the classification by the algorithm was correct and "No" denotes the classification was wrong. GR represents good responders and PR represents poor responders

The SVM classifier misclassified one sample (out of six) in the first group of paired samples, with a correct classification rate of 83% (95% CI=36%, 100%) (Table 2). The only misclassified sample was from a patient (#410) who was classified as a GR based on histologic response but was predicted to be a PR by the multigene classifier. Interestingly, this patient initially presented with localized disease but eventually developed recurrent disease in the lungs 25 months after completion of therapy, suggesting that there were resistant cells present in the IB that were recognized by the multigene classifier, and presumably these resistant cells metastasized to the lungs prior to DS, and subsequently gave rise to the recurrent tumor. Ironically, the multigene predictor classified this patient's DS sample (452) as a GR, implying that either the DS sample used in our analysis was not representative of the primary tumor in that it did not contain the resistant cells, or that the resistant cells had already metastasized before DS, and therefore were no longer detectable in the primary tumor.

In the second group of independent IB samples, the classifier correctly predicted eight out of eight of the samples (100% correct, 95% CI=63%, 100%). These eight

Table 2 Classification of IB samples (paired and independent) using SVM classifier (see legend of Table 1)

Tumor ID	Histologic response	Concordance with histologic response	
		Paired	Independent
410	GR	No	
197	PR	Yes	
207	PR	Yes	
278	GR	Yes	
289	PR	Yes	
345	GR	Yes	
204	PR		Yes
274	PR		Yes
299	GR		Yes
464	PR		Yes
479	PR		Yes
481	PR		Yes
545	GR		Yes
654	GR		Yes

samples included five PRs and three GRs. These results further indicate that the gene expression signature of the resistant cells in the DS samples was already present in the IB samples at the time of diagnosis. Our results are consistent with the notion proposed by Ramaswamy et al[15] that the metastatic signature of metastatic tumors is already present in the primary tumor.

Conclusions

The high accuracy of our multigene classifier in identifying GR and PR from two separate groups of IB samples suggests that response to chemotherapy can potentially be predicted at the time of diagnosis. However, because of the limited number of samples used in the study, the classifier and chemoresistant signature need to be validated in a larger multi-institutional study. If validated, this can significantly impact the design of future therapeutic studies of osteosarcoma, in which intensified therapy could be given at the time of diagnosis to those patients who are predicted to be poor responders to standard therapy, in order to improve their outcome. Validation of such molecular signatures is now underway in collaboration with the Children's Oncology Group by analyzing initially the archival cases enrolled in the Biology Protocol (~150) and subsequently, the cases that are currently being enrolled in the joint European and North American Osteosarcoma Study (EURAMOS). It should be emphasized that such chemoresistance signatures are naturally therapy-dependent and therefore, should be identified and validated based on patients who are treated identically. In addition, because genomic profiling data are by nature of high dimensionality, and multiple testing is necessary for the discovery steps,

Molecular Classification of Osteosarcoma 465

robust and reliable signatures could only be identified and validated in studies with large sample size such as that of the EURAMOS study (1400).

Acknowledgements This work was supported by NIH grants CA88126, CA97874, CA109467, and CA114757, as well as grants from the John S. Dunn Research Foundation, the Robert J. Kleberg, Jr. and Helen C. Kleberg Foundation, the Gillson Longenbaugh Foundation and Cancer Fighters of Houston, Inc.

References

1. Ochi K, Daigo Y, Katagiri T, et al. Prediction of response to neoadjuvant chemotherapy for osteosarcoma by gene-expression profiles. *Int J Oncol.* 2004;24:647-655.
2. Mintz MB, Sowers R, Brown KM, et al. An expression signature classifies chemotherapy-resistant pediatric osteosarcoma. *Cancer Res.* 2005;65:1748-1754.
3. Man TK, Chintagumpala M, Visvanathan J, et al. Expression profiles of osteosarcoma that can predict response to chemotherapy. *Cancer Res.* 2005;65:8142-8150.
4. Link MP, Gebhardt MC, Meyers PA. In: Pizzo P, Poplack D, editors. Principles and Practice of Pediatric Oncology. 4th ed. Philadelphia: Lippincott-Williams & Wilkins; 2002. p. 1051-1089
5. Provisor AJ, Ettinger LJ, Nachman JB, et al. Treatment of nonmetastatic osteosarcoma of the extremity with preoperative and postoperative chemotherapy: a report from the Children's Cancer Group. *J Clin Oncol.* 1997;15:76-84.
6. Meyers PA, Heller G, Healey J, et al. Chemotherapy for nonmetastatic osteogenic sarcoma: the Memorial Sloan-Kettering experience. *J Clin Oncol.* 1992;10:5-15.
7. Baldini N, Scotlandi K, Barbanti-Brodano G, et al. Expression of P-glycoprotein in high-grade osteosarcomas in relation to clinical outcome. *N Engl J Med.* 1995;333:1380-1385.
8. Bacci G, Longhi A, Ferrari S, et al. Prognostic significance of serum alkaline phosphatase in osteosarcoma of the extremity treated with neoadjuvant chemotherapy: recent experience at Rizzoli Institute. *Oncol Rep.* 2002;9:171-175.
9. Gorlick R, Huvos AG, Heller G, et al. Expression of HER2/erbB-2 correlates with survival in osteosarcoma. *J Clin Oncol.* 1999;17:2781-2788.
10. Bielack SS, Kempf-Bielack B, Delling G, et al. Prognostic factors in high-grade osteosarcoma of the extremities or trunk: an analysis of 1,702 patients treated on neoadjuvant cooperative osteosarcoma study group protocols. *J Clin Oncol.* 2002;20:776-790.
11. Davis AM, Bell RS, Goodwin PJ. Prognostic factors in osteosarcoma: a critical review. *J Clin Oncol.* 1994;12:423-431.
12. Feugeas O, Guriec N, Babin-Boilletot A, et al. Loss of heterozygosity of the RB gene is a poor prognostic factor in patients with osteosarcoma. *J Clin Oncol.* 1996;14:467-472.
13. Franzius C, Bielack S, Flege S, et al. Prognostic significance of (18) F-FDG and (99 m) Tc-methylene diphosphonate uptake in primary osteosarcoma. *J Nucl Med.* 2002;43: 1012-1017.
14. Ulaner GA, Huang HY, Otero J, et al. Absence of a telomere maintenance mechanism as a favorable prognostic factor in patients with osteosarcoma. *Cancer Res.* 2003;63:1759-1763.
15. Ramaswamy S, Ross KN, Lander ES, Golub TR. A molecular signature of metastasis in primary solid tumors. *Nat Genet.* 2003;33:49-54.

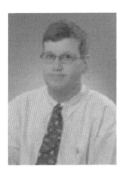

Current Concepts on the Molecular Biology of Osteosarcoma

Richard Gorlick

Abstract Despite the knowledge of many of the genetic alterations present in osteosarcoma, its complexity precludes placing its biology into a simple conceptual framework. In contrast to many other malignancies, multiple genetic and environmental factors can all lead to the development of osteosarcoma which is defined phenotypically rather than molecularly. Despite the many factors capable of leading to its development, osteosarcoma is a rare malignancy that is relatively homogeneous in its clinical behavior and chemotherapy response. It remains unknown whether the clinical features of osteosarcoma are defined by the cell of origin, the genetic events leading to transformation, the timing of those events or factors related to differentiation into an osteoblastic phenotype. Identifying new treatment approaches has generally been through empiric and screening approaches. In this presentation the genetic alterations present in osteosarcoma, issues related to the cell of origin and bone differentiation will be reviewed along with the recent results of preclinical drug screening.

Grant Support: Supported by the Foster Foundation, the Swim Across America Foundation, and Cure Search Foundation.

Introduction

Osteosarcoma is defined pathologically by its production of osteoid.[1-4] Producing bony matrix is a cellular behavior or a phenotype, not a genetic marker. Considerable variability exists in the predominant matrix produced, described as the histologic subtype, but the presence of even a small area of osteoid in association with a malignant spindle cell is sufficient to make the diagnosis. Cytogenetics, specific molecular probes and immunohistochemistry are not typically used to assist in making the diagnosis.[1-4] Despite this phenotypic definition, the clinical behavior of

---

R. Gorlick (✉)
The Albert Einstein College of Medicine of Yeshiva University, The Children's Hospital at Montefiore, 3415 Bainbridge Avenue, Rosenthal 3rd floor, Bronx, NY, 10467, USA
e-mail: rgorlick@montefiore.org

high grade osteosarcoma is remarkably homogeneous. Histologic subtype does not influence the chemotherapy utilized or the tendency of the disease to metastasize early in its natural history or to a great extent chemotherapy response or prognosis.[3,4]

All sarcomas can be broadly characterized into those that are genetically complex and those that have relatively simple karyotypes in association with a recurrent chromosomal translocation.[5] Osteosarcoma is a prototypical member of the former, and larger group of sarcomas. As is characteristic of these group of sarcomas, p53 is frequently altered but not prognostic, there is an association with a variety of etiologic factors and each tumor is associated with a large number of genetic alterations many of which are recurrent in different tumors but at the same time variable.[5]

Unlike adult tumors that are predominantly of epithelial origin, osteosarcoma does not have an obvious multi-step progression. Low grade osteosarcomas are not believed to be the precursor lesions of the high grade osteosarcomas that occur in children and adolescents. The equivalent of a premalignant dysplastic lesion or a carcinoma in situ is not known to exist for osteosarcoma as is the case with most pediatric malignancies. In defining the molecular pathogenesis of osteosarcoma, the first lesion that can be analyzed is already a fully malignant cancer. This fact coupled with these tumors' molecular complexity makes it extremely difficult to define the molecular features essential in the tumor's pathogenesis.[6-9] Despite these difficulties, a considerable amount is known about osteosarcoma's pathogenesis which will be reviewed.

Genetic Alterations Involved in Osteosarcoma Pathogenesis

Despite its genetic complexity, numerous clues exist as to the processes and genetic pathways that may be associated with the formation of osteosarcoma, including mouse models of osteosarcoma, human predisposition syndromes, etiologic-environmental factors and studies of genetic alterations in tumors. In contrast to most cancers, too many models rather than too few produce osteosarcoma. Given the rarity of osteosarcoma, many of these genetic events may not be clinically relevant or alternatively the development of osteosarcoma is restricted or limited by mechanisms which are not understood at present. Factors/models which provide clues as to the etiology of osteosarcoma are summarized in Table 1.

Perhaps the most compelling data potentially defining osteosarcoma's pathogenesis are humans with germ-line genetic alterations that lead to a predisposition for osteosarcoma. In individuals with hereditary retinoblastoma, which is associated with a germ-line mutation in the Rb gene, secondary malignancies are common, and 40% of these malignancies will be an osteosarcoma.[10,11] Supportive of the Rb gene's involvement in osteosarcoma is the frequent derangement of this pathway in tumor specimens.[12-14] On the other hand, the vast majority of Rb gene abnormalities are inherited in an autosomal dominant manner and have high penetrance.[15] Hence,

Current Concepts on the Molecular Biology of Osteosarcoma

Table 1 Models which provide clues as to the etiology of osteosarcoma

Human predisposition models	Hereditary Retinoblastoma (Rb)
	Li–Fraumeni syndrome (p53)
	Rothmund–Thomson (RecQL4)
	Werner syndrome (WRN)
Murine predisposition models	p53 knock out mouse
	SV40 Tag transgenics
	Myc transgenics
	Fos transgenics
	Parathyroid hormone
Epidemiology	Radiation
	Bone turnover – Paget's Disease
	Growth

the lack of a history of prior retinoblastoma in the vast majority of patients who are diagnosed with sporadic osteosarcoma suggests that germ-line alterations of Rb in this patient population is not common. Low penetrance Rb mutations have been reported but their incidence among patients with sporadic osteosarcoma is not known. Similarly, in Li–Fraumeni syndrome with germ-line alterations in p53, malignancy is frequent and approximately 10% of these are osteosarcomas, the second most common tumors that develop.[16,17] In a manner analogous to the Rb gene, the p53 pathway is frequently deranged in tumors, but in a study of germ-line p53 abnormalities among patients with sporadic osteosarcoma, only 3% were found to harbor unsuspected alterations.[18,19]

The data supporting the RecQL4 and WRN genes' involvement in the pathogenesis of osteosarcoma is somewhat more limited. In the context of Rothmund–Thomson Syndrome, mutation of RecQL4 is associated with osteosarcoma development.[20] In sporadic osteosarcomas, RecQL4 is rarely altered, suggesting that it does not play a role in the pathogenesis of these tumors.[21] Werner syndrome, a result of an abnormality in the WRN gene, is associated with genetic instability and a general malignancy predisposition. Although they develop osteosarcomas, these tumors comprise less than 10% of the cancers that develop.[22]

A large number of murine models develop osteosarcoma. These include p53 knock out mice, fos, myc and SV40 transgenic mice as well as parathyroid hormone and radiation exposed mice.[23–28] All of these models produce malignant spindle cell tumors which produce osteoid; hence, tumor is pathologically defined as osteosarcoma, but it is unclear which model(s) accurately recapitulates the human disease. Many of these genetic alterations functionally inactivate the p53 and Rb genes or drive bone proliferation as the common feature. It has been suggested by many investigators that these are appropriate models for chemoprevention and treatment studies. This is extremely controversial in the context of osteosarcoma. The clinical utility or even interest in chemo-preventive factors for this disease is not established, given its rarity. In addition, a model of osteosarcoma, which is derived from a monogenic event, may not sufficiently represent the heterogeneity of this disease, limiting its usefulness as a model for testing chemotherapy efficacy.

A number of epidemiologic factors are associated with the development of osteosarcoma. These include the much discussed but somewhat controversial association with growth linked both through correlations with the most rapid periods of growth and height in humans as well as canines.[1-4] Although these are not genetic events, these have provided support that the growth hormone-insulin like growth factor axis is involved in osteosarcoma pathogenesis. Although epidemiologic factors such as radiation exposure, which is a nonspecific mutagen, and Paget's disease, which results in bone proliferation, are not associated with clear genetic alterations leading to osteosarcoma, they will be mentioned here as being associated with an osteosarcoma predisposition for completeness' sake.[1-4]

The most consistent feature across human predisposition syndromes, murine predisposition syndromes and analyses of human tumors are alterations of the Rb and p53 tumor suppressor pathways (Fig. 1). In human tumors, virtually all osteosarcomas have inactivation of these pathways, which is accomplished by a variety of typically nonoverlapping mechanisms. As an example, inactivation of the p53 tumor suppressor genes can be accomplished by p53 mutation, MDM2 amplification, COPS3 amplification and INK4 locus deletion.[18,19,26,27] If the percentages of each of these derangements in human tumors are combined (most studies have revealed these alterations to be in large part nonoverlapping), virtually 100% of tumors will have inactivation of the p53 tumor suppressor pathway. This is true for the Rb gene as well. What this suggests is that inactivation of these pathways may be essential for the development of osteosarcoma. This does not necessarily establish these events as the first step in

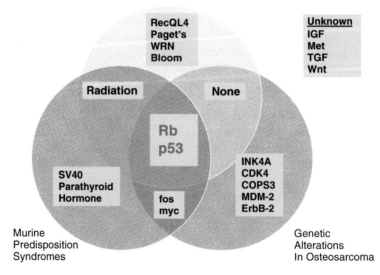

Fig. 1 Human predisposition syndromes, engineered murine models and analysis of osteosarcoma tissue all provide clues as to the etiology of osteosarcoma. Loss of the tumor suppressor genes Rb and p53 are the only events that are involved in osteosarcoma in all of these three systems

Current Concepts on the Molecular Biology of Osteosarcoma

the tumor's pathogenesis as other events may drive the development of these abnormalities and serve as the initiating genetic event.

Cell of Origin

Osteosarcoma has traditionally been believed to arise from an osteoblast, but the data supporting that assertion is rather limited.[1,2] Several lines of evidence suggest that osteosarcoma has a more pluripotent potential and may, in fact, arise from a more primitive precursor. Normal osteoblasts are derived from a mesenchymal stem cell. Mesenchymal stem cells are cells which can differentiate into bone, cartilage, muscle, stroma, fat and fibrous tissue in a manner not unlike hematopoiesis. The presence of osteoid has led to the traditional viewpoint that the tumor is derived from osteoblasts. It has repeatedly been reported that great variability exists in the histological patterns seen in this tumor and in the degree of osteoid production; so, extensive review of the pathologic material may be required to demonstrate tumor osteoid. It is also known that these tumors are capable of differentiating toward fibrous tissue, cartilage, or bone and can have chondroblastic, fibroblastic and osteoblastic components, suggesting that the cell of origin may be more pluripotent than an osteoblast.[1,2] Tumors with various patterns of differentiation are traditionally referred to as histologic subtypes. It is well recognized that many tumors have mixed patterns. It is also known that the histologic subtype does not impact in a major way on chemotherapy response or outcome, and the patients are treated identically irrespective of subtype, suggesting that these various patterns of differentiation are reflective of a single clinical disease.[1-4] At present, the factors associated with an osteosarcoma having a particular histologic appearance are poorly understood. Osteosarcoma could arise from a mesenchymal stem cell which acquires patterns of osteoblastic differentiation during transformation. Similarly, osteosarcoma may arise from an osteoblast and the pluripotent capacity can be acquired through de-differentiation during the transformation process. Both the acquisition and loss of differentiation properties can be observed in the development of hematopoietic malignancies. Even if one accepted osteoblasts as the cell of origin of osteosarcoma, these cells exist at various stages of maturity, and in various pools including the bone marrow, in growth plates and the periosteum, with it being unclear which pool serves as the usual cell of origin. Identifying the cell of origin and the molecular basis of osteosarcoma is likely to be of critical clinical importance.

Redundancy

In osteosarcoma, numerous studies have been undertaken to characterize the genetic abnormalities present in tumor samples. Osteosarcomas have tremendous chromosomal complexity with numerous whole chromosome alterations as well as a large number of regions with consistent genetic gains and losses. Each of these sites has been characterized to a variable extent and a large list of genes frequently altered in osteosarcoma has emerged. A partial list of genes which may be altered in osteosarcoma include Rb, INK4A, CDK4, p53, MDM2, COPS3, MYC, FOS, MET, IGF-1R, PDGF, HER2, ErbB-4, TERT, ALT, TGF, BMP, WNT, LRP5, CXCR4, ezrin, fas, VEGF, MDR1, RFC, DHFR, and MAPK7.[5] Space and likely reader interest preclude going through each of these genes in detail, but several points may be worth discussing. Investigators have demonstrated that only a few genetic elements are necessary to transform a normal cell into a cancer as only a few fundamental processes need to be deranged. To become a cancer, a normal cell needs a signal to progress through the cell cycle, a loss of checkpoint control, telomere length stabilization and loss of contact inhibition/dependence.[29] Osteosarcoma clearly does not need all of the alterations it possesses to achieve these tasks, and many genetic events are likely to be bystander effects related, perhaps, to genetic instability. This is, perhaps, no more evident in osteosarcoma's expression of growth factor receptors. Osteosarcoma has been reported to express IGF, VEGF, HER2, ErbB-4, PTHR and HGF among others.[30–38] Many of these pathways are redundant, and expression of a growth factor alone is not sufficient to establish the pathway as being involved in the tumor's proliferation or behavior. This is exemplified in a recently published manuscript from our laboratory, describing PDGF as being expressed in osteosarcoma, but imatinib mesylate, which targets this receptor as not appearing to be a relevant therapy for osteosarcoma.[39] This suggests that PDGF, although expressed, has limited functional relevance in this context. As an additional point, it may be necessary to consider osteosarcoma in the context of its environment in order to understand the relevant signals. Interaction with osteoclasts may be an important component of osteosarcomas clinical behavior.[38] Only by studying osteosarcoma in the context of this environment will these influences be adequately assessed.

The Potential Clinical Relevance of Osteosarcoma Biology Studies

Recent progress in improving the survival of osteosarcoma patients has been limited (Fig. 2). It is hoped that an increased understanding of biology will translate into clinical benefit. The clinical goals of osteosarcoma research include identifying prognostic factors which may serve as a basis for stratification of therapy and helping to prioritize clinical trials of new therapeutic agents.

It must be acknowledged that thus far no biologically based validated prognostic factors have been identified. The failure to identify prognostic factors can be explained in a variety of potential ways (Table 2). A factor must be measured in a sufficiently standardized manner and remain prognostic across a prospective

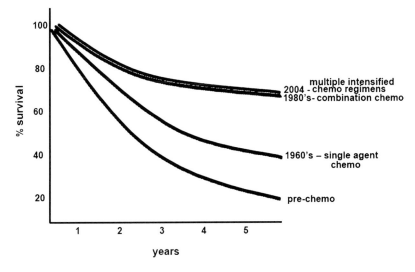

Fig. 2 Cartoon of osteosarcoma survival by era. *Highlighted* is that recent progress in improving the survival of osteosarcoma has been limited

Table 2 Potential reasons for failure to validate prognostic factors

Limited power of single institutional retrospective studies
Different patient populations
Insufficiently robust prognostic factors
Differences in tissue handling in multi-institutional studies
Differences in tissue processing in multi-institutional studies
Changes in method
Changes in interpretation
Other factors not identified

multi-institutional study in order to be clinically relevant. Only factors identified as part of large multi-institutional biology studies are likely to meet these criteria. For biology efforts to be successful, the establishment and maintenance of large clinically annotated banks of tissue will be critical. A successful model for such an effort comes from the Children's Oncology Group Osteosarcoma tumor bank. The biology study was initiated in 1998 and all OS patients aged ≤40 years were eligible for participation. Part of its success can potentially be attributed to the fact that specimen collection was centralized and predominantly performed through an impartial National Cancer Institute funded group, the Cooperative Human Tissue Network. Access to tissue was through an application process and was open to all investigators. Through this effort, the largest reported bank of osteosarcoma related biological materials has been established, and a large number of studies using this material are under way.

Approaches to Identify Therapeutic Targets

The value of chemotherapy in the treatment of high grade osteosarcoma is no longer disputed, and its value is established definitively in the context of a randomized clinical trial.[1-4] Supporting its effectiveness is the consistent prognostic value of response to neoadjuvant chemotherapy. As chemotherapy has had a dramatic effect on the outcome of osteosarcoma, it is perhaps intuitive to assume that genetic alterations which produce drug resistance would be associated with inferior chemotherapy response and patient survival. Hence, studying drug resistance genes may be a manner in which prognostic factors could be defined, without necessarily deciphering the issues of pathogenesis. Along these lines, perhaps the most extensively studied prognostic marker is the expression of p-glycoprotein.[40] p-Glycoprotein is a transmembrane ATP-dependent efflux pump protein encoded by the multi-drug resistance (MDR1) gene, which is responsible for the efflux of numerous chemotherapeutic agents from the malignant cell. In the context of osteosarcoma, the most important drug which can be effluxed by p-glycoprotein is doxorubicin, although etoposide is also a substrate.[40] Despite its extensive study, use of p-glycoprotein or MDR1 expression as a prognostic marker remains controversial.[41] High dose methotrexate with leucovorin rescue is a major component of current protocols for the treatment of osteosarcoma. High-dose methotrexate is vastly more effective than conventional dose methotrexate in the treatment of osteosarcoma – a finding that is not observed in other malignancies treated with methotrexate, implying a mechanism of intrinsic methotrexate resistance within osteosarcoma tumor cells. In experimental systems, resistance to methotrexate can occur through a variety of mechanisms, including impaired intracellular transport of the drug via the reduced folate carrier, upregulation of dihydrofolate reductase, and diminished intracellular retention due to decreased polyglutamylation. Our laboratory has reported studies that have demonstrated that impairment of drug influx as a result of decreased expression and mutations in the reduced folate carrier gene are the major basis of intrinsic resistance: 65% of osteosarcoma tumor samples were found to have decreased reduced folate carrier expression at the time of initial biopsy. In contrast, dihydrofolate reductase overexpression was seen relatively infrequently at initial biopsy – in only 10% of tumor samples, compared with 62% of the tumors examined at the time of definitive surgery or relapse, suggesting DHFR overexpression as the major mechanism of acquired methotrexate resistance in osteosarcoma.[42,43] These are being explored as potential prognostic factors in the context of the Children's Oncology Group osteosarcoma biology study. Other potential mechanisms of drug resistance include alterations in multidrug resistance associated protein (MRP) expression, topoisomerase II, glutathione S-transferases, DNA repair, DNA damage response, drug metabolism or inactivation, and reduced intracellular delivery, some of which are being assessed as prognostic factors.[5]

As had been suggested previously many genetic alterations occur in osteosarcoma that are not central to the tumor's pathogenesis or maintenance. One approach to deciphering critical events may be through laboratory assessments of complete pathways rather than single gene assessments. If alterations in a growth factor receptor result in activation of a signal transduction cascade and downstream activation, the pathway may be more relevant to the tumor. Ultimately, improved bioinformatic analyses of oligonucleotide expression arrays may allow the identification of signatures related to pathway activation, but at present these approaches have difficulty in doing so in the context of osteosarcoma which may be another reflection of the tumor's heterogeneity.[44] Targeted analyses of several proteins/genes in a given pathway either through functional studies or phospho-specific western blots have been among the more successful approaches for analyzing osteosarcoma.

The Pediatric Preclinical Testing Program

A tremendous clinical need is the rapid identification of new therapies which are effective in the treatment of osteosarcoma. In order to do so, increasing emphasis is being placed on preclinical laboratory studies of chemotherapy effectiveness in various tumor model systems. The rationale for this approach includes the following: If a drug targets a pathway, which is central to a tumor's viability ("gene addicted"), we would expect it to be efficacious; as long as normal cells were less dependent upon the pathway, a therapeutic index should exist; although few drugs are developed specifically for sarcomas, pathways central to some sarcomas may overlap with those of more common cancers; and numerous new drugs exist but there are too few osteosarcoma patients to test them all clinically. The Pediatric Preclinical Testing Program is one such effort underway to facilitate the introduction of new, active agents into clinical trials for all childhood cancers. With a consortium of laboratories in the United States and abroad, the Pediatric Preclinical Testing Program is able to quickly screen a large number of agents using in vitro and in vivo models. Preclinical testing may potentially predict the activity of new agents, in patients with childhood cancers, allowing the rational design of clinical trials utilizing new agents which can presumably lead to the identification of active agents more rapidly. Some believe that the value of the preclinical testing needs to be validated as accurately representing responses in human clinical trials prior to utilizing the information as a means of prioritizing clinical trials. Others believe that, in the absence of other data, preclinical testing should be used as a basis of prioritization as it is more likely to be predictive than intuitive or random selection of new agents for clinical trials in osteosarcoma. Regardless of how this data is utilized, the Pediatric Preclinical Testing Program has generated a large amount of data, which has rapidly been published. The group has evaluated several standard and novel agents including: cyclophosphamide, vincristine, topotecan, 19D12 (Anti-IGF-1R antibody), AZD2171 (a specific inhibitor of VEGF-receptor), AZD6244 (MEK1/2 inhibitor), bortezomib (proteosome inhibitor), ABT-263 (a Bcl-2 inhibitor), MLN8237 (aurora A kinase inhibitor), rapamycin, vorinostat (histone deacetylase inhibitor), lapitinib (EGFR and ErbB2 inhibitor) and sunitinib.[45-55] Thus far, of all of the novel agents tested; 19D12, AZD2171 and rapamycin have been among the most effective for the treatment of osteosarcoma. In this section the focus has been on the Pediatric Preclinical Testing Program, but this is not meant to diminish the clear importance of other models, such as spontaneously arising osteosarcoma in canines. It is anticipated that the canine model will be covered in more detail within other reviews.

Conclusion

Despite having a great deal of data characterizing osteosarcoma, we have little molecular understanding of its nature because of its genetic complexity, redundancy and our inability to simplify the system. This does not diminish our enthusiasm for an increased biological understanding of osteosarcoma, which will lead to clinical advances. Developing the resources to make these biology studies possible, along with new laboratory approaches for studying osteosarcoma, holds much promise for the future.

References

1. Dorfman HD, Czerniak B. Bone cancers. *Cancer*. 1995;75:203-210.
2. Huvos A. *Bone Tumors: Diagnosis, Treatment and Prognosis*. 2nd ed. WB Saunders: Philadelphia; 1991.
3. Gorlick R, Bernstein ML, Toretsky JA, et al. Bone Tumours. In: Holland J, Frei E, eds. *Cancer Medicine*. 7th ed. Hamilton, ON: BC Decker; 2006:2019-2027.
4. Meyers PA, Gorlick R. Osteosarcoma. *Pediatr Clin N Am*. 1997;44:973-989.
5. Ladanyi M, Gorlick R. The molecular pathology and pharmacology of osteosarcoma. *Pediatr Pathol Mol Med*. 2000;19:391-413.
6. Man T-K, Lu X-Y, Jaeweon K, et al. Genome-wide array comparative genomic hybridization reveals distinct amplifications in osteosarcoma. *BMC Cancer*. 2004;4:45.
7. Lau CC, Harris CP, Lu X-Y, et al. Frequent amplification and rearrangement of chromosomal bands 6p12-p21 and 17p11.2 in osteosarcomas. *Genes Chromosomes Cancer*. 2004;39:11-21.
8. Bayani J, Zielenska M, Pandita A, et al. Spectral karyotyping identifies recurrent complex rearrangements of chromosomes 8, 17, and 20 in osteosarcomas. *Genes Chromosomes Cancer*. 2003;36:7-16.
9. Nellissery MJ, Padalecki SS, Brkanac Z, et al. Evidence for a novel osteosarcoma tumor-suppressor gene in the chromosome 18 region genetically linked with Paget disease of bone. *Am J Hum Genet*. 1998;63:817-824.
10. Wong FL, Boice JD, Abramson DH, et al. Cancer incidence after retinoblastoma: radiation dose and sarcoma risk. *JAMA*. 1997;278:1262-1267.
11. Draper GJ, Sanders BM, Kingston JE. Second primary neoplasms in patients with retinoblastoma. *Br J Cancer*. 1986;53:661-671.
12. Wadayama B, Toguchida J, Shimizu T, et al. Mutation spectrum of the retinoblastoma gene in osteosarcomas. *Cancer Res*. 1994;54:3042-3048.
13. Benassi MS, Molendini L, Gamberi G, et al. Alteration of pRb/p16/cdk4 regulation in human osteosarcoma. *Int J Cancer*. 1999;84:489-493.

14. Hansen MF, Koufos A, Gallie BL, et al. Osteosarcoma and retinoblastoma: a shared chromosomal mechanism revealing recessive predisposition. *Proc Natl Acad Sci U S A*. 1985;82:6216-6220.
15. Harbour JW. Molecular basis of low-penetrance retinoblastoma. *Arch Ophthalmol*. 2001;119:1699-1704.
16. Li FP, Fraumeni JF Jr, Mulvihill JJ, et al. A cancer family syndrome in twenty-four kindreds. *Cancer Res*. 1988;48:5358-5362.
17. Malkin D, Li FP, Strong LC, et al. Germline p53 mutations in a familial syndrome of breast cancer, sarcomas, and other neoplasms. *Science*. 1990;250:1233-1238.
18. Lonardo F, Ueda T, Huvos AG, Healey J, Ladanyi M. p53 and MDM2 alterations in osteosarcomas: Correlation with clinicopathologic features and proliferative rate. *Cancer*. 1997;79:1541-1547.
19. McIntyre JF, Smith-Sorensen B, Friend SH, et al. Germline mutations of the p53 tumor suppressor gene in children with osteosarcoma. *J Clin Oncol*. 1994;12:925-930.
20. Wang LL, Gannavarapu A, Kozinetz CA, et al. Association between osteosarcoma and deleterious mutations in the RECQL4 gene in Rothmund–Thomson syndrome. *J Natl Cancer Inst*. 2003;95:669-674.
21. Nishijo K, Nakayama T, Aoyama T, et al. Mutation analysis of the RECQL4 gene in sporadic osteosarcomas. *Int J Cancer*. 2004;111:367-372.
22. Goto M, Miller RW, Ishikawa Y, Sugano H. Excess of rare cancers in Werner syndrome (adult progeria). *Cancer Epidemiol Biomarkers Prev*. 1996;5:239-246.
23. Jacks T, Remington L, Williams BO, et al. Tumor spectrum analysis in p53-mutant mice. *Curr Biol*. 1994;4:1-7.
24. Grigoriadis AE, Schellander K, Wang ZW, Wagner ER. Osteoblasts are target cells for transformation in c-fos transgenic mice. *J Cell Biol*. 1993;122:685-701.
25. Jain M, Arvanitis C, Chu K, et al. Sustained loss of a neoplastic phenotype by brief inactivation of MYC. *Science*. 2002;297:102-104.
26. Yan T, Wunder JS, Gokgoz N, et al. COPS3 amplification and clinical outcome in osteosarcoma. *Cancer*. 2007;109:1870-1876.
27. Knowles BB, McCarrick J, Fox N, Solter D, Damjanov I. Osteosarcomas in transgenic mice expressing an alpha-amylase-SV40 T-antigen hybrid gene. *Am J Pathol*. 1990;137:259-262.
28. Vahle JL, Sato M, Long GG, et al. Skeletal changes in rats given daily subcutaneous injections of recombinant human parathyroid hormone (1-34) for 2 years and relevance to human safety. *Toxicol Pathol*. 2002;30:312-321.
29. Hahn WC, Counter CM, Lundberg AS, Beijersbergen RL, Brooks MW, Weinberg RA. Creation of human tumour cells with defined genetic elements. *Nature*. 1999;400:464 468.
30. Baserga R, Peruzzi F, Reiss K. The IGF-1 receptor in cancer biology. *Int J Cancer*. 2003;107:873-877.
31. Benini S, Baldini N, Manara MC, et al. Redundancy of autocrine loops in human osteosarcoma cells. *Int J Cancer*. 1999;80:581-588.
32. Burrow S, Andrulis IL, Pollak M, Bell RS. Expression of insulin-like growth factor receptor, IGF-1, and IGF-2 in primary and metastatic osteosarcoma. *J Surg Oncol*. 1998;69:21-27.
33. Ferracini R, Renzo MFD, Scotlandi K, et al. The Met/HGF receptor is overexpressed in human osteosarcomas and is activated by either a paracrine or autocrine circuit. *Oncogene*. 1995;10:739-749.
34. Gorlick R, Huvos AG, Heller G, et al. Expression of HER2/erbB-2 correlates with survival in osteosarcoma. *J Clin Oncol*. 1999;17:2781-2788.
35. Kaya M, Wada T, Akatsuka T, et al. Vascular endothelial growth factor expression in untreated osteosarcoma is predictive of pulmonary metastasis and poor prognosis. *Clin Cancer Res*. 2000;6:572-577.
36. Hughes DP, Thomas DG, Giordano TJ, Baker LH, McDonagh KT. Cell surface expression of epidermal growth factor receptor and her-2 with nuclear expression of her-4 in primary osteosarcoma. *Cancer Res*. 2004;64:2047-2053.

37. Jung ST, Moon ES, Seo HY, Kim JS, Kim GJ, Kim YK. Expression and significance of TGF-beta isoform and VEGF in osteosarcoma. *Orthopedics*. 2005;28:755-760.
38. Yang R, Hoang BH, Kubo T, et al. Over-expression of parathyroid hormone Type 1 receptor confers an aggressive phenotype in osteosarcoma. *Int J Cancer*. 2007;121:943-954.
39. Kubo T, Piperdi S, Rosenblum J, et al. Platelet-derived growth factor receptor as a prognostic marker and a therapeutic target for imatinib mesylate therapy in osteosarcoma. *Cancer*. 2008;112(10):2119-2129.
40. Baldini N, Scotlandi K, Barbanti-Brodano G, et al. Expression of p-glycoprotein in high-grade osteosarcomas in relation to clinical outcome. *N Engl J Med*. 1995;333:380-1385.
41. Schwartz CL, Gorlick R, Teot L, et al. Multiple Drug Resistance in Osteogenic Sarcoma (INT0133). *J Clin Oncol*. 2007;25:2057-2062.
42. Guo W, Healey JH, Meyers PA, et al. Mechanisms of methotrexate resistance in osteosarcoma. *Clin Cancer Res*. 1999;5:621-627.
43. Yang R, Sowers R, Mazza B, et al. Sequence alterations in the reduced folate carrier are observed in osteosarcoma tumor samples. *Clin Cancer Res*. 2003;9:837-844.
44. Mintz MB, Sowers R, Brown KM, et al. An expression signature classifies chemotherapy-resistant pediatric osteosarcoma. *Cancer Res*. 2005;65:1748-1754.
45. Houghton PJ, Morton CL, Tucker C, et al. The pediatric preclinical testing program: Description of models and early testing results. *Pediatr Blood Cancer*. 2007;49:928-940.
46. Whiteford CC, Bilke S, Greer BT, et al. Credentialing preclinical pediatric xenograft models using gene expression and tissue microarray analysis. *Cancer Res*. 2007;67:32-40.
47. Maris JM, Courtright J, Houghton PJ, et al. Initial Testing (Stage 1) of the VEGFR Inhibitor AZD2171 by the Pediatric Preclinical Testing Program. *Pediatr Blood Cancer*. 2008;50:581-587.
48. Tajbakhsh M, Houghton PJ, Morton CL, et al. Initial testing of cisplatin by the pediatric preclinical testing program. *Pediatr Blood Cancer*. 2008;50:992-1000.
49. Houghton PJ, Morton CL, Kolb EA, et al. Initial testing (stage 1) of the mTOR inhibitor rapamycin by the pediatric preclinical testing program. *Pediatr Blood Cancer*. 2008;50:799-805.
50. Kolb EA, Gorlick R, Houghton PJ, et al. Initial testing of dasatinib by the pediatric preclinical testing program. *Pediatr Blood Cancer*. 2000;50:1198-1206.
51. Lock R, Carol H, Houghton PJ, et al. Initial testing (stage 1) of the BH3 mimetic ABT-263 by the pediatric preclinical testing program. *Pediatr Blood Cancer*. 2008;50:1181-1189.
52. Kolb EA, Gorlick R, Houghton PJ, et al. Initial testing (stage 1) of a monoclonal antibody (SCH 717454) against the IGF-1 receptor by the pediatric preclinical testing program. *Pediatr Blood Cancer*. 2008;50(6):1190-1197.
53. Hernan C, Morton CL, Houghton PJ, et al. Pediatric Preclinical Testing Program (PPTP) evaluation of the topoisopmerase I inhibitor topotecan. *Proc AACR*. 2008;710:710. [abstract].
54. Houghton PJ, Morton CL, Maris JM, et al. Pediatric Preclinical Testing Program (PPTP) evaluation of the Aurora A kinase inhibitor MLN8237. *Proc AACR*. 2008;49:710. [abstract].
55. Smith MA, Morton CL, Maris JM, et al. Pediatric Preclinical Testing Program (PPTP) evaluation of the MEK 1/2 inhibitor AZD6244 (ARRY-142886). *Proc AACR*. 2008;49:710. [abstract].

How the NOTCH Pathway Contributes to the Ability of Osteosarcoma Cells to Metastasize

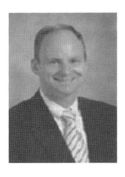

Dennis P.M. Hughes

Abstract Controlling metastasis is the key to improving outcomes for osteosarcoma patients; yet our knowledge of the mechanisms regulating the metastatic process is incomplete. Clearly Fas and Ezrin are important, but other genes must play a role in promoting tumor spread. Early developmental pathways are often recapitulated in malignant tissues, and these genes are likely to be important in regulating the primitive behaviors of tumor cells, including invasion and metastasis. The Notch pathway is a highly conserved regulatory signaling network involved in many developmental processes and several cancers, at times serving as an oncogene and at others, behaving as a tumor suppressor. In normal limb development, Notch signaling maintains the apical ectodermal ridge in the developing limb bud and regulated size of bone and muscles. Here, we examine the role of Notch signaling in promoting metastasis of osteosarcoma, and the underlying regulatory processes that control Notch pathway expression and activity in the disease.

We have shown that, compared to normal human osteoblasts and non-metastatic osteosarcoma cell lines, osteosarcoma cell lines with the ability to metastasize have higher levels of Notch 1, Notch 2, the Notch ligand DLL1 and the Notch-induced gene Hes1. When invasive osteosarcoma cells are treated with small molecule inhibitors of γ-secretase, which blocks Notch activation, invasiveness is abrogated. Direct retroviral expression has shown that Hes1 expression was necessary for osteosarcoma invasiveness and accounted for the observations. In a novel orthotopic murine xenograft model of osteosarcoma pulmonary metastasis, blockade of Hes1 expression and Notch signaling eliminated spread of disease from the tibial primary tumor. In a sample of archival human osteosarcoma tumor specimens, expression of Hes1 mRNA was inversely correlated with survival ($n=16$ samples, $p=0.04$). Expression of the microRNA 34 cluster, which is known to downregulate DLL1, Notch 1 and Notch 2,

---

D.P.M. Hughes (✉)
Children's Cancer Hospital, University of Texas M.D. Anderson Cancer Center,
1515 Holcombe Blvd, Houston, TX, 77030-4009, USA
e-mail: dphughes@mdanderson.org

was inversely correlated with invasiveness in a small panel of osteosarcoma tumors, suggesting that this family of microRNAs may be responsible for regulating Notch expression in at least some tumors. Further, exposure to valproic acid at therapeutic concentrations induced expression of Notch genes and caused a 250-fold increase in invasiveness for non-invasive cell lines, but had no discernible effect on those lines that expressed high levels of Notch without valproic acid treatment, suggesting a role for HDAC in regulating Notch pathway expression in osteosarcoma. These findings show that the Notch pathway is important in regulating osteosarcoma metastasis and may be useful as a therapeutic target. Better understanding of Notch's role and its regulation will be essential in planning therapies with other agents, especially the use of valproic acid and other HDAC inhibitors.

Introduction

Regulation of Notch Pathway Signaling

The Notch cascade is a signaling pathway essential to the development of multiple organ systems whose essential features have been preserved evolutionarily throughout eukaryotic development.[1] Originally discovered and named for a characteristic wing abnormality found in drosophila with mutations of the Notch gene, Notch pathway members now are known to be responsible for numerous developmental functions in worms, insects, lower vertebrates and mammals, including humans.[2]

In humans, the Notch pathway consists of two families of ligands, the Jagged and Delta-like ligands, and four receptors: Notch1, Notch2, Notch3 and Notch4 (see Fig. 1 for a schematic diagram of Notch pathway signaling).[3] Upon binding ligand, the Notch receptors are activated via a two-step proteolytic cleavage, first by ADAM10,[4] which cleaves away the extracellular domain, and then by gamma-secretase,[5] which cleaves in the middle of the transmembrane domain. Once gamma-secretase cuts the receptor, there are not sufficient lipophilic amino acid residues to hold the receptor in the plasma membrane, and the intracellular domain of Notch (ICN) is liberated to float free in the cytosol.[1] There, a nuclear localization signal mediates transport of ICN to the nucleus. Once in the nucleus, ICN, in cooperation with the mastermind-like (MAML) protein, displaces co-repressor elements from CSL, also known as RBP-Jκ, allowing transcription of CSL target genes. Notch also promotes transcription of some genes, such as DELTEX1, in a CSL independent fashion. CSL target genes include basic helix-loop-helix transcription factors of the Hairy/Enhancer of Split (HES) and the Hes-related repressor proteins (HERP) families. The specific genes activated by ICN vary among different tissues, and most of these genes are, themselves, transcription modulators with targets that may vary by tissue type. Thus, the effect of Notch pathway activity may be highly variable between different tissues.

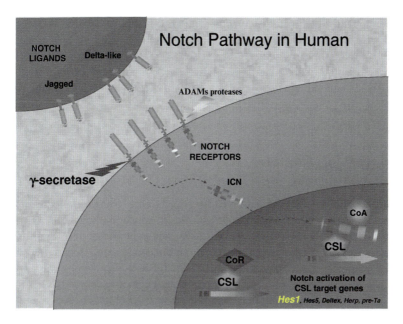

Fig. 1 Schematic Representation of Notch Pathway Signaling in Humans: The cell-surface components of the Notch pathway include two families of ligands: the Jagged and Delta-like ligands. There are four receptors, termed Notch1, Notch2, Notch3 and Notch4. Upon binding ligand, these receptors are subject to a two-step proteolytic cleavage, first by ADAM10, then by γ-secretase, which cuts in the transmembrane region. Once this region is cut, the intracellular domain of the Notch receptor (ICN) floats free into the cytosol, when a nuclear localization signal mediates translocation into the nucleus. In the nucleus, ICN displaces co-repressor elements (CoR) from the transcription factor CSL, converting it from a transcriptional repressor to a transcription activator. This binding, which requires co-activating elements (CoA) such as the Mastermind-like protein, activates transcription of Notch target genes, including the Hairy and Enhancer of Split (HES) family, Deltex, the HERP family and other factors. Most of these proteins also are transcription modifiers

Notch in Normal Bone and Limb Development

Notch pathway signaling is critical to normal bone development, both for osteoblasts[6–8] and osteoclasts.[9,10] Tezuka and colleagues have shown that ICN promotes the development of osteoblasts from mesenchymal stem cells,[8] and Dallas et al. localized ADAM 10 to sites of active bone formation.[11] Over-expression of Delta in animal models blocks the maturation of chondrocytes[12] and the development of osteoclasts[9] from bone marrow progenitors. Over-expression of Notch1 in stromal cells increases expression of RANKL and OPG and inhibits M-CSF expression, resulting in a lack of support to developing osteoclasts.[10] Notch pathway signaling is responsible both for regulating apoptosis that controls development of the apical ectodermal ridge[13] and for dorsal-ventral limb patterning,[14] as well as regulating muscle mass development during limb formation.[15]

Mutations of Notch pathway members are responsible for several known mutant phenotypes in mice and humans. The Pudgy Mouse results from a mutation in DLL3,[16–18] while murine syndactylism arises from a mutation in a different Notch ligand.[19] A similar mutation in human DLL3 causes about 60% of inherited Jarcho-Levin Syndrome (Spondylocostal Dysplasia).[20] Mutations of Jag1 cause Alagille syndrome and butterfly vertebrae.[21–24]

Notch in Cancer

Signaling pathways, important in early organogenesis and development, often exhibit aberrant expression and important roles in cancer pathogenesis; so, it is not surprising that the Notch pathway would have important effects in several cancers.[25] The first evidence for Notch functioning as an oncogene came from a translocation in a T-cell acute lymphoblastic leukemia (T-ALL), in which Notch1 was expressed under the direction of the T cell receptor promoter.[26] Subsequent studies showed that Notch pathway signaling in early bone marrow development suppresses B cell and myeloid development and promotes T cell development.[27,28] Following these investigations, Dr. Patrick Zweidley-McKay and colleagues showed that Notch functions as a tumor suppressor for B-cell lineage acute leukemias, from early Pre-B ALL through mature B-cell ALL phenotypes.[29] Recently, he has shown a similar effect for myeloid malignancies.[30] Currently, oncogenic functions for Notch have been identified in non-small-cell lung cancer, breast cancer, colon cancer and melanoma.[25,31–37] Conversely, Notch signaling has a tumor-suppressor effect in small-cell lung cancer, basal cell carcinoma, squamous cell carcinoma and neural crest-derived cancers.[33,38,39] Since Notch is important in making cell fate decisions, promoting the growth of some cell types while suppressing other types, the duality of effects of Notch signaling in cancer makes sense. However, in all of the examples given, Notch functions as a complete oncogene or tumor suppressor, essentially affecting all aspects of malignant behavior equally. Our observations in osteosarcoma are the first evidence that Notch signaling can act on a single aspect of malignant behavior (metastasis) without affecting the others.[40] This difference allows the opportunity to identify those Notch-driven signals that are important in promoting metastasis.

Experimental Evidence

Notch Pathway Expression in Osteosarcoma

We have shown that Notch pathway family members are expressed in primary and established osteosarcoma cell lines and patient-derived samples.[40] Using mRNA isolated from invasive osteosarcoma cell lines OS 187,[41] COL,[42] the non-metastatic line Saos-2 and its metastatic subline LM7,[43,44] we performed RT-PCR analysis for the Notch ligand *dll1*, *Notch1*, *Notch2*, *Notch3*, *Notch4* and the Notch target genes *Hes1*, *Hes5*, *Deltex1* and *Herp2* (Fig. 2, adapted[40]). Normal human osteoblast cells served as a control. We draw particular attention to Saos-2 and its metastatic subline LM7 because LM-7 was derived from the serial passage of Saos-2 cells through murine lungs, without any other genetic or pharmacologic manipulation.[44] Thus, we expected that any differences in Notch pathway expression between the two lines would directly reflect metastatic potential. Compared to the non-metastatic line, LM-7 had increased expression of *dll1*, *Notch1*, *Notch2* and *Hes1* (Fig. 2). *Notch4*, which can act to oppose signaling by the other Notch pathway genes through competition for signaling cofactors, was higher in Saos-2 than in LM-7. The invasive primary osteosarcoma lines OS 187 and COL had similar expression of these genes, with variable expression of *Notch3*, *Hes5*, *Deltex1* and *Herp2*. Samples of freshly derived metastatic osteosarcoma had Notch pathway gene expression that was similar to OS 187.[40] Hes1 is a transcriptional repressor whose expression in most circumstances is completely dependent upon Notch-mediated activation of CSL. As this was the primary Notch target gene upregulated in LM-7 cells and the only Notch target genes expressed by all invasive cells tested, we reasoned that *Hes1* might be the effector gene whose expression could be driving metastasis.

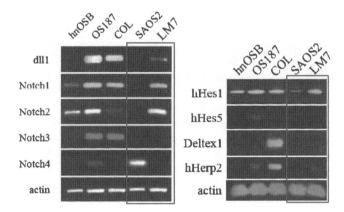

Fig. 2 RT_PCR Analysis of Notch Pathway and Notch Target Genes from Osteosarcoma Cell Lines: RNA was isolated from normal human osteoblast cells (hnOSB) and osteosarcoma cells OS 187, COL and SAOS2, as well as the metastatic subline of SAOS2, LM-7. RT-PCR was performed for the Notch ligand dll1, Notch 1-4 and the Notch target genes Hes1, Hes5, Deltex1, and Herp2. Actin was used for loading and quality control. The red box highlights the differences that arose between the non-metastatic SAOS2 cells and the metastatic subline LM-7 as a result of serial selection for metastasis to lung. Compared to non-metastatic parental cells, LM-7 has upregulated Notch1, Notch2 and Hes1. The expression in OS 187 and COL cells, which also are metastatic lines, is similar to LM-7

Gamma-Secretase Inhibitors Block Osteosarcoma Invasiveness

Notch-mediated activation of CSL target gene transcription is completely dependent upon the two part proteolytic cleavage of the Notch protein, first by ADAM10,[4] then by γ-secretase.[5] Because of its central role in cleaving the β-amyliod protein that promotes Alzheimer's disease, small molecule inhibitors of γ-secretase (GSI) have been developed by several pharmaceutical companies.[45] While these compounds have not yet become new treatments for dementia, they can provide insights into signaling events in which γ-secretase plays a key role.[36]

To determine what impact Notch pathway signaling might have upon osteosarcoma cells, we cultured primary and established osteosarcoma cell lines in Compound E, a GSI that is effective at approximately 1 nM. In the range from 0.1 to 1 nM, this GSI titratibly reduced the expression of Hes1 in osteosarcoma cells at both the mRNA and protein levels.[40] GSI treatment had no effect, however, upon cell proliferation or in vitro tumorigenesis (soft agar colony formation) for any osteosarcoma line tested (Fig. 3a, b). In contrast, GSI titratibly reduced invasion of OS 187 cells into matrigel (Fig. 3c), and the reduced invasion corresponded to a reduction of Hes1 expression at both the mRNA and protein levels.[40] The non-metastatic cell line Saos-2 does not invade matrigel readily, while the metastatic subline derived from it, LM-7, does (Fig. 3d). Treatment with GSI reduces the invasiveness of LM-7 nearly to the level of the non-invasive parental line (Fig. 3d), indicating that the invasiveness selected for serial passage through murine lungs requires γ-secretase for the processing of signals promoting this behavior.

Direct Manipulation of Notch Pathway Components Alters Invasiveness

The impact of GSI upon OS invasion suggested that Hes1 expression drives invasion, but many signaling pathways can be affected by GSI.[5,36,45,46] To directly assess the impact of Notch and Hes1 on OS invasion, we enforced expression of Notch pathway genes to up- or down-regulate Hes1 in OS cells, and then measured the ability of these cells to invade matrigel in vitro. Using the invasive cell line OS 187, we transduced cells with retroviral expression vectors encoding a constitutively active *Notch1* intracellular domain (ICN1), a dominant negative form of the Mastermind-like gene MAM (dnMAM), Hes1 or the empty vector (MIgR1). Transduction with either ICN1 or Hes1 increased matrigel invasion three- to eightfold, while inhibiting Notch-mediated Hes1 expression with dnMAM reduced invasion by more than 50% (Fig. 4, taken from ref.[40]). For the non-invasive line Saos-2, ICN1 and Hes1 transduction caused similar increases, but Notch inhibition with dnMAM did not significantly reduce invasion, presumably because Hes1 levels are already low in this line. Transduction with dnMAM did reduce invasion of the metastatic subline LM-7.

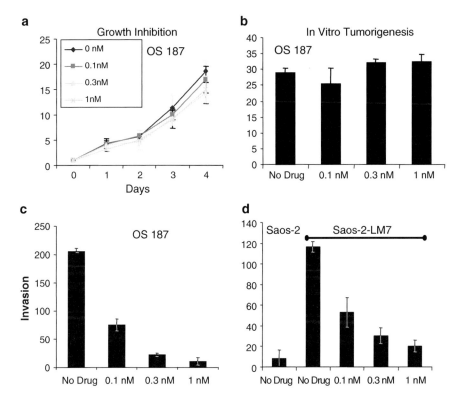

Fig. 3 In Vitro Effects of γ-Secretase Inhibition on Notch Pathway Activation: Osteosarcoma cell lines OS 187, Saos-2 or LM-7 were treated with a g-secretase inhibitor (Compound E, or GSI) at the concentrations indicated. The compound completely inhibits g-secretase at a concentration of 1 nM. (**a**) Cells were cultured in GSI for 4 days, and cells quantified daily. Histograms represent the average of three samples at each dose and time-point. Media and drug were refreshed daily. (**b**) Histograms represent average colony formation in soft-agar culture after 14 days exposure to the drug concentrations listed. (**c**) Matrigel invasion assay: OS-187 cells were plated atop matrigel in traswell cultures using 10% FBS as a chemo-attractant. After 48 h culture in the GSI drug concentrations listed, cells migrating to the underside of the transwell were counted. Histograms represent average of three wells from this representative experiment. GSI almost completely eliminated matrigel invasion. (**d**) Matrigel invasion assay: Saos-2 cells do not invade matrigel. LM-7 cells are highly invasive when not exposed to GSI. GSI-mediated inhibition of Notch pathway signaling reduces invasion to nearly the level of the non-invasive parental cells. Data are represented as in (**c**).

Based on these observations, we expected that Notch-mediated expression of Hes1 was the primary pathway being blocked by GSI when that treatment reduces invasion of OS cells in vitro. To prove the importance of Hes1 expression in this process, we evaluated the ability of enforced expression of Hes1 to rescue OS cells from GSI treatment (Fig. 5, taken from ref. [40]). The invasion of untransduced cells was severely impaired by GSI treatment, as shown in Fig. 3. However, OS cells transduced with ICN1 or Hes1 did not have a significant change in invasion when

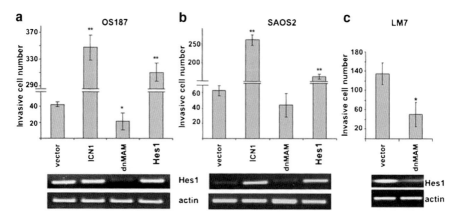

Fig. 4 Effects of Manipulation of Notch Signaling on Osteosarcoma Invasiveness in vitro. (**a–c**) *top*, relative invasiveness in vitro of O S187 cells (1 x 10[4] per well; (**a**), SAOS2 cells (1.5 x 10[5] per well; (**b**), and LM7 cells (5 x 10[4] per well; (**c**) transduced with *ICN1*, *dnMAM*, or *HES1*. Note: the input of cells for each cell line was adjusted to give roughly equal number of invading cells for each vector control sample. Histograms depict the quantified invasiveness. **, $P<0.005$; *, $P<0.05$. Bottom, gel depicts PCR analysis of *HES1* and *actin* in the transduced cells

treated with GSI, indicating that Hes1 expression was downstream of the critical role played by GSI.

Notch inhibition Reduces Metastasis in an Orthotopic Xenograft Model of Osteosarcoma

Invasiveness is considered essential for sarcoma metastasis, but invasion into matrigel in the laboratory is a highly artificial condition that may not accurately assess metastatic potential in vivo. We wished to measure the impact of Notch pathway signaling and Hes1 expression using an in vivo model. An ideal model for assessing metastasis in vivo would involve using cells grown in tissue culture, allowing for genetic modification in vitro. These cells would be used to create a primary tumor in an orthotopic location, from which metastatic tumors arise in the same anatomic sites seen in spontaneous human disease. The models commonly used to study metastasis in murine xenografts were limited for our purposes. The LM-7 model created by Dr. Kleinerman at the Children's Cancer Hospital[43,44] is very good for assessing lung trophism, but does not make primary orthotopic tumors. The KRIB cell line will make primary orthotopic tumors from which metastases arise, but KRIB has been transduced with oncogenic Ras, a mutation that has never been reported in osteosarcoma.[47] Because the signaling properties of KRIB have been genetically altered, we did not feel that this cell line would make a good model for our purpose.

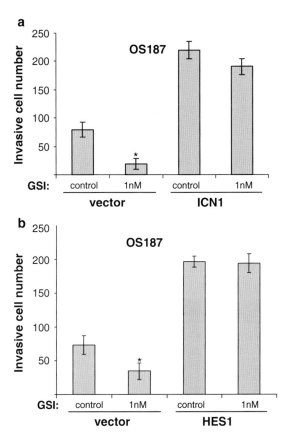

Fig. 5 Effects of GSI (1 nmol/L) on in vitro invasiveness of OS187 cells transduced with empty vector, ICN1 (*, $P<0.05$), and HES1 (*, $P<0.05$). GSI (1 nmol/L) significantly suppressed invasion of OS187 cells transduced with empty vector. However, OS187 cells transduced with ICN1 (**a**) or HES1 (**b**) are resistant to GSI treatment. Data are displayed as in Fig. 3c

To study metastasis in vivo, we established a new orthotopic xenograft model using OS 187 cells. 200,000 of these cells injected into the tibia of a NOD/SCID/IL-2Rγ-deficient mouse reliably produced primary tumors within 4 weeks. From these tumors, microscopic metastatic nodules developed within 6 weeks in almost all the mice. We injected mice with OS 187 cells transduced with either dnMAM, to inhibit the Notch pathway, or the empty vector. After 6 weeks, mice in both groups had similar primary tumors (Fig. 6a). In the lungs, however, we saw a dramatic difference in micrometastases between the two groups. The vector control mice had an average of 15 tumors identified per section of lung, while the Notch-inhibited dnMAM mice developed only one nodule (Fig. 6b). The dnMAM nodules appeared smaller as well (Fig. 6c). Thus, inhibition of Notch-mediated Hes1 expression also abrogated metastasis in our novel orthotopic xenograft model, confirming the essential role of Hes1 in osteosarcoma metastasis.[40]

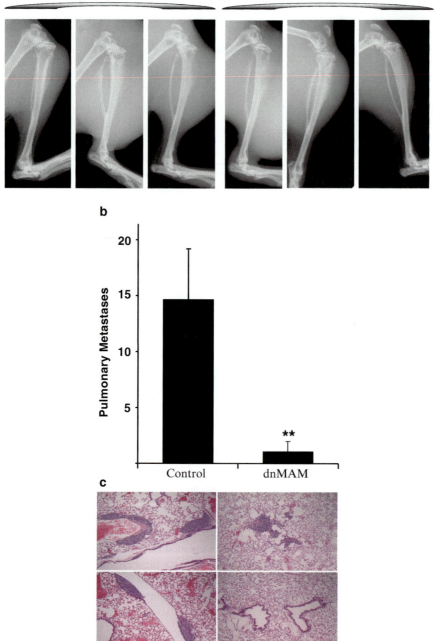

Fig. 6 Notch Inhibition Blocks Metastasis in vivo: OS 187 cells were transduced either with control vector (MigR1) or vector containing dominant negative Mastermind-Like (dnMAM), a dominant negative inhibitor of Notch pathway signaling. Tumor cells were injected into the tibia of immuno-compromised mice and allowed to grow into "primary" tumors, from which spontaneous metastases arose. (**a**) Six weeks after injection, both groups had similar primary tumors, as shown by plain

Hes-1 Expression Is Associated with Reduced Survival in OS Patients

For Hes1 expression to be identified as a key protein driving metastasis in osteosarcoma, we would expect to see evidence for differential expression of Hes1 between patients that do well with osteosarcoma and those who eventually die from metastasis. To make a preliminary evaluation of the hypothesis that Hes1 is essential for metastasis, we assembled a panel of 56 archival tumor samples obtained from patients treated at the University of Michigan's sarcoma center. These experiments were conducted in collaboration with Dr. Dafydd Thomas, MD, PhD, of the University of Michigan Medical Center. These tumors represented material from 37 individuals, since multiple tumors had been removed from some patients. To obtain a uniformly treated group of tumors for this initial analysis, we examined only primary, untreated tumors from patients who presented in 1989 or later and received chemotherapy with a backbone of cisplatin and doxorubicin. These restrictions reduced the number of evaluable tumor to 16 samples. To obtain a comparison sample of osteosarcoma cells with known behavior, we also extracted RNA from a sample of OS 187 osteosarcoma cells that had been fixed and embedded in paraffin 4 years prior to extraction. The expression of Hes1 in these samples was assessed by Q-PCR.

All values were normalized first to GAPDH as an internal control for RNA concentration and quality, using our previously described methods. The value generated by this method, however, is an inverse log value, such that higher levels of expression of the gene result in increasingly small, and eventually negative numbers. To generate values in which increasing concentrations of Hes1 result in increasingly positive numbers, all ΔCt-ΔCt values were subtracted from a single constant to generate a range of values between 0 and 20, where the highest values now represented the highest levels of Hes1 expression. The samples were then divided based upon outcome, with long-term survivors compared to patients who died from progressive disease. The average Hes1 values for the two groups were similar (9.1 for survivors, 11.6 for those dead of disease), and both groups had a mean Hes1 value greater than that observed for OS-187 (7.9). However, the group that died from progressive disease had no samples below the value observed for OS 187, suggesting that patients with low Hes1 levels may have a good overall prognosis (Fig. 7). These results must be verified with a larger sample of patients, and that analysis should use a more sophisticated statistical approach such as Kaplan–Meier graphing with Log-Rank analysis. This sample size is not adequate for that more detailed analysis. Still, these data are consistent with the hypothesis that Notch-mediated expression of Hes1 promotes a metastatic phenotype and more frequent death from disease in patients.

Fig. 6 (continued) radiographs. (**b**) Lung metastases were assessed from formalin-fixed, paraffin-embedded whole lung preparations sectioned vertically and stained with H&E. *Top panel*: average number of lung metastases visualized from one section of lung in each treatment group. *Bottom panel*: representative H&E sections of lung from each treatment group. ** indicates $p < 0.005$; $n = 3$ mice per experiment

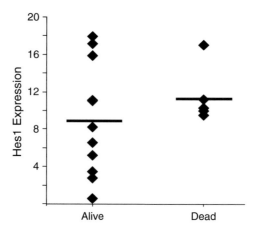

Fig. 7 Hes1 Expression in Archival Osteosarcoma Tumor Samples: RNA was extracted from archival pre-treatment tumor samples from 16 patients with osteosarcoma. Quantitative, real-time PCR was used to measure expression of Hes1, normalized to GAPDH expression. Scatter plot depicts relative Hes1 expression in arbitrary units. Analysis compares levels measured from surviving patients from that observed in patients who were dead from disease. Horizontal line shows the average value in each group

Valproic Acid Induces Notch Pathway Expression and Invasion in Osteosarcoma

It is not clear what mechanism(s) are responsible for regulating Notch pathway expression in osteosarcoma, though we have preliminary evidence that epigenetic mechanisms may play an important role. We have preliminary experiments suggesting that differential expression of microRNAs may play an important role (data not shown). One key epigenetic mechanism affecting gene expression is the acetylation of histones, which can control opening or compacting of specific regions of DNA, making these regions either available or unavailable for the transcription machinery.[37] While the regulation of gene expression by histone deacetylase (HDAC) is complex and remains an active area of investigation, this mechanism is already being exploited for cancer therapy. Small molecule inhibitors of the enzyme complex histone deacetylase (HDACi) are being developed and have some therapeutic benefit for several diseases, especially when used in combination with either radiation therapy or traditional chemotherapy.[48] A role for HDACi in osteosarcoma therapy has not yet been established, and our understanding of the field is still expanding.

In fact, the use of HDACi therapeutically predates the functional understanding of HDAC. One of the commonly used drugs for treating seizures in children and adults, valproic acid, or valproate, had recently been shown to act as an HDACi.[49,50] Researchers in brain tumor therapy have been using valproate as a radiosensitizer for children with brain tumors undergoing radiation treatment for their diseases.[51]

Because of its ability to synergize with radiation,[52] we have begun exploring the use of valproate for osteosarcoma patients receiving XRT at the Children's Cancer Hospital at M.D. Anderson Cancer Center.

In the summer of 2007, Greenblatt and colleagues published a report showing that carcinoid cell lines, when exposed to valproic acid, upregulated Notch pathway expression and activity.[53] We were unsure if a similar effect would be observed for osteosarcoma; but clearly, since Notch-mediated expression of Hes1 apparently drives metastasis in osteosarcoma, we deemed it important to determine if valproic acid promotes osteosarcoma metastasis.

To assess Notch pathway expression in osteosarcoma cells as a function of valproate exposure, we treated OS 187 cells, which can metastasize (see Fig. 6b, c) and Saos-2 cells, which do not, with increasing concentrations of valproate. After 48 h, RNA was isolated and expression of the Notch target gene Hes1 was assessed by RT-PCR (Fig. 8a). For the invasive line, OS 187, Hes1 was already present in untreated cells, and no apparent upregulation of Hes1 was observed with exposure to 1, 2 or 4 micromolar valproate. For the non-invasive Saos-2 cells, on the other hand, little Hes1 was observed in untreated cells, consistent with our previous reports. Hes1 was upregulated in these cells with exposure to 1, 2 or 4 micromolar valproate, however, similar to the effect described for the carcinoid cells. Quantitative real-time PCR analysis of Hes1 confirmed these findings (data not shown). Given these effects of valproate on Hes1 expression, we thought it important to know the impact of valproate on proliferation and invasion for these cells.

To assess the impact of valproate on proliferation, OS-187 and Saos-2 cells were exposed to 1, 2 or 4 micromolar valproate for up to 3 days, and cell yield was assessed daily. For the non-metastatic Saos-2 cells, cell yield was decreased only moderately by valproate exposure, and this decrease only achieved significance at a concentration of 4 micromolar, which is not really achievable in patients (Fig. 8b). By contrast, there was dramatic reduction in cell yield for the metastatic OS 187 cells, and we observed significant reduction in cell number for this cell line with concentrations of as little as 0.3 micromolar, equivalent to 50 mg/deciliter, the lower limit of the therapeutic range for patients (data not shown).

To assess directly if the increased Hes1 expression observed in Saos-2 cells exposed to valproate would induce increased invasiveness, we treated Saos-2 cells to 0.3, 0.6, 1, 2 or 4 micromolar valproate for 48 h, then assessed their ability to invade matrigel. As expected from their Hes1-negative state, untreated Saos-2 cells did not invade in matrigel. By contrast, Saos-2 cells exposed to 0.3 micromolar valproate increased their measured invasiveness 250-fold (Fig. 8c). Higher concentrations led to reduced levels of measured invasiveness, presumably due to the reduced cell yields measured at these concentrations compared to 0.3 micromolar valproate. OS 187 cells did not demonstrate increased invasion with valproate exposure, presumably due to the dramatic loss of tumor cells induced by valproate (data not shown).

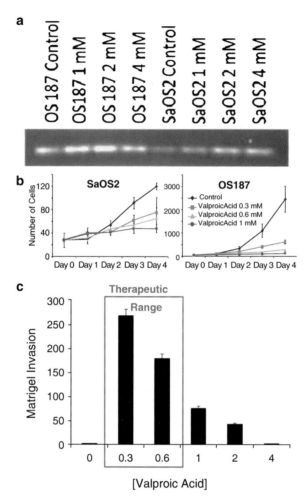

Fig. 8 Effect of Valproate on Notch Pathway Expression and Osteosarcoma Invasiveness: (**a**) Osteosarcoma cell lines OS 187 and Saos-2 were treated with 1, 2, or 4 millimolar valproic acid for 48 h and RNA isolated from surviving cells. RT-PCR for the Notch target gene Hes1 shows upregulation in Saos-2 but not Os 187 cells. (**b**) Osteosarcoma cells were cultured in valproate at the concentrations indicated for 4 days. Graphs represent average cell yield on each day at each concentration. Reduced cell yield was much more apparent for OS 187 than for Saos-2 cells. (**c**) Saos-2 cells were exposed to valproate at the concentrations indicated for 48 h, then assayed for matrigel invasion as per Fig. 3c. The red box highlights the therapeutic range for valproate

Discussion

Given the similarities between normal limb development at the cellular level and the cellular behaviors involved in metastasis, it is perhaps not surprising that there are regulatory pathways in common between these processes. The mechanics of cell migration are similar to the mechanics of metastasis, so dysregulation of the regulatory mechanisms responsible for early limb development might logically lead to recapitulation of those same behaviors in neoplastic tissue derived from limb bud tissues or mesenchymal stem cells. Indeed, such a dysregulation is precisely what we have demonstrated for the Notch pathway in osteosarcoma. The impact of enforced expression of Hes1 via retrovirus, upon invasion in vitro, either through constitutive ICN1 expression or through transduction with Hes1 itself, was a clear indication of the importance that Hes1 plays in this process. As this constitutive activation also rescues osteosarcoma invasion through inhibition by γ-secretase, we conclude that Hes1 accounts for the majority of the effect that γ-secretase has upon osteosarcoma invasion.

To prove the role of Notch pathway signaling in osteosarcoma, it was essential to show an effect using a good in vivo model. Our recent manuscript[40] is the first report of our newly developed xenograft model for osteosarcoma metastasis. We found this model to be beneficial because it assesses all aspects of the process of metastasis: migration of cells outward from the primary tumor, separation and travel via hematogenous spread, implantation in the lungs, invasion through the basement membrane to establish a new nidus of metastatic tumor, and vasculogenesis and angiogenesis for that metastatic tumor. Our data clearly show that Notch expression, and Hes1 in particular, are essential to that process. Our preliminary data regarding Hes1 expression in archival tumors support this interpretation.

The mechanisms regulating Notch pathway expression are unclear, but our data with valproate suggest that epigenetic regulatory mechanisms will be important.[37] Exposure to an HDACi for osteosarcoma cells with low expression both induced Notch pathway expression and increased invasion. These data are quite concerning for treatments of patients with non-metastatic disease and suggest that patients with non-metastatic osteosarcoma should not be treated with valproate. One would even recommend that, should a patient with a seizure disorder be diagnosed with osteosarcoma, that patient perhaps should be transitioned to a different anti-seizure medication.

The role of HDACi in metastatic disease, especially when used as a radiosensitizer[52] or chemosensitizer,[54] is less clear. In our hands, valproate did not appear to increase Notch pathway expression in those cells that already have high levels of the gene, and HDACi, or at least valproate, was directly toxic to cells in vitro, even at fairly low levels. As such, there may well be an important role for HDACi in therapy for metastatic osteosarcoma, as these tumors appear to have Notch pathway expression at baseline and may benefit from treatment. The current poor salvage rate for recurrent disease and extrapulmonary metastasis[55,56] reinforces the need to explore new therapeutic options in the most desperate cases. However, if valproate treatment would cause residual cells to have increased metastatic potential, any benefit from the direct toxicity of valproate and impact of sensitization may be quite short-lived. Clearly further research is indicated.

Finally, the role of Hes1 in promoting metastasis in osteosarcoma affords an opportunity to better understand the mechanisms of metastasis that may be operating in all solid tumors. As discussed above, where Notch has been shown to play a role in other solid tumor models, it affects all aspects of malignant behavior, including proliferation, survival and spreading.[25,32,33,36] In our study, though, the role of Hes1 appears to be limited exclusively to the process of metastasis.

The process of metastasis is incompletely understood, and should continue to be an area of major investigation for all solid tumors. It seems likely that common mechanisms will be used by most, if not all, solid tumors. By studying the mechanisms by which Hes1 promotes metastasis, we may be able to identify new mechanisms and regulatory control points for metastasis. Since controlling metastasis is the key to improving survival in osteosarcoma and most other solid tumors, a better understanding of how Hes1 regulates osteosarcoma metastasis may identify new therapeutic targets, not just for children with bone cancer, but for many cancer victims.

Acknowledgments The research presented in this chapter was supported by the Physician-Scientist Program of the University of Texas M.D. Anderson Cancer Center and by a fellowship award from the Jori Zemel Children's Bone Tumor Foundation. I am grateful for their support.

References

1. Artavanis-Tsakonas S, Rand MD, Lake RJ. Notch signaling: cell fate control and signal integration in development. *Science*. 1999;284(5415):770-776.
2. Greenwald I. LIN-12/Notch signaling: lessons from worms and flies. *Genes & Dev*. 1998;12(12):1751-1762.
3. Gridley T. Notch signaling and inherited disease syndromes. *Hum Mol Genet*. 2003;12(Suppl_1):R9-R13. %R 10.1093/hmg/ddg052.
4. Hartmann D, et al. The disintegrin/metalloprotease ADAM 10 is essential for Notch signalling but not for {alpha}-secretase activity in fibroblasts. *Hum Mol Genet*. 2002;11(21):2615-2624. %R 10.1093/hmg/11.21.2615.
5. Fortini M. Gamma-secretase-mediated proteolysis in cell-surface-receptor signalling. *Nat Rev Mol Cell Biol*. 2002;3(9):673-684.
6. Schnabel M, et al. Differential expression of Notch genes in human osteoblastic cells. *Int J Mol Med*. 2002;9(3):229-232.
7. Sciaudone M, et al. Notch 1 impairs osteoblastic cell differentiation. *Endocrinology*. 2003;144(12):5631-5639.
8. Tezuka K, et al. Stimulation of osteoblastic cell differentiation by Notch. *J Bone Miner Res*. 2002;17(2):231-239.
9. Yamada T, et al. Regulation of osteoclast development by Notch signaling directed to osteoclast precursors and through stromal cells. *Blood*. 2003;101(6):2227-2234.
10. Bai S, et al. Notch1 regulates osteoclastogenesis directly in osteoclast precursors and indirectly via osteoblast lineage cells. *J Biol Chem*. 2007;M707000200 (%R 10.1074/jbc. M707000200).
11. Dallas DJ, et al. Localization of ADAM10 and Notch receptors in bone. *Bone*. 1999;25(1):9-15.
12. Crowe R, Zikherman J, Niswander L. Delta-1 negatively regulates the transition from prehypertrophic to hypertrophic chondrocytes during cartilage formation. *Development*. 1999;126(5):987-998.
13. Francis JC, Radtke F, Logan MP. Notch1 signals through Jagged2 to regulate apoptosis in the apical ectodermal ridge of the developing limb bud. *Dev Dyn*. 2005;234(4):1006-1015.
14. Irvine KD, Vogt TF. Dorsal-ventral signaling in limb development. *Curr Opin Cell Biol*. 1997;9(6):867-876.

How the NOTCH Pathway Contributes to the Ability of Osteosarcoma Cells

15. Schuster-Gossler K, Cordes R, Gossler A. Premature myogenic differentiation and depletion of progenitor cells cause severe muscle hypotrophy in Delta1 mutants. *Proc Natl Acad Sci USA*. 2007;104(2):537-542. %R 10.1073/pnas.0608281104.

16. Dunwoodie SL, et al. Axial skeletal defects caused by mutation in the spondylocostal dysplasia/pudgy gene Dll3 are associated with disruption of the segmentation clock within the presomitic mesoderm. *Development*. 2002;129(7):1795-1806.

17. Kusumi K, et al. The mouse pudgy mutation disrupts Delta homologue Dll3 and initiation of early somite boundaries. *Nat Genet*. 1998;19(3):274-278.

18. Kusumi K, et al. Dll3 pudgy mutation differentially disrupts dynamic expression of somite genes. *Genesis*. 2004;39(2):115-121.

19. Sidow A, et al. Serrate2 is disrupted in the mouse limb-development mutant syndactylism. *Nature*. 1997;389(6652):722-725.

20. Bulman MP, et al. Mutations in the human delta homologue, DLL3, cause axial skeletal defects in spondylocostal dysostosis. *Nat Genet*. 2000;24(4):438-441.

21. Ponio JB-D, et al. Biological function of mutant forms of JAGGED1 proteins in Alagille syndrome: inhibitory effect on Notch signaling. *Hum Mol Genet*. 2007;16(22):2683-2692. %R 10.1093/hmg/ddm222.

22. Yuan ZR, et al. Mutational analysis of the Jagged 1 gene in Alagille syndrome families. *Hum Mol Genet*. 1998;7(9):1363-1369. %R 10.1093/hmg/7.9.1363.

23. Li L, et al. Alagille syndrome is caused by mutations in human Jagged1, which encodes a ligand for Notch1. *Nat Genet*. 1997;16(3):243-251.

24. Turnpenny PD, et al. Abnormal vertebral segmentation and the Notch signaling pathway in man. *Dev Dyn*. 2007;236(6):1456-1474.

25. Allenspach E, et al. Notch signaling in cancer. *Cancer Biol Ther*. 2002;1(5):466-476.

26. Ellisen L, et al. TAN-1, the human homolog of the Drosophila notch gene, is broken by chromosomal translocations in T lymphoblastic neoplasms. *Cell*. 1991;66(4):649-661.

27. Pear W, et al. Exclusive development of T cell neoplasms in mice transplanted with bone marrow expressing activated Notch alleles. *J Exp Med*. 1996;183(5):2283-2291.

28. Reizis B, Leder P. Direct induction of T lymphocyte-specific gene expression by the mammalian Notch signaling pathway. *Genes & Dev*. 2002;16(3):295-300.

29. Zweidler-McKay PA, et al. Notch signaling is a potent inducer of growth arrest and apoptosis in a wide range of B-cell malignancies. *Blood*. 2005;106(12):3898-3906.

30. Sutphin RM, et al. Notch agonists: emerging as a feasible therapeutic approach in AML. *Blood* (ASH Annual Meeting Abstracts) 2006; 108(11): 1419.

31. Collins B, Kleeberger W, Ball D. Notch in lung development and lung cancer. *Semin Cancer Biol*. 2004;14(5):357-364.

32. Nickoloff B, Osborne B, Miele L. Notch signaling as a therapeutic target in cancer: a new approach to the development of cell fate modifying agents. *Oncogene*. 2003;22(42):6598-6608.

33. Radtke F, Raj K. The role of Notch in tumorigenesis: oncogene or tumour suppressor? *Nat Rev Cancer*. 2003;3(10):756-767.

34. Shou J, et al. Dynamics of Notch expression during murine prostate development and tumorigenesis. *Cancer Res*. 2001;61(19):7291-7297.

35. Bailey JM, Singh PK, Hollingsworth MA. Cancer metastasis facilitated by developmental pathways: sonic hedgehog, Notch, and bone morphogenic proteins. *J Cell Biochem*. 2007;102(4):829-839.

36. Shih I-M, Wang T-L. Notch signaling, {gamma}-secretase inhibitors, and cancer therapy. *Cancer Res*. 2007;67(5):1879-1882. %R 10.1158/0008-5472.CAN-06-3958.

37. Dominguez M. Interplay between Notch signaling and epigenetic silencers in cancer. *Cancer Res*. 2006;66(18):8931-8934. %R 10.1158/0008-5472.CAN-06-1858.

38. Proweller A, et al. Impaired Notch signaling promotes de novo squamous cell carcinoma formation. *Cancer Res*. 2006;66(15):7438-7444. %R 10.1158/0008-5472.CAN-06-0793.

39. Kunnimalaiyaan M, Chen H. Tumor suppressor role of Notch-1 signaling in neuroendocrine tumors. *Oncologist*. 2007;12(5):535-542. %R 10.1634/theoncologist.12-5-535.

40. Zhang P, et al. Critical role of Notch signaling in osteosarcoma invasion and metastasis. *Clin Cancer Res.* 2008;14(10):2962-2969. %R 10.1158/1078-0432.CCR-07-1992.
41. Hughes DPM, et al. Cell surface expression of epidermal growth factor receptor and her-2 with nuclear expression of her-4 in primary osteosarcoma. *Cancer Res.* 2004;64(6):2047-2053.
42. Hughes DPM, et al. Essential erbB family phosphorylation in osteosarcoma as a target for CI-1033 Inhibition. *Pediatr Blood Cancer.* 2006;46(5):614-623.
43. Jia S, et al. Eradication of osteosarcoma lung metastases following intranasal interleukin-12 gene therapy using a nonviral polyethylenimine vector. *Cancer Gene Ther.* 2002;9(3):260-266.
44. Jia S, et al. Eradication of osteosarcoma lung metastasis using intranasal gemcitabine. *Anticancer Drugs.* 2002;13(2):155-161.
45. Pollack S, Lewis H. Secretase inhibitors for Alzheimer's disease: challenges of a promiscuous protease. *Curr Opin Investig Drugs.* 2005;6(1):35-47.
46. Vidal GA, et al. Presenilin-dependent {gamma}-secretase processing regulates multiple ERBB4/HER4 activities. *J Biol Chem.* 2005;280(20):19777-19783. 10.1074/jbc.M412457200.
47. Berlin O, et al. Development of a novel spontaneous metastasis model of human osteosarcoma transplanted orthotopically into bone of athymic mice. *Cancer Research.* 1993;53(20):4890-4895.
48. Bali P, et al. Activity of suberoylanilide hydroxamic acid against human breast cancer cells with amplification of her-2. *Clin Cancer Res.* 2005;11(17):6382-6389. 10.1158/1078-0432.CCR-05-0344.
49. Phiel CJ, et al. Histone deacetylase is a direct target of valproic acid, a potent anticonvulsant, mood stabilizer, and teratogen. *J Biol Chem.* 2001;276(39):36734-36741. %R 10.1074/jbc.M101287200.
50. Gurvich N, et al. Histone deacetylase is a target of valproic acid-mediated cellular differentiation. *Cancer Res.* 2004;64(3):1079-1086. %R 10.1158/0008-5472.CAN-03-0799.
51. Li X-N, et al. Valproic acid induces growth arrest, apoptosis, and senescence in medulloblastomas by increasing histone hyperacetylation and regulating expression of p21Cip1, CDK4, and CMYC. *Mol Cancer Ther.* 2005;4(12):1912-1922. %R 10.1158/1535-7163.MCT-05-0184.
52. Zaskodova D, et al. Effect of valproic acid, a histone deacetylase inhibitor, on cell death and molecular changes caused by low-dose irradiation. *Ann N Y Acad Sci.* 2006;1091(1):385-398. %R 10.1196/annals.1378.082.
53. Greenblatt DY, et al. Valproic acid activates Notch-1 signaling and regulates the neuroendocrine phenotype in carcinoid cancer cells. *Oncologist.* 2007;12(8):942-951. %R 10.1634/theoncologist.12-8-942.
54. Catalano MG, et al. Valproic acid, a histone deacetylase inhibitor, enhances sensitivity to doxorubicin in anaplastic thyroid cancer cells. *J Endocrinol.* 2006;191(2):465-472. %R 10.1677/joe.1.06970.
55. Kempf-Bielack B, et al. Osteosarcoma relapse after combined modality therapy: an analysis of unselected patients in the Cooperative Osteosarcoma Study Group (COSS). *J Clin Oncol.* 2005;23(3):559-568. 10.1200/JCO.2005.04.063.
56. Bacci G, et al. Treatment and outcome of recurrent osteosarcoma: experience at Rizzoli in 235 patients initially treated with neoadjuvant chemotherapy. *Acta Oncol.* 2005;44(7):748-755.

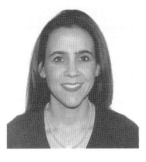 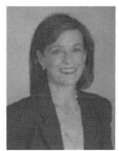

The Role of Fas/FasL in the Metastatic Potential of Osteosarcoma and Targeting this Pathway for the Treatment of Osteosarcoma Lung Metastases

Nancy Gordon and Eugenie S. Kleinerman

Abstract Pulmonary metastases remain the main cause of death in patients with Osteosarcoma (OS). In order to identify new targets for treatment, our laboratory has focused on understanding the biological properties of the tumor microenvironment that contribute to or interfere with metastasis. Dysfunction of the Fas/FasL signaling pathway has been implicated in tumor development, and progression. Here we describe the status of Fas expression in murine nonmetastatic K7 and metastatic K7M2 cells and human nonmetastatic SAOS and LM2 and metastatic LM6 OS cells. We demonstrated that Fas expression correlates *inversely* with metastatic potential. Pulmonary metastases from patients were uniformly Fas$^-$ supporting the importance of Fas expression to the metastatic potential. Since FasL is constitutively expressed in the lung, our data suggests that Fas$^+$ tumor cells undergo apoptosis and are cleared from the lung. By contrast, Fas$^-$ tumor cells evade this host defense mechanism and form lung metastases. We confirmed these findings by blocking the Fas pathway using Fas Associated Death Domain Dominant-Negative (FDN). Fas$^+$ cells transfected with FDN were not sensitive to FasL, showed delayed clearance and formed lung metastases. Fas$^+$ cells were also able to form lung metastases in FasL-deficient mice. Using our mouse model systems, we demonstrated that aerosol treatment with liposomal 9-Nitrocamptothecin and Gemcitabine (chemotherapeutic agents known to upregulate Fas expression) increased Fas expression and induced tumor regression in wild type mice. Lung metastases in FasL deficient mice did not respond to the treatment.

N. Gordon (✉)
Division of Pediatrics, Children's Cancer Hospital, University of Texas M. D. Anderson Cancer Center, 1515 Holcombe Boulevard, Unit #87, Houston, TX, 77030-4009, USA
e-mail: ngordon@mdanderson.org

We conclude that Fas is an early defense mechanism responsible for clearing invading Fas+ tumor cells from the lung. Fas− cells or cells with a nonfunctional Fas pathway evade this defense mechanism and form lung metastases. Therapy that induces Fas expression may therefore be effective in patients with established OS lung metastases. Aerosol delivery of these agents is an ideal way to target treatment to the lung.

Introduction

The lung is the most common site of metastatic spread in patients with osteosarcoma (OS). While combination chemotherapy and surgery has resulted in a disease-free survival rate of 60–65%, this cure rate has not changed for over 20 years.[1–9] Pulmonary metastases remain the major cause of death in these patients. Our laboratory has therefore focused on understanding the biologic properties in the tumor microenvironment that support and contribute to OS cell growth in the lung with the goal of identifying new targets for therapy. Altering the tumor microenvironment may be a reasonable therapeutic approach for the treatment of OS as metastases are usually limited to the lung and are the leading cause of death.

Fas and its ligand FasL are cell surface receptors which belong to the TNF receptor family. Interaction of the Fas receptor on cells with FasL results in ligand-mediated cell death.[10–13] Two different apoptosis-signaling pathways have been identified. The type I pathway involves Caspase 8 with subsequent activation of Caspase 3. The type II or mitochondrial pathway involves Caspase 9 (Fig. 1). While Fas is constitutively expressed on T cells, B cells and in numerous tissues, the constitutive expression of FasL is limited to the testes, small intestine, anterior chamber of the eye, and the lung.[14,15] Fas/FasL induced cell death is a critical regulator of immune homeostasis and is required for the maintenance of peripheral tolerance.[10] Deletion of activated T cells and inflammatory cells at the end of an immune response is mediated by this pathway. Constitutive expression of FasL in tissues, therefore, creates an immunotolerant microenvironment as B cells and activated T cells, which express Fas, are eliminated upon entering the organ. Constitutive expression of FasL prevents a massive immune response which can damage these organs. Indeed, herpes eye infections in FasL-deficient mice resulted in large immune cell infiltration into the anterior chamber of the eye resulting in blindness. By contrast wild-type mice showed a short controlled immune response, clearing the infection without sequelae.[14,16–19] Fas-mediated cell death has also recently been implicated as a regulator of tumor development, out-growth and progression. Downregulation of Fas or impaired Fas signaling have been correlated with tumor progression.[10,12,20–22]

The organ microenvironment can influence the success or failure of metastatic cells to survive and grow at distant sites. As OS metastasizes almost exclusively to the lung and lung epithelium constitutively expresses FasL, we investigated whether the expression of Fas on OS cells correlated with their metastatic potential. For these investigations, we used two different OS mouse models. The first is a human OS mouse model[23] where parental SAOS cells were injected i.v. into mice, a lung metastasis harvested and those cells reinjected i.v. (LM2 subline). This process was repeated five additional times to create the very metastatic LM6 and LM7 sublines.

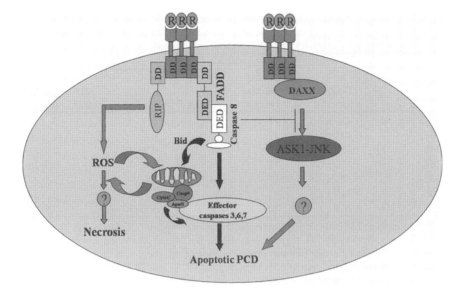

Fig. 1 Apoptosis signaling pathways triggered by interaction of Fas receptor on cells with FasL. The Type I pathway, involves Caspase 8 with subsequent activation of Caspase 3 and apoptosis. The Type II or mitochondrial pathway involves Caspase 9

Specific characteristics of the parental and LM2–LM7 cell lines are depicted in Table 1. The second is the K7M2 mouse OS model created in a similar fashion. The parental K7 cells are poorly metastatic compared with the K7M2 variant.[24,25]

Role of Fas in the Metastatic Potential of OS Cells in the Lung

As FasL is constitutively expressed on lung epithelium, our hypothesis was that tumor cells expressing the Fas receptor with a functional Fas signaling pathway will be eliminated by the engagement of the FasL expressed in the lung. These Fas+ cells would therefore be unable to form lung metastases. Fas− OS cells, by contrast, would escape this host defense mechanism and form lung metastases (Fig. 2). Indeed, the poorly metastatic parental SAOS cells expressed high levels of Fas and Fas cell surface protein while the metastatic sublines LM6 and LM7 showed low to no Fas expression (Fig. 3a, b). Similarly, the metastatic K7M2 cells showed a lower intensity of cell surface Fas compared with the nonmetastatic K7 cells (Fig. 3c). LM6, LM7 and K7M2 lung nodules were Fas− by immunohistochemistry,[26–28] as were lung nodules from patients with OS.[29] Furthermore, transfection of the Fas gene into LM7 cells inhibited their ability to form lung metastases following i.v. administration while control transfection had no effect on metastatic potential.[26,30] These data support our hypothesis that Fas expression correlates inversely with the ability of OS cells to form lung metastases.

If Fas-mediated cell death is responsible for clearing OS cells from the lung and inhibiting tumor growth in this organ, Fas+ cells with a blocked Fas signaling pathway

Table 1 Metastatic characteristics of the SAOS parental and LM sub lines. No lung metastases were seen 17 weeks following the i.v. injection of SAOS parental or LM2 cells. LM3–LM7 sub lines all form lung metastases. LM7 is the most metastatic subline

Cell line	Doubling time (h)[a]	Lung metastases[b] Time of sacrifice (weeks)	Incidence[c]	Median no (range)	Diameter (mm)
SAOS parental	45.7±3.3	17	0	0	0
LM2	43.6±4.2	17	0	0	0
LM3	44.1±2.6	17	2/5	0 (0–1)	0.5–1.0
LM4	40.0±0.9	17	3/4	9 (0–100)	0.5–2.0
LM5	37.2±3.8	17	4/4	88 (7–>200)	0.5–5.0
LM6	34.9±1.4	12	9/9	92 (30–>200)	0.5–5.6
LM7	26.8±1.3	10	12/12	100 (30–>200)	0.5–7.0

[a]SAOS parental or LM cells (3×10^3) were plated and incubated at 37°C for 24, 48, 72 and 96 h. The cells were labeled with [^{3}H]-thymidine during the last 24 h of incubation. Doubling time was calculated using the following formula: time × log 2/log (n/n_0) where n_0 is the cpm of cells incubated for 24 h and n is the cpm of cells incubated for 48, 72 and 96 h. It was expressed as the average of three independent experiments.

[b]Nude mice were injected with 1×10^6 of the indicated cells. Mice injected with SAOS, LM1, LM2, LM3, LM4 or LM5 were sacrificed 17 weeks later. Mice injected with LM6 and LM7 cells were sacrificed earlier because of signs of distress. The lungs were removed, fixed and tumor nodules were counted and measured.

[c]Number of tumor-positive mice/number of inoculated mice.

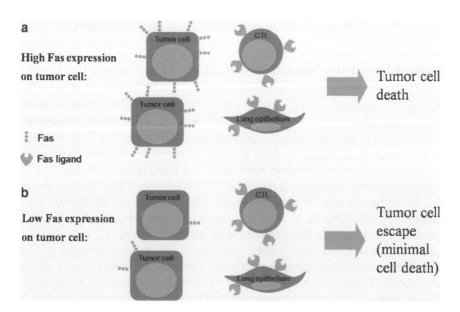

Fig. 2 Fas expression correlates inversely with the metastatic potential of OS cells to the lung. (**a**) Fas⁺ tumor cells enter the lung and undergo apoptosis triggered by FasL constitutively expressed by lung endothelium. (**b**) Tumor cells with low or no Fas expression evade this host defense mechanism

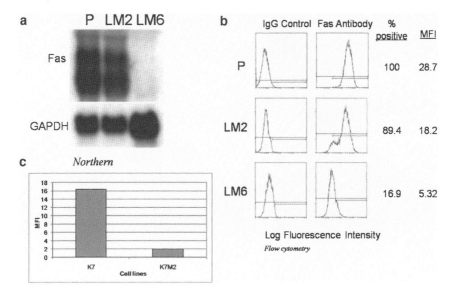

Fig. 3 Fas expression correlates inversely with the metastatic potential of human and murine OS cells. (**a**) Northern blot analyses shows high Fas expression in poorly metastatic parental SAOS-2 and LM2 cells and no Fas expression in the metastatic LM6 cells. (**b**) Flow cytometry confirms higher cell surface Fas protein expression in parental SAOS-2 and LM2 cells compared with LM6 cells. (**c**) Higher Fas expression in poorly metastatic parental K7 cells compared with the metastatic K7M2 cells

will not be susceptible to this clearance mechanism and should form lung metastases when injected intravenously. To test this hypothesis, we inhibited the Fas signaling pathway in Fas+ nonmetastatic K7 OS cells by transfecting these cells with Fas associated death-domain dominant negative (FDN). FDN blocks apoptosis in both type I and type II cells by inhibiting Caspase 8 at the DISC complex (Fig. 4). K7/FDN cells were not sensitive to FasL-induced cell death. Fas receptor expression in these cells was unaffected. We demonstrated that K7/FDN cells were retained in the lung compared to control-transfected K7/neo cells.[31] Two days after i.v. injection, there were five times the number of K7/FDN cells in the lung compared with the control-transfected cells. K7/FDN cells formed numerous large pulmonary metastases while the lungs from mice injected with K7/neo cells were clear (Fig. 5). The K7/FDN tumors were Fas+ by immunohistochemistry with some Fas− cells as well.[31] The important finding here is that blocking the Fas signaling pathway resulted in retention of Fas+ cells in the lung and the subsequent development of Fas+ tumor nodules.

The absence of FasL in the tumor microenvironment should also allow Fas+ OS cells to form lung metastases (Fig. 6). To address this question, Fas+ nonmetastatic K7 cells were injected i.v. into FasL-deficient mice. All of the mice developed lung metastases.[31] The immunohistochemistry analysis of these nodules revealed both Fas+ and Fas− cells.[31]

The K7M2 subline contains both Fas+ and Fas− cells. However, the lung nodules formed following i.v. or intrabone injection into wild-type Balb/c mice are all Fas−. If constitutive FasL in the lung is responsible for clearing Fas+ cells, then K7M2

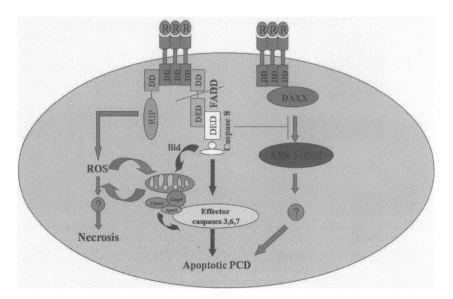

Fig. 4 Blocking the Fas signaling pathway with Fas Associated Death Domain Dominant-Negative (FDN) to inhibit FasL-induced cell death. FDN blocks apoptosis in both type I and type II cells by inhibiting C8 at the DISC complex

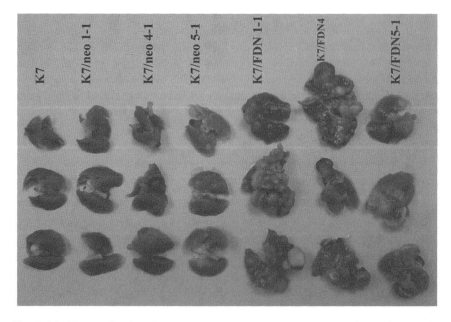

Fig. 5 Blocking the Fas signaling pathway alters the metastatic potential of Fas+ K7 cells. K7 cells were transfected with FDN or control vector (neo) and injected i.v. into mice. The mice were sacrificed 4 weeks later and lung metastases were quantified. K7/FDN cells induced numerous large pulmonary metastases compared with K7/neo and K7 cells

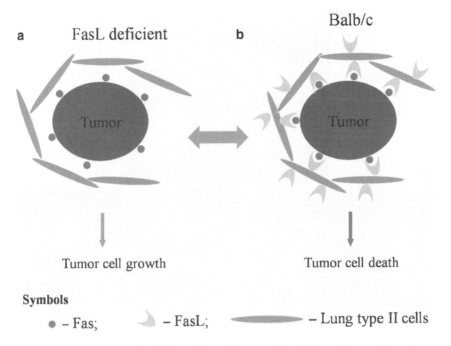

Fig. 6 (a) Absence of FasL in the lung microenvironment allows Fas+ cells to survive and grow. (b) By contrast, constitutive FasL in the lung of wild-type Balb/c mice binds to the cell surface Fas activating the Fas pathway which leads to apoptosis

cells injected into FasL-deficient mice should form heterogeneous lung metastases comprised of both Fas+ and Fas− cells as the Fas+ will not be eliminated (Fig. 6). Indeed, we demonstrated this phenomenon,[28] (Fig. 7). K7M2 nodules in FasL deficient mice contained areas of Fas+ as well as Fas− cells within the same lung (Fig. 7b). By contrast, wild-type BALB/c mice injected with K7M2 cells developed only Fas− lung nodules (Fig. 7a). Taken together, these data confirm our hypothesis that FasL is responsible for eliminating the Fas+ OS cells once they enter the lung. These data were the first to demonstrate that the expression of Fas and the presence of a functional Fas signaling pathway contributes to the ability of OS cells to form lung metastases. We were also the first to demonstrate that the pulmonary microenvironment plays a critical role in the metastatic potential of OS cells.

Therapeutic Effect of Aerosol Therapy on Established OS Lung Metastases

Having demonstrated that Fas expression is a critical determinant for OS cell growth in the lung, we next determined whether upregulating Fas expression in established Fas− OS lung nodules would result in tumor regression. Our hypothesis

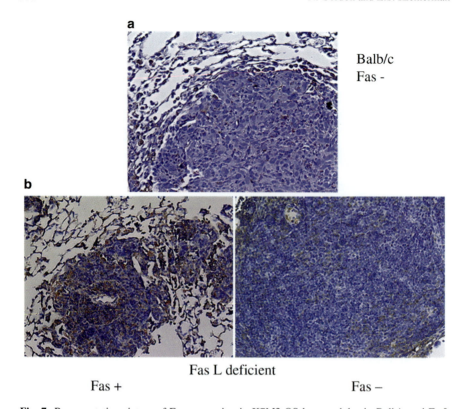

Fig. 7 Representative picture of Fas expression in K7M2 OS lung nodules in Balb/c and FasL deficient mice. K7M2 cells were injected i.v. into Balb/c and FasL deficient mice. The mice were sacrificed 2 weeks later, lungs were resected and stained for Fas expression. (**a**) K7M2 OS lung metastases from Balb/c mice were Fas⁻. (**b**) K7M2 OS lung metastases from FasL deficient mice showed heterogeneous Fas expression with areas of Fas⁺ and Fas⁻ cells within the same lung

was that agents that stimulate the reexpression of Fas in Fas⁻ lung nodules would result in tumor cell apoptosis induced by the FasL-expressing lung cells (Fig. 8). We demonstrated that both gemcitabine and liposomal 9-nitrocamptothecin (L-9NC) increased Fas expression in LM7 and K7M2 cells in vitro.[27,28,32] For in vivo analysis of efficacy, we elected to deliver these chemotherapy agents via the aerosol route. Aerosol technology has several advantages over systemic therapy. The agent is delivered directly to the organ where the tumor is growing avoiding dilution in the bloodstream. Aerosol administration avoids the first pass metabolic degradation in the liver and GI tract. This allows the achievement of high pulmonary drug concentrations with minimal systemic exposure resulting in decreased or minimal systemic toxicity. Finally, the drug is uniformly distributed throughout the lung. As OS metastasizes almost exclusively to the lung, aerosol therapy makes sense and is appealing. We demonstrated that the administration of aerosol L-9NC, initiated 8 weeks following tumor cell injection, or aerosol gemcitabine initiated 3 days after tumor cell injection, induced Fas expression in

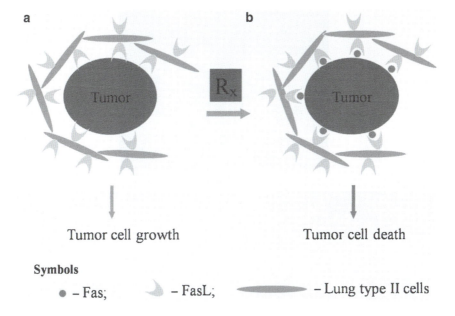

Fig. 8 Therapy induced expression of Fas on Fas⁻ tumor cells. (**a**) Fas⁻ tumor cells are not eliminated from the lung. (**b**) Treatment of Fas⁻ lung metastases with agents that stimulate the reexpression of Fas will result in tumor cell apoptosis induced by the FasL expressing lung cells

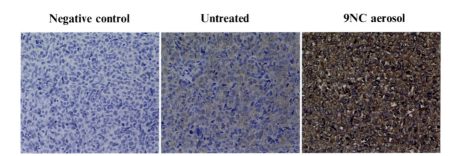

Fig. 9 Fas expression in LM7 lung metastases following aerosol liposome-9NC. Nude mice with established pulmonary metastases were treated with aerosol liposome-9NC daily for 6 weeks. The mice were sacrificed, the lungs were sectioned and evaluated by IHC for Fas expression. Brown staining represents positive Fas expression. Untreated pulmonary metastases were Fas⁻ whereas those treated with aerosol L-9NC were Fas⁺

established OS lung nodules (Fig. 9), tumor cell apoptosis (Fig. 10), and tumor regression.[27,28,32] To confirm that the effect of aerosol chemotherapy was mediated in part by the constitutive FasL in the lung, the in vivo aerosol therapy studies were repeated in FasL-deficient mice. No therapeutic affect was seen when FasL deficient mice were treated with aerosol Gemcitabine.[28] Although aerosol Gemcitabine induced Fas expression in the pulmonary nodules, these nodules continued to proliferate in size and number.[28] These data indicate that targeting the

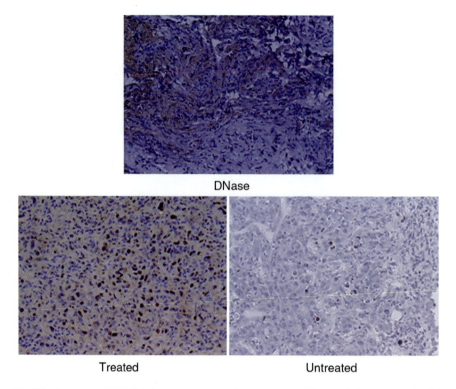

Fig. 10 Apoptosis of K7M2 OS lung metastases after treatment with aerosol Gemcitabine. Balb/c mice with established pulmonary metastases were treated with aerosol Gemcitabine and sacrificed after 2 weeks. Sections were analyzed for TUNEL as a marker of apoptosis. Brown staining represents apoptosis. Increased apoptosis was observed in the pulmonary metastases from Gemcitabine treated mice compared with those from control untreated mice

Fas pathway is a therapeutic opportunity for treating patients with established OS lung metastases and that the efficacy of aerosol chemotherapy may be closely linked to the microenvironment in the lung.

Summary

The metastatic process is complicated, involving multiple steps and factors that contribute to the ability of cancer cells to degrade the extracellular matrix in the primary tumor site, escape into the circulation, travel through the bloodstream from the local site to a distant organ, survive in the new organ microenvironment, and finally to initiate new vasculature to bring the needed oxygen and nutrients to support tumor growth in the new environment. The microenvironment itself can be a key factor in either permitting or inhibiting tumor cell survival and growth.

We have demonstrated that Fas$^+$ OS cells are rapidly cleared from the lung while Fas$^-$ cells remain. OS lung nodules are uniformly Fas$^-$. Inhibiting the Fas signaling pathway interferes with the clearance of Fas$^+$ OS cells resulting in the formation of Fas$^+$ lung metastases. Similarly, the lack of FasL in the host microenvironment allowed Fas$^+$ nonmetastatic cells to induce pulmonary metastases.[28,31]

We were the first to demonstrate that the Fas pathway plays a critical role in the metastatic potential of OS cells and that the lung microenvironment can influence treatment efficacy of OS lung metastases. Based on our data, we hypothesize that Fas is an early defense mechanism responsible for clearing invading Fas$^+$ tumor cells from the lung. Fas$^-$ cells or cells with a blocked or nonfunctional Fas pathway can evade FasL-induced cell death and go on to form lung metastases. Our data also suggest that inducing the expression of Fas can result in tumor regression, which is mediated by the FasL lung microenvironment. Identifying agents that enhance Fas expression in lung metastases or restore Fas signaling pathway activity may have therapeutic potential for patients with established unresponsive lung metastases. Our data also suggest that delivery of these agents by the aerosol route should be considered.

Acknowledgements We are very grateful to Joyce Furlough for her clerical assistance. This work was supported in part by NCI grant CA42992 (ESK) and NIH Core grant CA16672.

References

1. Marina N, et al. Biology and therapeutic advances for pediatric osteosarcoma. *Oncologist.* 2004;9(4):422-41.
2. Meyers PA, et al. Chemotherapy for nonmetastatic osteogenic sarcoma: The Memorial Sloan-Kettering experience. *J Clin Oncol.* 1992;10(1):5-15.
3. Kager L, et al. Primary metastatic osteosarcoma: Presentation and outcome of patients treated on neoadjuvant Cooperative Osteosarcoma Study Group protocols. *J Clin Oncol.* 2003;21(10):2011-8.
4. Verschraegen CF, et al. Feasibility, phase I, and pharmacological study of aerosolized liposomal 9-nitro-20(S)-camptothecin in patients with advanced malignancies in the lungs. *Ann N Y Acad Sci.* 2000;922:352-4.
5. Khanna C, et al. The membrane-cytoskeleton linker ezrin is necessary for osteosarcoma metastasis. *Nat Med.* 2004;10(2):182-6.
6. Ferguson WS, Goorin AM. Current treatment of osteosarcoma. *Cancer Invest.* 2001;19(3):292-315.
7. Goorin AM, et al. Phase II/III trial of etoposide and high-dose ifosfamide in newly diagnosed metastatic osteosarcoma: A pediatric oncology group trial. *J Clin Oncol.* 2002;20(2):426-33.
8. Goorin AM, et al. Presurgical chemotherapy compared with immediate surgery and adjuvant chemotherapy for nonmetastatic osteosarcoma: Pediatric Oncology Group Study POG-8651. *J Clin Oncol.* 2003;21(8):1574-80.
9. Bruland OS, Pihl A. On the current management of osteosarcoma: A critical evaluation and a proposal for a modified treatment strategy. *Eur J Cancer.* 1997;33(11):1725-31.
10. Owen-Schaub L, et al. Fas and Fas ligand interactions in malignant disease. *Int J Oncol.* 2000;17(1):5-12.
11. Nagata S. Apoptosis by death factor. *Cell.* 1997;88(3):355-65.

12. Owen-Schaub LB, et al. Fas and Fas ligand interactions suppress melanoma lung metastasis. *J Exp Med.* 1998;188(9):1717-23.
13. Algeciras-Schimnich A, et al. Molecular ordering of the initial signaling events of CD95. *Mol Cell Biol.* 2002;22(1):207-20.
14. Ferguson TA, Griffith TS. A vision of cell death: Insights into immune privilege. *Immunol Rev.* 1997;156:167-84.
15. Lee HO, Ferguson TA. Biology of FasL. *Cytokine Growth Factor Rev.* 2003;14(3-4):325-35.
16. Green DR, Ferguson TA. The role of Fas ligand in immune privilege. *Nat Rev Mol Cell Biol.* 2001;2(12):917-24.
17. Ferguson TA, Green DR. Fas-ligand and immune privilege: The eyes have it. *Cell Death Differ.* 2001;8(7):771-2.
18. Griffith TS, et al. Fas ligand-induced apoptosis as a mechanism of immune privilege. *Science.* 1995;270(5239):1189-92.
19. Griffith TS, et al. CD95-induced apoptosis of lymphocytes in an immune privileged site induces immunological tolerance. *Immunity.* 1996;5(1):7-16.
20. Moller P, et al. Expression of APO-1 (CD95), a member of the NGF/TNF receptor superfamily, in normal and neoplastic colon epithelium. *Int J Cancer.* 1994;57(3):371-7.
21. Hill LL, et al. Fas ligand: A sensor for DNA damage critical in skin cancer etiology. *Science.* 1999;285(5429):898-900.
22. Zornig M, et al. Loss of Fas/Apo-1 receptor accelerates lymphomagenesis in E mu L-MYC transgenic mice but not in animals infected with MoMuLV. *Oncogene.* 1995;10(12):2397-401.
23. Jia SF, Worth LL, Kleinerman ES. A nude mouse model of human osteosarcoma lung metastases for evaluating new therapeutic strategies. *Clin Exp Metastasis.* 1999;17(6):501-6.
24. Khanna C, et al. Metastasis-associated differences in gene expression in a murine model of osteosarcoma. *Cancer Res.* 2001;61(9):3750-9.
25. Khanna C, et al. An orthotopic model of murine osteosarcoma with clonally related variants differing in pulmonary metastatic potential. *Clin Exp Metastasis.* 2000;18(3):261-71.
26. Worth LL, et al. Fas expression inversely correlates with metastatic potential in osteosarcoma cells. *Oncol Rep.* 2002;9(4):823-7.
27. Koshkina NV, Kleinerman ES. Aerosol gemcitabine inhibits the growth of primary osteosarcoma and osteosarcoma lung metastases. *Int J Cancer.* 2005;116(3):458-63.
28. Gordon N, et al. Corruption of the Fas pathway delays the pulmonary clearance of murine osteosarcoma cells, enhances their metastatic potential, and reduces the effect of aerosol gemcitabine. *Clin Cancer Res.* 2007;13(15 Pt 1):4503-10.
29. Gordon N, et al. Fas expression in lung metastasis from osteosarcoma patients. *J Pediatr Hematol Oncol.* 2005;27(11):611-5.
30. Lafleur EA, et al. Increased Fas expression reduces the metastatic potential of human osteosarcoma cells. *Clin Cancer Res.* 2004;10(23):8114-9.
31. Koshkina NV, et al. Fas-negative osteosarcoma tumor cells are selected during metastasis to the lungs: The role of the Fas pathway in the metastatic process of osteosarcoma. *Mol Cancer Res.* 2007;5(10):991-9.
32. Koshkina NV, et al. 9-Nitrocamptothecin liposome aerosol treatment of melanoma and osteosarcoma lung metastases in mice. *Clin Cancer Res.* 2000;6(7):2876-80.

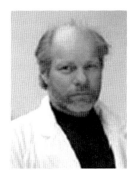

Bone Marrow Micrometastases Studied by an Immunomagnetic Isolation Procedure in Extremity Localized Non-metastatic Osteosarcoma Patients

Øyvind S. Bruland, Hanne Høifødt, Kirsten Sundby Hall, Sigbjørn Smeland, and Øystein Fodstad

Abstract Hematogenous spread of tumor cells is an early event in osteosarcoma and present in the majority of patients at primary diagnosis. Eradication of such micrometastases by adjuvant combination chemotherapy is crucial for survival. However, a survival plateau of 60-70% was reached over two decades ago, above which it seems difficult to further advance with the currently available therapies.

In this study we have, by an immunomagnetic isolation procedure, examined the presence and prognostic impact of disseminated tumor cells in bone marrow aspirates taken at primary diagnosis in a cohort of 41 non-metastatic patients with extremity localized, high-grade osteosarcoma.

Introduction

One characteristic feature of osteosarcoma (OS) is the early hematogenous spread of tumor cells in a majority of patients. The successful eradication of micrometastases (MM) by adjuvant combination chemotherapy is crucial for survival.[1] A survival plateau of 60-70% was reached over two decades ago,[2] above which it still seems difficult to advance with the current diagnostic and therapeutic armamentarium.

OS displays considerable heterogeneity in metastatic capacity and chemosensitivity,[2-6] Historical evidence has revealed that as many as 20% of OS patients without overt lung metastasis detected at primary diagnosis were in fact cured by surgery alone.[2,7] In the group of patients who would otherwise relapse, approximately 50% have chemosensitive tumors and are cured by the adjuvant therapy.[2] It would be important to identify two subgroup of patients; i.e. (a) those not having MM disease – and spare them from the toxic post-operative adjuvant chemotherapy currently given to all, and (b) the cohort of 30-40% having chemore-

---

Ø.S. Bruland (✉)
Faculty of Medicine, University of Oslo and Dept. of Oncology, The Norwegian Radium Hospital, N-0310, Oslo, Norway
e-mail: oyvind.bruland@medisin.uio.no

sistant MM who currently succumb to their disease. In this group, the most aggressive combination of chemotherapy is justified, and novel therapies should be explored, ideally instituted already in the primary/neo-adjuvant setting.

Risk-adapted therapy and individualized treatment has significantly improved the outcome in other cancers.[8,9] Unfortunately, it has thus far not been possible at the time of primary diagnosis to identify OS patients that belong to the different risk groups, and improved methods are needed to further advance the survival and/ or reduce long-term toxicity from chemotherapy.

In several other cancers, the presence of MM; i.e. disseminated tumor cells (DTC) detected in bone-marrow (BM) or peripheral blood, is convincingly shown to have a negative prognostic impact.[10-15] We have previously reported our first experience on DTC in 60 patients with primary bone sarcomas, 49 of whom had OS.[16] In the present paper, we have updated the follow up time and disease related events among the 22 patients that presented with extremity localized, non-metastatic, high grade OS at clinical presentation in this first series. In addition, BM aspirates from another 19 OS-patients treated at our institution have been collected. Hence, in the current study we have examined the presence and prognostic impact of DTC in BM at primary diagnosis in a cohort of 41 patients with extremity localized, high-grade OS without evidence of metastases at primary diagnosis.

Background

It has long been a goal to identify MM in OS patients. In two theses from The Mayo Clinic, a tritiated thymidine labeling method was explored,[17,18] and researchers at our institution used a technique employing Millipore filters in the vein draining the primary tumor.[19,20]

More recently, improved methods have been developed to detect DTCs in several types of cancer.[21,22] Our Institution has pioneered the development of an immunomagnetic procedure (Fig. 1) permitting rapid isolation of tumor cells present in samples of peripheral blood and BM aspirates from cancer patients.[14,16,23,24]

To our knowledge, the only recent publication on DTC in OS is our first series of 60 patients with suspected bone sarcoma[16] studied by the immunomagnetic detection assay mentioned above. Forty-nine of the patients had OS, and of these 63% had tumor cells in BM. Only four (8%) were positive in peripheral blood also. None of the 38 control BM samples were positive, including 11 from patients with suspected bone sarcoma at the time of sampling who later were found not to have OS.[16] Among the 22 patients with extremity localized, non-metastatic, high-grade OS, none of the 10 DTC-negative patients did relapse, whereas four of the 12 DTC-positive did. Information was available on the histological response to pre-operative chemotherapy in 15 of these 22 patients. None of the three patients in the BM-negative group who had a poor response to chemotherapy did relapse, whereas two of the four poor responders in the BM-positive cohort, died of disease.[16] We further characterized the immunomagnetically isolated cells by the use of fluores-

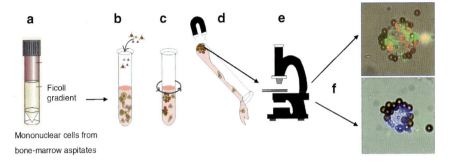

Fig. 1 Mononuclear cells are obtained by density gradient centrifugation of heparinized bone-marrow aspirates (A). Paramagnetic iron-containing monodisperse beads – Dynabeads[R] pre-incubated with monoclonal antibodies binding to cell surface markers are added (B). Incubation for 30 min on ice during constant rotation (C). A magnetic field is applied, and the supernatant is decanted (D). Rosettes are scored in a microscope (E). The technique also allows for detecting several cell surface epitopes simultaneously – by adding fluorescent latex-microbeads coated with other monoclonal antibodies that used for the rosetting step (F), see also ref.[16]

cent latex microparticles with surface-bound antibodies targeting different membrane markers (see Fig. 1F). In cases with numerous OS cells in BM, attempts to grow the isolated cells in vitro were successful in 2/8 attempts, and in 2/5 cases s.c. injected rosettes produced tumors with OS characteristics in nude mice,[16] proving the malignant properties of the selected DTCs in these cases.

Materials and Methods

We have now obtained mononuclear cells (MNC) from iliacal crest aspirated bone-marrow, as previously described,[16] in a total of 41 patients with localized extremity OS. See www.ssg-org.net for the consecutive clinical protocols SSG-II, SSG-VIII, ISG/SSG-I and SSG XIV describing the various chemotherapy combinations given.

Twenty-two were males and 19 were females. Anatomical sites of the primary tumor were: Femur – 19, tibia – 10, humerus – 10 and fibula – 2. All the patients were studied at primary diagnosis and were free of overt metastases as assessed by CT of the chest and ^{99m}Tc MDP bone scintigraphy. Patients with a minimum follow up of 2 years were included in this study.

Two monoclonal antibodies (Mabs) were used for the immunomagnetic study. TP-3 detects an epitope on an OS-associated cell surface antigen with homology to the bone izoenzyme of alkaline phosphatase.[25–28] The high affinity Mab 9.2.27 (obtained from Dr. R. Reisfeld, Scripps Research Institute, La Jolla, CA) was originally developed against melanoma.[29] This Mab recognizes a cell surface epitope on the high molecular weight melanoma-associated antigen, and is also shown to bind some subgroups of sarcoma, including OS.[30] Both Mabs have previously been shown to be non-reactive with MNC in peripheral blood and bone marrow from normal donors.[16,26,30]

The rapid and simple procedure for immunomagnetic detection of cancer cells in BM-samples has a sensitivity of approximately 2 target cells in 2×10^7 MNC, depending on the affinity of the monoclonal antibody used and the number of antigen epitopes expressed in a particular target cell population.[24] Briefly, iron containing, super-paramagnetic monodisperse particles with a diameter of 4.5 μm, coated with polyclonal sheep anti-mouse IgG (Dynabeads SAM-450, Invitrogen AS, Oslo, Norway), are pre-incubated with one of the tumor-associated Mabs and washed before the isolation procedure is performed (Fig. 1). Typically, 60 μg of purified Mab is added to 30 mg (4×10^8 beads) of Dynabeads. SAM-450 Dynabeads alone are used as negative control. Approximately 2×10^7 isolated MNC are re-suspended in one ml PBS with 1% human serum albumin (HSA) in a plastic tube, and immunobeads are added in a concentration of 0.5:1 to the total number of cells. After incubation of the mixture under rotation for 30 min, the cells are diluted with PBS + 1% HSA, and the tube is put in a magnet holder (Dynal, Oslo, Norway). Cells reactive with the Mabs bind the beads as rosettes, and cell-bead rosettes are trapped on the wall of the test tube. The supernatant, containing unbound cells, is decanted. The remaining positive fraction in a volume of approximately 200 μl is placed on ice, and a 20 μl aliquot is examined for rosettes (Fig. 1) by microscopy, using a Zeiss Axioscope (Carl Zeiss, Jena, Germany). A sample containing at least two cells with five or more TP-3 or 9.2.27 beads attached as a rosette is regarded as positive.

Results

In this series of 41 OS-patients, the age at diagnosis ranged from 8 to 51 years, with a mean age of 16 years. DTC's were detected in 26 of the 41 patients (63%) with a mean follow up of 73 months. Among the 15 patients (seven males and eight females) that did not have micrometastases isolated from their bone-marrow aspirate – hereafter called micrometastasis negative (MM-) – none have experienced an OS-related event following adjuvant chemotherapy. Mean follow up for this cohort was 92 months. One patient died of acute leukemia nine years following the diagnosis of OS. The remaining 14 are all NED. In this MM- group, five had a primary tumor of malignancy grade 3 and 10 had OS of grade 4.

The 26 OS-patients (15 males and 11 females) in the micrometastasis positive (MM+) cohort had a significantly worse outcome (log rank $p = 0.038$ – see Fig. 2). A total of seven OS-related events were observed. Despite the fact that a higher percentage of patients had grade 4 tumors (23 out of 26 tumors) in this MM + cohort, two events were seen in patients with grade 3 OS – one of these patients is DOD and one ALVM. The remaining five events were observed in patients with grade 4 tumors; three are DOD, one ALVM and one in CR2 following a local relapse that was treated by amputation. The median follow up among MM + patients was 69 months.

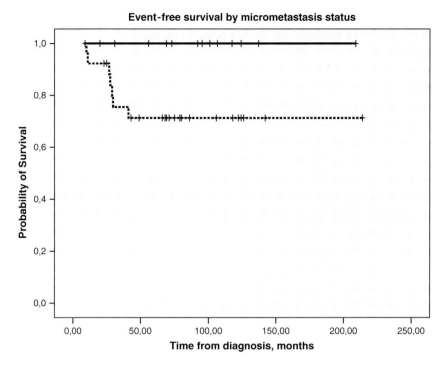

Fig. 2 Survival of 41 osteosarcoma patients by micrometastasis status, 15 micrometastasis negative patients: *whole line*. 26 micrometastasis positive patients: *dotted line*. Log rank $p=0.038$

Discussion and Future Perspectives

Experience on the prognostic impact of MM in primary bone sarcoma is so far sparse, but it has also been reported in Ewing sarcoma and other pediatric sarcomas.[31–33]

Recently, improved methods enabling molecular characterization of MM by recombinant DNA-technology has been reported.[34] This should allow the definition of novel targets for therapy.[16,35–39] Ideally, an adjuvant therapy should be tailored and based on properties of the MM, not of the primary tumor.

Summary

In conclusion, a very high fraction of classical OS patients had malignant cells in BM at primary diagnosis, and a significant correlation between the presence of DTCs and disease progression was found. The data demonstrate the clinical potential of this immunomagnetic method. Attempts to subgroup OS-patients for more individualized treatment based on the presence of MM cells should be studied in a larger cohort of patients. Molecular characterization of isolated MM could identify cellular pathways as a basis for targeted adjuvant therapies.

References

1. Malawer MM, Helman LJ, O'Sullivan B. Sarcomas of bone. In: Devita VT, Hellman S, Rosenberg SA, eds. *Cancer – Principles & Practice of Oncolog*. 7th ed. Philadelphia: Lippincott-Raven Publishers; 2005:1638-1686.
2. Bruland OS, Pihl A. On the current management of osteosarcoma. A critical evaluation and a proposal for a modified treatment strategy. *Eur J Cancer*. 1997;33(11):1725-1731.
3. Huvos AG. Osteogenic sarcoma. In: Huvos AG, ed. *one Tumors. Diagnosis, treatment and prognosis*. Philadelphia: WB Saunders; 1991:85-155.
4. Dahlin D, Unni K. Osteogenic sarcoma of bone and its important recognizable varieties. *Am J Surg Pathol.*. 1977;1:61-72.
5. Sæter G, Bruland ØS, Follerås G, et al. Extremity and non-extremity high-grade osteosarcoma The Norwegian Radium Hospital experience during the modern chemotherapy era. *Acta Oncol*. 1996;35(Suppl 8):129-134.
6. Aksnes LH, Hall KS, Folleraas G, et al. Management of high-grade bone sarcomas over two decades: the Norwegian Radium Hospital experience. *Acta Oncol*. 2006;45(1):38-46.
7. Cade S. Osteogenic sarcoma: a study based on 133 patients. *J R Coll Surg Edinb*. 1955;1: 79-111.
8. Tournade MF, Com-Nougué C, Voûte PA, et al. Results of the Sixth International Society of Pediatric Oncology Wilms' Tumor Trial and Study: a risk-adapted therapeutic approach in Wilms' tumor. *J Clin Oncol*. 1993;11(6):1014-1023.
9. Larson S, Stock W. Progress in the treatment of adults with acute lymphoblastic leukemia. *Curr Opin Hematol*. 2008;15(4):400-407.
10. Mansi JL, Gogas H, Bliss JM, et al. Outcome of primary-breast-cancer patients with micro-metastases: a long-term follow-up study. *Lancet.*. 1999;354(9174):197-202.
11. Pantel K, Cote RJ, Fodstad O. Detection and clinical importance of micrometastatic disease. *J Natl Cancer Inst*. 1999;91(13):1113-1124.
12. Wiedswang G, Borgen E, Kaaresen R, et al. Detection of isolated tumor cells in bone marrow is an independent prognostic factor in breast cancer. *J Clin Oncol*. 2003;21:3469-3478.
13. Pantel K, Muller V, Auer M, et al. Detection and clinical implications of early systemic tumor cell dissemination in breast cancer. *Clin Cancer Res*. 2003;9(17):6326-6334.
14. Brunsvig PF, Flatmark K, Aamdal S, et al. Bone marrow micrometastases in advanced stage non-small cell lung carcinoma patients. *Lung Cancer*. 2008;61(2):170-176.
15. Braun S, Vogl FD, Naume B, et al. A pooled analysis of bone marrow micrometastasis in breast cancer. *N Engl J Med*. 2005;353(8):793-802.
16. Bruland OS, Høifødt H, Saeter G, Smeland S, Fodstad O. Hematogenous micrometastases in osteosarcoma patients. *Clin Cancer Res*. 2005;11(13):4666-4673.
17. Carlson MJ. Circulating sarcoma cells: the incidence of ^{3}thymidine labeling in the peripheral blood of normal and sarcoma patients. Thesis – University of Minnesota 1978.
18. Kaiser TE. The detection of tritiated thymidine labeled cells in the peripheral blood of sarcoma patients and the nature of these cells bearing prognostic significance for sarcoma patients. Thesis – University of Minnesota 1985.
19. Foss PO, Messelt OT, Efskind J. Isolation of cancer cells from blood and thoracic duct lymph by filtration. *Surgery*. 1963;53(2):241-246.
20. Foss PO, Brennhovd IO, Messelt OT, Efskind J, Liverud K. Invasion of tumor cells into the bloodstream caused by palpation or biopsy of the tumor. *Surgery*. 1966;59(5):691-695.

21. Ghossein RA, Bhattacharya S. Molecular detection and characterisation of circulating tumour cells and micrometastases in solid tumours. *Eur J Cancer.* 2000;36(13):1681-1694.
22. Taback B, Chan AD, Kuo CT, et al. Detection of occult metastatic breast cancer cells in blood by a multimolecular marker assay: Correlation with clinical stage of disease. *Cancer Res.* 2001;61:8845-8850.
23. Flatmark K, Bjørnland K, Johannessen HO, et al. Immunomagnetic detection of micrometastatic cells in bone marrow of colorectal cancer patients. *Clin Cancer Res.* 2002;8(2):444-449.
24. Faye R, Aamdal S, Høifødt HK, et al. Immunomagnetic detection and clinical significance of micrometastatic tumor cells in malignant melanoma patients. *Clin Cancer Res.*2004;15:4134-4149.
25. Bruland ØS, Fodstad Ø, Funderud S, Pihl A. New monoclonal antibodies specific for human sarcomas. *Int J Cancer.* 1986;38:27-31.
26. Bruland ØS, Fodstad Ø, Stenwig E, Pihl A. Expression and characteristics of a novel human osteosarcoma-associated cell surface antigen. *Cancer Res.* 1988;48:5302-5309.
27. Bruland ØS, Fodstad Ø, Skretting A, Pihl A. Selective radiolocalization of two radiolabelled anti-sarcoma monoclonal antibodies in human osteosarcoma xenografts. *Br J Cancer.* 1987;56:21-25.
28. Bruland ØS, Aas M, Fodstad Ø, et al. Immunoscintigraphy of bone sarcomas. Results in five patients. *Eur J Cancer.* 1994;30:1484-1489.
29. Morgan AC Jr, Galloway DR, Reisfeld RA. Production and characterization of a monoclonal antibody to a melanoma specific glycoprotein. *Hybridoma.* 1981;1:27-36.
30. Godal A, Bruland OS, Haug E, Aas M, Fodstad O. Unexpected expression of the 250 kD melanoma-associated antigen in human sarcoma cells. *Br J Cancer.* 1986;53:839-841.
31. Fagnou C, Michon J, Peter M, et al. Presence of tumor cells in bone marrow but not in blood is associated with adverse prognosis in patients with Ewing's tumor. *J Clin Oncol.* 1998;16:1707-1711.
32. Athale UH, Shurtleff SA, Jenkins JJ, et al. Use of reverse transcriptase polymerase chain reaction for diagnosis and staging of alveolar rhabdomyosarcoma, Ewing sarcoma family of tumors, and desmoplastic small round cell tumor. *J Pediatric Hematol/Oncol.* 2001;23/2:99-104.
33. Schleiermacher G, Peter M, Oberlin O, et al. Increased risk of systemic relapse associated with bone marrow micrometastasis and circulating tumor cells in localized Ewing tumor. *J Clin Oncol.* 2003;21(1):85-91.
34. Tveito S, Maelandsmo GM, Hoifodt HK, Rasmussen H, Fodstad Ø. Specific isolation of disseminated cancer cells: a new method permitting sensitive detection of target molecules of diagnostic and therapeutic value. *Clin Exp Metastasis.* 2007;24(5):317-321.
35. Baldini N, Scotlandi K, Barbanti-Brodano G, et al. Expression of P-glycoprotein in high-grade osteosarcoma in relation to clinical outcome. *N Engl J Med.* 1995;333:1380-1385.
36. Gorlick R, Anderson P, Andrulis I, et al. Biology of childhood osteogenic sarcoma and potential targets for therapeutic development: meeting summary. *Clin Cancer Res.* 2003;5442/9:5442-5453.
37. Serra M, Scotlandi K, Reverter-Branchat G, et al. Value of P-glycoprotein and clinicopathologic factors as the basis for new treatment strategies in high-grade osteosarcoma of the extremities. *J Clin Oncol.* 2003;21(3):536-542.
38. Valabrega G, Fagioli F, Corso S, et al. ErbB2 and bone sialoprotein as markers for metastatic osteosarcoma cells. *Br J Cancer.* 2003;88:396-400.
39. Serra M, Reverter-Branchat G, Maurici D, et al. Analysis of dihydrofolate reductase and reduced folate carrier gene status in relation to methotrexate resistance in osteosarcoma cells. *Ann Oncol.* 2004;15:151-160.

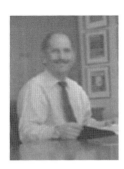 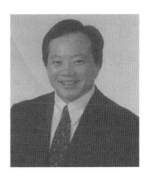

Strategies to Explore New Approaches in the Investigation and Treatment of Osteosarcoma

Su Young Kim and Lee J. Helman

Abstract Studies in osteosarcoma over the past 40 years have led to a steady improvement in the overall outcome of patients with osteosarcoma. In the year 2008, we can expect greater than 60% overall survival for newly diagnosed non-metastatic appendicular osteosarcoma. However, to achieve this current outcome, many patients are treated with aggressive cytotoxic chemotherapy and ultimately are not cured, and some patients who would be curable even without this aggressive approach are likely treated and cured. And finally, patients presenting with metastatic disease and those whose tumors recur after standard approaches continue to do very poorly. We believe that in order to continue to make progress in the treatment of this disease, we must achieve two main objectives. Firstly, we must find biomarkers that prospectively and accurately identify newly diagnosed non-metastatic patients who will not be cured with current modalities.

We hope that the achievement of this goal will allow for innovative clinical studies in this high-risk population while not jeopardizing those patients who currently are cured using the available treatment approaches, and ultimately accelerate progress toward curing more patients. Secondly, we must develop entirely new approaches to the treatment of metastatic and recurrent osteosarcoma. Our approach has been to develop models of highly aggressive and less aggressive osteosarcoma, and to use these models to identify genetic alterations and signaling pathways that distinguish the two phenotypic behaviors. We have identified plasma membrane-cytoskeletal linker protein, ezrin, as one pathway that identifies aggressive biological behavior in mouse and dog osteosarcoma. Using ezrin as the initial discriminator, we have high ezrin expression to activation of mTOR signaling, suggesting a possible novel target for therapy of aggressive osteosarcoma. We have also linked β4 integrin signaling to metastatic behavior that also appears to be linked to mTOR signaling. Most recently, we have identified a critical relationship between mTOR signaling and the IGF I signaling pathway that may help point the way to combination target-

---

L.J. Helman (✉)
Center for Cancer Research, National Cancer Institute, National Institutes of Health, 31, Center Drive MSC-2440, Bethesda, MD, 20892-2440, USA
e-mail: helmanl@mail.nih.gov

ing therapy aimed at blocking both mTOR and IGF signaling in these tumors. Finally, we have proposed a novel clinical trial design to begin to test agents targeted at recurrent, metastatic disease, and this also will be discussed.

Introduction

The five-year survival rates for patients with localized osteosarcoma have dramatically improved from less that 15% in the 1950s to greater that 60% since the 1980s.[1,2] This improvement was achieved with the introduction and adoption of adjuvant/neo-adjuvant systemic chemotherapy for all patients treated for localized disease. Since the vast majority of patients treated prior to the use of systemic chemotherapy died of pulmonary metastases, it can be concluded that the adoption of systemic therapy dramatically reduces the likelihood of systemic relapse in this disease for those patients who appear to present with localized tumor, by eliminating micrometastatic disease. Unfortunately, progress since the mid 1980s has been minimal with 5-year survival rates still in the 60–70% range.[3] Furthermore, progress in the outcome of osteosarcoma patients presenting with metastatic disease has been much more disappointing, with only 25% of patients surviving long term, and this has not changed in the past 50 years.[4] Thus, while progress has been real, our ability to make continued improvement in the outcome of patients with osteosarcoma has been challenged.

We have therefore focused our attention on developing new approaches to complement our current therapeutic modalities, with the belief that a better understanding of the biology of osteosarcoma and the biology of pulmonary metastases will identify novel targets that will ultimately translate into more effective therapies. This report will focus on what we have learned recently regarding the underlying biology of osteosarcoma and the biology of metastases in this disease, with a focus on the latter. The therapeutic implications of these findings will also be discussed.

Genetic Alterations in Osteosarcoma

Chromosomal Abnormalities

Osteosarcoma falls into the category of sarcomas that are characterized by non-specific genetic alterations and complex unbalanced karyotypes.[5] Thus, the presence of a complex disordered karyotype is the hallmark genetic feature of these tumors, and reflects marked telomere dysfunction. Current data suggests that the mechanism of telomere lengthening in osteosarcomas (like other sarcomas with complex karyotypes) appears to be through the alternative lengthening of the telomeres (ALT) pathway, in contradistinction to most epithelial tumors where telomerase

Strategies to Explore New Approaches in the Investigation   519

activation is responsible for abnormalities of telomeres.[6] However, in a small study of osteosarcoma cell lines, no mutations in telomere stability genes were noted.[7] In a study of 62 patient samples of osteosarcoma, investigators reported that tumors without evidence of telomere maintenance had improved survival.[8] A subsequent study also suggested that expression of telomerase itself in osteosarcoma primary tumor specimens was associated with a poor outcome.[9] Taken together, it seems likely that telomere dysfunction plays a significant role in the underlying pathophysiology of this tumor, although it is not yet obvious how such dysfunction could be targeted for therapy.

Genetic Abnormalities

Several genetic predisposition syndromes are associated with osteosarcoma, thus linking the specific abnormalities associated with these syndromes to osteosarcoma. Hereditary retinoblastoma is caused by germ-line mutations in the tumor suppressor gene RB, which is known to function by blocking entry of cells into the DNA synthesis (S) phase of the cell cycle.[10] Patients with hereditary retinoblastoma are known to have an approximately 100-fold increased risk of developing osteosarcoma, thus strongly implicating RB abnormalities with osteosarcoma. Indeed, loss of heterozygosity of the RB gene has been reported in almost 50% of cases of sporadic osteosarcoma, making it the most frequent genetic abnormality in these tumors.[11–13] There have also been reports suggesting that RB alterations in osteosarcoma lead to a less favorable prognosis.[11,12] However, not all studies have confirmed this finding.[13] In summary, alterations in the RB pathway appear to be the most frequent genetic alterations seen in osteosarcomas, but it is not clear how such alterations can be targeted at this time.

The Li-Fraumeni syndrome is a hereditary cancer predisposition syndrome that is associated with germ-line mutations in the p53 gene, which is known to function as a sensor of DNA damage or cellular stress.[10] Patients with the Li-Fraumeni syndrome are known to have an excess risk of osteosarcoma. Like the case in hereditary retinoblastoma, mutations in p53 occur in approximately 20–40% of cases of sporadic osteosarcoma.[14] While there are no current therapies directly targeting mutant p53, a number of approaches are being developed that attempt to use mutant p53 as an "Achilles heel" where the inability to sense DNA damage could ultimately lead to specific cell death in tumor cells.

Rare constitutional mutations in members of the RecQ family of DNA helicases lead to Werner syndrome and Rothmund-Thomson syndrome.[15] DNA helicases function to unwind DNA and are thought to maintain DNA integrity. Both syndromes are associated with an increased risk of osteosarcoma. However, despite intensive ongoing investigations, there does not yet appear to be an association of mutations of RecQ helicases in sporadic cases of osteosarcoma.[16]

Activation of Growth Factor Signaling Pathways

Most cancers have been found to have an activation of various growth factor signaling pathways involving a variety of tyrosine and serine/threonine kinases, and osteosarcomas appear to be no exception. These pathways are becoming increasingly important, as many new therapeutic agents are being developed to specifically alter kinase signaling in tumors. While many carcinomas harbor mutations or amplifications in a specific kinase-signaling molecule leading to constitutive activation of the enzyme, these have not been demonstrated in osteosarcomas. Nevertheless, several growth factor pathways appear to be activated and suggest potential novel targets for treatment.

Insulin-Like Growth Factors

A role for Insulin-like growth factors (IGF), particularly IGF-I in osteosarcoma has long been suspected because of the role IGF-I plays in normal bone growth. Early data suggested that inhibition of the Growth Hormone (GH)/IGF-I axis prevented metastatic behavior in a mouse model of osteosarcoma.[17] Subsequently, it was shown that human osteosarcoma cell lines appear to require IGF-I for growth.[18] In addition, a significant proportion of osteosarcoma tumor samples expressed IGF-I and its receptor.[19] Based on these, and other findings linking the IGF-I signaling pathway with the biology of osteosarcoma, an early clinical trial aimed at blocking circulating levels of IGF-I was reported several years ago using a somatostatin analog to block the GH/IGF-I axis.[20] Although no clinical activity was reported, only a 50% reduction in serum IGF-I levels was obtained. It was therefore unclear whether an effect would have been observed if a higher level of suppression could have been achieved. However, with the recent development of specific inhibitors of the IGF-I receptor, additional trials of this approach in osteosarcoma appear to be warranted.

Src Kinase

Src kinase is a member of a family of non-receptor tyrosine kinases, many of which are activated during proliferation and metastases of human cancers.[21] Among the many targets of Src kinase is paxillin, a scaffolding molecule that regulates the organization of the actin cytoskeleton at focal adhesions.[22] Recently, using human osteosarcoma cell lines of high and low metastatic potential, investigators found that phosphorylation of paxillin by Src kinase was associated with the metastatic phenotype, suggesting that the Src/paxillin axis contributed directly to the metastatic potential of human osteosarcoma.[23] Unpublished studies from our laboratory have shown that 95% of osteosarcoma samples had high-level expression of phosphorylated Src or phosphorylated paxillin. Both of these findings are of clinical relevance, since a number of small molecule inhibitors of src family kinases are currently making their way through clinical trials.

Modulation of Cell Surface Receptors

Integrins make up a family of cell surface receptors that are responsible for mediating interactions between cells and the extracellular matrix. To date, 18α and 8β subunits have been identified and these subunits dimerize to form at least 25 different integrin heterodimers, many of which are crucial in the regulation of adhesion, migration, proliferation, survival and metastasis.[24] Our laboratory has recently utilized immunohistochemistry to demonstrate that 35 of 35 osteosarcoma patient samples expressed β4 integrin, the majority at high levels (submitted for publication). Further studies have shown that shRNA mediated knockdown of β4 integrin in the metastatic human osteosarcoma cell line MNNG/HOS resulted in dramatic attenuation of metastatic lung nodules in immunocompromised mice. Similar results were obtained using dominant negative β4 integrin constructs. Interestingly, these mutant constructs did not affect the growth of primary tumors in xenografts, suggesting a specific role of β4 integrin in the metastatic cascade. Furthermore, we have also demonstrated that there is a direct interaction between β4 integrin and ezrin (submitted for publication).

Ezrin is a membrane-cytoskeleton linker protein that was first identified based on differential expression between highly metastatic and poorly metastatic murine osteosarcoma cell lines.[25] Similar to the experiments with β4 integrin, antisense RNA mediated knockdown of ezrin resulted in complete suppression of metastatic lung nodules in mouse models. Utilization of ex vivo imaging approaches indicated that ezrin provided an early survival advantage to metastatic osteosarcoma cells that reached the lung (submitted for publication). High expression of ezrin was associated with a significantly shorter disease free interval in pediatric patients with osteosarcoma.[25] In addition, the risk for recurrence was 80% greater for patients with high ezrin expression in their primary tumors.

Additional experiments then showed that inhibition of ezrin resulted in decreases in both 4EBP1 and S6K. The importance of these findings is that both of these genes are downstream of the mammalian target of rapamycin (mTOR), which is downstream of ezrin. mTOR is a serine/threonine kinase that is a central regulator of cell growth, proliferation and metabolism in response to environmental and nutritional cues.[26] Many different mechanisms lead to the activation of the mTOR pathway in cancer cells. Although rapamycin has been used as an immunosuppressive agent for quite some time, it was only after the finding that rapamycin inhibited the growth of murine and human cancer cell lines in tissue culture and in xenograft models that it came under investigation as an anti-cancer agent. There are four mTOR inhibitors: rapamycin itself and three analogs, AP23573, CCI-779 and RAD001, all of which are currently being tested in clinical trials.[27,28] In addition, we have shown that mice bearing primary osteosarcoma tumors that were treated with either rapamycin or CCI-779 had significantly fewer lung nodules and markedly prolonged survival.[29] Unlike the genes described previously, the relationship between mTOR activation and overall survival in osteosarcoma has not yet been examined.

In total, the above examples point to an important role for the pathway that begins with β4 integrin on the cell surface, utilizes the linker protein ezrin and signals through mTOR, in the process of metastases. In all cases, inhibition of any of the above genes resulted in a decrease in the metastatic phenotype. The important questions that remain to be answered are the different mechanisms by which these genes mediate the metastatic cascade.

Chemokines are another area of interest in osteosarcoma metastases. Chemokines are small chemotactic cytokines that play important roles in many physiological processes. Their importance in metastatic disease was first described in breast cancer.[30] Muller et al found that the chemokine receptor, CXCR4, was expressed at high levels in primary tumors but at low levels in normal breast tissue. Its corresponding ligand, CXCL12, was expressed at high levels in lymph nodes, lung, bone marrow and liver, all of which are sites at which breast cancer metastasizes. The chemokine model of metastasis hypothesizes that tumor cells that express high levels of a chemokine receptor have a higher likelihood of binding its corresponding ligand at the target organ, and when that event occurs, it triggers the metastatic cascade (Fig. 1). Laverdiere et al have shown that patients who had low CXCR4 expression had a 90% survival rate.[31] Conversely, patients with high CXCR4 expression had only 15% survival. The finding that treatment of mice with a

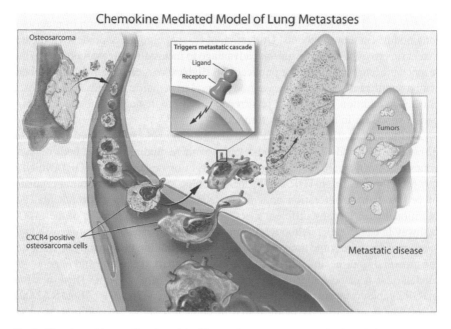

Fig. 1 The chemokine mediated model of lung metastases. At a certain time during tumorigenesis, osteosarcoma cells that are positive for the chemokine receptor CXCR4, enter the circulation. When they encounter a vascular bed, such as the lung, that has an abundant level of the ligand CXCL12, there is a higher chance that the receptor will bind the ligand. The coupling of ligand to the receptor triggers a cascade that allows the cancerous cells to attach to the normal tissue, invade, survive and finally proliferate, thereby leading to the formation of metastatic tumors

Strategies to Explore New Approaches in the Investigation 523

CXCR4 antagonist decreased the number of metastatic osteosarcoma lung nodules also supports the chemokine model of metastasis.[32]

In our laboratory, we have also shown that CXCR4 is expressed in almost all osteosarcoma cell lines, although at low levels.[33] In vitro, we have shown that CXCR4 inhibition resulted in decreased adhesion to extracellular matrix proteins, decreased migration and decreased invasion through a matrigel layer.[33] We also developed a novel ex vivo luciferase-based imaging technique to examine harvested, luciferin bathed lung samples, immediately following the intravenous injection of luciferase tagged osteosarcoma cells. Using this technique, we determined that CXCR4 inhibition reduced the number of cells that remained adherent to the cell surface immediately after their arrival in the lungs. In vivo treatment of mice with a CXCR4 antagonist resulted in a twofold decrease in lung nodules. However, this result was only obtained when the cells were pre-treated with the antagonist. These findings confirmed our earlier finding that direct ligand/receptor inhibition was the most likely factor in subsequent development of metastases.

In total, these findings suggested that CXCR4 inhibition may play an important role in preventing metastatic disease. However, a theoretical concern must be addressed for any therapy that is aimed at chemokine inhibition. For osteosarcoma, it is assumed that micro-metastatic disease is present at the time of diagnosis. If cells have already reached the lung, then the utility of an agent whose role is to prevent the cell from binding to its metastatic target organ is called into question. One would have to hypothesize that osteosarcoma cells remain in circulation for months, or even years, after removal of the primary tumor, or that they remain in a state of dormancy in organs other than the target of the eventual metastatic site. Unless either of these conditions is true, even if chemokine directed therapy is initiated on the day of diagnosis of osteosarcoma, it may prove to be ineffective.

Modeling the Metastatic Cascade

The steps that are required for a cancer cell to spread are complex. At a minimum, the cell must have the genetic components to be able to enter the systemic circulation. Once the cell is in the blood, it must be able to evade immune cells and survive the tortuous route that cells must traverse, including high volume flow pressures and small diameter capillaries. Once the cell is able to reach its target organ, it must then stop, extravasate, invade, adhere, survive and proliferate, eventually resulting in gross metastatic nodules.

The models that are currently available can only effectively measure the final step in this process, namely gross metastatic nodules. But experiments in our laboratory suggest that CXCR4 acts very early in the metastatic process, allowing for physical interactions immediately after arrest in the capillary. Other experiments also suggest that ezrin provides a survival advantage, giving the cells more likelihood of proliferative capability. In addition, inhibition of $\beta 4$ integrin, ezrin or mTOR, all of which are part of a common pathway, resulted in suppression of metastases. However, it is possible that dysregulation of different genes in a common pathway may affect different steps in the metastatic process. It is therefore imperative that we perfect the tools that will be required to dissect the stages of metastases.

The process of developing more refined models to highlight the different steps in the metastatic cascade is ongoing. In vitro, many laboratories are currently developing three-dimensional tissue culture models to answer some of these questions. The matrix for these systems has ranged from nanofibers, to collagen layers, to matrigel extracts. Labeling of cell lines with fluorophores of different wavelengths is one method that allows for distinction between cancer cells and stromal cells or other cell types of interest (Fig. 2). These types of models will allow for visualization and eventual dissection of the events that occur when a tumor cell contacts a cell in the target organ. The ability to easily manipulate the cells, in addition to the milieu they are grown in, will lead to many advances in this field.

Ex vivo analysis of harvested organs at various time points following the introduction of metastatic cells will also allow for more refined identification of the different stages of metastases. The ability to analyze samples serially, or for prolonged periods of time, will be instrumental in defining what happens during the early stages of metastases. One of these methods, is described in the chapter by Khanna et al.

In vivo analysis of mice has been successful in revealing the number of metastatic nodules as an endpoint for the metastatic cascade. The development of luminescent

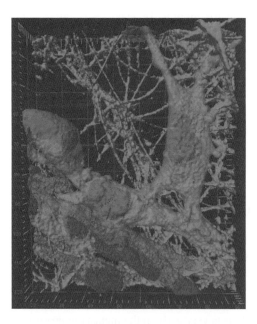

Fig. 2 A reconstruction of a three-dimensional tissue culture system containing osteosarcoma cells (*green*), fibroblasts (*red*) and nuclei (*blue*). Cells were plated in a nanofiber-based (*pink*), matrigel-coated matrix and allowed to grow for 24 h followed by confocal microscopy imaging. Software reconstruction allowed for three-dimensional visualization of the fields

Strategies to Explore New Approaches in the Investigation 525

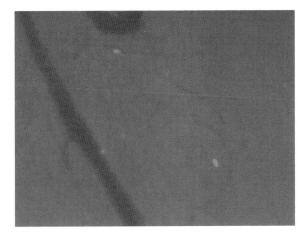

Fig. 3 Fluorescent microscopy demonstrates three single osteosarcoma cells (*green*) in the lung parenchyma, minutes after injection of CMFDA-labeled osteosarcoma cells into the tail vein of a nude mouse, followed by a bolus of Texas-red dextran (red) to visualize the vessels. Time-lapse microscopy allowed for visualization of blood flow (*black*) in the vessels of a live anesthetized mouse. A black and white camera was used for imaging followed by green color rendering of the white fluorescent signal

and fluorescent technology has greatly increased the types of experiments that can be performed in vivo by providing a surrogate marker of the disease burden. Our studies have shown that we can detect a faint luminescent signal prior to the development of grossly visible or palpable metastatic nodules in the lung. Advances in this field are progressing very quickly, and there are a plethora of dyes and markers that span the wavelength spectra, including those in the near infrared range. Coupled with advances in microscopy, the impact of these refinements will greatly advance how we think about metastases. One pilot experiment in our laboratory utilized time-lapse microscopy of anesthetized mice injected with green osteosarcoma cells and red dextran to visualize blood vessels. We were able to detect single cells immediately after their arrival in the lung, and we are currently working to synchronize timed ventilation to timed imaging in an attempt to perform time lapse imaging of a single cell in vivo (Fig. 3). One goal of these types of studies is to visualize what occurs to a single cell when it arrives at its target organ and then to continue to monitor that cell to see if it invades, adheres, proliferates or interacts with other cells.

Therapeutic Implications

The discussions for both metastatic osteosarcoma and recurrent osteosarcoma are very similar. Both are associated with a very poor survival rate of only 25%.[2-4] Attempts at intensification of chemotherapy to target the tumor have resulted in almost no improvement in either group. And in both cases, lack of surgical resection of the tumor leads to an even lower survival rate. We will concentrate on recurrent osteosarcoma, but the same arguments can also be used as the developmental base for clinical trials in patients with metastases.

Approximately 33% of patients who have completed therapy for osteosarcoma will have a recurrence. In large retrospective analyses performed by the Cooperative Osteosarcoma Study Group and the Rizzoli Institute, the only patients who survived long-term were those who achieved complete surgical removal of recurrent tumor.[4,34] Specifically, 291 patients did not achieve surgical remission, and none of these patients survived long-term. In contrast, 512 patients achieved surgical remission and the 5-year overall survival rates were 38% and 30% in the two studies. These patients received either multi-agent, single agent or no chemotherapy, but they shared the common feature that everyone had achieved a second surgical remission. Conversely, for those treated with chemotherapy or radiation therapy only without surgery, there were no survivors.

The above statistics demonstrate several important points to consider in clinical trials. First, and fortunately, there are very few patients who relapse. Secondly, there has been very little uniformity on how they have been treated. Therefore, it is difficult to calculate a true historical survival rate, and even more difficult to calculate what increase in survival advantage will be significant. As models of metastases improve, we will be able to add to the growing number of genes that are important in this process. Active agents for these biological targets are being, or will be, developed. As these agents become available for clinical testing, it is important that concepts of how best to test these agents be available.

For recurrent osteosarcoma, we know that the number of patients will be small to begin with.[4,34] The most rigorous trial would be a randomized, placebo-controlled study using a homogenous patient population, such as those who have achieved complete surgical remission of recurrent disease. Our calculations suggest that in this patient population, in order to detect a 33% increase in overall survival of a test drug versus a placebo, enrollment of over 300 patients would be required (using a two-sided alpha of 0.05 and 82% power). Accrual of 30 patients per year may require the enrollment of every patient in the United States, and even then, the study would last a minimum of 10 years. One compromise is to lower the statistical threshold. For example, the same study using a one-sided alpha of 0.1 would only require enrollment of 88 patients. The time to completion would be significantly reduced. However, the inability to obtain the consensus statistical significance may require a definitive subsequent trial.

Obviously, neither of these options is optimal, but such choices may have to be made in order to complete a clinical trial. One element that can help clinicians develop optimal clinical trials is for researchers to identify which genes are involved in what steps of metastases and recurrence. This will provide the first step to allow for the identification of a homogenous patient population who are most likely to benefit in a clinical trial.

References

1. Dahlin DC, Coventry MB. Osteogenic sarcoma: a study of six hundred cases. *J Bone Joint Surg Am.* 1967;49A:101-110.
2. Bielack SS, Kempf-Bielack B, Delling G, et al. Prognostic factors in high-grade osteosarcoma of the extremities or trunk: an analysis of 1,702 patients treated on neoadjuvant Cooperative Osteosarcoma Study Group protocols. *J Clin Oncol.* 2002;20:776-790.
3. Meyers PA, Schwartz CL, Krailo M, et al. Osteosarcoma: a randomized, prospective trial of the addition of ifosfamide and/or muramyl tripeptide to cisplatin, doxorubicin, and high-dose methotrexate. *J Clin Oncol.* 2005;23:2004-2011.
4. Kempf-Bielack B, Bielack SS, Jurgens H, et al. Osteosarcoma relapse after combined modality therapy: an analysis of unselected patients in the Cooperative Osteosarcoma Study Group (COSS). *J Clin Oncol.* 2005;23:559-568.
5. Sandberg AA, Bridge JA. Updates on the cytogenetics and molecular genetics of bone and soft tissue tumors: osteosarcoma and related tumors. *Cancer Genet Cytogenet.* 2003;145:1-30.
6. Keith WN, Evans TRJ, Glasspool RM. Telomerase and cancer: time to move from a promising target to a clinical reality. *J Pathol.* 2001;195:404-414.
7. Savage SA, Stewart BJ, Liao JS, et al. Telomere stability genes are not mutated in osteosarcoma cell lines. *Cancer Genet Cytogenet.* 2005;160:79-81.
8. Ulaner GA, Huang HY, Otero J, et al. Absence of a telomere maintenance mechanism as a favorable prognostic factor in patients with osteosarcoma. *Cancer Res.* 2003;63:1759-1763.
9. Sanders RP, Drissi R, Billups CA, et al. Telomerase expression predicts unfavorable outcome in osteosarcoma. *J Clin Oncol.* 2004;22:3790-3797.
10. Strahm B, Malkin D. Hereditary cancer predisposition in children: genetic basis and clinical implications. *Int J Cancer.* 2006;119:2001-2006.
11. Wadayama BI, Toguchida J, Shimizi T, et al. Mutation spectrum of the retinoblastoma gene in osteosarcomas. *Cancer Res.* 1994;54:3042-3048.
12. Feugeas O, Guriec N, Babin-Boilletot A, et al. Loss of heterozygosity in the RB gene is a poor prognostic factor in patients with osteosarcoma. *J Clin Oncol.* 1996;14:467-472.
13. Heinsohn S, Evermann U, Stadt UZ, et al. Determination of the prognostic value of loss of heterozygosity at the retinoblastoma gene in osteosarcoma. *Int J Oncol.* 2007;30:1205-1214.
14. Wunder JS, Gokgoz N, Parkes R, et al. TP53 mutations and outcome in osteosarcoma: a prospective, multicenter study. *J Clin Oncol.* 2005;23:1483-1490.
15. Wang LL. Biology of osteogenic sarcoma. *Cancer J.* 2005;11:294-305.
16. Nishijo K, Nakayama T, Aoyama T, et al. Mutation analysis of the RECQL4 gene in sporadic osteosarcomas. *Int J Cancer.* 2004;111:367-372.
17. Pollak M, Sem AW, Richard M, et al. Inhibition of metastatic behavior of murine osteosarcoma by hypophysectomy. *J Natl Cancer Inst.* 1992;84:966-971.
18. Pollak M, Polychronakos C, Richard M. Insulin like growth factor I: a potent mitogen for human osteogenic sarcoma. *J Natl Cancer Inst.* 1990;82:301-305.
19. Burrow S, Andrulis IL, Pollak M, et al. Expression of insulin-like growth factor receptor, IGF-1, and IGF-2 in primary and metastatic osteosarcoma. *J Surg Oncol.* 1998;69:21-27.
20. Mansky PJ, Liewehr DJ, Steinberg SM, et al. Treatment of metastatic osteosarcoma with the somatostatin analog OncoLar: significant reduction of Insulin-like Growth Factor-1 serum levels. *J Pediatr Hematol Oncol.* 2002;24:440-446.
21. Yeatman TJ. A renaissance for Src. *Nat Rev Cancer.* 2004;4:470-480.
22. Webb DJ, Donais K, Whitmore LA, et al. FAK-Src signalling through paxillin, ERK and MLCK regulates adhesion disassembly. *Nat Cell Biol.* 2004;6:154-161.
23. Azuma K, Tanaka M, Uekita T, et al. Tyrosine phosphorylation of paxillin affects the metastatic potential of human osteosarcoma. *Oncogene.* 2005;24:4754-4764.
24. Hood JD, Cheresh DA. Role of integrins in cell invasion and migration. *Nat Rev Cancer.* 2002;2:91-100.

25. Khanna C, Wan X, Bose S, et al. The membrane-cytoskeleton linker ezrin is necessary for osteosarcoma metastasis. *Nat Med*. 2004;10:182-186.
26. Faivre S, Kroemer G, Raymond E. Current development of mTOR inhibitors as anticancer agents. *Nat Rev Drug Discov*. 2006;5:671-688.
27. Chawla SP, Sankhala KK, Chua V, et al. A phase II study of AP23573 (an mTOR inhibitor) in patients (pts) with advanced sarcomas. *J Clin Oncol*. 2005;23(suppl):9068.
28. Chawla SP, Tolcher AW, Staddon AP, et al. Updated results of a phase II trial of AP23573, a novel mTOR inhibitor, in patients (pts) with advanced soft tissue or bone sarcomas. *J Clin Oncol*. 2006;24(suppl):9505.
29. Wan X, Mendoza A, Khanna C, Helman LJ. Rapamycin inhibits ezrin-mediated metastatic behavior in a murine model of osteosarcoma. *Cancer Res*. 2005;65:2406-2411.
30. Muller A, Homey B, Soto H, et al. Involvement of chemokine receptors in breast cancer metastasis. *Nature*. 2001;410:50-56.
31. Laverdiere C, Hoang BH, Yang R, et al. Messenger RNA expression levels of CXCR4 correlate with metastatic behavior and outcome in patients with osteosarcoma. *Clin Cancer Res*. 2005;11:2561-2567.
32. Perissinotto E, Cavalloni G, Leone F, et al. Involvement of chemokine receptor 4/stromal cell-derived factor 1 system during osteosarcoma tumor progression. *Clin Cancer Res*. 2005;11:490-497.
33. Kim SY, Lee CH, Midura BV, et al. Inhibition of the CXCR4/CXCL12 chemokine pathway reduces the development of murine pulmonary metastases. *Clin Exp Metastasis*. 2008;25:201-211.
34. Bacci G, Briccoli A, Longhi A, et al. Treatment and outcome of recurrent osteosarcoma: experience at Rizzoli in 235 patients initially treated with neoadjuvant chemotherapy. *Acta Oncol*. 2005;44:748-755.

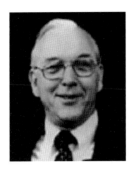

History of Orthopedic Oncology in the United States

Progress from the Past, Prospects for the Future

William F. Enneking

Abstract Orthopedic oncology in the United States has its roots in European medicine of the 1800s in which sarcomas were first classified on the basis of their gross characteristics (1804) and amended on the basis of their histologic features (1867). Surgical management, local excision, with unacceptable mortality gave way to amputation in the 1870s and remained so, until limb-sparing resection was cautiously embarked upon in the mid 1900s. Nonsurgical adjuvant was first devised in the 1880s (as Coley's toxins) but remained largely ineffective until the advent of chemotherapy in the 1970s. The combination of these in the last 30 years, together with vastly improved staging and reconstructive techniques has led to the current preponderance of limb-salvaging surgery and greatly improved survival rates. Their application has been greatly enhanced by the development of Orthopedic oncology fellowships, formation of Orthopedic oncology societies, and the institution of federally funded regional cancer centers with the formation of multidisciplinary sarcoma treatment teams.

History of Orthopedic Oncology in the United States

Like so many of our endeavors, the seeds of Orthopedic oncology as it is today were planted in Europe. The term *sarcoma*, derived from the Greek meaning *fleshy excrescence*, was apparently first used by John Abernathy in 1804 in his paper entitled *Attempts to Form a Classification of Tumours According to Their Anatomical Structure*.[1] Illustrations from publications early in the nineteenth century showed the type of clinical material available to Abernathy (Figs. 1 and 2). His classification was based entirely on the gross characteristics of the various

W.F. Enneking (✉)
Departments of Orthopaedics and Pathology, College of Medicine, University of Florida, Gainesville, FL, USA
e-mail: billkingfisher@aol.com

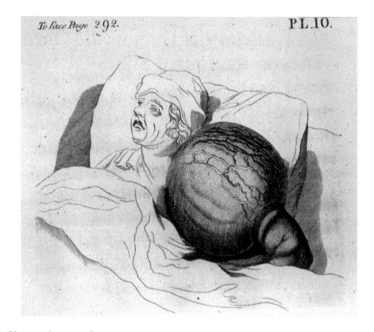

Fig. 1 Untreated sarcoma[1]

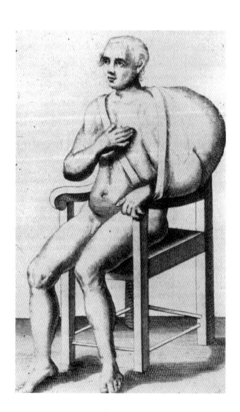

Fig. 2 Large tumor[1]

History of Orthopedic Oncology in the United States

lesions, and he distinguished sarcomas from gumma, tuberculosis, and exostosis by their firm, fleshy feel. Astley Cooper,[2] in 1818, affirmed this classification and noted that in a substantial number of cases, "tumors of a similar kind form in other parts of the body during their progress (Figs. 3 and 4) so also when the affected limb has been amputated a similar disease will occur at a future period, and in organs of the greatest importance to life;" i.e., the first description of subsequent pulmonary metastasis after amputation.[2] Alexis Boyer in 1805[3] introduced the term *osteosarcoma*, while Guillaume Dupuytren in 1847[4] first described its demographics and natural history in some detail. Joseph Recamier introduced the term *metastasis* in 1829.[5] and explained the difference between primary bone and soft tissue lesions and those which involved bone secondarily, i.e., sarcomas vs. metastatic carcinomas. Thus, when in 1829 Jean Cruveilhier[6] published his magnificent 2-volume work on pathologic anatomy, replete with colored illustrations (that no publisher could afford today), a substantial amount of information about sarcomas, as we now understand them, had been accumulated, without the benefit of either the microscope or the X-ray.

Hermann Lebert of Zurich (Fig. 5) is credited with the first description of the microscopic anatomy of bone tumors in 1854 (Fig. 6)[7]. From this point on, all papers dealing with bone and soft tissue tumors would be accompanied by descriptions of the cellular structures of the lesions. The first comprehensive classification of bone tumors based on their histologic features was published by Rudolf Virchow in 1867.[8] Unfortunately, these advances in understanding did little to ameliorate the desperate situation of patients with such tumors. Treatment of patients in those times was delayed until the case was so far advanced that excision or amputation promised only palliation.

In 1879 Samuel Gross of Philadelphia (Fig. 7), published a paper entitled *Sarcoma of the Long Bone Based Upon a Study of One Hundred and Sixty-five Cases* in which he advocated early amputation despite the then operative mortality of 30% because limb-salvaging resection had, in his experience, inevitably led to local recurrence, distant metastasis, and death.[9] Despite the aggressive approach taken with regard to bone tumors after this pivotal paper, survival rates did not significantly improve.

In 1883, on the basis of a serendipitous observation, the first attempt at a nonsurgical adjuvant treatment of bone tumors was devised by William B. Coley of New York Hospital (Fig. 8). He encountered a patient whose inoperable round cell sarcoma of the neck spontaneously regressed after he accidentally contracted erysipelas. When 7 years later the patient was found alive and well, Coley began to inoculate patients with sterilized suspensions of streptococci. He later extended the use of *Coley's Toxins*, as the method had come to be known, following definitive surgery for a variety of sarcomas. In 1914, he reported the results in 90 cases (Fig. 9).[10] Following his death in the 1936, his daughter, not a physician, collected and published the longer-term results, until in 1934, the American Medical Association stated "Coley's toxins are the only effective systemic treatment for cancer." His work formed the basis for the development of the now exciting field of tumor necrosing factors.

Fig. 3 Large tumor[2]

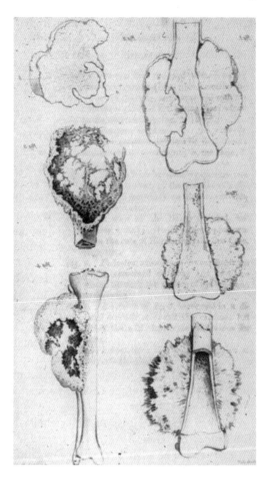

A landmark was Roentgen's discovery of X-rays in 1895.

They were quickly used in both the diagnosis and treatment of bone tumors.

In 1909 Ernest Codman (Fig. 10), Boston-born and bred, described the radiographic characteristics of the periosteal reaction to malignant tumors that, to this day, is know as *Codman's triangle*.[11] He subsequently described *Codman's tumor of the shoulder*, as chondroblastoma was known in that time.[12] Codman was a founder of the American College of Surgeons and, working through this organization, founded the first *Bone and Soft Tissue Sarcoma Registry*, which collected and disseminated information on the diagnosis and treatment of bone tumors. This material was subsequently presented to the Armed Forces Institute of Pathology in 1953 and provided the nucleus for that institution which has done much to enlarge our pathologic database.

At about the same time, James Ewing, the first Professor of Pathology at Cornell Medical College in New York, conducted careful studies of bone tumors. In his textbook

Fig. 4 Large tumor[2]

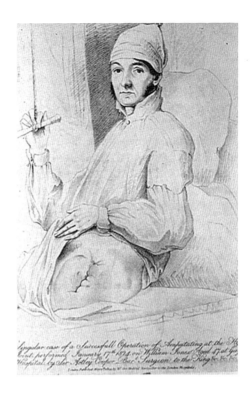

Fig. 5 Herman Lebert

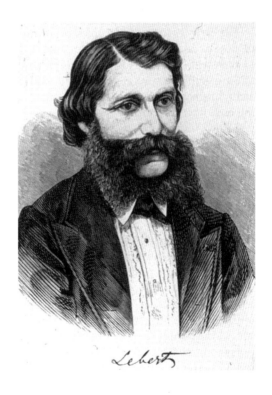

of pathology, he described the tumor that bears his eponym.[13] Ewing became a founder of the American Cancer Society, and his monumental contributions were recognized by his designation as the *Man of the Year* by *Time Magazine* in 1931 (Fig. 11). As a result of these studies, Ewing's growing bias against surgical treatment of bone tumors extended to even biopsy. In 1922, he wrote "clinical history, Roentgen-ray findings, and the response to therapeutic tests with radiation or radium can provide the diagnosis in the great majority of cases. The therapeutic test is, at the same time, the best treatment for a large portion of bone sarcomas."[14] However, the almost universal mortality of tumors treated by radiation equaled the dismal record of amputation. These failures of both surgery and radiation therapy fostered the development of the first preoperative adjuvant protocol, a combination of preoperative radiation followed by amputation 6 months later in those patients who had not developed metastases in the interval. Popularized by Sir Stafford Cade, a British radiotherapist, and Albert Ferguson, a radiologist at the New York Orthopedic Dispensary, its aim was to avoid unnecessary mutilating amputation at all costs.[15] This defeatist attitude persisted throughout the interval between the first and second World Wars and provided the background of skepticism that greeted the reports of 20% 5-year survival after exarticulation that subsequently appeared in the 1950s.[16,17] Ewing's observations were enlarged upon in an extensive monograph on bone tumors published under the aegis of the fledgling American Cancer Society by Charles Geshickter and Murray Copeland in 1931.[18] This monograph, which served as the landmark for the 1930s and 1940s, was based upon the material collected at the Johns Hopkins.

The early 1940s were occupied by World War II, but shortly after the cessation of hostilities, detailed pathologic studies by Henry Jaffe (Fig. 12) and Lewis Lichtenstein from the Hospital for Joint Disease in New York provided a "disease of the month" for several years. Their work established the definition, delineation, and refinement of numerous benign, quasi-benign, and malignant lesions, clarifying both their diagnostic criteria and natural history.[19] Jaffe's text entitled *Tumor and Tumor-like Conditions of Bone* became the bible for the orthopedic oncologists of that era (Fig. 13).[19]

Capitalizing on this knowledge, surgeons in scattered centers, led by the pioneering work of Dallas Phemeister (Fig. 14) and Howard Hatcher (Fig. 15) at the University of Chicago, began to explore limb-salvaging resection in lieu of amputation.[20] Both had studied with Virchow's pupil, Erdheim, in Vienna, and they stressed on obtaining adequate surgical margins in carefully selected cases whose pathologic characteristics made resection, in light of the reconstructive technology of that era, a practicality. Their work established the principles of limb-salvaging surgery as they are practiced today.

The 1950s saw a decade of the gathering of detailed data on the recently defined lesions from many centers. Prominent in this effort was the Armed Forces Institute of Pathology (AFIP), under the direction of Lent Johnson and Jack Ivins (Fig. 16) and David Dahlin (Fig. 17) of the Mayo Clinic. Analysis of the mounting data began to furnish guidelines for the treatment of individual lesions and allowed in-depth extension of the surgical principles established by Phemeister and Hatcher.

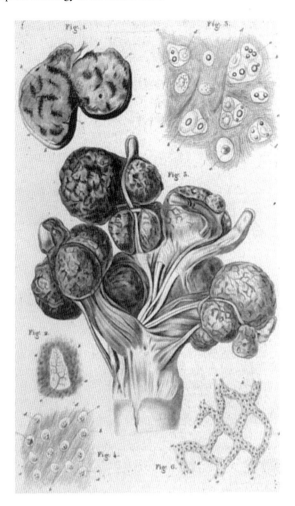

Fig. 6 Microscopic anatomy from bone tumor[7]

In the twenty-first century, there has been an explosion in the understanding of these diseases by developments in biochemical and histochemical markers, ultrastructural morphology, and the beginnings of the unraveling of the mysteries of oncogenetics, immunologic interactions between host and neoplasm, and environmental influences on the genesis of neoplasms, to mention but a few.

The historical perspective of oncologic surgical procedures is equally fascinating. Although there have been accounts of excision of benign exostoses prior to the introduction of anesthesia and aseptic surgical technique, surgical treatment, as we know it today, began in the last quarter of the nineteenth century. Successful curettage followed by packing of the cavity with iodoform gauze for giant cell tumor was reported by Krause in 1889,[21] and in 1898, Hinds[22] first described curettage plus a physical adjuvant in the form of cauterization with zinc chloride. Phenol as a supplement

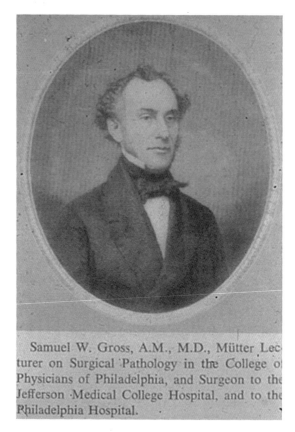

Fig. 7 Samuel N. Gross. Reproduced with permission from Enneking WF. *Clinical Orthopedics and Related Research* 2000;374:15-124

to curettage was described by Joseph Bloodgood in 1902 (Fig. 18), and later in 1912, he advocated subsequent filling of the cavity with autogenous bone chips.[23]

Until the 1960s, curettage and autogenous bone grafting was widely practiced for the treatment of most benign bone tumors. Following the extensive report in 1970 by Goldenberg, Bonfiglio, and Campbell[24] that curettage was associated with an unacceptably high recurrence rate, there was a swing to more aggressive resection with the attendant reconstructive problems and morbidity, as the price to pay for the greatly reduced recurrence rate. In 1965, Marcove et al[25] showed that liquid nitrogen could be used to extend the margins of conservative curettage as a less disabling means of reducing recurrence. Because of the complications of the method, it has been largely replaced by methyl methacrylate, described in 1976 by Person and Wouters[26] in the Netherlands, as the most widely used physical adjuvant. In combination with improvements in staging, imaging, and surgical technique, its widespread use has led to a return to curettage as the procedure of choice for the majority of benign lesions.

Fig. 8 William B. Coley

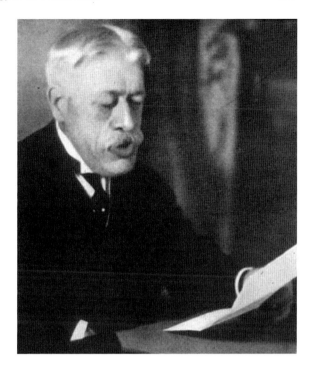

Following the pre-Civil War advocacy of primary amputation for malignant bone tumors, it remained the principal surgical treatment for more than 100 years. However, episodic anecdotes describing limb salvage began to appear even earlier In 1876 in London, Morris[27] reported resection of the distal two-thirds of the radius and ulna for a malignant giant cell tumor. In 1895, Mikulicz[28] published two resection/arthrodeses of the knee for distal femoral lesions, although he was dismayed by the disability that accompanied the shortening of the limb (Fig. 19). In 1908, Lexer[29] described the use of osteoarticular homogenous, now termed allogeneic, bone grafts to reconstruct joint defects produced by tumor resection. In the following year, Tikoff, in Russia, carried out a resection of the scapula and proximal humerus for a malignant tumor of the scapula in lieu of an interscapular-thoracic or forequarter amputation. This procedure was later refined by Linberg.[30] Imagine, if you can, such a procedure with the available technologies of more than a 100 years ago! In 1922, Sauerbruch,[31] in The Netherlands, described *Umkipp plastic* or a "turn-up plasty," in which the tibia was turned up into the defect produced by resection of the entire femur (Figs. 20 and 21). This procedure, the forerunner of modern rotationplasty, is still used to salvage failed total-femoral devices. In 1929, Juvara[32] first described a method of massive autogenous grafting to preserve the functional length of the extremity after a resection/arthrodesis for a distal femoral lesion (Fig. 22). These isolated efforts were first coordinated into a systematic approach to limb salvage by Phemeister. His article entitled *Conservative Bone*

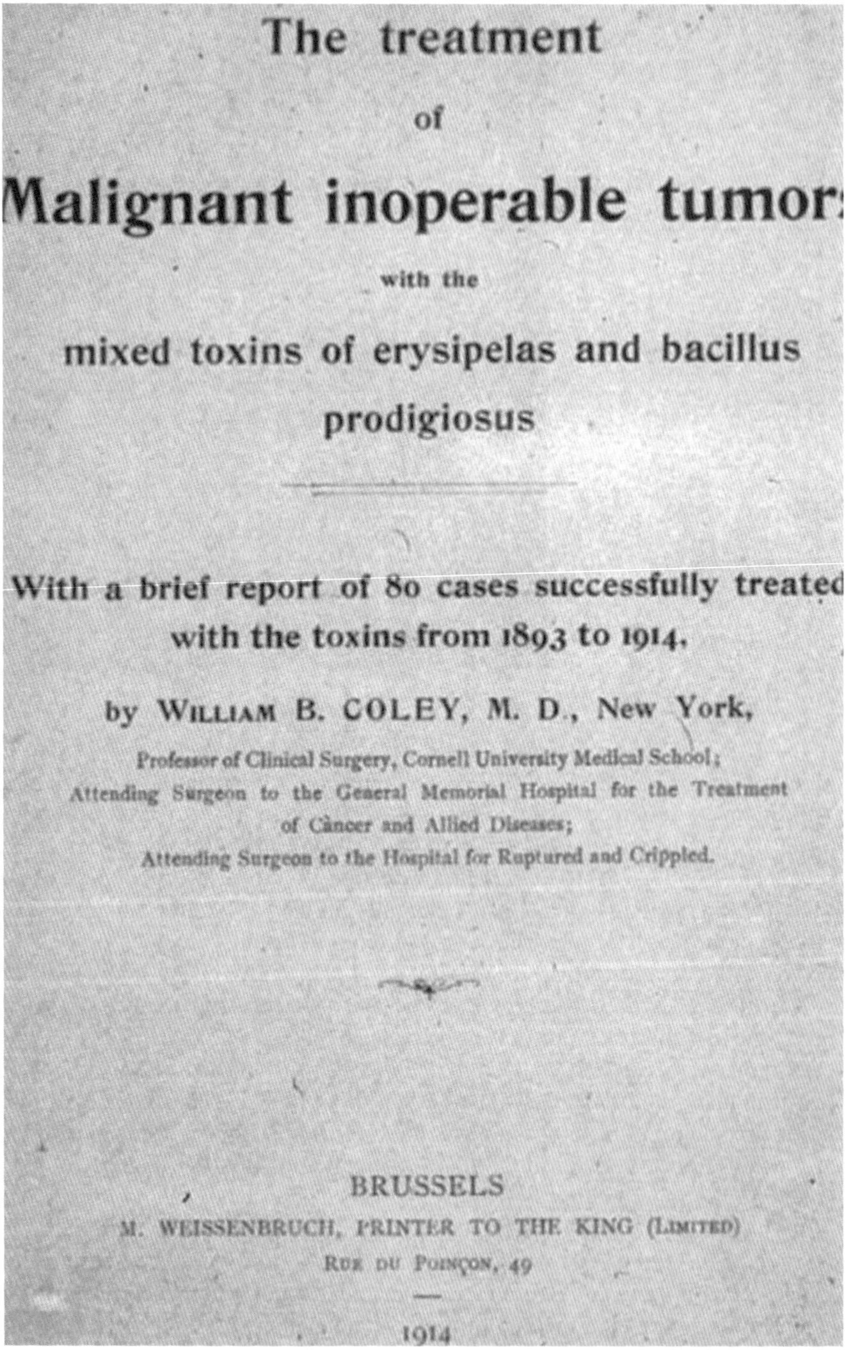

The treatment

of

Malignant inoperable tumors

with the

mixed toxins of erysipelas and bacillus prodigiosus

With a brief report of 80 cases successfully treated
with the toxins from 1893 to 1914.

by WILLIAM B. COLEY, M. D., New York,

Professor of Clinical Surgery, Cornell University Medical School;
Attending Surgeon to the General Memorial Hospital for the Treatment
of Cancer and Allied Diseases;
Attending Surgeon to the Hospital for Ruptured and Crippled.

BRUSSELS

M. WEISSENBRUCH, PRINTER TO THE KING (LIMITED)
RUE DU POINÇON, 49

1914

Fig. 9 Face sheet of Coley's publication[10]

Fig. 10 Earnest Codman

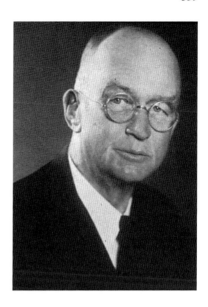

Fig. 11 James Ewing

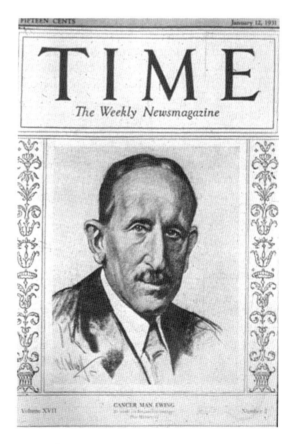

Fig. 12 Henry Jaffe

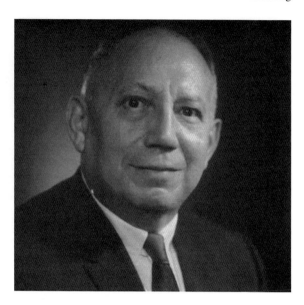

Surgery in the Treatment of Bone Tumors is often cited as a classic in the field of limb salvage[20] (Fig. 23). In it he demonstrated how careful selection of low-grade, and occasionally high-grade, malignancies could provide low-risk candidates for limb-salvaging resection.

In the early 1970s, dramatic changes in diverse fields combined to revolutionize the surgical treatment of malignant bone tumors: (1) the development of chemotherapy; (2) improvements in diagnostic radiographic techniques; (3) advances in reconstructive surgery; (4) improvements in orthopedic oncologic surgical expertise; and (5) establishment of multidisciplinary oncologic referral centers. The following is a brief look at how each of these developments has influenced the field of orthopedic oncology.

Chemotherapy

In 1972, adriamycin was first reported by Cortes et al,[33] from the Roswell Park Cancer Hospital in Buffalo, New York, to be effective in delaying the growth of metastatic osteosarcoma (Fig. 24). Soon, clinical trials were begun to evaluate its use postoperatively in suppressing the development of pulmonary metastases. Because of the relative rarity of the tumor, early reports from the MD Anderson in Houston, the Dana Farber Institute in Boston, and Memorial Sloan Kettering in New York were based on small groups of patients. Larger multi-institutional groups were formed to increase patient accrual – the first such being the South West

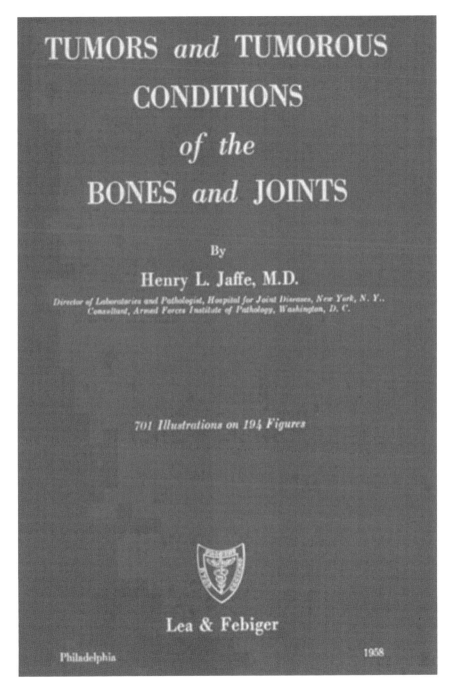

Fig. 13 Face sheet of Jaffe's publication[19]

Fig. 14 Dallas Phemeister

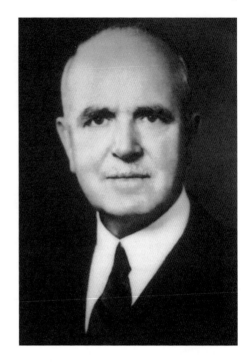

Fig. 15 Howard Hatcher

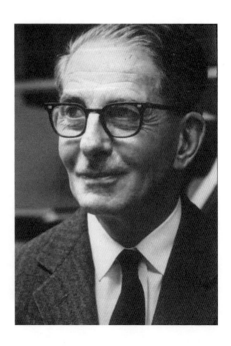

Fig. 16 Jack Ivins

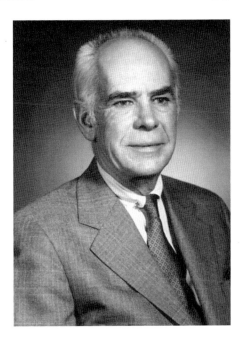

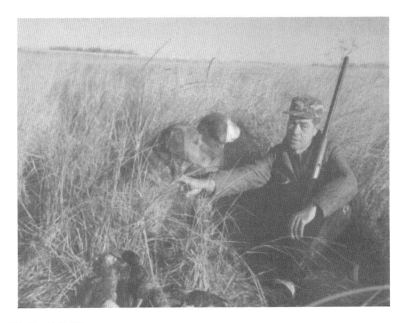

Fig. 17 David Dahlin

Fig. 18 Joseph Bloodgood

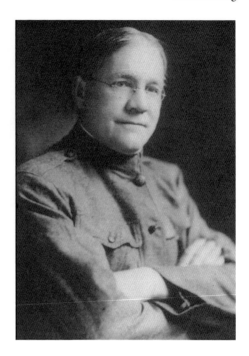

Fig. 19 Resection arthrodesis of knee[28]

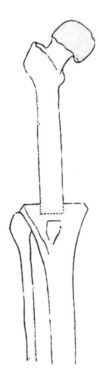

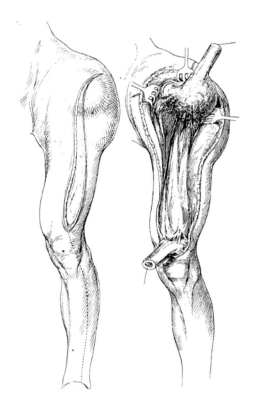

Fig. 20 Procedure in "turn-up plasty," (*Umkipp plastic*) forerunner of modern rotationplasty[31]

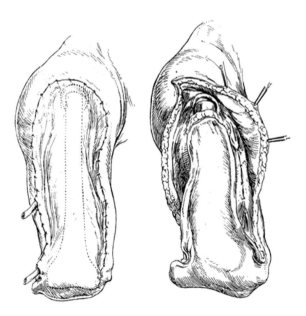

Fig. 21 Procedure in "turn-up plasty," (*Umkipp plastic*) forerunner of modern rotationplasty[31]

546 W.F. Enneking

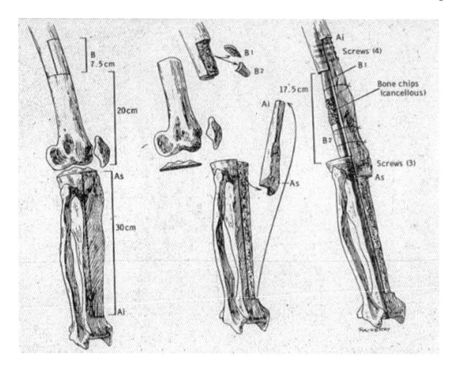

Fig. 22 Massive autogenous grafting[32]

CONCLUSIONS

These experiences warrant the conclusion that in carefully selected cases resection of bone sarcoma and repair of the defect with a bone graft is a justifiable procedure which may save an extremity and carries only slightly more risk to life than does amputation. Also in cases in which for any reason amputation

Fig. 23 Cited in *Conservative Bone Surgery in the Treatment of Bone Tumors*[20]

Oncology Group headed by Wataru Sutow of the MD Anderson Hospital (Fig. 25). By the mid 1960s, it was evident that postoperative chemotherapy was associated with a doubling in crude survival rates from the historical controls.

With the introduction of new drugs and an exponential leap in the number and expertise of medical oncologists, survival rates inched upwards during the 1970s, and orthopedists began to embark on limb-salvaging procedures in lieu of amputation in the hope that the heretofore high local recurrence rates would be improved by postoperative chemotherapy. By the early 1980s, preoperative or neoadjuvant chemotherapy had been introduced, and the dramatic response to the primary lesion in some tumors led to an avalanche of limb-salvaging protocols. In 1981 at the first International Symposium on Limb Salvage (ISOLS), held in Rochester, Minnesota, 532 resections were reported with a local recurrence rate of 18% and a surgical failure rate in reconstruction of 15% for an overall failure rate of 1 in 3 attempts. At the end of the decade, in 1989 at St. Malo, France, more than 2,500 resections were reported with a combined local recurrence and surgical failure rates of 1 in 10 attempts – a remarkable decrease in the short span of one decade. Studies from around the world documented that chemotherapy had made possible a new era of limb-salvaging surgery for malignant tumors that carried no more risk than amputation and yielded disease-free survival rates three times as high as those prior to chemotherapy.[34]

Radiographic Imaging

In the 1950s, diagnostic radiology (Fig. 26) was the mainstay of preoperative diagnosis, and the identification of a bone tumor was the indication for an immediate open biopsy. Following histologic confirmation of the diagnosis, a surgical plan – usually amputation – was immediately carried out. All teaching stressed the need for close cooperation among the radiologic, pathologic, and surgical triad, early biopsy, and swift surgical intervention. In the 1960s, the development of radioisotope scanning and angiography (Fig. 27) laid the foundation for preoperative selection of low-risk candidates for limb-salvage. The development of computerized tomography (Fig. 28) in the 1970s and magnetic resonance imaging (Fig. 29) in the 1980s advanced preoperative staging from an art to a science. They have brought preoperative planning from a resolution of centimeters to millimeters and significantly reduced the morbidity of biopsy and resection. These advances are in large measure responsible for the reduction in local recurrences after limb-salvaging procedures by fostering better patient selection and more accurate operative design.

Advances in Reconstructive Surgery

The first attempts at reconstruction of large defects created by tumor resection utilized autogenous bone grafts. In 1912, Bloodgood[23] described this use of the articular surface of the patella and a sliding tibial bone graft to replace the proximal

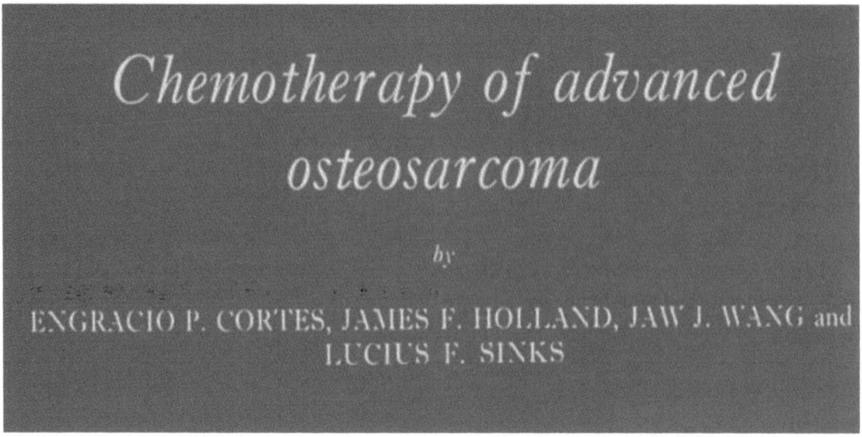

Chemotherapy of advanced osteosarcoma

by

ENGRACIO P. CORTES, JAMES F. HOLLAND, JAW J. WANG and LUCIUS F. SINKS

Fig. 24 Face sheet of publication by Cortes et al[33]

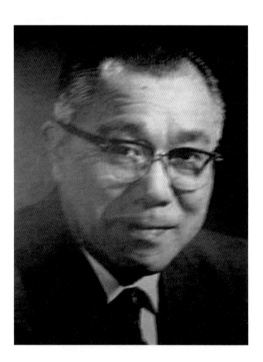

Fig. 25 Wataru Sutow

tibia after resection of a giant cell tumor (Fig. 30). At about the same time, Eric Lexer[29] first described the use of allogeneic osteoarticular allografts to reconstruct tumor defects. The first large series of osteoarticular allografts was reported after World War II by Volkov in Russia.[35] Carlos Ottolenghi (Fig. 31) of Argentina summarized, in 1972, his 40 years of experience in osteoarticular allografting.[36]

History of Orthopedic Oncology in the United States

The first extensive modern bone bank in North America for large segmental reconstruction was established by the US Navy during World War II.

The first series of osteoarticular allografts in the United States was reported by Frank Parrish (Fig. 32) from the MD Anderson Hospital, in 1968.[37] Although these authors reported occasional long-term successes, a high incidence of complications, late disintegration of joint surfaces, and resorption of the grafts more often than not defeated the reconstructive efforts. More recently, improved results have been reported by Czitrom et al[38], by employing fresh articular cartilage and by Mankin et al in Boston, by using cryopreservation of banked allogeneic grafts.[39] Their work has fostered the rapidly expanding use of massive allografts in North America.

The use of conventional autogenous grafts, the mainstay of biologic reconstruction until the 1970s, was constrained by the inadequate stock available for reconstructing large segmental or osteoarticular defects. In 1972, Wilson,[40] summarizing the biomechanical shortcomings of massive autogenous grafts that had been used to reconstruct large bone effects, emphasized these problems. However, technical improvements in microscopic surgery in the 1970s, led to a rebirth in interest in autogenous grafts in the form of vascularized grafts. This interest, however, was far from new. The value of preserving the circulation of a bone graft had been recognized long before. In 1887, Anton Von Eiselberg[41] published a method of incorporating a bone graft into a pedicled skin graft (Fig. 33).

An intriguing attempt to utilize a direct vascular pedicle for a bone graft was reported by Phelps[42] in New York, in 1881. The technique was used to reconstruct a tibial defect after generous excision of a congenital pseudarthrosis of the tibia. He fixed a pedicled bone graft from the proximal ulna of a dog into a boy's tibial defect, with an intramedullary rod (Fig. 34). The boy and dog were immobilized together in plaster but remained united for only 6 days, at which time the pedicle was prematurely divided because of inability to maintain immobilization of the parties. No details were provided on the outcome. The concept of free, rather than pedicled, vascularized autogenous grafts began with the demonstration of the feasibility of vascular anastomosis by Alexis Carrel[43] in 1912, for which he received the Nobel Prize.

The concept, however, did not come to fruition until the technical development of microvascular surgery, in the 1970s. Currently, vascularized grafts, with their ability to hypertrophy and to flourish in compromised beds and with their resistance to the consequences of chemotherapy, have earned for themselves a place of respect, in the oncologist's reconstructive armamentarium. The prospect of successfully combining these principles, a vascularized allogeneic osteoarticular allograft, or even a whole limb is, indeed, fascinating. The groundwork, of course, had already been laid. Saints Cosmos and Damian (Fig. 35) are said to have attempted such a procedure in the fifteenth century.[44]

Paul Bert, a student of Claude Bernard, demonstrated in 1862 successful parabiosis – the surgical production of Siamese twins – in rodents (Fig. 36).[45] Others have demonstrated successful allogeneic limb transplants in rodents using clinically unacceptable methods of immunosuppression.[46] Nevertheless, the seeds have been

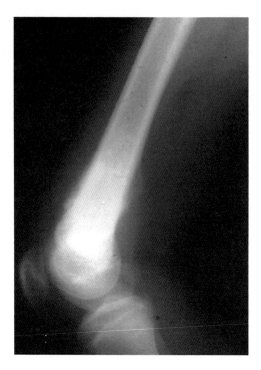

Fig. 26 Radiograph osteosarcoma. Scelortic tumor infiltration of distal femur. Codman`s triangle present. Cortex and periosteum infiltrated and eroded by tumor. Soft tissue swelling noted

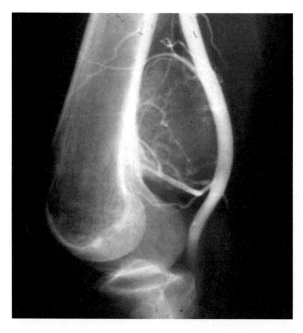

Fig. 27 Angiogram synovial sarcoma. Large tumor on posterior surface with neovasculrity

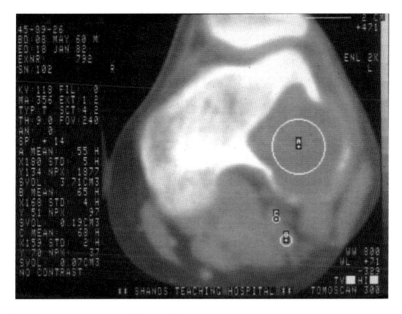

Fig. 28 Computed tomogram of giant cell tumor

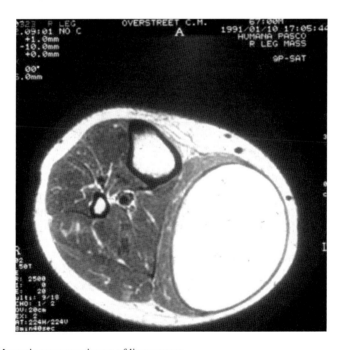

Fig. 29 Magnetic resonance image of liposarcoma

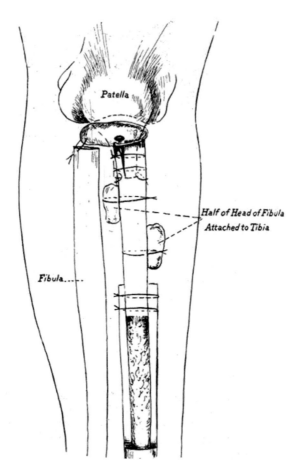

Fig. 30 Articular surface of patella and sliding tibial bone graft to replace proximal tibia after resection[23]

sown, are currently germinating in various laboratories, and will undoubtedly achieve clinical fruition in our lifetime.

A third major reconstructive advance has been the use of prosthetic implants. In 1940, Austin Moore (Fig. 37) in Columbia, South Carolina, performed a reconstruction of the proximal femur after resection of a Stage 3 giant cell tumor, with a metallic prosthesis (Fig. 38). To my knowledge, this was the first such procedure in North America and, perhaps, the world.[47] Moore tested the ability of the device made of a cobalt-steel alloy which he named *vitallium,* to withstand corrosion by burying it in his garden for 6 months before resurrecting it for implantation. Since that modest beginning, several generations of devices and techniques have been developed.

The early attempts were, in the main, palliative, in patients who had refused amputation, adopting devices designed for other purposes that were, by current

Fig. 31 Carlos Ottolenghi

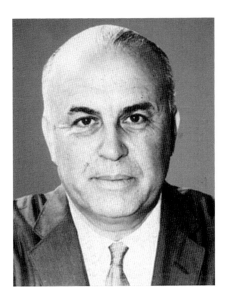

Fig. 32 Frank Parrish

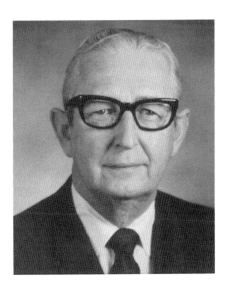

standards, bio-mechanically unacceptable (Fig. 39). However, in the 1970s, with the suddenly rising rates in survival, serious attention was given to designing devices for such purposes. Customized replacements (Fig. 40) pioneered by John Scales[48] in Great Britain, and the development of ingenious modular implants have led to an explosion in the field. Perusing the data from the various limb-salvage symposia, it is evident that in the 1980s, the majority of limb-salvage procedures

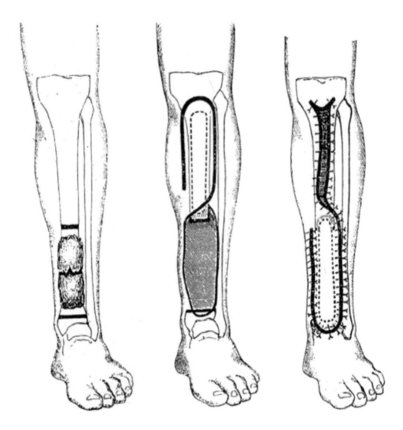

Fig. 33 Incorporating bone graft into pedicled skin graft[41]

were reconstructed prosthetically rather than biologically, while in the 1990s, the reconstructions had been equally divided between the two approaches.

Recently there have been reports of combining prosthetic and biologic techniques – prostheses encased in allografts for better muscle attachment, and biomechanically more sound prosthetic fixation, as well as combinations of vascularized autograft and free allografts for improved rates of union and repair.[34] In fact, a series of prostheses have been designed to replace biologic growth – the so called expanding prostheses. Although the introduction was met with a large dose of skepticism, the oft-cited comparison between reaching the moon and developing enduring prosthetic bones and joints does not seem valid any more.

Surgical Experience

Not the least of the factors that have contributed to these advances has been the increase in surgical expertise. Perusing the historical accounts in this, as in any surgical field, one is struck by the constant reference to a few giants. Until the emergence of

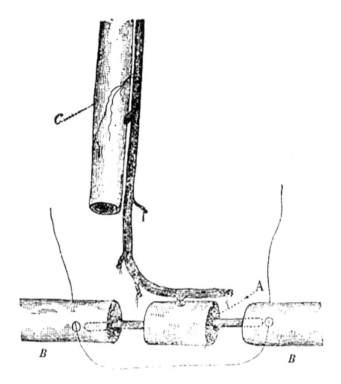

Fig. 34 Vascular pedicled bone graft from the proximal ulna of a dog into a boy's tibial defect with an intramedullary rod[42]

Orthopedics as a specialty, care of sarcomas was in the hands of surgeons-in-general who were usually interested in tumors of all systems. Phemeister,[20] for example, made significant contributions in gall bladder disease and esophageal surgery, in addition to his better-known contributions to musculoskeletal surgery. The bone services of all the major cancer hospitals in the 1960s were staffed by general surgeons. In fact, as recently as 1970, Higgenbothom, a noted sarcoma surgeon at Memorial in New York, wrote that "by training and disposition, oncologic surgery of the musculoskeletal system best be left to general surgeons and kept away from orthopedists." With the advent of limb salvage and the prerequisite expertise in reconstructive skeletal technology, the reins passed to orthopedic oncologists.

But it was not until 1977 that the first orthopedist was appointed to serve as full-time director of the bone service at Memorial; Eugene Mindell became the first full-time orthopedist at the Roswell Park in 1990; and John Murray became the first full-time orthopedist in charge of the bone service at the MD Anderson in 1991 (Fig. 41). However, prior to this, orthopedists in various centers had begun to focus their practices and interests on tumor surgery. Although not formally trained, they recognized the principles of oncologic surgery, particularly as they differed from traditional orthopedic thinking and practice. As they began to publish their experiences and findings, a small informal group formed the nucleus of what became, at its first meeting in Boston in 1977, the Musculoskeletal Tumor Society. One of the requirements for membership was the successful completion of postresidency fellowship, although at that time there were probably no more than three in the United States. Today, there are more than two hundred fellowship-trained orthopedic oncologists with an annual intake of about ten fellows per year amongst the current

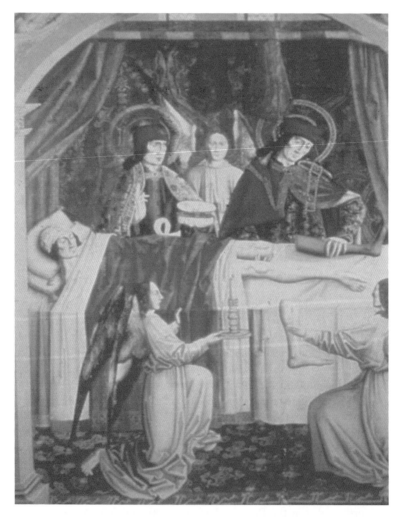

Fig. 35 Saints Cosmos and Damian[44]
Cosmos and Damian appeared to Deacon Justinian who worked in the Basilica of Saints Cosmos and Damian in Rome carrying their instruments and salves and amputated his diseased leg after he had fallen asleep in the church. They replaced the leg from the body of a Moor who had died on that day

History of Orthopedic Oncology in the United States 557

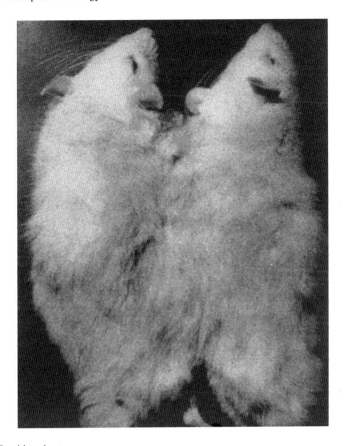

Fig. 36 Parabiosed rats

fellowship programs. In addition, the proceedings of the biannual International Limb Salvage Symposia have been published, and gradually these procedures and techniques have found their way into standard orthopedic surgical teaching and texts. Quite clearly, through their membership and cooperative studies, the Musculoskeletal Tumor Society and its offspring, the International Limb Salvage Symposia, have been prime movers in the development of surgical expertise in this field.

Development of Sarcoma Referral Centers

Prior to World War II, centers for cancer treatment were randomly scattered about the landscape, with few of them having identifiable bone or sarcoma services. During the administration of Richard Nixon, (Fig. 42) stimulated by his proclaimed *"war on cancer,"* regional cancer treatment centers, for the most part clustered

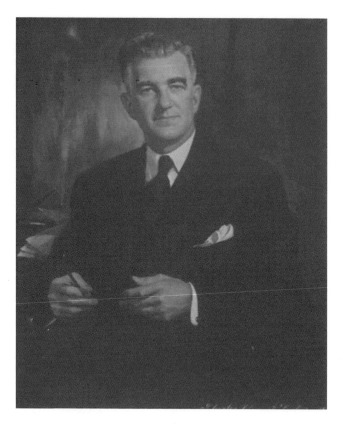

Fig. 37 Austin Moore

about academic institutions, were established with the support of the National Cancer Institute, the National Institutes of Health, and the American Cancer Society. As these centers became established, teams of pathologists, radiologists, surgeons, oncologists, and radiation therapists were formed in various areas of neoplasia, focused usually on one system – i.e., breast, prostate, renal, gastrointestinal, lung, and so on. The establishment of these centers went hand-in-hand with the evolution of staging systems, establishment of professional societies, and the formation of inter-institutional study groups. Amongst the last services to be recognized in these centers were the sarcoma treatment teams. However, with the growing number of oncologic trained orthopedists as their nucleus, sarcoma treatment teams have been formed across the country. This pattern has had a profound effect on the referral patterns for the management of bone and soft tissue sarcomas. Now the patient, whose sarcoma is suspected by a community based orthopedist, usually is promptly referred to a regional center for staging, biopsy, and definitive surgical and adjuvant

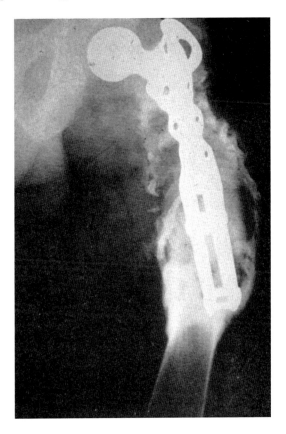

Fig. 38 Radiograph of Moore's prosthesis

treatment. The results of this far-sighted approach of 40 years ago are evident all about us. It was the right program, in the right place, at the right time! To it must go, together with technical and professional advances, the credit for the rapid rise in survival rates and the increase in the quality of these patients' lives.

Current History

So where are we in the twenty-first century? This estimate can best be gleaned from the data provided by the biannual symposia of the International Society of Limb Salvage covering the past 25 years. The Organization has convened in various parts of the globe (Fig. 43). The number of patients reported at the meetings is presented in Fig. 44. The data is admittedly soft, but the number of patients is large enough to

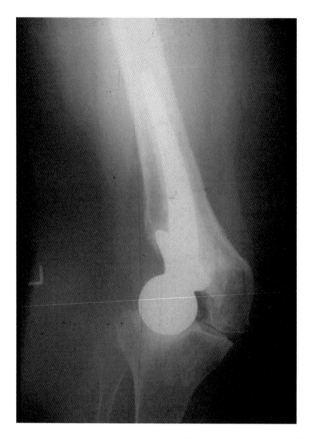

Fig. 39 Thompson hip prosthesis used to reconstruct distal femoral condyle (1957)

indicate the current situation. Approximately 5/6 of sarcoma patients are low risk candidates for limb salvage procedures rather than amputation (Fig. 45). The 5-year survival rates for limb salvage patients had risen to approximately two-thirds by the early 1990s and have not appreciably increased during the past 15 years (Fig. 46). This parallels the survival rate for amputation. The incidence of local recurrence decreased from 18% in 1981 to less than 10% by the early 1990s but with longer follow-up has slowly risen and remains at 15% (Fig. 47). This is considerably larger than the 3% for comparable amputation.

Approximately one fourth of limb salvage procedures have a significant surgical complication compromising function (Fig. 48). This is considerably greater than the less than 5% for amputation.

The satisfactory functional outcomes for limb salvage procedures are approximately double that of amputation – two of three against one of three (Fig. 49). However, the psychosocial assessments in terms of education, occupation, limitation of activity,

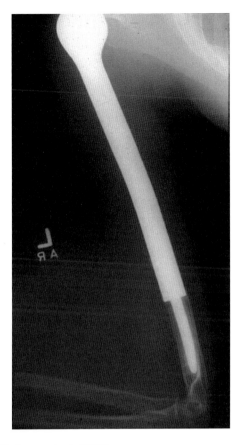

Fig. 40 Customized Scales prosthesis (1985)

pain, emotional distress, social interaction, self image, and rehabilitation show no significant differences between patients treated by limb salvage and amputation (Fig. 50). With the remarkable advances in customized prosthetic capabilities, in many instances amputees may out-perform the more fragile reconstructed limbs (Fig. 51). The world's record for the 100 meter dash by female athletes is less than 2 s behind that of normal athletes (Fig. 52). Figure 53 demonstrates that both the limb salvage patient on the right, whose X-ray of his reconstructed leg is in the middle panel, and the above-knee amputee on the left, are successful triathlon competitors. In contrast, more sedentary patients such as this schoolteacher with her reconstructed arm often have greater capabilities than those with shoulder disarticulations (Fig. 54). And as this young family shows, the mother whose osteosarcoma was resected and lower extremity reconstructed at age fifteen, has realized the benefits of her limb-salvaging management (Fig. 55).

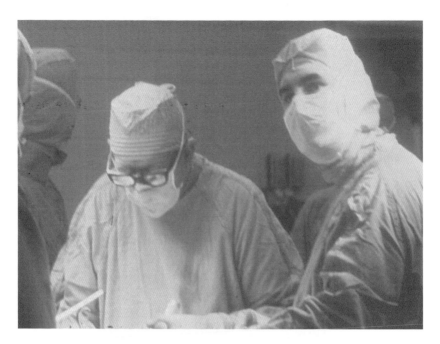

Fig. 41 John Murray (center) in operating room

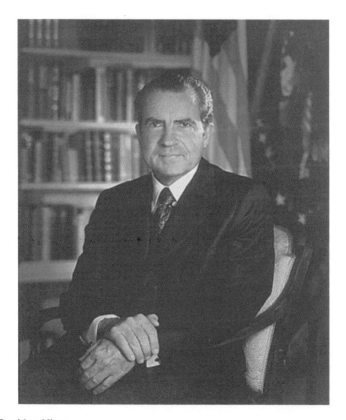

Fig. 42 President Nixon

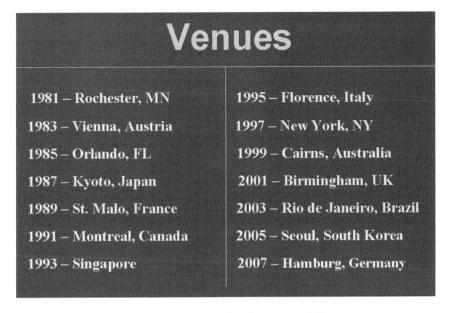

Fig. 43 Venues of the International Society of Limb Salvage (ISOLS)

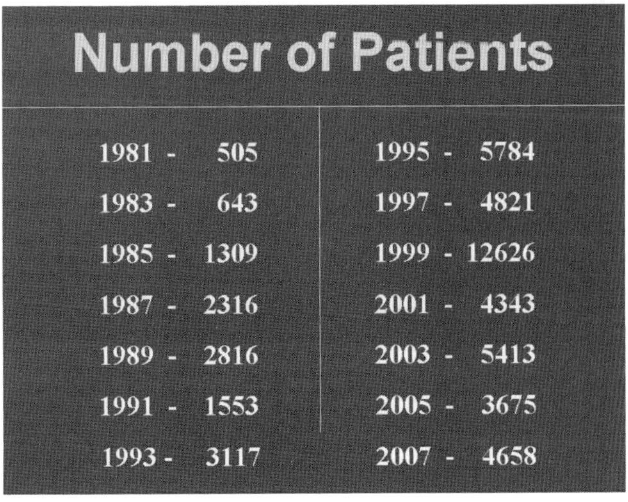

Fig. 44 Data Base of the International Society of Limb Salvage (ISOLS)

Limb Salvage vs. Amputation
Incidences
L.S. AMP
Adult 85 % 15 %
Child 75 % 25 %

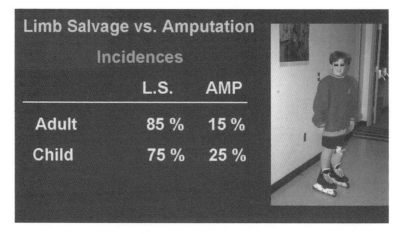

Fig. 45 Incidence of Limb Salvage vs. Amputation. Data reported at the International Society of Limb Salvage (ISOLS)

Survival: 5 Years
1981 - 225 / 505 44%
1983 - 328 / 643 51%
1985 - 825 / 1309 63%
1987 - 1343 / 2316 58%
1989 - 1913 / 2816 68%
1991 - 1025 / 1553 66%
1993 - 2182 / 3117 70%
1995 - 3986 / 5784 69%
1997 - 3278 / 4821 68%
1999 - 5704 / 8034 71%
2001 - 3190 / 4343 73%
2003 - 3936 / 5413 69%
2005 - 2646 / 3675 72%
2007 - 3210 / 4658 70%

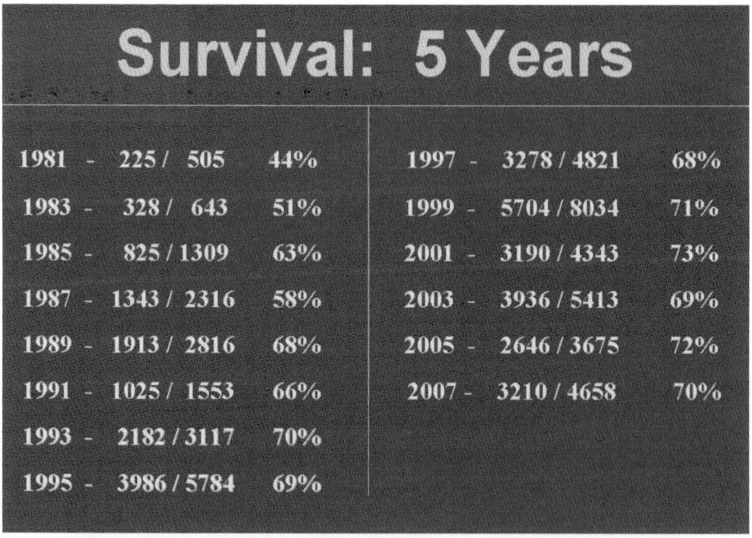

Fig. 46 Survival the International Society of Limb Salvage (ISOLS). Data reported at the International Society of Limb Salvage (ISOLS)

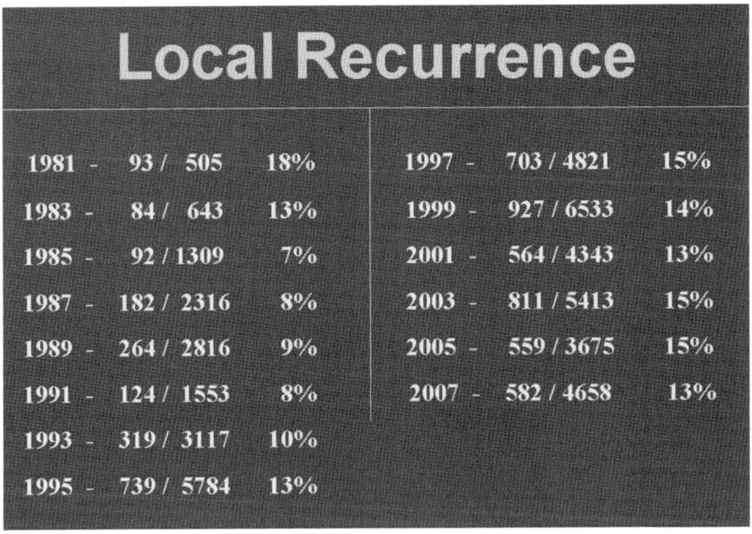

History of Orthopedic Oncology in the United States 565

1981	93 / 505	18%	1997	703 / 4821	15%
1983	84 / 643	13%	1999	927 / 6533	14%
1985	92 / 1309	7%	2001	564 / 4343	13%
1987	182 / 2316	8%	2003	811 / 5413	15%
1989	264 / 2816	9%	2005	559 / 3675	15%
1991	124 / 1553	8%	2007	582 / 4658	13%
1993	319 / 3117	10%			
1995	739 / 5784	13%			

Fig. 47 Local recurrence data reported at the International Society of Limb Salvage (ISOLS)

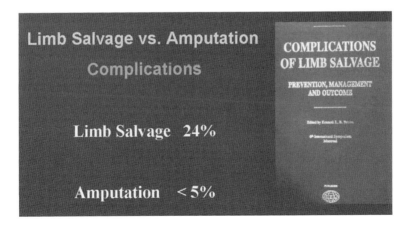

Fig. 48 Complications. Data reported at the International Society of Limb Salvage (ISOLS)

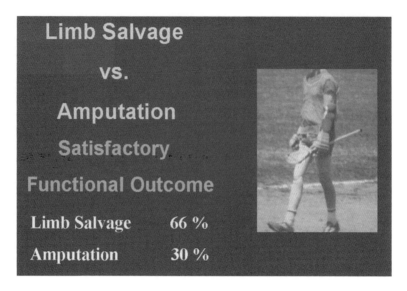

Fig. 49 Functional outcome. Data reported at the International Society of Limb Salvage (ISOLS)

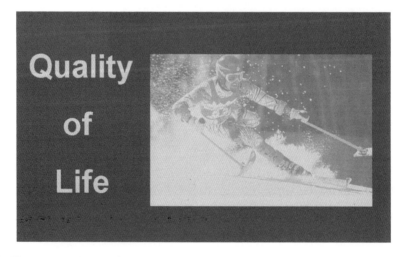

Fig. 50 Amputee adept at skiing

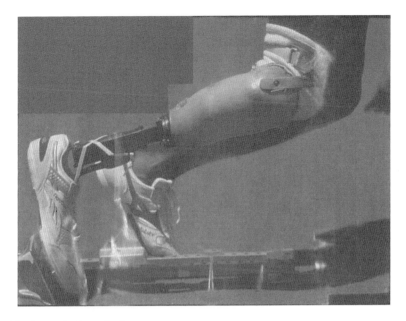

Fig. 51 Customized prosthesis

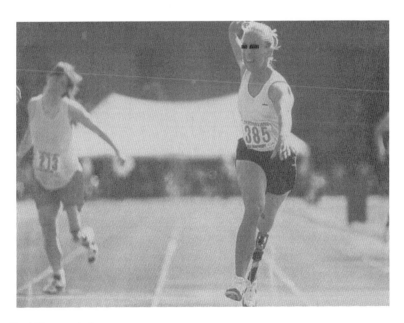

Fig. 52 100 meter dash

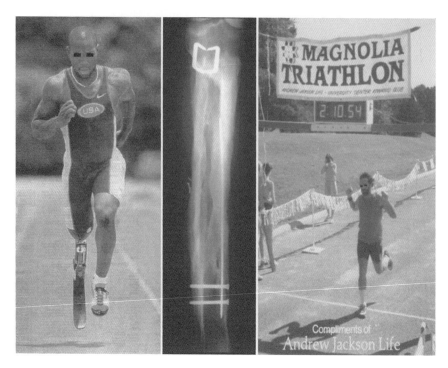

Fig. 53 Triathlon competitors

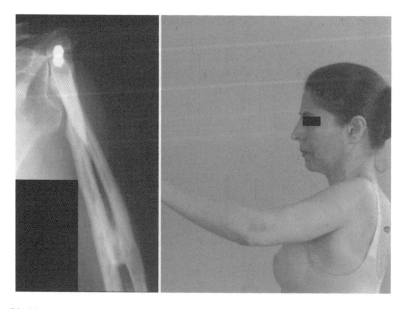

Fig. 54 Limb salvage – upper extremity

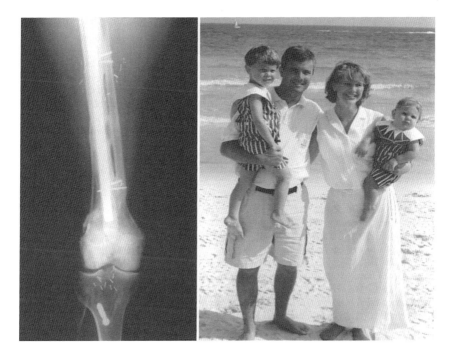

Fig. 55 Limb salvage – lower extremity

References

1. Abernathy J. *Surgical Observations on Tumors*. London: Longman and Rees; 1804.
2. Cooper A, Travers B. *Surgical Essays, Part I*. 3rd ed. London: Cox and Son; 1818:169-223.
3. Boyer A. *The Lectures of Boyer Upon Disease of the Bone*. Philadelphia: James Humphreys; 1805:182-186.
4. Dupuytren G. *On Injuries and Diseases of Bones* [Le Gros Clark F, Trans.]. London: Sydenham Society; 1847:418.
5. Recamier JC. *Recherches sur le Traitment du Cancere par la Compression Methodique*. Paris: Gabon; 1829.
6. Cruveilhier J. *Anatomie Pathologique Kdu Corps Humaine*. Paris: JB Baillier; 1829.
7. Lebert H. *Physiologie Pathologiques des Recherches Cliniques, on Experimentales et Microscopiques, etc*. Paris: JB Bailliere; 1845.
8. Virchow R. *Die Krankenhaften Gewulstewulste*. Berlin: Hirschwald; 1867:170-384.
9. Gross SW. Sarcoma of the long bones: Based on a study of one hundred sixty-five cases. *Am J Med Sci*. 1879;8:338-377.
10. Coley W. *The Treatment of Malignant inoperable Tumors with the Mixed Toxins of Erysipelas and Bacillus Prodigiosus*. Brussels: W Eisenbruch; 1914.
11. Codman EA. The Use of the X-ray and Radiation in Surgery. In: Keen WB, ed. *Surgery, Its Principles and Practice by Various Authors*. Philadelphia: WB Saunders; 1909:1170.
12. Codman EA. *The Shoulder*. Thomas Todd Co, Printers: Boston; 1934.
13. Ewing J. *Neoplastic Diseases*. Philadelphia: WB Saunders Co; 1919.
14. Ewing J. An analysis of radiation therapy in cancer. *Trans Coll Phys Philadelphia*. 1922;44:190-235.

15. Ferguson AB. Treatment of osteogenic sarcoma. *J Bone Joint Surg.* 1940;22:92-96.
16. Coly BL, Harrold CC Jr. An analysis of fifty-five cases of osteogenic sarcoma with survival for five years or more. *J Bone Joint Surg.* 1950;32A:307-310.
17. Coventry MB, Dahlin DC. Osteogenic sarcoma: A critical analysis of 430 cases. *J Bone Joint Surg.* 1957;39A:741-757.
18. Geshickter CE, Copeland MM. Tumors of Bone. *Am J Cancer* New York City, 1931.
19. Jaffe HL. *Tumors and Tumorous Conditions of the Bone and Joints.* Philadelphia: Lea & Febiger; 1958.
20. Phemister DB. Conservative surgery in the treatment of bone tumors. *Surg Gynecol Obstet.* 1940;70:355-364.
21. Krause F. Uber die Behandlund der Schaligen Myelogenen Sarkome (Myeloide, Riesen-zellenmark-sarkome Durch k Aus Raumung Anstart Durch Amputation. *Verb Dtsch Ges Chir.* 1889;18:198-202.
22. Hinds F. Case of myeloid sarcoma of the femur treated by scraping. *Br Med J.* 1898;1:555.
23. Bloodgood J. The conservative treatment of giant cell sarcoma with the study of bone transplantation. *Ann Surg.* 1912;56:210-239.
24. Goldenberg RR, Campbell CP, Bonfiglio M. Giant cell tumor of bone. An analysis of two hundred and eighteen cases. *J Bone Joint Surg.* 1970;52A:619-664.
25. Marcove RC, Wers LD, Vagharwalla MR, et al. Cryosurgery in the treatment of giant cell tumors of bone: A report of 52 consecutive cases. *Clin Orthop.* 1978;34:275-289.
26. Person BM, Wouters HW. Curettage and acrylic cementation in surgery of giant cell tumors of bone. *Clin Orthop.* 1976;120:125-133.
27. Morris H. Conservative surgery. *Lancet.* 1876;1:440.
28. Mikulicz J. Ueber Ausgedehnte Resectionen der langen Rohrenknochen Weten Maligner Geschwulste. *Arch Klin Chir.* 1895;50:60-75.
29. Lexer E. Die Vervendung der freien Knochenplastikk nebst Versuchen udber Glenk-versteifung und Gelenktransplantation. *Arch Klin Chir.* 1908;86:939-954.
30. Linberg BE. Interscapulo-thoracic resection for malignant tumors of the shoulder joint region. *J Bone Joint Surg.* 1928;10:344-349.
31. Sauerbruch F. Die Extripatipn des Femur mit Umkipp-Plastik des Unterschenkels. *Dtsch Zeit Chir.* 1922;169:1-12.
32. Juvara E. Reconstitution de la tige osseuse femorotibbiale. *Bull Mem Soc Nat Chir.* 1929;55:541-556.
33. Cortes EP, Holland JF, Wang JJ, et al. Amputation and adriamycin in primary osteo-sarcoma. *N Engl J Med.* 1974;291:998-1000.
34. Enneking WF. *Limb Salvage in Musculoskeletal Oncology.* Churchill Livingstone: New York; 1987.
35. Volkov V. Allotransplantation of joints. *J Bone Joint Surg.* 1970;52B:49-53.
36. Ottolenghi CE. Massive osteo and osteo-articular bone grafts: Technic and results in 62 cases. *Clin Orthop.* 1972;87:156-164.
37. Parish FF. Treatment of bone tumors by total excision and replacement with massive autologous and homologous grafts. *J Bone Joint Surg.* 1968;48A:968-990.
38. Czitrom AA, Keating S, Gross AE. The viability of articular cartilage in fresh osteo-chondoral grafts after clinical transplantation. *J Bone Joint Surg.* 1990;72A:574-581.
39. Mankin HJ, Fogelson FJ, Thrasher DZ, et al. Massive resection and allograft transplantation in the treatment of malignant bone tumors. *N Engl J Med.* 1976;294:247-255.
40. Wilson PD Jr. A clinical study of the biomechanical behaviour of massive bone transplants used to reconstruct large bone defects. *Clin Orthop.* 1972;87:81-109.
41. von Eiselsberg A. Zur heilungkgrosser defecte der tibia durch gestielte haut-periost-knochenlappen. *Arch Klin Chir.* 1887;55:435-444.
42. Phelps AM. Transplantation of tissue from lower animals to man. *Med Rec.* 1881;39:221-225.
43. Carrel A. Results of transplantation of blood vessels, organs and limbs. *J Am Med Assoc.* 1908;51:162-167.

History of Orthopedic Oncology in the United States

44. Peltier LF. Patron saints of medicine. *Clin Orthop.* 1997;334:374-379.
45. Bert P. *Greffe Animale Parapproache [De Deux Jeunes Rats Albinos Dequinze Jours].* Paris: Impr Coson; 1862.
46. Burchardt H, Glowczewskie FP, Enneking WF. Short-term immuno-supression with fresh segmental fibular allografts in dogs. *J Bone Joint Surg.* 1981;63A:411-415.
47. Moore AT, Bohlman HR. Metal hip joint: A case report. *J Bone Joint Surg.* 1943;25:88-92.
48. Scales JT, Waite ME, Wright KW. Intramedullary fixation of "custom made" major endoprostheses with special reference to the bone response. *Eng Med.* 1984;13:185-189.

Editorial Summation

What have we learned, where do we stand and where do we go from here?

The conference, including questions presented to the speakers, and the chapters appearing herein provided an extensive overview of our current understanding of osteosarcoma: epidemiology, and etiology were reviewed and an opportunity was provided to examine the management of this disease in different institutions. This included clinical, radiological, and pathological investigation and treatment with chemotherapy and surgery and, in selected cases, radiotherapy. Nursing and physical as well as occupational therapy were addressed, and factors relating to the quality of life including information on external prostheses available for amputee patients were presented. However, despite "delving" into many therapeutic regimens and a plethora of scientific reports as well as presentations of several innovative concepts and investigations, suggestions for the immediate application of promising new clinical treatments to conquer osteosarcoma did not emerge.

The different therapeutic approaches were of interest and worthy of note. They varied in complexity and strategy. The elixir of agents was not always successful and a change to an alternative combination in some instances could prove highly rewarding. It should be recognized that in the heterogeneous group "nonclassical osteosarcoma" comprising more than 40% of an unselected patient population, the prognosis is often dismal.

Notwithstanding the results in general were similar and essentially no major change in survival has occurred over the past 30 years. However, major advances in surgical techniques currently secure limb salvage in the vast majority of osteosarcoma patients. Furthermore, advances in supportive care have improved patients' quality of life over the years, both during treatment and thereafter.

The intelligent and innovative reader will readily acknowledge that the information provided will permit him/her to utilize or design protocols to suit the needs of their patient's varied circumstances. Deployment of less complicated protocols yielding similar results was of interest in this context. Also of note was the demonstration that in this age of instant electronic communication successful international collaboration (EURAMOS) is a viable possibility.

Novel strategies and new effective chemotherapeutic agents appeared an urgent dominant theme to further improve the outlook. The absence of such provided provocative questions and a stimulus to undertake additional scientific investigation and therapeutic research. The following enquiries arising from our review and questions from the participants may be considered a springboard for possible further fruitful clinical and scientific studies. These are but a few of the many questions and comments raised in our review and by the participants in the treatment and investigation of osteosarcoma:

- What is the role of second-line chemotherapy in addition to thoracotomy in patients relapsing with lung metastases?
- Is neoadjuvant/preoperative versus postoperative adjuvant chemotherapy (only) mandatory in all cases?
- Is there an impact of age distribution ("pediatric age" should be defined) when analyzing results from various trials/collaborative groups/countries/continents?
- What are the pros/cons for implementing a risk-adapted treatment strategy?
- Is there an impact on survival from dose intensities of each individual drug (or two to three of the most active) versus overall dose intensity/toxicity using four drugs?
- Does the lower jaw osteosarcoma carry a different tumor biology – are micrometastases frequent? Hence, is there a need for adjuvant chemotherapy?
- What is the role of radiotherapy as an ultimate resort for relapsed patients?
- Is there any role for the use of weekly cisplatin as a radiation sensitizer in the primary multimodal treatment strategy?
- Is there a role for implementation of novel targeted treatment principles?
- How can we avoid clinical studies which involve "end-stage" patients only and, hence, draw wrong conclusions on effect or lack of effect?
- Are there methods to determine the presence of pulmonary micrometastases: functional imaging, including PET, radio-guided techniques, or molecular pathology?
- What is the role of immunotherapy (if any)?
- Can the caliber of limb salvage prostheses be improved to prevent complications?
- Is biological reconstruction in limb salvage superior to mechanical internal prostheses?
- Does local recurrence or infection in limb salvage patients invariably result in amputation?
- Are there new strategies to treat residual microscopic disease at the surgical margins?
- Is a change in chemotherapy required if the tumor responds poorly to preoperative treatment. Does this depend on the degree of tumor necrosis?
- What other scientific studies are required to conquer the disease?

Editorial Summation

A Final Comment

The conference (like many others) had both weak and strong points. The authors and organizers apologize for any unintended weak points and perceived deficits; fortunately, there seem to have been few. The evaluations were overwhelmingly positive and enthusiastic and participants were extremely generous with their accolades. This was due entirely to the caliber of the proffered material and presentations by the speakers. One dominant fact emerged: in the mid-century of the past era, the diagnosis of osteosarcoma was contemplated with fear and despair. The discovery that high-dose methotrexate and adriamycin were effective in the disease generated hope to physicians and patients. Investigations raised the expectation of new strategies in treatment. Expectation soon turned Hope into Reality. It is in this spirit that the editors reviewed the content of the conference and elected to present some of the comments and questions raised by participants and their critique. The burden of Hope to discover a complete cure is reflected in the Progress of the Past and demonstrates Realistic Prospects for the Future.

Norman Jaffe
Øyvind S. Bruland
Stefan Bielack

Index

A

Absolute neutrophil count (ANC), 321
Acellular tumor-produced matrix, 77
Active immunotherapy, in osteosarcoma, 449–451
Adjuvant chemotherapy, 220–221, 232–233
  chemotherapy, 221–223
  controversy, 223–230
  in dogs, 443
  MIOS ramifications, 232
  multi-institutional osteosarcoma study, 230–232
  in osteosarcoma, 277–278
  treatment, 233–234
Adolescence osteosarcoma
  imaging techniques
    conventional radiography, 35–41
    extended diagnostic and therapeutic, 42–51
  rehabilitation
    current occupational-therapy, 376, 378–379
    current physical-therapy, 372–376
    discharge recommendations, 381–382
    future perspectives, 382
    interdisciplinary rehabilitation team, 368–369
    occupational-therapy and physical-therapy interventions, 379–381
    rehabilitation therapy, historical perspectives, 369–372
Adolescent and pediatric patients
  prosthetics, 395–396
    foot, 402–407
    knee, 408–409
    liners, 412
    lower extremity design, 400–402
    personal care and hygiene, 418
    principles, 396–398
    prosthesis care, 417–418
    socket accommodation, 409–412
    suspensions, 412–414
    upper extremity, 398–400
    Van Ness rotationplasty, 414–417
  surgical treatment (*see also* Osteosarcoma pulmonary metastases)
    evaluation, 186–188
    future perspectives, 199
    historical background, 185–186
    outcomes, 194–198
    surgical resection, 188–194
Adoptive immunotherapy, 453–454
Adriamycin and dacarbazine (ADIC), 357
Adriamycin, in metastatic osteosarcoma treatment, 540
Aerosol gemcitabine, role, 205, 505
Aerosol therapy, in OS lung metastases treatment, 503–506
AFIP. *See* Armed Forces Institute of Pathology
African Americans, osteosarcoma incidence, 7
Alkylating agents exposure, in osteosarcoma occurrence, 26
Allogeneic osteoarticular allografts, in tumor defects reconstruction, 548
Allografts transplantation, usage, 136–137. *See also* Skeletal reconstruction
Alternative lengthening of the telomeres (ALT), 518–519
American Society of Clinical Oncology, 232
Amoureaux, role, 448
Amputation, for osteosarcoma treatment, 141, 276, 372
Aneurysmal bone cysts and osteosarcoma, 100–103
Angiogram synovial sarcoma, 550
Angiography, in osteosarcoma diagnosis, 42
Anthracyclines usage and osteosarcoma, 26
Area under the curve (AUC), 50

Armed Forces Institute of Pathology, 534
ASCO. *See* American Society of Clinical
    Oncology

B

Bacillus Calmette-Guerin (BCG), 449
Barium, in lung tissue marking, 192
Benign lung lesions, histology, 170–171
Biological constructs, for osteosarcoma
    treatment, 134–138. *See also*
    Skeletal reconstruction
Biologic reconstruction techniques, usage, 328
Biopsy, for osteosarcoma treatment, 73,
    126–127. *See also* Skeletal
    reconstruction
Bleomycin, cyclophosphamide, dactinomycin
    (BCD), 291, 310, 357
Bloom syndrome, 24
Bone abnormalities and OS, 24
Bone and joint cancers, incidence rate, 5
Bone and limb development, notch pathway
    signaling, 481–482
Bone cancer treatment, amputation, 424
Bone cysts and ostersarcoma, 119–120
Bone graft, in pedicled skin graft, 554
Bone-marrow (BM), 510
    micrometastases, immunomagnetic
        isolation procedure, 509–510
        background, 510–511
        future perspectives, 513
        materials and methods, 511–512
        outcomes, 512–513
Bone replacement, for osteosarcoma
    treatment, 138–139. *See also*
    Skeletal reconstruction
Bone resections, types, 129–130
Bone scintigraphy, usage, 171
Bone-seeking radioisotope, usage, 160–161
Bone transportation, application, 139. *See also*
    Skeletal reconstruction
Bone trauma and osteosarcoma, 28
Bone tumor. *See* Osteosarcoma (OS)
5′-Bromodesoxyuridine (BUdR), 161

C

Cade method, in osteosarcoma treatment, 276
Calendars, in OS patients treatment, 386–387.
    See also Nursing, in OS patients
    treatment
Canadian Sarcoma Group (CSG), 264
Cancer, notch pathway signaling, 482

Cancer rehabilitation, goals, 369
Canine osteosarcoma, 440
    bone growth, 440
    and human osteosarcoma, 440
    lytic lesions, 441
    metastastatic progression, 443
    risk factors, 439
Carboplatin drug, 253
Cell surface receptors, modulation, 521–523
Centers for Disease Control and Prevention
    (CDC), 8
Chemokines, in osteosarcoma metastases, 522
Chemotherapy
    agents, 340
    analysis, COSS protocol, 150–151
    in dogs, 443
    EOI in osteosarcoma treatment, 269–270
    era, 277–281
    extra pulmonary metastases, 205
    late effects, 283–284
    limitation, 255–257
    in metastases osteosarcoma, 205 (*see also*
        Pulmonary metastases, in
        osteosarcoma)
    in multimodality treatment of
        osteosarcoma, 322–323
        dose intensity and acute toxicity,
            329–330
    in neoadjuvant COSS, 292
    neoadjuvant, in osteosarcoma, 278–281
    nurse role, 388–389
    in orthopedic oncology, 540–547 (*see also*
        Orthopedic oncology, in United
        States)
    in osteosarcoma, 51–54
        adjuvant, 277–278
        neoadjuvant, 278–281
        side effect, 432
    preoperative, 462–464
    for primary pulmonary metastases,
        176–177
    in pulmonary metastases, 205
Chemotherapy, effect evaluation, 76–77
Childhood osteosarcoma
    imaging techniques
        conventional radiography, 35–41
        extended diagnostic and therapeutic,
            42–51
    multimodality therapy in Turkey
        characteristics and variables evaluation,
            323–324
        complications in treatment, 329–330
        follow-up, 325

outcomes, 325–329, 334–336
patients and methods, 321–322
response assessment, 324
survival, outcome and prognosis, 330–334
toxic effects and statistical analysis, 324–325
treatment, 322–323
Children's Cancer Group (CCG), 342
Chondroblastic osteosarcoma, 69, 82
Chondroblastoma and osteosarcoma, 90
Chondrosarcoma and osteosarcoma, 87–90, 105–106
Chromosomal aberrations and osteosarcoma, 20–24
Chromosomal abnormalities, in OS, 518–519
Cisplatin drug, 205, 245–251, 389, 391
Cisplatinum (cis-Pt) drug, 310
Clear cell chondrosarcoma and osteosarcoma, 106
Closed biopsy, usage, 73
Codman's triangle, definition, 532
Codman's tumor. *See* Chondroblastoma and osteosarcoma
Coley's toxins, in cancer treatment, 531. *See also* Orthopedic oncology, in United States
Color Doppler ultrasound, usage, 43
Compassionate Investigational New Drug (CIND), 254
Compound Covariate Predictor (CCP), 461
Computed tomogram, of giant cell tumor, 551. *See also* Orthopedic oncology, in United States
Computed tomography (CT)
in lung metastases detection, 166–167, 170–171, 181, 187
in osteosarcoma diagnosis, 42–43
Conservative Bone Surgery in the Treatment of Bone Tumors, 537, 540
Continuous relapse-free survival assessment, for OS, 358–360
Conventional autogenous grafts, usage, 549
Conventional osteosarcoma, 65–69
Conventional radiography, role, 34–41
Cooperative osteosarcoma study (COSS)
group, 175, 284
group analysis
material and methodologies, 149–152
outcomes, 152–161
and osteosarcoma, 289–290
aims, 290
local therapy, 302–303

mortality, 303–304
neoadjuvant, patients and methods, 291–294
outcomes of neoadjuvant, 294–302
prognostic factors, 304–306
recurrent disease treatment, 306
registration policy, 290
Cox proportional hazards model, 152
Cox regression analysis, role, 325
Cryopreservation techniques, application, 137. *See also* Skeletal reconstruction
CT-scanning, in pulmonary metastases, 170–171
Cuff suspension strap, for transtibial prostheses, 412–414
Cushion liner and prosthesis, 412. *See also* Prosthetics, in pediatric and adolescent amputees
Customized Scales prosthesis, 553, 561, 567
CXCR4
expression, 522
in metastatic disease prevention, 523
Cyclin-dependent kinase 4 (*CDK4*) genes, 21
Cyclophosphamide, in osteosarcoma, 251, 252

D
Dahlin's classification, of osteosarcoma, 67
Dedifferentiated chondrosarcoma and OS, 105–106
Dedifferentiated parosteal osteosarcoma, 72
Definitive surgery (DS), 460
Delayed-type hypersensitivity (DTH), 451
Department of Melanoma/Sarcoma Medical Oncology, 356
DFI. *See* Disease free intervals
Digital imaging, in osteosarcoma detection, 128
Dimethyldiethyl triazeno imidazole carboxamide, 245
Disarticulation. *See* Amputation, for osteosarcoma treatment
Disease free intervals, 194–196
Disease-free survival (DFS), 449
Disseminated tumor cells, 510
Distraction techniques, in bone transportation, 139
Down-sized modular prostheses, role, 131
Doxorubicin drug, 205, 245, 310
DTC. *See* Disseminated tumor cells
DTIC. *See* Dimethyldiethyl triazeno imidazole carboxamide
Dynamic contrast-enhanced MRI (DCE-MRI), usage, 49–50

E

EDTMP. *See* Ethylene diamine tetramethylene phosphonate
EFS. *See* Event-free survival
Elbow arthroplasty, for osteosarcoma treatment, 131. *See also* Skeletal reconstruction
Endoprostheses, limitation, 426
EOI. *See* European Osteosarcoma Intergroup
Ethylene diamine tetramethylene phosphonate, 149
Etoposide and ifosfamide, role, 343–345
European and North American Osteosarcoma Study (EURAMOS), 343–349, 464, 465
European Osteosarcoma Intergroup, 263, 341–342
   in osteosarcoma treatment, 263–264
    chemotherapy, dose intensity, 269–270
    conspectus, 273
    initial study, 264–265
    interval compression, 271
    second study, 265–269
    third study, 271–273
European Science Foundation (ESF), 339
Event-free survival, 282, 324, 450
Ewing sarcoma and osteosarcoma, 25–26, 111–113
Exoskeletal and endoskeletal prostheses design, 400, 402
Expanding prostheses, definition, 554. *See also* Orthopedic oncology, in United States
Extensive intraosseous tumor involvement, 138–139
Extracorporeal irradiation (ECI), 159
Extra pulmonary metastases in osteosarcoma. *See also* Osteosarcoma pulmonary metastases
   non-surgical treatment, 203–204
    chemotherapy, 205
    physical means, 205–208
    radiation therapy, 208
    thermal ablation, 208–211
Extraskeletal tumors, 38, 44
Ezrin protein, 521

F

Family-centered care, 386. *See also* Nursing, in OS patients treatment
Fas associated death-domain dominant negative (FDN), 501, 502
Fas/FasL, in osteosarcoma lung metastases treatment, 498–499
   aerosol therapy, 503–506
   role, 499–503
Fas signaling pathway, of FDN, 502
FDG-PET-scanning, of lung metastases, 171–172
Febrile neutropenia, treatment, 323
F-18-FDG-PET, in pulmonary metastases detection, 172
F-18-FDG-PET scans, for pulmonary metastases, 172
[18] F-fluorodeoxyglucose ([18] F-FDG), 34, 50–51
Fibroblastic osteosarcoma, 70–71, 82
Fibrous dysplasia and osteosarcoma, 90–100
Fibula, osteoblastic osteosarcoma in, 37, 68
Flash drive program, 388. *See also* Nursing, in OS patients treatment
Folic-acid antagonist 4-aminopteroyl-glutamic acid, role, 221
Foot prosthesis, 402–407
Fracture and osteosarcoma, 115–116

G

Gamma-secretase inhibitors, role, 484
Genetic aberrations and osteosarcoma, 20–24, 519
Genetic alterations, in osteosarcoma
   chromosomal abnormalities, 518–519
   genetic abnormalities, 519
Genetic predisposition, in osteosarcoma development, 26
Giant cell tumor
   computed tomogram, 551. *See also* Orthopedic oncology, in United States
   of bone and osteosarcoma, 113
Gnathic osteosarcomas, 38, 86
Granulocyte-macrophage colony-stimulating factor (GM-CSF), 254, 323, 329, 452–453
Growth factor signaling pathways, in osteosarcoma
   IGF, 520
   Src kinase, 520
Growth Hormone (GH), 520
γ–Secretase (GSI), 484, 485

H

Hairy/Enhancer of Split (HES), 480
Hamster osteosarcomas, 27

Index

Health care team and family-centered care, association, 386
Hereditary retinoblastoma, causes, 519
Hes1 expression, in OS, 489–490
Hes-related repressor proteins (HERP), 480
High-grade surface osteosarcoma, 72
Histologic analysis, of osteosarcoma, 76–82
Histone deacetylase (HDAC), 490
Human and canine osteosarcoma, comparison, 440
Human predisposition syndromes, 470
Human serum albumin (HSA), 512
Hygiene and prosthesis, 418. *See also* Prosthetics, in pediatric and adolescent amputees

I

ICAM. *See* Intercellular adhesion molecule
Ifosfamide and etoposide, role, 343–345
Ifosfamide drug, 252, 388, 389
Ilizarov method, application, 427
Image-guided radiotherapy (IGRT), 160
Imaging, in pulmonary metastases. *See also* Pulmonary metastases, in osteosarcoma
CT-scanning, 170–171
nuclear imaging, 171–172
Imaging techniques
in adolescence osteosarcoma
conventional radiography, 35–41
extended diagnostic and therapeutic, 42–51
in bone tumor diagnosis, 34 (*see also* Osteosarcoma (OS))
conventional radiography, 35–41
extended diagnostic and therapeutic modalities, 42–51
Immunomagnetic isolation, bone marrow micrometastases, 509–510
background, 510–511
future perspectives, 513
materials and methods, 511–512
outcomes, 512–513
Immunotherapy. *See also* Osteosarcoma (OS)
active, 449–451
adoptive immunotherapy, 453–454
definition, 447–448
future perspectives, 454–455
history, 448
immune stimulatory agents, 451–453
Independent Data Monitoring Committee (IDMC), 347

Inflammatory metachronous hyperostosis and ostersarcoma, 116–117
Initial biopsy (IB), 460
Innovative Therapy for Children with Cancer, 284
Insulin-like growth factors (IGF), 520
Intensity modulated RT (IMRT), 160
Intercalary bone defect, replacement, 133. *See also* Skeletal reconstruction
Intercellular adhesion molecule, 335, 450
Interdisciplinary rehabilitation team, for pediatric OS, 368–369
Intergroup Rhabdomyosarcoma Study Group (IRSG), 342
Interleukin-12 (IL-12), in osteosarcoma treatment, 453
International Limb Salvage Symposia, 557
International Paediatric Oncology Society (SIOP), 264
International Registry of Lung Metastases, 194
International Society of Limb Salvage
data base, 563
functional outcome, 566
local recurrence and complications, 565
survival, 564
International Symposium on Limb Salvage, 547
INT-0133, in OS treatment, 345–346
Intra-arterial chemotherapy, for OS treatment, 161
Intra-arterial cisplatin administration, advantage, 341
Intra-arterial therapy, role, 250
Intramedullary nail stabilization, usage, 138
Intraosseous osteosarcoma, 86
Intravenous radium 224 usage and osteosarcoma, 26
Investigational new drug (IND), 347
Ionizing radiation, in osteosarcoma occurrence, 25–26
Ipsilateral hemithorax and posterolateral thoracotomy, 190
IRLM. *See* International Registry of Lung Metastases
ISOLS. *See* International Society of Limb Salvage; International Symposium on Limb Salvage
Isomet saw, usage, 75
stanbul University Institute of Oncology (UIO), 320
ITCC. *See* Innovative Therapy for Children with Cancer

J

Jarcho-Levin Syndrome, 482
Jaw and skull osteosarcomas, 72

K

Kaplan–Meier method, 152, 324–325
K-Nearest Neighbor (K-NN), 461
Knee arthrodesis, 429

L

Lactic dehydrogenase (LDH), 321
Large segmental allografts, disadvantages,
137. *See also* Skeletal
reconstruction
Leave-One-Out Cross Validation, 461, 463
Lesions, in osteosarcoma mimicking, 85–86
Li-Fraumeni syndrome, 23, 469
and osteosarcoma, 519
Limb-salvage surgery, 422
conditions, 129
in osteosarcoma, 425–427
reoperation following, 427–429
Limb-salvaging management, 561
Limb sparing surgery, in dogs, 443
Limb-sparing tumor resection, for OS
treatment, 129–131, 372. *See also*
Skeletal reconstruction
Linear Discriminant Analysis (LDA), 461
Liposarcoma, magnetic resonance image, 551.
See also Orthopedic oncology, in
United States
Liposomal muramyl tripeptide phosphatidyl
ethanolamine, 254
in osteosarcoma treatment, 451–452
usage, 208
Liposomal 9-nitrocamptothecin, 504
Liquid nitrogen, usage, 536
L-MTP-PE. *See* Liposomal muramyl
tripeptide phosphatidyl
ethanolamine
L-9NC. *See* Liposomal 9-nitrocamptothecin
Local control, definition, 158
Local recurrence management, for OS
treatment, 142. *See also* Skeletal
reconstruction
Local transposition muscle flaps and free
tissue transfers, usage, 141
Log-rank test, usage, 152
LOOCV. *See* Leave-One-Out Cross Validation
Lung metastases, chemokine mediated
model, 522

Lung, OS cells, Fas/FasL role, 499–503
Lungs, prophylactic irradiation, 276–277
Lung tissue marking, barium, 192

M

Magnetic resonance image, of liposarcoma,
551. *See also* Orthopedic oncology,
in United States
Magnetic resonance imaging (MRI), 34, 322
Malignant bone cancers, types, 5
Malignant fibrous histiocytoma, 71–72
Malignant primary tumors, biopsy hazards, 73
Malignant tumors, 85
Mammalian target of rapamycin, 521–523
Massive autogenous grafting method, 537,
546, 549
Mastermind-like (MAML) protein, 480
Median sternotomy, usage, 190, 191
Medical Research Council (MRC), 346
Medication bags, in OS patients treatment,
387. *See also* Nursing, in OS
patients treatment
Memorial Sloan-Kettering Cancer Center, 170
Mesenchymal chondrosarcoma and
osteosarcoma, 106–111
Metachronous osteosarcoma, occurrence, 11
Metachronous pulmonary metastases,
treatment and prognosis, 179–180.
See also Osteosarcoma pulmonary
metastases
Metastatic cascade modeling, 523–525
Metastatic disease, detection, 168
Metastatic osteosarcoma, inpatient *vs.*
outpatient, 205–207. *See also*
Pulmonary metastases, in
osteosarcoma
Methotrexate drug, 205, 222, 227, 228, 232,
242–244, 389
Methotrexate-leucovorin (MTX-L), 242
Methotrexate (MTX) drug, 310
Meticulous pin care, role, 139
MFH. *See* Malignant fibrous histiocytoma
Micrometastases (MM), 509
Micrometastasis negative (MM-/+), 512
Microprocessor knee, 408
Microvascular surgical techniques, for
osteosarcoma treatment, 128. *See
also* Skeletal reconstruction
MIOS. *See* Multi-institutional Osteosarcoma
Study
Modular oncology prosthetic reconstruction
systems, 128

Index 583

Mononuclear cells (MNC), 511
MSKCC. *See* Memorial Sloan-Kettering Cancer Center
MSTS. *See* Musculoskeletal Tumor Society
mTOR. *See* Mammalian target of rapamycin
MTP-PE. *See* Muramyl tripeptide-phosphatidylethanolamine
Multiagent chemotherapy, for pediatric OS, 321
Multicentric trials for OS, outcomes, 320
Multi-drug resistance associated protein (MRP), 474
Multi-drug resistance (MDR1) gene, 474
Multigene classifier usage, in IB, 462–464
Multi-institutional Osteosarcoma Study, 230–232
Multimodality therapy, for childhood OS
  characteristics and variables evaluation, 323–324
  complications in treatment
    acute and late complications of surgery, 330
    chemotherapy dose intensity and acute toxicity, 329–330
  follow-up, 325
  outcomes, 325–329, 334–336
  patients and methods, 321–322
  response assessment, 324
  survival, outcome and prognosis, 330–334
  toxic effects and statistical analysis, 324–325
  treatment
    chemotherapy, 322–323
    surgery and radiotherapy, 323
Multimodal therapy, in primary pulmonary metastases, 175. *See also* Primary pulmonary metastases
Multiple intra operative factors, in soft tissue coverage, 140–141
Muramyl tripeptide-phosphatidylethanolamine, 448
Murine double minute 2 *(MDM2)*, 21
Murine predisposition syndromes, 470
Muscle-sparing thoracotomy, role, 189
Musculoskeletal Tumor Society, 129, 422–424
Myositis ossificans and ostersarcoma, 117–119

N
National Cancer Data Base Report, 9
National Cancer Institute Common Toxicity Criteria, 324
National Cancer Institute SEER Study, on osteosarcoma incidence, 7
National Vital Statistics System, 8
National Wilm's Tumor Study Group (NWTSG), 342
Nearest Centroid (NC), 461
Necrosis determination, in DS, 460
Needle biopsy, role, 73
Neoadjuvant and adjuvant chemotherapy combination, for OS treatment, 157–158
Neoadjuvant chemotherapy, for osteosarcoma, 148–149, 278–281
Neutron therapy, for osteosarcoma, 160
Non-metastatic osteosarcoma
  BM study, 509–510
    background, 510–511
    future perspectives, 513
    materials and methods, 511–512
    outcomes, 512–513
  treatment, 343
Nonmetastatic osteosarcoma, treatment, 275–276
  chemotherapy era, 277–281
  future perspectives, 284
  late effects of chemotherapy, 283–284
  postrelapse survival, 282–283
  prechemotherapy era, 276–277
  prognostic factors, 281–282
Nonmethotrexate regimen, adoption, 334
Nonsurgical adjuvant treatment, for bone tumors, 531
Non-surgical treatment. *See also* Osteosarcoma pulmonary metastases
  in osteosarcoma (*see also* Pulmonary metastases, in osteosarcoma)
    chemotherapy, 205
    physical means, 205–208
    radiation therapy, 208
    thermal ablation, 208–211
  of pulmonary and extra pulmonary metastases, 203–204
    chemotherapy, 205
    physical means, 205–208
    radiation therapy, 208
    thermal ablation, 208–211
North American Children's Oncology Group (COG), 342
Notch pathway signaling, 492–494
  in bone and limb development, 481–482
  in cancer, 482
  components, 484–486

584 Index

Notch pathway signaling (*cont.*)
  expression, 482–483
  gamma-secretase inhibitors, 484
  Hes1 expression, 489–490
  orthotopic xenograft model, 486–488
  regulation, 480–481
  valproic acid, 490–492
Nuclear imaging, of pulmonary metastases,
    171–172
Nursing, in OS patients treatment
  family-centered care, 386
  home chemotherapy, 388–389
  nursing practitioners, 392
  patient tools development
    calendars, 386–387
    flash drive, 388
    medication bags, 387
    medication schedules, 387
    one page summary, 386
  post operative pain
    nausea and vomiting, 391
    nutrition, 391–392
    oral mucocitis, 391
    progressive disease pain, 390–391
  symptom prevention and management,
    389–390

O

Occupational therapy, for pediatric and adult
    OS, 368–369
  complications, 371–372
  goal, 370
  and physical therapy, 379–381
  present practice, 376, 378–379
Onion skin appearance. *See* Ewing sarcoma
    and osteosarcoma
Open biopsy, usage, 73
Oral mucocitis and pain, 391. *See also*
    Nursing, in OS patients treatment
Orthopedic oncologists, role, 127
Orthopedic oncology, in United States
  chemotherapy, 540–547
  current history, 559–569
  history, 529–540
  radiographic imaging, 547
  reconstructive surgery, 547–554
  sarcoma referral centers development,
    557–559
  surgical experience, 554–557
Orthopedic techniques, in fracture
    management, 128
Orthotic devices, usage, 374, 379

Orthotopic xenograft model, in metastatis
    study, 486–488
Osseous metastases detection, bone
    scintigraphy, 171
Ossifying fibroma. *See* Fibrous dysplasia and
    osteosarcoma; Osteofibrous
    dysplasia and osteosarcoma
Osteoarticular allografts, role, 138
Osteoarticular resections, 130
Osteoblastic osteosarcoma, of fibula, 37, 68
Osteoblastoma and osteosarcoma, 113–115
Osteofibrous dysplasia and osteosarcoma,
    90–100
Osteoid, definition, 64
Osteoid osteoma and osteosarcoma, 113–115
Osteomyelits and osteosarcoma, 116
Osteosarcoma chemotherapy, inpatient *vs.*
    outpatient, 206–207. *See also*
    Osteosarcoma pulmonary metastases
Osteosarcoma lung metastases treatment
  Fas/FasL, 498–499
    aerosol therapy, 503–506
    role, 499–503
Osteosarcoma metastasis treatment,
    strategy, 204
Osteosarcoma (OS), 392–393, 422–423
  adolescence and childhood, imaging
    techniques
    conventional radiography, 35–41
    extended diagnostic and therapeutic,
      42–51
  in animals and human, 439–445
  biological behavior, 220–221
  and bone abnormalities, 24
  canine osteosarcoma, 440
  categories, 34
  cell of origin, 471
  cell surface receptors, modulation,
    521–523
  challenges, 459
  chemotherapy, 340–341
  clinical relevance, 472–473
  COSS group analysis, 148–149, 289–290
    aims, 290
    local therapy, 302–303
    material and methodologies, 149–152
    mortality, 303–304
    neoadjuvant, patients and methods,
      291–294
    outcomes, 152–161
    outcomes of neoadjuvant, 294–302
    prognostic factors, 304–306
    recurrent disease treatment, 306

Index

registration policy, 290
in dogs, 441
environmental factors
  alkylating agents exposure, 26
  ionizing radiation, 25–26
  perinatal factors, 27
  trauma, 28
  viruses, 27–28
EOI perspective, 263–264
  chemotherapy, dose intensity, 269–270
  conspectus, 273
  initial study, 264–265
  interval compression, 271
  second study, 265–269
  third study, 271–273
EURAMOS investigators, 343–349
expression profiling, 460–462
functional outcomes, 423–424
  amputation, 424–425
  economic considerations, 429–430
  limb-salvage surgery, 425–427
  reoperation following limb salvage, 427–429
gamma-secretase inhibitors, 484
genetic alterations
  chromosomal abnormalities, 518–519
  genetic abnormalities, 519
genetic and familial factors, 20–24
growth factor signaling pathways
  IGF, 520
  Src kinase, 520
Hes1 expression, 489–490
historical evolution, 315
host factors, 19–20
immunotherapy, 447–448
  active, 449–451
  adoptive immunotherapy, 453–454
  future perspectives, 454–455
  history, 448
  immune stimulatory agents, 451–453
limb sparing surgery, 443
local recurrence, 56–57
in mammals, 439–440
management
  biopsy, 73
  conventional osteosarcoma, 65–69
  histologic analysis, 76–82
  osteosarcoma variants, 69–73
  specimen preparation, 75–76
  therapy evaluation, 73–75
metastatic cascade modeling, 523–525
mimicking conditions, 85–87
  differential diagnosis, 87–105

miscellaneous tumors, 111–120
nontraditional osteoid-producing
  entities, 105–111
multigene classifier usage, 462–464
multimodality protocol for childhood
  characteristics and variables evaluation,
    323–324
  complications in treatment, 329–330
  follow-up, 325
  outcomes, 325–329, 334–336
  patients and methods, 321–322
  response assessment, 324
  survival, outcome and prognosis,
    330–334
  toxic effects and statistical analysis,
    324–325
  treatment, 322–323
neoadjuvant chemotherapy, 148–149
notch pathway components, 484–486
notch pathway expression, 482–483
nurse in treatment
  family-centered care, 386
  home chemotherapy, 388–389
  nursing practitioners, 392
  symptom prevention and management,
    389–390
orthotopic xenograft model, 486–488
pathogenesis, genetic alterations, 468–471
patient tools development
  calendars, 386–387
  flash drive, 388
  medication bags, 387
  medication schedules, 387
  one page summary, 386
pediatric and adult, 356–362
  current occupational-therapy, 376,
    378–379
  current physical-therapy, 372–376
  discharge recommendations, 381–382
  future perspectives, 382
  interdisciplinary rehabilitation team,
    368–369
  occupational-therapy and physical-
    therapy interventions, 379–381
  rehabilitation therapy, historical
    perspectives, 369–372
Pediatric Preclinical Testing Program,
  475–476
post operative pain
  nausea and vomiting, 391
  nutrition, 391–392
  oral mucocitis, 391
  progressive disease pain, 390–391

Osteosarcoma (OS) (*cont.*)
- post-therapy complications, 54–56
- preoperative assessment, 126–129
- present treatment outcomes, 341–343
- primary osteosarcoma
  - incidence, 4–7
  - mortality, 8
  - survival rate, 8–10
- prognostic markers, 460
- psychosocial and professional outcomes, 430–432
- redundancy, 471–472
- response monitoring for chemotherapy, 51–54
- risk factors, 17–18
- SSG in treatment, 309–310, 315–317
  - clinical trials, 312
  - conspectus, 317
  - ISG/SSG I, 310
  - outcomes, 312–315
  - SSG II, 310
  - SSG VIII, 310
  - SSG XIV, 311
- surgical strategies for primary, 125–126
  - biological constructs, 134–138
  - bone replacement, 138–139
  - limb-sparing tumor resection, 129–131
  - prosthetic arthroplasty, 131–134
  - rotationplasty and amputation, 141
  - soft tissue management, 140–141
  - surveillance, 142
- therapeutic implications, 525–526
- therapeutic targets, 474–475
- therapy, late effects, 432
- treatment
  - carboplatin, 253
  - chemotherapy regimens, 254–255
  - cisplatin, 245–251
  - conpadri/compadri series, 240–241
  - doxorubicin, 245
  - future perspectives, 257
  - limitation of chemotherapy, 255–257
  - L-MTPPE, 254
  - methotrexate, 242–244
  - oxazaphosphorines, 251–253
  - samarium, 253
  - trimetrexate, 253
- treatment induced, 10
- treatment of nonmetastatic, 275–276
  - chemotherapy era, 277–281
  - future perspectives, 284
  - late effects of chemotherapy, 283–284
  - postrelapse survival, 282–283
  - prechemotherapy era, 276–277
  - prognostic factors, 281–282
- valproic acid, 490–492

Osteosarcoma protocol, 311

Osteosarcoma pulmonary metastases, 165
- adjuvant chemotherapy, 220–221, 232–233
  - chemotherapy, 221–230
  - denouement, 233–234
  - MIOS, 232
  - multi-institutional osteosarcoma, 230–232
- future perspectives for detection, 181
- location and frequency, 168–169
- non-surgical treatment, 203–204
  - chemotherapy, 205
  - physical means, 205–208
  - radiation therapy, 208
  - thermal ablation, 208–211
- in pediatric and adolescent patients, surgical treatment
  - evaluation, 186–188
  - future perspectives, 199
  - historical background, 185–186
  - outcomes, 194–198
  - surgical resection, 188–194
- primary pulmonary metastases treatment
  - chemotherapy, 176–177
  - multimodal therapy, 175
  - prognostic factors, 175–176
  - surgery, 176
- recurrence
  - risk factors, 179
  - survival data, 177–178
- role of imaging
  - CT-scanning, 170–171
  - implications, 172–174
  - nuclear imaging, 171–172
- survey, 166–168
- treatment and prognosis of metachronous, 179–180

Osteosarcomatosis, 38

Osteosarcoma variants, 69–73

Outpatient therapy, recommendation, 381

Overall survival (OS), definition, 324

Oxazaphosphorines drug, 251–253

P

Paget's disease and osteosarcoma, 24

Pain, in OS patients, 390. *See also* Nursing, in OS patients treatment
- post operative
  - nausea and vomiting, 391

nutrition, 391–392
oral mucocitis, 391
progressive disease pain, 390–391
Palonosetron drug, 389
Parosteal osteosarcoma, 72
Passive prosthesis, role, 400
Patella Tendon Bearing Socket
(PTB socket), 409
Patients tool, development, 386
calendars, 386–387
flash drive, 388
medication schedules and bags, 387
Paxillin phosphorylation, Src kinase, 520
PCNA. *See* Proliferating cell nuclear
antigen
Pediatric and Adolescent Osteosarcoma
Symposium, 165
Pediatric and adolescent patients
prosthetics, 395–396 (*see also* Prosthetics,
in pediatric and adolescent
amputees)
foot, 402–407
knee, 408–409
liners, 412
lower extremity design, 400–402
personal care and hygiene, 418
principles, 396–398
prosthesis care, 417–418
socket accommodation, 409–412
suspensions, 412–414
upper extremity, 398–400
Van Ness rotationplasty, 414–417
surgical treatment (*see also* Osteosarcoma
pulmonary metastases)
evaluation, 186–188
future perspectives, 199
historical background, 185–186
outcomes, 194–198
surgical resection, 188–194
Pediatric and adult osteosarcoma, comparison,
356–362
Pediatric Oncology Group (POG), 341
Pediatric osteosarcoma
rehabilitation
current occupational-therapy, 376,
378–379
current physical-therapy, 372–376
discharge recommendations, 381–382
future perspectives, 382
interdisciplinary rehabilitation team,
368–369
occupational-therapy and physical-
therapy interventions, 379–381

rehabilitation therapy, historical
perspectives, 369–372
Pediatric Preclinical Testing Program,
475–476
Pediatric sarcoma, PET detection, 171–172
Pegfilgrastim drug, 389
Pelvic resections, limitation, 139
Peoperative angiogram study, for
osteosarcoma patients, 75
Percutaneous biopsy techniques, for
osteosarcoma treatment, 127
Periacetabular resections, construction, 139.
See also Skeletal reconstruction
Perinatal factors, in osteosarcoma
development, 27
Periosteal osteosarcomas, 38, 40, 41, 72
Periprosthetic infections, frequency,
426–427
p53 gene, 22
P-glycoprotein, expression, 282
Phemeister, role, 555
Physical therapy intervention, for pediatric and
adult OS, 368
complications, 371–372
goal, 370
and occupational-therapy, 379–381
present practice, 372–376
Planned dose intensity, definition, 329–330
Planned duration, definition, 330
Plate fixation. *See* Intramedullary nail
stabilization, usage
Polycentric knees, 408–409
Positron emission tomography (PET)
and CT scans
advantage, 187
in bone detection, 208
Posterolateral thoracotomy, 189
Postinduction chemotherapy assessment, for
osteosarcoma treatment, 127
Postrelapse survival (PRS), 282
Prenatals, x-rays exposure, 27
Preoperative chemotherapy
advantage, 340–341
clinical response, 324
in IB, 462–464 (*see also* Osteosarcoma
(OS))
in multimodality treatment of
osteosarcoma, 325–327
response, 79, 335
usage, 320
Preoperative radiotherapy, for
osteosarcoma, 160
Primary cancers and osteosarcoma, 10–11

Primary osteosarcomas, 34, 35, 38
  incidence, 4–7
  mortality, 8
  preoperative assessment, 126–129
  surgical strategies
    biological constructs, 134–138
    bone replacement, 138–139
    limb-sparing tumor resection, 129–131
    prosthetic arthroplasty, 131–134
    rotationplasty and amputation, 141
    soft tissue management, 140–141
    surveillance, 142
  survival rate, 8–10
Primary osteosarcoma treatment,
    radiotherapy, 320
Primary pulmonary metastases. *See also*
    Osteosarcoma pulmonary
    metastases
  involvement site, 168
  treatment and outcome
    chemotherapy, 176–177
    multimodal therapy, 175
    prognostic factors, 175–176
    surgery, 176
Prognostic factors, for OS local control,
    155–157
Prognostic markers, of osteosarcoma, 460
Proliferating cell nuclear antigen, 335
Prophylactic irradiation, of lungs, 320
Prophylactic lung irradiation (PLI), 160
Prosthetic arthroplasty, for osteosarcoma
    treatment, 131–134. *See also*
    Skeletal reconstruction
Prosthetics, in pediatric and adolescent
    amputees, 395–396
  foot, 402–407
  knee, 408–409
  liners, 412
  lower extremity design, 400–402
  personal care and hygiene, 418
  principles, 396–398
  prosthesis care, 417–418
  socket accommodation, 409–412
  suspensions, 412–414
  upper extremity, 398–400
  Van Ness rotationplasty, 414–417
Proximal fibular epiphysis transfer, usage,
    135. *See also* Skeletal
    reconstruction
Proximal tibia, osteosarcoma, 229
Pulmonary metastasectomy
  advantage, 188
  reports, 186

Pulmonary metastases, in osteosarcoma, 165
  future perspectives for detection, 181
  location and frequency, 168–169
  non-surgical treatment, 203–204
    chemotherapy, 205
    physical means, 205–208
    radiation therapy, 208
    thermal ablation, 208–211
  in pediatric and adolescent patients,
      surgical treatment
    evaluation, 186–188
    future perspectives, 199
    historical background, 185–186
    outcomes, 194–198
    surgical resection, 188–194
  primary pulmonary metastases treatment
    chemotherapy, 176–177
    multimodal therapy, 175
    prognostic factors, 175–176
    surgery, 176
  recurrence
    risk factors, 179
    survival data, 177–178
  role of imaging
    CT-scanning, 170–171
    implications, 172–174
    nuclear imaging, 171–172
  survey, 166–168
  treatment and prognosis of metachronous,
      179–180

R
Radiation-induced osteosarcomas, 10,
    25–26, 73
Radiation therapy
  in metastases osteosarcoma, 208 (*see also*
      Pulmonary metastases, in
      osteosarcoma)
  of pulmonary metastases, 208
Radiofrequency ablation, 194, 208
Radiographic imaging, of bone tumor, 547
Radiography, in osteosarcoma diagnosis,
    34–41
Radiologic imaging, of osteosarcoma
    treatment, 126
Radionuclide bone scan, in osteosarcoma
    diagnosis, 42
Radiotherapy
  analysis, COSS protocol, 149–150
  in multimodality treatment of
      osteosarcoma, 334–335
Rb gene, 468, 469, 519

Index 589

Received Dose Intensity (RDI), 270, 330
Received duration, definition, 330
Reconstructive surgery, advances, 547–554
RECQL4 gene, 24
Recurrent metastases, involvement sites, 169
Recurrent osteosarcoma, 56–57, 526
Rehabilitation, for pediatric and adolescence
  osteosarcoma
    current occupational-therapy, 376,
      378–379
    current physical-therapy, 372–376
    discharge recommendations, 381–382
    future perspectives, 382
    historical perspectives, 369–372
    interdisciplinary rehabilitation team,
      368–369
    occupational-therapy and physical-therapy
      interventions, 379–381
Relapsed osteosarcoma, second line
  chemotherapy, 179–180. *See also*
  Osteosarcoma pulmonary
  metastases
Relapse-free interval (RFI), 282
Relative dose intensity, definition, 329
Remission-free survival (RFS), 452
Residual viable tumor tissue, identification, 50
Retinoblastoma and osteosarcoma
  development, 21, 22
Retinoblastoma susceptibility gene *(RB1)*, 21
RFA. *See* Radiofrequency ablation
Rotationplasty, for osteosarcoma treatment, 141
Rothmund–Thomson (RecQL4) gene, 469
Rothmund–Thomson syndrome, 23–24

S
Samarium drug, 253
Samarium-153-EDTMP, usage, 160–161
SARC. *See* Sarcoma Alliance for Research
  through Collaboration
Sarcoma Alliance for Research through
  Collaboration, 284
Sarcoma, derivation, 529. *See also* Orthopedic
  oncology, in United States
Sarcoma referral centers, development,
  557–559
Scandinavian Sarcoma Group, 284, 309
  in osteosarcoma treatment, 309–310,
    315–317
    clinical trials, 312
    conspectus, 317
    ISG/SSG I, 310
    outcomes, 312–315

SSG VIII, 310
SSG XIV, 311
Scandinavian Sarcoma Group (SSG), 342
SCID. *See* Severe combined immune
  deficiency
Seattle foot, advantage, 405
Secondary osteosarcoma, 34, 38
Secondary radiation-induced bone sarcoma,
  25–26
Second line chemotherapy, relapsed
  osteosarcoma, 179–180
Segmental allograft and prosthesis,
  advantages, 138
Segmental graft methods, usage, 138
Selective popliteal arteriogram, in
  osteosarcoma, 48
Severe combined immune deficiency, 448
Silesian belt, usage, 414
Simian virus 40 (SV40), 28
Skeletal reconstruction, in osteosarcoma
  treatment
    biological constructs, 134–138
    bone replacement, 138–139
    prosthetic arthroplasty, 131–134
    soft tissue management, 140–141
Socket, usage, 417
Sock management, 410, 411
Soft tissue coverage, 140–141
Solid Ankle Cushion Heel foot, 402–407
Sox-9 expression in chondrosarcoma, 110
Specimens preparation, goal, 75
SPSS software, role, 294
Src kinase, 520
SSG. *See* Scandinavian Sarcoma Group
Standard magnetic resonance imaging, usage,
  43, 47
Support Vector Machine (SVM), 461, 463
Surface osteosarcomas, 38
Surgical biopsies, for osteosarcoma
  treatment, 126
Surgical strategies
  for primary osteosarcomas (*see also*
    Osteosarcoma (OS))
    biological constructs, 134–138
    bone replacement, 138–139
    limb-sparing tumor resection, 129–131
    prosthetic arthroplasty, 131–134
    rotationplasty and amputation, 141
    soft tissue management, 140–141
    surveillance, 142
  in primary pulmonary metastases, 176
    (*see also* Primary pulmonary
      metastases)

Surgical strategies (*cont.*)
of pulmonary metastases (*see also*
Pulmonary metastases, in
osteosarcoma)
evaluation, 186–188
future perspectives, 199
historical background, 185–186
outcomes, 194–198
surgical resection, 188–194
Surveillance, Epidemiology and End Results
(SEER) Cancer Statistics Review, 5
Synovial sarcoma and osteosarcoma, 111
Systemic chemotherapy, in osteosarcoma
treatment, 339

T

T-ALL. *See* T-cell acute lymphoblastic
leukemia
T-cell acute lymphoblastic leukemia, 482
Telangiectatic osteosarcoma and
osteosarcoma, 71, 101, 103–105
Therapy evaluation in osteosarcoma, goal,
73–75
Thermal ablation, in metastases osteosarcoma,
208–211. *See also* Pulmonary
metastases, in osteosarcoma
Thoracoscopic interventions, for pulmonary
metastases, 173
Thoracoscopy, advantage, 191, 193
Thorotrast, in osteosarcoma development, 26
TILs. *See* Tumor-infiltrating lymphocytes
Transfemoral prosthesis
polycentric knee, 407
and SACH foot, 406, 407
suspension, 414
suspension suction socket, 415
Transfemoral prosthesis, suspension, 414
Transfemoral suspension method, role, 414
Transtibial prosthesis, socket, 409–412
Transverse thoracosternotomy, 190
Trimetrexate drug, 253
Trouper foot, advantage, 406
Tumor-infiltrating lymphocytes, 448
Turkey, multimodality therapy for childhood OS
characteristics and variables evaluation,
323–324
complications in treatment
acute and late complications
of surgery, 330
chemotherapy dose intensity and acute
toxicity, 329–330
follow-up, 325

outcomes, 325–329, 334–336
patients and methods, 321–322
response assessment, 324
survival, outcome and prognosis, 330–334
toxic effects and statistical analysis, 324–325
treatment
chemotherapy, 322–323
surgery and radiotherapy, 323
Turkish Pediatric Oncology Group Tumor
Registry data, 320
Turn-up plasty, procedure, 537, 545

U

Umkipp plastic, procedure, 537, 545
Unicameral bone cyst, 119
Unilateral lung disease, approach, 173–174
United Kingdom Children's Cancer Study
Group (UKCCSG), 264
United States
childhood and adolescent cancer, 4–5
orthopedic oncology
chemotherapy, 540–547
current history, 559–569
history, 529–540
radiographic imaging, 547
reconstructive surgery, 547–554
sarcoma referral centers development,
557–559
surgical experience, 554–557
osteosarcoma, 4–5
Upper extremity prostheses, 398–400
U.S. Cancer Statistics Working Group, on
osteosarcoma incidence, 6, 19

V

VAC. *See* Vincristine, dactinomycin
(actinomycin D), and
cyclophosphamide
Valproic acid, in notch pathway expression,
490–492
Van Ness rotationplasty limb salvage surgery,
414–417. *See also* Prosthetics, in
pediatric and adolescent amputees
Vascularized fibular graft, usage, 135, 137. *See
also* Skeletal reconstruction
Vascular pedicle technique, in bone graft, 549
VATS. *See* Video-assisted thoracoscopy
Video-assisted thoracoscopy, 173
Vincristine, dactinomycin (actinomycin D),
and cyclophosphamide, 241
Vincristine drug, 222

Index 591

Viral infection and osteosarcoma, 27–28
Vitallium device, role, 552

W
Wedge resection, 193
Werner syndrome (WRN) gene, 469

X
X-rays exposure in prenatal
and osteosarcoma, 27

Z
Zoledronate drug, 205